Handbook
of Veterinary
Neurology

Handbook
of Veterinary
Neurology

Fourth Edition

Michael D. Lorenz, D.V.M.

Professor and Interim Dean
College of Veterinary Medicine
Oklahoma State University
Stillwater, Oklahoma

Joe N. Kornegay, D.V.M., Ph.D.

Professor and Dean
College of Veterinary Medicine
University of Missouri
Columbia, Missouri

SAUNDERS

An Imprint of Elsevier

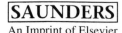

SAUNDERS

An Imprint of Elsevier

11830 Westline Industrial Drive
St. Louis, Missouri 63146

NOTICE

Companion animal practice is an ever-changing field. Standard safety precautions must be followed, but as
new research and clinical experience broaden our knowledge, changes in treatment and drug therapy may
become necessary or appropriate. Readers are advised to check the most current product information provided by the manufacturer of each drug to be administered to verify the recommended dose, the method and
duration of administration, and contraindications. It is the responsibility of the licensed prescriber, relying on
experience and knowledge of the patient, to determine dosages and the best treatment for each individual
patient. Neither the publisher nor the author assumes any liability for any injury and/or damage to persons or
property arising from this publication.

Previous editions copyrighted 1997, 1993, 1983

1004802747

International Standard Book Number 0-7216-8986-8

Publishing Director: Linda Duncan
Senior Editor: Liz Fathman
Associate Developmental Editor: Shelly Dixon
Publishing Services Manager: Pat Joiner
Project Manager: David Stein
Designer: Bill Drone

Printed in China

Last digit is the print number: 9   8   7   6   5   4   3   2   1

We dedicate this edition to our friend and colleague, Dr. John Oliver. John has inspired both of us in our veterinary medical careers to pursue the truth, to accept criticism, and to be honest with our colleagues and students. We thank him for his ability to mentor young faculty members and for his contributions to academic veterinary medicine and the discipline of neurology.

Preface

The fourth edition of *Handbook of Veterinary Neurology* continues the same problem-oriented format used in previous editions. We emphasize lesion localization throughout the book, since one cannot diagnose what is wrong if one does not know where the lesion(s) is (are) located.

We continue our efforts to make the text simple and easy to use by students and practitioners. Numerous algorithms are included that diagram the logic necessary to localize lesions and to formulate diagnostic plans. Numerous tables are included that organize diseases for quick reference when formulating diagnostic plans. Each chapter has been extensively reviewed and new diseases have been added.

We thank Ray Kersey, who patiently guided our revisions. Shelly Dixon and David Stein provided valuable help in editing the text.

Finally, we thank all of you, our colleagues, for making a fourth edition necessary.

Michael D. Lorenz
Joe N. Kornegay

Contents

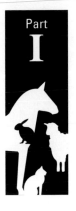

Fundamentals

Neurologic History and Examination

The objectives in the management of a patient with a problem that may be related to the nervous system are to (1) determine that the problem is caused by a lesion in the nervous system, (2) localize the lesion in the nervous system, (3) estimate the extent of the lesion in the nervous system, (4) determine the cause or the pathologic process or both, and (5) estimate the prognosis with no treatment or with various alternative methods of treatment.

Many diseases are poorly defined and may be accompanied by a complex combination of clinical signs and laboratory data. Diagnosis of these diseases may seem impossible. Weed demonstrated the value of starting the diagnostic process by independently listing and analyzing all the patient's problems.[1] A minimum set of data (minimum database) is necessary to solve any medical problem. The minimum database may be modified because of risk, cost, or accessibility, as balanced against the severity of the disease. Priorities should be established for collecting data that evaluate the most probable causes of a problem. Tests for rare diseases and those that are dangerous are reserved until last.

Weed's problem-oriented system is eminently suited for neurologic diagnosis. The steps necessary for the management of a neurologic problem are listed in Table 1-1.

MINIMUM DATABASE

The initial evaluation of a patient, including a history and a physical examination, usually provides evidence that a neurologic problem is present (Table 1-2). Some problems are difficult to classify, for example, syncope versus convulsions or weakness (loss of muscle strength) versus paresis (loss of neural control). The initial physical examination of every patient should include a screening neurologic examination designed to detect the presence of any neurologic abnormality. The screening examination is described later in this chapter under Neurologic Examination.

The minimum database recommended for an animal with a neurologic problem is listed in Table 1-3. Because chemistry panels are usually available at less cost than individual tests, selection of tests is usually not necessary. Otherwise, the selection of chemistry profiles should be based on the problems presented. Additions to the database are recommended for specific problems.

PROBLEM LIST

A problem list is formulated from information obtained from the minimum database. For each problem, a diagnostic plan is formulated. A diagnostic plan for a neurologic problem includes the following steps:

1. The level of the lesion is localized with a neurologic examination. Confirmation of the lesion may require survey or contrast radiography.
2. The extent of the lesion is estimated both longitudinally and transversely (e.g., L4-6 spinal cord segments, left side). The neurologic examination provides most of this information, but ancillary diagnostic procedures may be of assistance.
3. The cause of the pathologic process is determined. The history is most useful for establishing the class of disease (neoplasia, infectious disease, trauma, and so forth). Laboratory, radiographic, or electrophysiologic tests are usually required to substantiate the diagnosis. From this information, the clinician can establish a prognosis with and without appropriate therapy, based on information available about the disease (see Table 1-1).

This chapter describes the history and neurologic examination. An in-depth discussion of the organization and function of the nervous system and application to clinical signs and lesion localization is presented in Chapter 2.

Table 1-1 **Plan for Neurologic Diagnosis**

Collect minimum database
Identify problems
Identify one or more problems related to nervous
  system
Localize level of lesion
Estimate extent of lesion within that level
List most probable causes (rule-outs or differential
  diagnosis)
Construct diagnostic plan to determine cause or
  pathologic lesion
Determine prognosis with and without therapy

Modified from Oliver JE Jr: Localization of lesions in the
nervous system. In Hoerlein BF, editor: *Canine neurology*,
3rd ed. Philadelphia, 1978, WB Saunders.

TAKING THE HISTORY

Traditionally, the history is taken by the veterinarian. Paraprofessional personnel assist the process by obtaining a *defined database* that is used in conjunction with a problem-oriented medical record system.[1] If one establishes a minimum base of necessary information about every patient or about every patient with a certain problem, then one can obtain that information in a number of ways.

Owner-supplied History

A basic history can be obtained by use of a well-designed questionnaire. The receptionist gives the questionnaire to the client, who completes it in the reception area. A paraprofessional (veterinary technician, nurse) can assist the client in answering difficult questions. The general medical history is available for review by the veterinarian, who notes significant items that may need further clarification. Problem-specific owner histories can be used to supplement the general history.

Role of the Veterinarian

The veterinarian should review most of the important parts of the history with the client. Misinterpretation of terminology, a course of events, or clinical signs occurs frequently. The veterinarian may need to rephrase questions several times before receiving a meaningful answer.

Table 1-2 **Clinical Problems in the Nervous System**

Problem	Localization
Usually of CNS Origin	
1. Convulsions	Cerebrum, diencephalon
2. Altered mental status	Cerebrum, limbic system
a. Stupor or coma	Brainstem reticular formation
b. Abnormal behavior	Limbic system
3. Paresis, paralysis, proprioceptive deficit	See Tables 2-2 to 2-4
4. Ataxia	
a. Head tilt, nystagmus	Vestibular system
b. Intention tremor, dysmetria	Cerebellum
c. Proprioceptive deficit, no head involvement	Spinal cord
5. Hypesthesia, anesthesia	See Figures 1-32 to 1-35; CN V
Possibly of CNS Origin	
1. Syncope	Usually cardiovascular, metabolic
2. Weakness	See Figure 2-7 and Table 2-3; metabolic or muscular
3. Lameness	Orthopedic: see Table 2-1
4. Pain, hyperesthesia	
a. Generalized	Thalamus, meningitis
b. Localized	See Figures 1-32 to 1-35; CN V
5. Blindness	
a. Pupils normal	Occipital cortex (contralateral)
b. Pupils abnormal	Retina, optic nerve, optic chiasma
6. Hearing deficit	
a. No vestibular signs	Cochlea
b. Vestibular signs	CN VIII, labyrinth
7. Anosmia	Nasal passages, CN I
8. Urinary incontinence	Pudendal/pelvic nerves, spinal cord, brainstem (see Chapter 13)

Modified from Oliver JE Jr: Localization of lesions in the nervous system. In Hoerlein BF, editor: *Canine neurology,* 3rd ed.
Philadelphia, 1978, WB Saunders.

Table 1-3 **Minimum Database: Neurologic Problem**

History
Physical examination
Neurologic examination
Clinical pathology
    CBC
    Urinalysis
    Chemistry profile
        BUN levels
        ALT levels
        Calcium levels
        Alkaline phosphatase levels
    Fasting blood glucose levels
    Total serum protein levels
    Albumin levels

CBC, Complete blood count; *BUN,* blood urea nitrogen; *ALT,* alanine aminotransferase.
Modified from Oliver JE Jr: Localization of lesions in the nervous system. In Hoerlein BF, editor: *Canine neurology,* 3rd ed. Philadelphia, 1978, WB Saunders.

The manner in which a question is phrased is important. Questions that imply negligence or ignorance on the part of the client may lead to defensive answers. Questions that suggest a correct answer may lead the client to interpret events incorrectly. All questions should be framed so that the answer "I don't know" is an acceptable alternative; otherwise, the client may hypothesize rather than relate facts.[2]

Neurologic History

Signalment

The species, breed, age, and sex of the patient may provide important clues to the diagnosis. Although few diagnoses can be positively ruled in or out on the basis of the signalment, many diseases are more or less likely to occur among certain groups of animals.

The prevalence of some diseases varies greatly among species and breeds. Many infectious diseases are species specific, such as canine distemper, feline infectious peritonitis, and equine protozoal encephalomyelitis. Known inherited diseases must be considered, especially in cases involving young animals. The Appendix lists many of the diseases with a species or breed predilection. Infectious diseases are listed in Chapter 15.

Young animals are more likely to have congenital and inherited disorders and infectious diseases. Older animals are likely to have degenerative and neoplastic diseases. Although these criteria are not absolute, the probability is much greater that a seizuring 8-year-old brachycephalic dog will have a neoplasm of the central nervous system (CNS) rather than a congenital anomaly. In the preliminary assessment, and sometimes in the final assessment, a diagnosis is an ordering of probabilities.

Sign-Time Graph

Construction of a sign-time graph is useful for evaluating the course of a disease (Figure 1-1). The sign-time graph plots the severity of clinical signs (on the vertical axis) against time (on the horizontal axis). A complete history allows the clinician to construct a graph that has no major gaps.[3] The sign-time graph is not usually drawn and entered on the case record. Rather, it is a useful tool for the clinician to construct mentally.

The time of onset of some problems may be exact (e.g., an automobile accident), or it may be difficult to determine, as in the case of neoplastic disease. The first time the client recognizes a problem must be taken as the starting point. Sometimes seemingly unrelated episodes may be the earliest signs and are recognized as such only as the complete history unfolds. For example, an animal with degenerative spinal cord disease may have been observed to stumble or to have difficulty with stairs for some time before clear manifestations of paresis were evident.

The course of the disease as revealed by the sign-time graph provides important information about the cause of the disease (see Figure 1-1). Slowly progressive diseases with an unrelenting course are immediately distinguished from acute diseases. The first step in making an etiologic diagnosis is classifying the problem as *acute* or *chronic* and *progressive* or *nonprogressive*. With this information, the problem logically falls into a group of diseases (Figures 1-1 and 1-2 and Table 1-4). The neurologic examination can further narrow the choice of diseases by indicating whether the problem is *focal* or *diffuse* (see Figure 1-2). After a

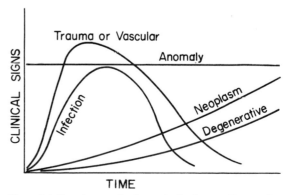

Figure 1-1 Sign-time graph of neurologic diseases. Progression of metabolic, nutritional, and toxic diseases is variable, depending on the cause.

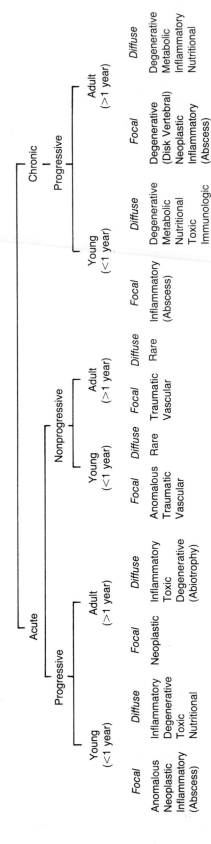

Figure 1-2 Classification of neurologic diseases in approximate order of frequency.

Table 1-4 Checklist for Differential Diagnosis

Category of Disease	Examples
D = Degenerative	Primary degeneration
	Storage disease
	Demyelinating diseases
	Neuronopathies
	Intervertebral disk disease
	Spondylosis
	Spondylopathies
A = Anomalous	Congenital defects
M = Metabolic	Nervous system disorders secondary to an abnormality of other organ systems (e.g., hypoglycemia, uremia)
N = Neoplastic	All tumors
Nutritional	All nutritional disorders
I = Idiopathic	Epilepsy
	Facial paralysis
	Vestibular syndrome
Immune	Myasthenia gravis (acquired)
	Polyradiculoneuritis
Inflammatory	Infectious diseases
	Immune mediated
T = Traumatic	Physical injury
Toxic	Exposure to all toxic agents (may include tetanus and botulism)
V = Vascular	Infarcts
	Hemorrhage

general etiologic or pathologic diagnosis is considered, the diagnostic plan can be established so that one can investigate each probable cause (see discussion of diagnostic methods in Chapter 4).

Neurologic Signs

Signs that are likely to be associated with an abnormality of the nervous system are listed in Table 1-2 and described in depth in Chapter 2.

Seizures nearly always indicate a problem in the forebrain, although the problem may be secondary to a metabolic or toxic condition. Differentiation between seizures and syncope may be difficult and may require wording the questions carefully and interpreting the answers even more carefully.

Stupor and coma are manifestations of abnormal cerebral or brainstem function. Behavioral changes may be caused by primary brain abnormalities or may be secondary to environmental factors.

Paresis and paralysis, signs of primary motor dysfunction, are caused by a neurologic abnormality. Lameness of musculoskeletal origin is differentiated from these signs by the neurologic examination.

Sensory deficits such as loss of proprioception or hypesthesia (decreased sensation) are always a result of an abnormality in the nervous system.

Pain may be related to neural lesions. For example, nerve-root irritation may cause localized pain and lameness, sometimes called *root signature*. The client's observations may be helpful in localizing the animal's pain. A careful physical and neurologic examination is essential to verify the signs.

Visual deficits may be caused by an abnormality of the eye or of the nervous system. Ocular and neurologic examinations are necessary to make a diagnosis. Historical information may be deceptive in the case of visual abnormalities. Animals in their usual surroundings may function normally even though they may be completely blind.

Deficits in hearing usually are not recognized unless they are bilateral. Bilateral hearing loss is usually caused by abnormalities of the inner ear. Brain lesions causing deafness are rare.

Loss of sense of smell (*anosmia*) is rarely recognized except in working dogs. Anorexia occasionally may be associated with anosmia.

PROGNOSIS

Providing the owner with a reasonably accurate prognosis is an essential part of clinical neurology. The prognosis is influenced by many variables. The major variables are the location, extent, and cause of the lesion.

The clinical course provides significant insight into the prognosis. Slowly progressive diseases such as neoplastic or degenerative conditions have a much poorer prognosis than those that have passed peak severity and are improving (see Figure 1-1).

Clinical signs are also valuable clues to prognosis. Spinal cord compression produces signs that vary with increasing compression (Figure 1-3). The signs are not related to the location of the tracts in the spinal cord but do correlate with the diameter of the fibers. With spinal cord compression, large fibers lose function before small fibers are affected. Functional recovery is possible until pain sensation is lost. An animal with no response to a painful stimulus for more than 48 hours has a low probability of recovery. Animals that do recover frequently have severe motor deficits.

The duration of the lesion is also a significant factor in prognosis because nervous tissue tolerates injury for only a short time. Spinal cord compression has been studied more thoroughly than most CNS injuries. Spinal cord compression severe enough to abolish voluntary motor function but not severe enough to abolish the response to a painful stimulus is associated with a reasonably good prognosis for recovery if decompression is achieved within 5 to 7 days. The longer the duration of compression, the slower the recovery.

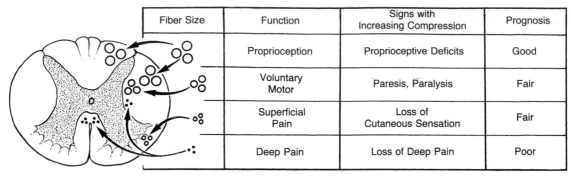

Fiber Size	Function	Signs with Increasing Compression	Prognosis
	Proprioception	Proprioceptive Deficits	Good
	Voluntary Motor	Paresis, Paralysis	Fair
	Superficial Pain	Loss of Cutaneous Sensation	Fair
	Deep Pain	Loss of Deep Pain	Poor

Figure 1-3 Progression of signs in spinal cord compression.

The location and character of the lesion are also important. An infarction of the spinal cord can range from mild to severe. Equally severe lesions have different prognoses, depending on the location. For example, an animal with an infarct primarily affecting gray matter at the L1 segment, with intact sensation to the pelvic limbs, has a reasonably good prognosis. The same degree of injury at the L5 segment is likely to produce permanent dysfunction because of destruction of the lower motor neurons supplying the femoral nerve.

THE NEUROLOGIC EXAMINATION

In the neurologic examination, the clinician systematically evaluates the functional integrity of the various components of the nervous system. An in-depth description can be found in Chapter 2.

The examination can be conveniently divided into the following parts: observation; palpation; examination of postural reactions, spinal reflexes, and cranial nerve responses; and sensory evaluation (Table 1-5). In every complete physical examination, each of these categories is investigated to assess any problem possibly related to the nervous system. An abbreviated neurologic examination might include the items marked with an asterisk in Table 1-5. Positive findings on any of these tests indicate the need for a more complete neurologic examination. Neurologic responses of neonatal dogs are outlined in Table 1-6.

The neurologic examination is usually described as a complicated process that is wholly separate from the physical examination. In reality, much of the neurologic examination is done as a routine part of the physical examination. The examiner need only be aware of what is being observed. The addition of a few extra steps completes the examination. A brief description of integration of the neurologic examination with the physical examination of a small animal patient is presented as an example. This is followed by detailed discussion of each of the components. The process of completing the neurologic examination differs depending on the examiner's routine in a physical examination.

Table 1-5 Neurologic Examination

I. Observation[*]
  Mental status
  Posture
  Movement
	Thoracic limb
	  Extensor carpi
	    radialis
	    muscle

II. Palpation[*]
  Integument
  Muscles
  Skeleton
	Triceps
	    brachii
	    muscle
	  Biceps brachii
	    muscle

III. Postural Reactions
  Proprioceptive
    positioning[*]
  Wheelbarrowing
  Hopping[*]
  Extensor postural
    thrust
  Hemistanding and
    hemiwalking
  Placing (tactile)
  Placing (visual)
  Sway test
  Tonic neck
	Flexor[*]
	  Extensor thrust
	  Perineal[*]
	  Crossed extensor
	  Extensor toe
	
	V. Cranial Nerves
	  Olfactory
	  Optic[*]
	  Oculomotor[*]
	  Trochlear
	  Trigeminal[*]
	  Abducent[*]
	  Facial[*]
	  Vestibulocochlear[*]

IV. Spinal Reflexes
  Myotatic
    Pelvic limb
      Quadriceps
      femoris
      muscle[*]
    Cranial tibial
      muscle
    Gastrocnemius
      muscle
	Glossopharyngeal[*]
	  Vagus[*]
	  Accessory
	  Hypoglossal[*]
	
	VI. Sensation
	  Touch
	  Hyperesthesia[*]
	  Superficial pain[*]
	  Deep pain†

[*]Included in a screening examination.
†If superficial pain is absent.

Table 1-6 **Neurologic Evaluation of the Neonatal Dog**

Response(s) Tested	Expected Response		
	Strong (Age in Days)	Weak, Variable (Age in Days)	Absent or Adultlike (Age in Days)
Motor			
Crossed extensor reflex	1-16	16-18	18+ (absent)
Magnus	1-17	17-21	21+ (absent)
Neck extension posture	Flexion 1-4	Hyperextension 4-21	Normotonia 21+
Forelimb placing	4+	2-4	0-2 (absent)
Hindlimb placing	8+	6-8	0-6 (absent)
Forelimb supporting	10+	6-19	0-6 (absent)
Hindlimb supporting	15+	11-15	0-11 (absent)
Standing on all limbs	21+	18-21	1-18 (absent)
Body righting (cutaneous)	1+	0-1	—
Sensory			
Rooting reflex	0-14	14-25	25+ (absent)
Nociceptive withdrawal reflex	0-19	19-23	23+ (adult)
Panniculus reflex	0-19	19-25	25+ (adult)
Reflex urination	0-22	22-25	25+ (absent)
Visual and Auditory			
Blinking response to light	16+	4-16	0-4 (absent)
Visual orientation	25+	20-25	0-20 (absent)
Auditory startle reflex	24+	15-24	0-15 (absent)
Sound orientation	25+	18-25	0-18

Modified from Fox MW: The clinical behavior of the neonatal dog. *J Am Vet Med Assoc* 143:1331-1335, 1963.

The Efficient Neurologic Examination

A simple numeric grading scheme may be used to record results of the examination. This scheme is provided in the case histories at the end of each chapter. Grades are assigned as follows: 0 = no response (reflex, reaction); +1 = a decreased response; +2 = a normal response; +3 = an exaggerated response; and +4 = a myotatic reflex with clonus.

1. *Observation.* Completed while taking the history.
2. *Palpation:* Usually done early in a physical examination.
3. *Postural reactions:* Require special tests. Hopping and proprioceptive positioning of each limb are usually all that are necessary. Proprioceptive positioning can be done during palpation; when the examiner's hand reaches the foot, the foot is knuckled under and the response observed.
4. *Spinal reflexes:* Require special tests. Quadriceps (knee jerk), extensor carpi radialis, and flexion reflexes are adequate. If gait and postural reactions are normal, spinal reflexes are usually normal.
5. *Cranial nerves (CN):* Can be examined during the general physical examination when the head is examined. While observing the head, the examiner notes symmetry of the face (CN VII) and symmetry of eye position and pupils (CN III, IV, VI, and sympathetic nerves). A menacing gesture is made at each eye, provoking a blink (CN II and VII). The medial and lateral canthus is touched on each eye, provoking a blink (CN V—ophthalmic [medial] and maxillary [lateral] branches; CN VII). The examiner turns the head from side to side, observing conjugate eye movements (CN III, IV, VI, and VIII) and then shines a light in each eye, observing the pupillary light reflex (CN II and III). The nose and lower jaw are touched or pinched, eliciting facial or behavioral movements (CN V—maxillary and mandibular; CN VII). The temporal and masseter muscles are palpated and the mouth opened, with the examiner noting jaw tone (CN V—mandibular). With the patient's mouth open, while assessing mucous membranes and tonsils, the examiner notes symmetry of the larynx and pharynx and touches the pharynx, causing a gag reflex (CN IX and X). The examiner observes symmetry of the tongue and, as the mouth is closed, rubs the nose; most animals will lick, illustrating symmetry of tongue movements (CN XII). During palpation of the animal, the trapezius and brachiocephalicus muscles are

observed for atrophy (CN XI). The only cranial nerve not tested is CN I—olfactory, which can be assessed by an aversive response to alcohol. It is not tested unless a forebrain deficit is suspected. This assessment of cranial nerves adds less than 2 minutes to the usual examination of the head.

6. *Sensory examination:* Hyperesthesia may have been detected during palpation. Response to pain can be assessed during flexion reflex testing and cranial nerve evaluation. Areas of suspicion are pursued last to avoid upsetting the animal early in the examination. Testing for deep pain is done only if the animal is not responsive to superficial stimulation.

The complete neurologic examination adds only a minimum amount of time to the total physical examination.

COMPONENTS OF THE NEUROLOGIC EXAMINATION

Observation

During every physical examination, the veterinarian should observe the animal's *mental status, posture*, and *movement*. The animal should be allowed to move around the examination room or in an open area while the history is being taken.[4-6]

Mental Status

Technique. The examiner can obtain a general impression of the animal's level of consciousness and behavior by observing its response to environmental stimuli or to people. Natural variations such as the aggressive curiosity of puppies, the indifference of older hounds, and the withdrawal of cats must be recognized as normal behavior. Overt aggression and fear-biting usually can be recognized.

Anatomy and Physiology. Consciousness is a function of the cerebral cortex and the brainstem.

Sensory stimuli from the body, such as touch, temperature, and pain, and from outside the body, such as sight, sound, and odors, provide input to the reticular formation. Consciousness is maintained by diffuse projections of the reticular formation to the cerebral cortex (Figure 1-4). This arousal system is termed the *reticular activating system.*[7] A common cause of decreased levels of consciousness is a disruption of the pathways between the reticular formation and the cerebral cortex. The limbic system, consisting of portions of the cerebrum and diencephalon, constitutes the substrate for behavior.

Assessment. An animal's mental status may be recorded as alert, depressed, stuporous, or comatose depending on its level of consciousness (see Chapter 12). Behavioral changes may include aggression, fear, withdrawal, and disorientation. Other signs related to abnormal behavior include yawning, head pressing, compulsive walking, circling, and "stargazing."

Depression in an animal is characterized by a conscious but inactive state. The animal is relatively unresponsive to the environment and tends to sleep when undisturbed. Depression may be caused by systemic problems such as fever, anemia, or metabolic disorders. When associated with primary brain problems, depression usually indicates diffuse cerebral cortex disease.

Stupor is exemplified by an animal that tends to sleep when undisturbed. Innocuous stimuli such as touch or noise may not cause arousal, but a painful stimulus causes the animal to awaken. Stupor usually is associated with partial disconnection of the reticular formation and the cerebral cortex, as in diffuse cerebral edema with herniation of the cerebrum causing compression of the brainstem.

Coma is a state of deep unconsciousness. The animal cannot be aroused even with painful stimuli, although simple reflexes may be intact. For example, pinching the foot produces a flexor reflex but does not cause arousal. Coma indicates

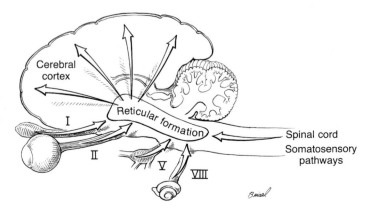

Figure 1-4 The ascending reticular activating system in the brainstem receives sensory information from the spinal cord and cranial nerves. It projects, through thalamic relays, diffusely to the cerebral cortex, thus maintaining consciousness.

complete disconnection of the reticular formation and the cerebral cortex. The most common cause in small animals is acute head injury with hemorrhage in the pons and the midbrain.[8] Animals that are unable to stand because of spinal cord dysfunction are alert.

Behavioral disorders are often functional, that is, related to environment and training. Primary brain disease, however, also can cause alterations in behavior. These are indicative of a cerebral or diencephalic lesion.

Posture

Technique. Abnormalities in posture may be noticed while the history is being recorded and the animal is free to move about. Further observations may necessitate moving the animal to different positions so that its ability to regain normal posture can be evaluated.

Anatomy and Physiology. Normal posture is maintained by coordinated motor responses to sensory inputs from receptors in the limbs and body, the visual system, and the vestibular system. Vestibular receptors sense alterations in the position of the animal's head in relation to gravity and detect motion. Sensory information is processed through the brainstem, cerebellum, and cerebrum. The cerebellum and vestibular system are especially important. The integrated output through motor pathways to the muscles of the neck, trunk, and limbs maintains normal posture. All domestic animals can maintain an erect posture shortly after birth; however, they vary in their ability to stand and walk.

Assessment

Head. The most common abnormality is a tilt or a twist to one side (Figure 1-5). Intermittent head tilt, especially if associated with rubbing of the ear, may be due to otitis externa or ear mites. A continuous head tilt with resistance to straightening of the head by the examiner is almost always due to vestibular system dysfunction (see Chapter 8). Signs range from tilting of the head (roll) or twisting of the head and neck (yaw) to twisting and rolling of the head, neck, and body. A yaw may indicate brainstem or cerebral disease; a roll is usually vestibular in origin. Both must be differentiated from spasms of cervical muscles caused by spinal cord or nerve root disease.

The head and neck may be held in a fixed position when cervical pain is present. Dogs with caudal cervical pain and weakness of the thoracic limb often arch their back and put their nose to the ground, apparently in an effort to keep weight off the thoracic limbs.

Trunk. Abnormal posture of the trunk may be associated with congenital or acquired lesions of

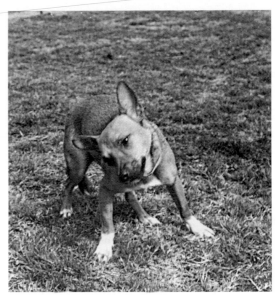

Figure 1-5 A dog with a head tilt and a broad-based stance, typical of vestibular disease.

the vertebrae or abnormal muscle tone from brain or spinal cord lesions. Deviations in vertebral contour consist of (1) *scoliosis*, lateral deviation; (2) *lordosis*, ventral deviation (swayback); and (3) *kyphosis*, dorsal deviation.

Limbs. Abnormal posture of the limbs includes improper positioning and increased or decreased extensor tone. A *wide-based stance* is common to all forms of ataxia (see Chapter 8) and is also seen in cases of generalized weakness. Proprioceptive or motor deficits may cause the animal to stand with a foot knuckled over (see Chapter 2). With lower motor neuron (LMN) or upper motor neuron (UMN) lesions, the animal often makes repeated attempts to reposition the limb. Uneven distribution of weight on the limbs may provide a clue to weakness or pain. Animals try to carry most of their weight on the thoracic limbs when the pelvic limbs are weak or painful and on the pelvic limbs when the thoracic limbs are affected.

Decreased tone in limb muscles is often associated with LMN lesions and causes abnormal posture. The limbs are positioned passively, often with the toes knuckled.

Decerebrate rigidity is characterized by extension of all four limbs and the trunk. It is caused by a lesion in the rostral brainstem (midbrain or pons). Opisthotonos may be associated with decerebrate rigidity if the rostral lobes of the cerebellum are damaged. Opisthotonos is dorsiflexion of the head and the neck.

Decerebellate rigidity is similar, but the pelvic limbs are usually flexed. It is seen only in association with an acute lesion of the cerebellum.

Increased tone in the extensor muscles is a sign of UMN disease (see Chapter 2). Partial lesions may produce an exaggerated straightness in the stifle and hock joints. *Decerebrate rigidity* is an extreme form of increased extensor tone. Increased tone in the forelimbs with flaccid paralysis of the hind limbs is called the *Schiff-Sherrington phenomenon* and is associated with spinal cord lesions between T2 and L4. Increased tone in both extensors and flexors is seen in tetanus and strychnine poisoning.

Movement

The animal should be observed for abnormal movements while resting and at gait. Careful observation is important because movement may be the most significant part of the neurologic examination, especially in large animals, in which postural reaction testing is more difficult.

Gait

Technique. The gait should be observed with the animal on a surface that offers adequate traction (carpet, synthetic turf, grass). Gaits vary among species and breeds, and the examiner must be knowledgeable of these differences. Some breeds of dogs have been selectively developed for characteristic gaits. Because of this breeding, neurologic diseases may have inadvertently been genetically selected. The gait should be observed from the side and while the animal is moving toward and away from the examiner. Each limb should be evaluated while the animal is walking and trotting. The animal should be turned in wide, tight circles and should be backed up. Large animals are walked up and down a slope and with the head and neck extended.[9] The examiner may exaggerate minimal abnormalities in gait by blindfolding the animal.

Anatomy and Physiology. The neural organization of gait and posture is complex, involving all levels of the nervous system. Limbs are maintained in extension for supporting weight by spinal cord reflexes. Stepping movements also are programmed at the spinal level (Figure 1-6). Organization of the various gaits used in normal locomotion occurs at the brainstem level in the reticular formation, probably in the subthalamic or pretectal areas. Removal of the input from the forebrain does not abolish the capacity for locomotion, including all normal gaits (trot, gallop, walk, and so forth). Cerebellar regulation of this system makes locomotion smooth and coordinated. Vestibular input maintains balance. Cerebral cortical input to the system is necessary for purposeful movement, voluntary control, and fine coordination, especially of learned movements.[10-12]

An animal with a cerebral cortex lesion is able to walk but does not have the precision of

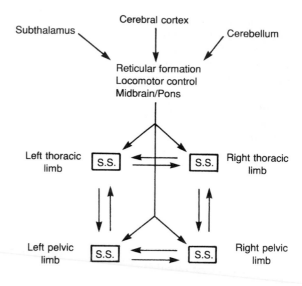

S.S. = Spinal stepping circuit in spinal cord

Figure 1-6 Schematic diagram of automatic control of locomotion. Spinal stepping reflexes are controlled by the brainstem centers for locomotion. Voluntary control is imposed from the cerebral cortex. The cerebellum and other areas coordinate the movements. *S.S.*, Spinal stepping circuit in spinal cord.

movement of a healthy animal. Postural reactions are abnormal. Severe rostral brainstem lesions (of the midbrain and the pons) cause decerebrate rigidity because the voluntary motor pathways that inhibit extensor muscle activity are lost. Lesions in the pons or the medulla abolish integrated locomotion. Acute lesions of the cerebellum produce rigidity, whereas chronic lesions produce ataxia and uncoordinated gait.

Assessment. Abnormalities of gait may include proprioceptive deficits, paresis, circling, ataxia, and dysmetria.

Proprioception, or position sense, is the ability to recognize the location of the limbs in relation to the rest of the body. A deficit appears as a misplacement or a knuckling of the foot that may not occur with every step. The proprioceptive pathways in the spinal cord are in the dorsal and dorsolateral columns and project to both the cerebellum (unconscious) and the cerebral cortex (conscious) (see the section on sensation in this chapter and Chapter 2).

Paresis is a deficit of motor function. Affected limbs have inadequate or absent voluntary motion, which may be described as *monoparesis*—paresis of one limb; *paraparesis*—paresis of both pelvic limbs; *tetraparesis* or *quadriparesis*—paresis of all four limbs; or *hemiparesis*—paresis of the thoracic and the pelvic limb on the same side.

The suffix *-plegia* may be used to denote complete loss of voluntary movements and is used by some to indicate both motor and sensory loss. In this text, *paresis* indicates partial deficit of motor function, whereas *paralysis* (*-plegia*) indicates a complete loss of voluntary movements. In general, the only difference in the two is the severity of the lesion; the localization is the same.

Paresis is caused by disruption of the voluntary motor pathways, which extend from the cerebral cortex through the brainstem to the lateral columns of the spinal cord. They continue to synapse on the LMN in each spinal cord segment that innervates the muscles. Paresis may be of the UMN or the LMN type (see Chapters 2 and 5 through 7).

A neurologic disease may cause an animal to circle. Circling may range from a tendency to drift in wide circles to forced spinning in a tight circle. Circling usually is not a localizing sign except that tight circles usually are caused by vestibular or caudal brainstem lesions and wide circles usually are caused by forebrain lesions. The direction of the circling is usually toward the side of the lesion, but exceptions occur, especially in lesions rostral to the midbrain. Twisting or head tilt associated with circling usually indicates involvement of the vestibular system (see Chapters 2 and 8).

Ataxia is a lack of coordination without spasticity, paresis, or involuntary movements, although each of these conditions may be seen in association with ataxia. Truncal ataxia is characterized by poorly controlled swaying of the body. Movement of the limbs is uncoordinated. The feet may be crossed or placed too far apart. Ataxia can be exaggerated by elevating the head or walking the animal on a slope. Ataxia may be caused by lesions of the cerebellum, the vestibular system, or the proprioceptive pathways (see Chapters 2 and 8).

Dysmetria is characterized by movements that are too long (hypermetria) or too short (hypometria). Goose-stepping is the most common sign of dysmetria. The stride may be abruptly stopped, forcing the animal to lurch from side to side. Dysmetria of the head and the neck may be most apparent when the animal tries to drink or eat and overshoots or undershoots the target. Dysmetria usually is caused by cerebellar or cerebellar pathway lesions and may be associated with ataxia and intention tremors (see Chapters 2 and 8).

Involuntary Abnormal Movement

Technique. Abnormal movements may occur when the animal is at rest or when it is moving and may be intermittent or continuous. The most frequently recognized movement disorders are tremors and myoclonus.

Assessment. A *tremor* is produced by alternating contractions of opposing groups of muscles. The oscillatory movements are small and rapid. Tremor should be characterized as an action (intention) tremor or one that occurs at rest. Tremor from neurologic causes must be differentiated from those induced by fatigue, fear, chilling, drug reactions, or primary muscle disease (see Chapter 10).

An *intention tremor* is one that is more pronounced when movements are initiated. It is an important sign of cerebellar disease. A *continuous tremor* usually is associated with an abnormality of the motor system.

Myoclonus is a coarse, jerking of muscle groups. Myoclonus associated with canine distemper encephalomyelitis is usually a rhythmic jerking of one muscle group, such as the flexors of the elbow or the temporal muscle. The myoclonus of distemper has been called chorea; however, chorea more accurately describes irregular, purposeless movements that are brief and that often change in location from one part of the body to the other. Two forms of myoclonus may be seen in the dog. In acute encephalitis, the lesion is probably related to destruction of areas in the basal nuclei. The more common chronic form is related to the interneurons or the LMN at the segmental level.[13] *Cataplexy* is a sudden, complete loss of muscle tone that causes the animal to fall limp. It is usually seen in association with narcolepsy (see Chapter 13). *Athetosis* is a "pillrolling" movement of the hands in people with Parkinson disease. A similar movement disorder has been produced in cats with lesions of the basal nuclei but has not been described in clinical patients.

Palpation

Technique. After the mental status, posture, and gait of the animal have been assessed, the physical examination is initiated. Careful inspection and palpation of the musculoskeletal and integumentary systems should be performed at one time or on a regional basis in conjunction with other parts of the examination. Comparison of one side with the other for symmetry is best done as one step in the examination.[14]

Assessment

Integument. Although the skin is not often involved in neurologic disease, careful inspection may reveal clues to the diagnosis. Scars may indicate previous trauma. Worn nails may be associated with paresis or with proprioceptive deficits. Coat and eye color may be related to a hereditary abnormality. For example, a white coat and blue eyes are associated with deafness in cats. A myelomeningocele may be palpated as it attaches to the skin in the lumbosacral region. The temperature of the extremities may be significantly lowered with arterial occlusion. Dermatomyositis is an inflammatory disease of the skin and muscle of collies and Shetland sheepdogs. Cutaneous lesions are present on the face, lips, and ears, and over bony prominences.

Skeleton. Careful palpation of the skeletal system may reveal *masses, deviation of normal contour, abnormal motion*, or *crepitation*. Tumors involving the skull or the vertebral column may be palpable as a mass. The spinous processes of the vertebrae should be palpated for irregularities of contour. Deviations may indicate a luxation, fracture, or congenital anomaly. Depressed or elevated skull fractures often can be palpated, especially in animals with minimal temporal muscle masses. Persistent fontanelles and suture lines in the skull may indicate hydrocephalus. Abnormal motion or crepitation may be detected in fractures and luxations. When vertebral luxations or fractures are suspected, manipulation should not be attempted because additional displacement may cause serious spinal cord damage. Peripheral nerve injuries may be associated with fractures of the long bones.

Muscles. Muscles are evaluated for *size, tone*, and *strength*. All muscle groups should be systematically palpated, starting with the head, extending down the neck and the trunk, and continuing down each limb.

Changes in muscle size may be apparent from observation as well as from palpation. Loss of muscle mass (*atrophy*) is the most frequent finding. Atrophy may indicate LMN disease or disuse. Criteria for differentiating the two are presented in Chapter 2. Localized muscle atrophy, which usually accompanies LMN disease, is an important localizing sign.

Muscle tonus is maintained through the spinal stretch (*myotatic*) reflex. Alterations in tone, either increased or decreased, can be detected by palpation and passive manipulation of the limb. Increased tone of the extensor muscles, a common finding in UMN disease, manifests as increased resistance to passive flexion of the limb (see Chapter 2 for an interpretation).

Muscle strength is difficult to evaluate even in the most cooperative patients. The extensor muscles can be evaluated during postural reactions such as hopping, in which the animal must support all of its weight on one limb (see the section on hopping in this chapter). The flexor muscles can be evaluated by comparing the relative strength of pull during a flexor reflex (see the section on the flexor reflex in this chapter). Loss of muscle strength is usually a sign of LMN disease but is occasionally observed with UMN disease.

Postural Reactions

The complex responses that maintain an animal's normal, upright position are known as *postural*. If an animal's weight is shifted from one side to the other, from front to rear, or from rear to front, the increased load on the supporting limb or limbs requires increased tone in the extensor muscles to keep the limb from collapsing. Part of the alteration in tone is accomplished through spinal reflexes, but for the changes to be smooth and coordinated, the sensory and motor systems of the brain must be involved.

Abnormalities of complex reactions such as the hopping reaction do not provide precise localizing information because lesions in any one of several areas of the nervous system may affect the reaction. The assessment of postural reactions, however, is an important part of the neurologic examination. Minimal deficits in the function of a key component such as the cerebral cortex may cause significant alterations in postural reactions that are not detected when one observes the gait.

Two major types of postural reactions are used. The first consists of hopping, wheelbarrowing, and extensor postural thrust; these require movement of the limb to correct for displacement of the body and differ only in which limbs are tested. Weight bearing occurs, and so weakness accentuates abnormality. The second type includes proprioceptive positioning and placing; these usually are performed with some support of the animal's weight. Therefore weakness has less influence on performance. Both types of reactions are useful. Because the pathways for the postural reactions are similar, interpretation is essentially the same for all reactions.

The following postural reactions are listed in a sequence convenient for performing an examination. In an initial screening examination, hopping and proprioceptive positioning reactions (Table 1-5) should be tested. If they are normal, abnormalities are unlikely to be found in the other reactions.

Proprioceptive Positioning Reaction (Foot/Limb Placement Test)

Technique. This reaction tests more than conscious proprioception: light touch and pressure are also evaluated. Although sensory functions are evaluated, the reactions described in this section also require motor responses. It is incorrect to assume that abnormalities observed are strictly due to proprioceptive dysfunction.

The simplest method of evaluation entails flexing the foot so that the dorsal surface is on the floor (Figure 1-7). The animal should return the foot to a normal position immediately. Most animals do

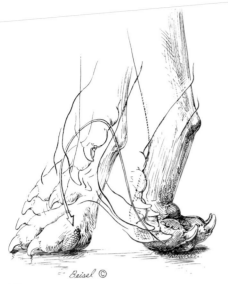

Figure 1-7 Proprioceptive positioning response. Conscious proprioceptive function is tested by placing the dorsal surface of the animal's foot on the floor. The animal should immediately replace it to the normal position. (From Green CE, Oliver JE: Neurologic examination. In Ettinger SJ (ed): *Textbook of veterinary internal medicine,* 2nd ed. Philadelphia, 1982, WB Saunders.)

not allow weight bearing to occur in the abnormal position. In large animals, the foot or hoof is placed on a sheet of cardboard that is slowly pulled laterally. As the limb reaches an abnormal position, the animal should reposition it for normal weight bearing. The first test is the most sensitive for proprioception in the distal extremity, whereas the second test is more sensitive for detecting abnormalities in the proximal portion of the limb. With either method, the examiner should test each foot separately.

Anatomy and Physiology. Proprioceptive information is carried in the dorsal columns and the spinomedullothalamic tract in the dorsolateral funiculus of the spinal cord, through the brainstem, to the sensorimotor cortex (Figure 1-8). The motor response is initiated by the cerebral cortex and is transmitted to the LMN in the spinal cord (see the section on sensation in this chapter).

Assessment. Because the proprioceptive pathways are sensitive to compression, abnormalities in proprioceptive positioning may occur before motor dysfunction can be detected (see Chapter 2). The response is abnormal if significant paresis exists, but other postural reactions such as hopping are also affected. Proprioceptive positioning is less useful in large animals because many do not respond. Observation of abnormal positioning of the limbs at rest may be interpreted similarly.[9] Some normal dogs will not reposition the paw after

it is knuckled over. In this situation, the hopping reaction should always be evaluated.

Hopping Reaction

Technique. The hopping reaction is the most predictive postural reaction. It evaluates all components involved in voluntary limb movements. Normal hopping responses require intact sensory receptors, peripheral nerves, ascending long tracts in the spinal cord and brainstem, sensory cortex, UMN systems, and integration with LMNs in the spinal cord (see Chapter 2).

The hopping reaction of the thoracic limbs is tested with one thoracic limb lifted from the ground (Figure 1-9). Although it is easy to pick up three limbs in small dogs and cats, this is not necessary in larger animals. The animal's pelvis should be supported sufficiently to increase weight bearing on the extended limb. As weight is increased on the extended limb, the ability of the animal to maintain full limb extension is assessed. The patient's weight is then shifted laterally, and initiation, movement, and support during hopping are assessed. Medial hopping is much more difficult, and more subtle abnormalities may be detected with this maneuver. Hopping of the pelvic limbs is accomplished by supporting the thorax and lifting one pelvic limb. Weight is shifted laterally on the extended limb and initiation, movement and support are assessed. A large animal such as a giant-breed dog, a horse, and a cow can be tested by lifting one limb and shifting the weight of the animal so that it hops on the opposite limb. Alternatively, large animals can be pulled by the tail or pushed laterally (*sway reaction*) to elicit movements similar to the hopping reaction.

Assessment. The hopping reaction is more sensitive than other postural reactions for detecting minor deficits. Poor initiation of the hopping reaction suggests sensory (*proprioceptive*) deficits, whereas poor follow-through suggests a motor system abnormality (*paresis*). Asymmetry is easily seen and helps to lateralize lesions.

Wheelbarrowing Reaction

Technique. The animal is supported under the abdomen with all of the weight on the thoracic limbs (Figure 1-10). The normal animal can walk forward and sideways with coordinated movements of both thoracic limbs. The examiner should not lift the pelvic limbs so high that the animal's posture is grossly abnormal. If movements appear normal, the maneuver is repeated with the head lifted and the neck extended. This position prevents visual compensation, making the animal mostly dependent on proprioceptive information. A tonic neck reaction, which causes slightly increased extensor

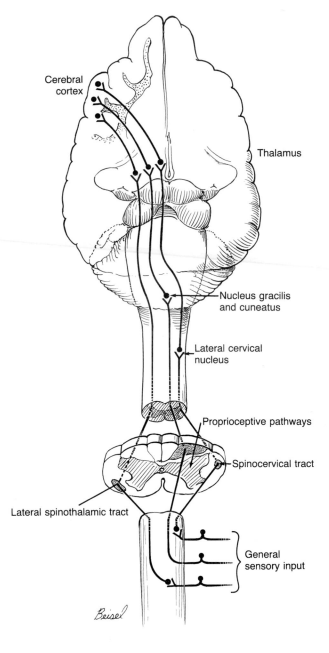

Figure 1-8 Somatic sensory innervation is transmitted to the brain through several pathways. Proprioception is a function of the spinomedullothalamic pathway (near the spinocervical tract) for the pelvic limbs and of the fasciculus cuneatus of the dorsal columns for the thoracic limbs. Pain is transmitted by several tracts (see also Figure 1-33), including the spinothalamic, spinocervical, and spinoreticular tracts and the dorsal columns.

tone in the forelimbs, is also elicited. When the neck is extended, subtle abnormalities of the thoracic limbs may be seen in animals that otherwise appear normal. *This reaction is especially useful for detecting compressive lesions in the caudal cervical region that largely cause paraparesis.*
Assessment. Weakness in the thoracic limbs may be detected when the wheelbarrowing reaction is tested because the animal is forced to carry most of its weight on two limbs while standing on only one limb while moving.

Slow initiation of movement may be a sign of proprioceptive deficit or of paresis that is caused by a lesion of the cervical spinal cord, the brainstem, or the cerebral cortex. Exaggerated movements (*dysmetria*) may indicate an abnormality of the cervical spinal cord, the caudal brainstem, or the cerebellum.

Extensor Postural Thrust Reaction

Technique. Extensor postural thrust is elicited by supporting the animal by the thorax caudal to the thoracic limb and lowering the pelvic limbs to the floor (Figure 1-11). When the limbs touch the floor, they should move caudally in a symmetric walking movement to achieve a position of support.

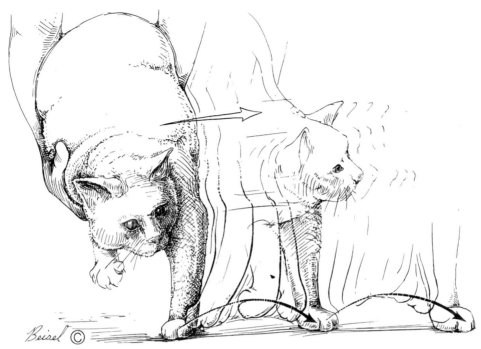

Figure 1-9 The hopping reaction. The normal animal responds to hopping by quickly replacing the limb under the body as it moves laterally. Large animals can be tested by picking up one limb and pushing the body laterally. (From Greenc CE, Oliver JE: Neurologic examination. In Ettinger SJ, editor: *Textbook of veterinary internal medicine,* 2nd ed. Philadelphia, 1982, WB Saunders.)

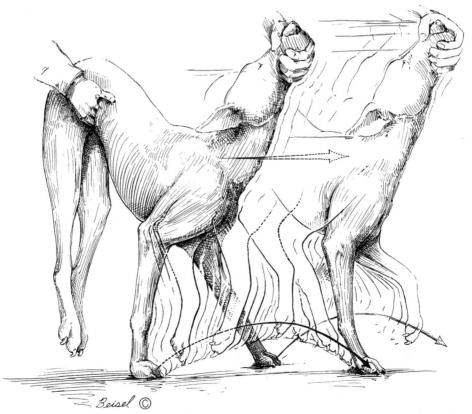

Figure 1-10 Wheelbarrowing with the neck extended. Wheelbarrowing is performed with the pelvic limbs elevated. The body should be in a position as close to normal as possible. The head may be elevated to accentuate abnormalities, as illustrated here. (From Greene CE, Oliver JE: Neurologic examination. In Ettinger SJ, editor: *Textbook of veterinary internal medicine,* 2nd ed. Philadelphia, 1982, WB Saunders.)

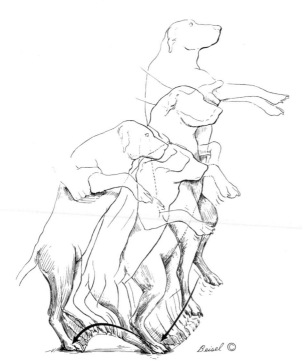

Figure 1-11 The extensor postural thrust reaction. The animal responds by stepping backward when its feet make contact with the floor. (From Greene CE, Oliver JE: Neurologic examination. In Ettinger SJ, editor: *Textbook of veterinary internal medicine,* 2nd ed. Philadelphia, 1982, WB Saunders.)

As the animal is lowered to the floor, it extends its limbs, anticipating contact. This is a vestibular reaction and may be lacking or uncoordinated in animals with lesions of the vestibular system.

Assessment. Asymmetric weakness, lack of coordination, and dysmetria can be seen in the extensor postural thrust reaction as in the wheelbarrowing reaction. Extensor postural thrust reaction is difficult or impossible to perform on larger animals.

Hemistanding and Hemiwalking Reactions

Technique. The thoracic and pelvic limbs on one side are lifted from the ground so that all of the animal's weight is supported by the opposite limbs. Forward and lateral walking movements are then evaluated.

Assessment. Abnormal signs may be seen in hemistanding and hemiwalking as in the other postural reactions. They are most useful in animals with forebrain lesions. These animals have relatively normal gaits but have deficits of postural reactions in both the thoracic and the pelvic limbs contralateral to the side of the lesion.

Placing Reaction

Technique. Placing is evaluated first without vision (*tactile placing*) and then with vision (*visual placing*). The examiner supports the animal under the thorax and covers its eyes with one hand or with a blindfold. The thoracic limbs are brought in contact with the edge of a table at or ventral to the carpus (Figure 1-12). The normal response is immediate placement of the feet on the table surface in a position that supports weight. Care must be taken not to restrict the movement of either limb. When one limb is consistently slower to respond, the animal should be held in the examiner's other hand to ensure that its movements are not being restricted.

Visual placing is tested by allowing the animal to see the table surface. Normal animals reach for the surface before the carpus touches the table. Peripheral visual fields can be tested by making a lateral approach to the table. The veterinarian can evaluate giant-breed dogs and large animals such as horses and cows by leading them over a curb or a step, with and without vision. Some dogs and cats that are accustomed to being held may ignore the table. These animals usually respond if they are held in a less secure or less comfortable position away from the body of the examiner.

Anatomy and Physiology. Tactile placing requires touch receptors in the skin, sensory pathways

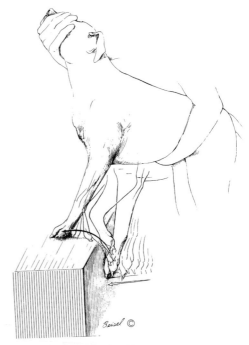

Figure 1-12 The tactile placing reaction is elicited with the animal's eyes covered. When the carpus makes contact with the edge of the surface, the animal should immediately place its foot on the surface. Similar responses can be elicited from large animals by leading them over a curb or up steps. (From Greene CE, Oliver JE: Neurologic examination. In Ettinger SJ, editor: *Textbook of Veterinary Internal Medicine,* 2nd ed. Philadelphia, 1982, WB Saunders.)

through the spinal cord and the brainstem to the cerebral cortex, and motor pathways from the cerebral cortex to the LMN of the thoracic limbs. Visual placing requires normal visual pathways to the cerebral cortex, communication from the visual cortex to the motor cortex, and motor pathways to the LMN of the forelimbs.[16]

Assessment. A lesion of any portion of the pathway may cause a deficit in the placing reaction. Normal tactile placing with absent visual placing indicates a lesion of the visual pathways. Normal visual placing with abnormal tactile placing suggests a sensory pathway lesion. Forebrain lesions produce a deficit in the contralateral limb. Lesions caudal to the midbrain usually produce ipsilateral deficits.

Tonic Neck Reaction

Technique. With the animal in a normal standing position, the head is elevated and the neck is extended. The normal reaction is a slight extension of the thoracic limbs and a slight flexion of the pelvic limbs. Lowering the head causes the thoracic limbs to flex and the pelvic limbs to extend. Turning the head to the side causes a slight extension of the ipsilateral thoracic limb and a slight flexion of the contralateral thoracic limb. The normal reactions are easy to remember if one considers the usual movements of an animal. For example, a cat about to jump onto a table extends the head and the neck, extends the thoracic limbs, and flexes the pelvic limbs. A dog crawling under a bed lowers the head and the neck and flexes the thoracic limbs as it extends the pelvic limbs for propulsion. A horse making a sharp turn leads with the head and the neck, plants the ipsilateral limb in extension, and flexes the contralateral limb to take a step.[17]

Tonic eye reactions also may be observed. They are discussed in the section on cranial nerves.

Assessment. The tonic neck reactions are initiated by receptors in the cranial cervical area and are mediated by brainstem reticular formation. The responses are subtle in normal animals and often are inhibited volitionally through cortical control.

Abnormalities in sensory (*proprioception*) or motor systems may produce abnormal reactions. Lesions in the cerebellum cause exaggerated tonic neck reactions. The tonic neck reactions are not usually helpful in detecting abnormality.

Spinal Reflexes

Examination of the spinal reflexes tests the integrity of the sensory and motor components of the reflex arc and the influence of descending motor pathways on the reflex. Three kinds of responses may be seen. *Absence* or *depression* of a reflex indicates complete or partial loss of either sensory or motor (LMN) components of the reflex; a *normal response* indicates that both sensory and motor components are intact; and an *exaggerated response* indicates an abnormality in the motor pathways (UMN) that normally have an inhibitory influence on the reflex or a deficit of the opposing muscles if paresis is also present.

The examination should be performed with the animal in lateral recumbency. Muscle tone, previously evaluated with the animal in a standing position, should be evaluated again at this time. The pelvic limbs are tested first. Passive manipulation of the limb assesses the degree of muscle tone, especially in the extensor muscles. Spreading the toes with slight pressure on the footpads elicits the extensor thrust reflex. The myotatic (stretch) reflexes then are evaluated. Routinely, only the knee jerk (quadriceps) reflex is tested. The cranial tibial and gastrocnemius muscles can also be evaluated, but the reflexes are more difficult to elicit and quantify. Next, the flexor reflex is tested by gently pinching the toes. To maintain cooperation of the patient, the examiner should apply the mildest stimulus that elicits a response. If flexion is induced by touching the foot, one need not crush the toe with a hemostat. The perineal reflex is a contraction of the anal sphincter in response to a touch, a pinprick, or a pinch in the perineal area. Flexion of the tail may occur simultaneously.

The most predictable myotatic reflex in the thoracic limb is elicited when the extensor carpi radialis muscle (tendons over the carpus in large animals) is struck, producing a slight extension of the carpus. The triceps and biceps reflexes are difficult to elicit and evaluate in many normal animals. After examining the limbs on one side, the veterinarian turns the animal and examines the opposite limbs.

Myotatic (Stretch) Reflexes

Quadriceps (Knee Jerk, Patellar) Reflex
Technique. With the animal in lateral recumbency, the limb is supported under the femur with the left hand (by a right-handed examiner) and the stifle is flexed slightly (Figure 1-13). The patellar ligament is struck crisply with the plexor. The response is a single, quick extension of the stifle.[18] The plexor is recommended for performing myotatic reflex testing, but other instruments such as bandage scissors may be used. Nose tongs or similar heavy instruments are useful for testing large animals. The examiner should use the same type of instruments in each examination to obtain consistent results.
Anatomy and Physiology. The myotatic or stretch reflexes are basic to the regulation of posture and movement. The reflex arc is a simple

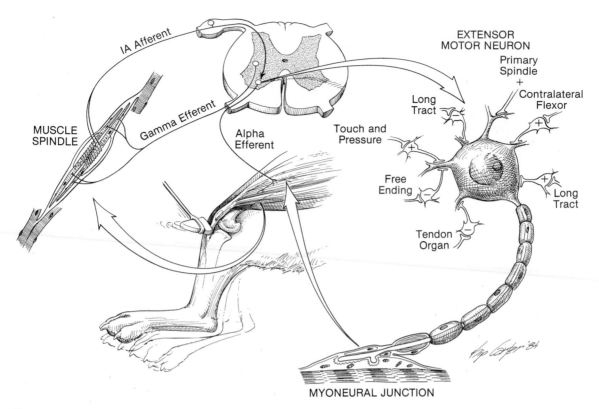

Figure 1-13 Myotatic (stretch) reflex. Percussion of the tendon or muscle stretches the muscle spindle. IA afferent fibers are activated and synapse directly on motor neurons of the muscle. The motor neuron discharges when a threshold level of excitation is reached. The level of excitation of the motor neuron is related to synapses from a variety of sources, as illustrated. The impulse travels down the axon (alpha efferent) to the neuromuscular junction, causing a release of acetylcholine. Acetylcholine binds to receptors on the muscle, causing depolarization and contraction of the muscle. Gamma motor neurons maintain tension on the muscle spindle regardless of the state of contraction of the muscle. (From Oliver JE, Hoerlein BF, Mayhew IG: *Veterinary neurology.* Philadelphia, 1987, WB Saunders.)

two-neuron (monosynaptic) pathway. The sensory neuron has a receptor in the muscle spindle and its cell body in the dorsal root ganglion. The motor neurons have their cell bodies in the ventral horn of the gray matter of the spinal cord. The axons form the motor components of peripheral nerves that end on the muscle (the neuromuscular junction) (see Figure 1-13).

The muscle spindle is the stretch receptor of the muscle. The spindle has three to five striated muscle fibers (intrafusal muscle fibers) at each end, with a nonstriated portion in the middle (see Figure 1-13). The spindles are located in the belly of the skeletal muscle (extrafusal muscle fibers). These sensory fibers are large and have a spiral ending, called the *primary ending*, around the nonstriated portion of each fiber. Small sensory fibers have secondary endings. Primary endings are of greatest importance in phasic responses (e.g., knee jerk). Secondary endings respond primarily to tonic activation (e.g., extensor thrust). The small intrafusal muscle fibers of the spindle are innervated by small (gamma) motor neurons.

Stretching a muscle depolarizes the nerve endings of the spindle, producing a burst of impulses in the sensory fibers. The sensory fibers directly activate the large (alpha) motor neuron in the spinal cord. The alpha motor neuron discharges impulses through its axon, causing a contraction of the extrafusal muscle fibers of the same muscle. Thus a sudden stretch of the muscle causes a reflex muscle contraction, as seen in the knee jerk reflex. A more tonic stretch of the muscle causes a slower discharge of sensory activity and a slower, steadier muscle contraction.

Contraction of the extrafusal muscle fibers causes relaxation of the intrafusal fibers because they are parallel. Loss of tension on the intrafusal fibers stops the sensory input from the spindle. To prevent this situation from occurring, gamma motor fibers adjust the length of the intrafusal fibers. Thus, tension is maintained on the spindle through the range of motion of the limb.

Gamma motor neuron activation of the intrafusal fibers also can stretch the primary spindle endings directly and thus can elicit a response indirectly in the alpha motor neuron. Alpha and gamma motor neurons are facilitated or inhibited by a variety of segmental and long spinal pathways. The output of the motor neurons is a summation of their facilitatory and inhibitory inputs. For example, the quadriceps motor neuron responds to a sudden stretch by a quick contraction (knee jerk) but can be blocked by voluntary inhibition (see Figure 1-13).

The spindle sensory fibers also facilitate interneurons in the spinal cord, which in turn inhibit motor neurons of antagonistic muscles. This activity is called *reciprocal innervation*. For example, spindle sensory fibers from the quadriceps muscle inhibit antagonistic flexor motor neurons, allowing the limb to extend. Spindle sensory fibers also contribute collaterals to ascending pathways, which provide information to the brain regarding activity in the muscles.

Assessment. The quadriceps reflex is the most reliably interpreted myotatic reflex. The reflex should be recorded as absent (0), depressed (+1), normal (+2), exaggerated (+3), or exaggerated with clonus (+4). Normal responses vary widely among species and among breeds within a species. In large dogs the response is less brisk than in small dogs. The examiner should become familiar with these natural variations.

Absence (0) of a myotatic reflex indicates a lesion of the sensory or motor component of the reflex arc—a LMN or segmental sign (see Chapter 2). Loss of the reflex in one muscle group suggests a peripheral nerve lesion, for example, a lesion of the femoral nerve. Bilateral loss of the reflex suggests a segmental spinal cord lesion affecting the motor neurons to both limbs located in spinal cord segments L4-6 in the dog. Differentiation between peripheral nerve and spinal cord lesions may require assessment of the sensory examination and the presence or absence of other neurologic signs.

Depression (+1) of the reflex has the same significance as absence of the reflex, except the lesion is incomplete. Depression of the reflex is more common with spinal cord lesions in cases in which some, but not all, of the segments (L4-6) are affected. Other reflexes also must be tested because generalized depression of reflexes may be seen in polyneuropathies or in abnormalities of the neuromuscular junction (botulism, tick paralysis).

Animals that are tense and keep the limb in extension commonly have depressed or absent reflexes. Sometimes the reflex is hard to elicit in normal dogs in the recumbent or nonrecumbent limb. You only have to elicit the normal reflex one time to be sure the reflex arc is intact.

Exaggerated reflexes (+3, +4) and increased tone result from loss of descending inhibitory pathways. *The voluntary motor pathways are facilitatory to flexor muscles and inhibitory to extensor muscles.* Damage to these pathways releases the myotatic reflex, causing an exaggerated reflex and increased extensor tone. Clonus (+4) is a repetitive contraction and relaxation of the muscle in response to a single stimulus. Clonus often is seen with chronic (weeks to months) loss of descending inhibitory pathways. Clonus has the same localizing significance as exaggerated reflexes. Bilateral exaggerated reflexes most often are associated with damage to descending inhibitory pathways cranial to the level of the reflex. *UMN injury causing exaggerated myotatic reflexes should also cause paresis.* If gait and postural reactions are normal, the "exaggerated reflex" is then likely to be examiner error or normal for the individual. Exaggerated reflexes should not be overinterpreted. If gait and postural reactions are normal, the only concern is that the reflex be at least normal.

Cranial Tibial Reflex

Technique. With the animal in lateral recumbency, the examiner tests the cranial tibial reflex. The belly of the cranial tibial muscle is struck with the plexor just distal to the proximal end of the tibia (Figure 1-14). The response is flexion of the hock.

Anatomy and Physiology. The cranial tibial muscle is a flexor of the hock and is innervated by the peroneal branch of the sciatic nerve (with origin in the L6-7 segments of the spinal cord in the dog).

Assessment. The cranial tibial reflex is more difficult to elicit in a normal animal than is the quadriceps reflex. Absent or decreased reflexes should be interpreted with caution. Exaggerated reflexes indicate a lesion cranial to the spinal cord segments L6-7.

Gastrocnemius Reflex

Technique. The gastrocnemius reflex is tested after the cranial tibial reflex. The tendon of the gastrocnemius muscle is struck with the plexor just dorsal to the tibial tarsal bone (Figure 1-15). Slight flexion of the hock is necessary for some tension of the muscle to be maintained. The response is extension of the hock.

Anatomy and Physiology. The gastrocnemius is primarily an extensor of the hock and is innervated by the tibial branch of the sciatic nerve (with origin in the L7-S1 segments of the spinal cord in the dog).

Assessment. The gastrocnemius reflex is interpreted in the same manner as the cranial tibial reflex but is even less reliable.

Extensor Carpi Radialis Reflex

Technique. The animal is in lateral recumbency while the reflexes of the thoracic limb are evaluated. The limb is supported under the elbow, with flexion of the elbow and the carpus maintained. The extensor carpi radialis muscle is struck with the plexor just distal to the elbow (Figure 1-16).

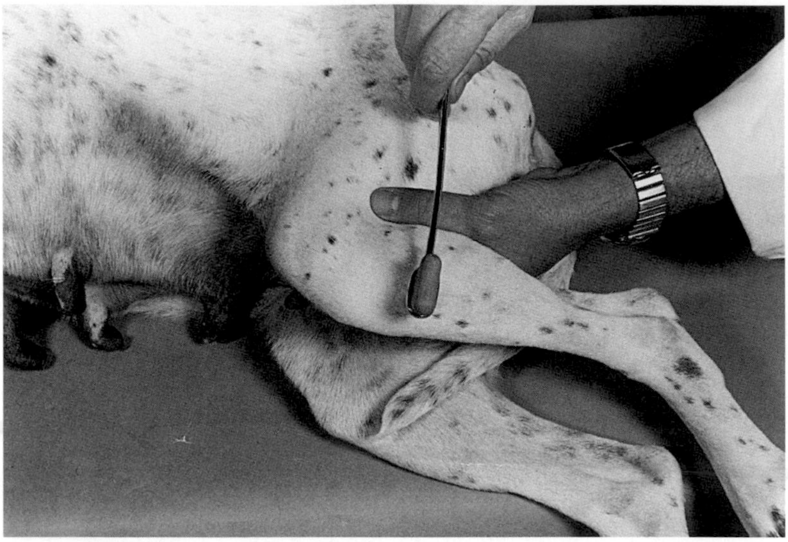

Figure 1-14 The cranial tibial reflex is elicited with the animal in lateral recumbency, with both stifle and hock slightly flexed. The cranial tibial muscle is percussed just distal to the stifle.

The response is a slight extension of the carpus. The carpus must be flexed, and the digits must not touch the floor or the other limb or the reflex will be mechanically inhibited.[17] The extensor tendons crossing the carpal joint are struck in large animals.

Anatomy and Physiology. The extensor carpi radialis is an extensor of the carpus and is innervated by the radial nerve (with origin in the C7-T1 segments of the spinal cord in the dog).

Assessment. The extensor carpi radialis reflex is more difficult to elicit than the quadriceps reflex but usually can be recognized in dogs. Absent or decreased reflexes should be evaluated with caution. Strong reflexes are usually exaggerated (+3) and indicate a lesion cranial to C7.

Triceps Reflex

Technique. The animal is held in the same position as that for the extensor carpi radialis reflex. The triceps brachii muscle is struck with the plexor just proximal to the olecranon (Figure 1-17). The response is a slight extension of the elbow or a visible contraction of the muscle. The elbow must be maintained in flexion for a response to be elicited.

Anatomy and Physiology. The triceps brachii muscle extends the elbow and is essential for weight bearing in the forelimb. Innervation is through the radial nerve (with the origin from spinal cord segments C7-T1 in the dog).

Assessment. The triceps reflex is difficult to elicit in the normal animal. Absent or decreased reflexes should not be interpreted as abnormal. Lesions of

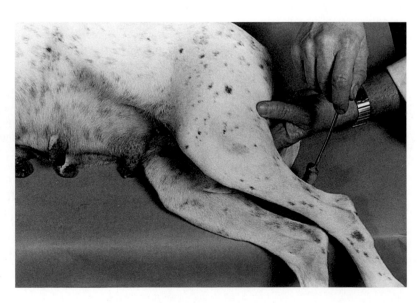

Figure 1-15 The gastrocnemius reflex is elicited with the animal in the same position as for testing of the cranial tibial reflex. The tendon of the gastrocnemius muscle is percussed proximal to the tarsus.

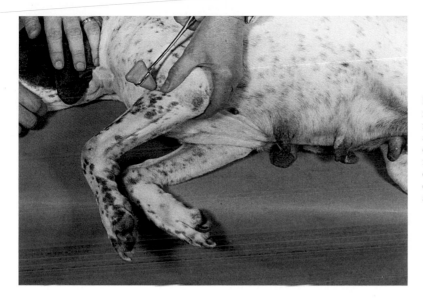

Figure 1-16 The extensor carpi radialis reflex is the most reliable myotatic reflex in the thoracic limb. With the animal in lateral recumbency and the elbow and carpus flexed, the extensor muscle group is percussed distal to the elbow. The digital extensor tendons can be percussed at the carpus in large animals.

the radial nerve can be recognized by a loss of muscle tone and an inability to support weight. Exaggerated reflexes are interpreted in the same way as for the extensor carpi radialis reflex.

Biceps Reflex
Technique. The index or middle finger of the examiner's hand that is holding the animal's elbow is placed on the biceps and the brachialis tendons cranial and proximal to the elbow. The elbow is slightly extended, and the finger is struck with the plexor (Figure 1-18). The response is a slight flexion of the elbow. Movement of the animal's elbow must not be blocked by the examiner's restraining hand.

Anatomy and Physiology. The biceps brachii and brachialis muscles are flexors of the elbow. They are innervated by the musculocutaneous nerve, which originates from spinal cord segments C6-8 in the dog.

Assessment. The biceps reflex is difficult to elicit in the normal animal. Absent or decreased reflexes should not be interpreted as abnormal. Flexion of the elbow on the flexor reflex provides a better assessment of the musculocutaneous nerve. An exaggerated (13) reflex is indicative of a lesion cranial to C6.

Flexor (Pedal, Withdrawal) Reflexes

Pelvic Limb
Technique. The animal is maintained in lateral recumbency, the same position as that for examination of the myotatic reflexes. A noxious stimulus is

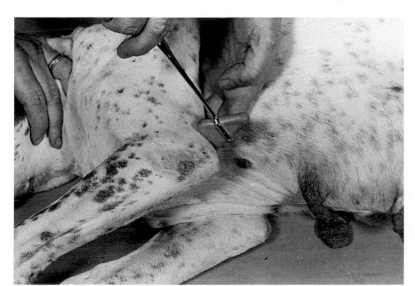

Figure 1-17 The triceps reflex is elicited with the animal in the same position as for the extensor carpi radialis reflex. The triceps tendon is percussed proximal to the elbow.

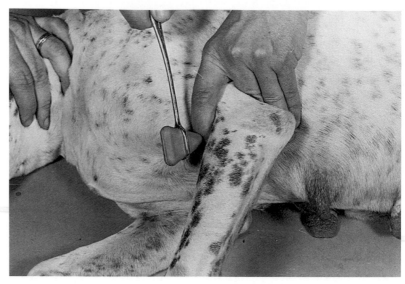

Figure 1-18 The biceps reflex is elicited with the elbow slightly extended. The examiner's finger is placed on the biceps tendon proximal to the elbow, and the finger is percussed.

applied to the foot. The normal response is a flexion of the entire limb, including the hip, stifle, and hock (Figure 1-19). The least noxious stimulus possible should be used. If an animal flexes the limb when the digit is touched, the digit need not be crushed. If a response is not easily elicited, a hemostat should be used to squeeze across a digit. Pressure should not be so great as to injure the skin. Both medial and lateral digits should be tested on each limb. The limb should be in a slightly extended position when the stimulus is applied to allow the limb to flex. The opposite limb also should be free to extend.[19]

Anatomy and Physiology. The flexor reflex is more complex than the myotatic reflex. The response involves all of the flexor muscles of the limb and thus requires activation of motor neurons in several spinal cord segments (see Figure 1-19).

The receptors for the flexor reflex are primarily free nerve endings in the skin and other tissues that respond to noxious stimuli such as pressure, heat, and cold. A stimulus that produces a sensory discharge in these nerves ascends to the spinal cord through the dorsal root. The sensory nerves from the digits of the pelvic limbs are primarily branches of the sciatic nerve, the superficial peroneal nerve on the dorsal surface, and the tibial nerve on the plantar surface. The sciatic nerve originates from spinal cord segments L6-S1. The medial digit is partially innervated by the saphenous nerve, a branch of the femoral nerve that originates from spinal cord segments L4-6. Interneurons are activated at these segments and at adjacent segments both cranially and caudally. The interneurons activate sciatic motor neurons, which stimulate flexor muscle contraction (see Figure 1-19). The net result is withdrawal of the limb from the noxious stimulus.

Inhibitory interneurons to the extensor motor neurons also are activated, resulting in decreased activity in the extensor muscles. Relaxation of the extensor muscles and contraction of the flexor muscles allow complete flexion of the limb.

The flexor reflex is a spinal reflex and does not require any activation of the brain. If an animal steps on a sharp piece of glass, it immediately withdraws the foot before consciously perceiving pain. If the spinal cord is completely transected cranial to the segments that are responsible for the reflex, the reflex is present even though the animal has no conscious perception of pain.

Assessment. Absence (0) or depression (+1) of the reflex indicates a lesion of L6-S1 segments or the branches of the sciatic nerve. Unilateral absence of the reflex is more likely the result of a peripheral nerve lesion, whereas bilateral absence or depression of the reflex is more likely the result of a spinal cord lesion. A normal (+2) flexor reflex indicates that the segments and the nerves are functional. An exaggerated (+3) flexor reflex rarely is seen with acute lesions of descending pathways. Chronic and severe descending pathway lesions may cause exaggeration of the reflex. This exaggeration is manifested as a sustained withdrawal after release of the stimulus. A *mass reflex* (+4) occasionally is seen as a sustained flexion of both pelvic limbs, with contraction of the tail and perineal muscles in response to a stimulus applied to only one limb. Exaggerated flexor reflexes usually reflect chronicity rather than severity of the lesion.

The crossed extensor reflex and the conscious perception of pain also are evaluated while the flexor reflex is performed, but these assessments are discussed later.

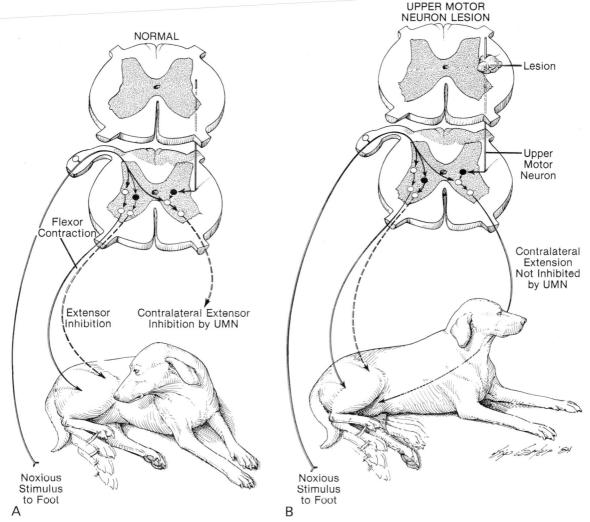

NORMAL

UPPER MOTOR
NEURON LESION

Lesion

Upper
Motor
Neuron

Flexor
Contraction

Contralateral
Extension
Not Inhibited
by UMN

Extensor
Inhibition

Contralateral Extensor
Inhibition by UMN

Noxious
Stimulus
to Foot

Noxious
Stimulus
to Foot

A

B

Figure 1-19 Flexor and crossed extension reflexes **A,**The animal is positioned in lateral recumbency and a noxious stimulus is applied to a digit. The limb is immediately withdrawn. Sensory fibers enter the spinal cord through the dorsal root to synapse on interneurons. Flexor motor neurons are activated, causing flexion of the limb. Simultaneously, inhibitory interneurons cause relaxation of the antagonistic extensor muscles. Other interneurons cross the spinal cord to activate contralateral extensor muscles—the crossed extensor reflex. **B,** The crossed extensor reflex is inhibited unless damage to UMN systems has occurred. Sensory fibers also project to the brain, causing a conscious awareness of pain and subsequently a behavioral reaction (A). The reflex is not dependent on a behavioral reaction. The behavioral reaction may be absent if sensory pathways are damaged. (From Oliver JE, Hoerlein BF, Mayhew IG: *Veterinary neurology.* Philadelphia, 1987, WB Saunders.)

Thoracic Limb

Technique. The thoracic limb flexor reflex is tested in the same manner as the pelvic limb flexor reflex. Cranial and palmar surfaces and medial and lateral digits should be tested.

Anatomy and Physiology. Branches of the radial nerve innervate the cranial surface of the foot and arise from spinal cord segments C7-T1. The medial palmar surface is innervated by the ulnar and median nerves, which originate from spinal cord segments C8-T1. The lateral palmar surface and most of the lateral digit are innervated by branches

of the ulnar nerve. The organization of the flexor reflex of the thoracic limb is similar to that previously described for the pelvic limb. Flexor muscles of the thoracic limb are innervated by the axillary, musculocutaneous, median, and ulnar nerves and by parts of the radial nerve. These nerves originate from spinal cord segments C6-T1, with small contributions from C5 and T2 in some animals.

Assessment. Depressed reflexes indicate a lesion of the C6-T1 segments of the spinal cord or the peripheral nerves. Exaggerated reflexes indicate a lesion cranial to C6.

Extensor Thrust Reflex

Technique. The reflex may be elicited with the animal in lateral recumbency (the same position as that for the myotatic reflex) or with the animal suspended by the shoulders with the pelvic limbs hanging free (Figure 1-20). The toes are spread, and slight pressure is applied between the pads. The response is a rigid extension of the limb.[20]

Anatomy and Physiology. The extensor thrust reflex is initiated by a stretching of the spindles in the interosseous muscles of the foot.[16] Simultaneously, the cutaneous sensory receptors are stimulated. The extensors predominate, forcing the limb into rigid extension. The sensory fibers are in the sciatic nerve (spinal cord segments L6-S1), and the response involves both femoral and sciatic nerves (spinal cord segments L4-S1). Excessive stimulation of the flexor reflex sensory fibers (e.g., with a noxious stimulus) causes the flexor reflex to predominate and withdrawal occurs.

The extensor thrust reflex is important for maintaining posture and is a component of more complex reactions such as hopping.[17]

Assessment. The extensor thrust reflex is difficult to elicit in normal animals, especially when they are in lateral recumbency. Elicitation of the reflex generally indicates a lesion cranial to L4.

Perineal (Bulbocavernosus, Anal) Reflex

Technique. The perineal reflex is elicited by light stimulation of the perineum with forceps. Painful stimuli usually are not necessary. The response is a contraction of the anal sphincter muscle and a flexion of the tail (Figure 1-21). One can obtain a similar response by squeezing the penis or the vulva (bulbocavernosus reflex). If the anal sphincter appears weak or if the response is questionable, the examiner can insert a gloved digit into the anus because minimal responses often can be felt in this manner.

Anatomy and Physiology. Sensory innervation occurs through the pudendal nerves and spinal cord segments S1-2 (sometimes S3) in the dog and the cat. Motor innervation of the anal sphincter also occurs through the pudendal nerves. Tail flexion is mediated through the caudal nerves. The organization of the reflex is similar to that of the flexor reflex.

Assessment. The perineal reflex is the best indication of the functional integrity of the sacral spinal cord segments and nerve roots. Evaluation of this reflex is especially important in animals with urinary bladder dysfunction (see Chapter 3). Absence (0) or depression (+1) of the reflex indicates a sacral spinal cord or pudendal nerve lesion.

Crossed Extensor Reflex

Technique. The crossed extensor reflex may be observed when the flexor reflex is elicited. The response is an extension of the limb opposite the stimulated limb.[19]

Anatomy and Physiology. The crossed extensor reflex is a part of the normal supporting mechanism of the animal. The weight of an animal in a standing position is evenly distributed among the limbs. If one limb is flexed, increased support is required of the opposite limb. The flexor reflex sensory fibers send collaterals to interneurons on the opposite side of the spinal cord, which excite extensor motor neurons (see Figure 1-19).

Assessment. The crossed extensor reflex generally is considered an abnormal reflex except in the standing position. In the normal recumbent animal, the extension response is inhibited through descending

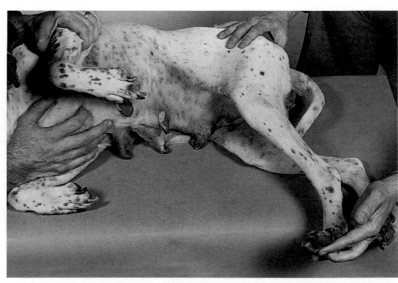

Figure 1-20 The extensor thrust reflex is elicited by spreading the phalanges.

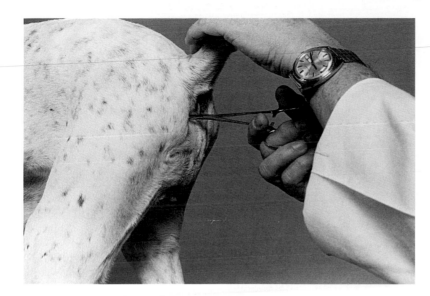

Figure 1-21 The perineal reflex is a contraction of the anal sphincter and a ventral flexion of the tail in response to tactile stimulation of the perineum.

pathways. Crossed extensor reflexes result from lesions in ipsilateral descending pathways, a sign of UMN disease. The crossed extensor reflex has been considered evidence of a severe spinal cord lesion. It is not a reliable indicator of the severity of the lesion, however. Animals that are still ambulatory may have crossed extensor reflexes, especially when the lesion is in the cervical spinal cord or the brainstem.

Extensor Toe (Babinski) Reflex

Technique. The animal is positioned in lateral recumbency (the same position as that for the myotatic reflex). The pelvic limb is held proximal to the hock, with the hock and the digits slightly flexed. The handle of the plexor or a forceps is used to stroke the limb on the caudolateral surface from the hock to the digits (Figure 1-22). The normal animal exhibits no response or a slight flexion of the digits. The abnormal response is an extension and a fanning of the digits.[21]

Anatomy and Physiology. The extensor toe reflex has been compared with the Babinski reflex in human beings.[22] The two reflexes are not strictly analogous because Babinski's reflex includes elevation and fanning of the large toe, which is not present in domestic animals; it is reported to be a sign of pyramidal tract damage in human beings. The extensor toe reflex has been produced by lesions in the brainstem.[22] It has been seen clinically in dogs with chronic UMN pelvic limb paresis.[21] Acute experimental lesions of the sensorimotor cortex, the dorsal columns, the lateral columns, or the ventral columns of the spinal cord have not produced an extensor toe reflex. Some investigators have considered this reflex to be an abnormal form of the flexor reflex.

Assessment. The extensor toe reflex has been observed in dogs with paralysis of the pelvic limbs associated with extensor hypertonus and exaggerated myotatic reflexes. In most cases clinical signs have been present for longer than 3 weeks. The reflex should be interpreted in the same manner as other exaggerated reflexes.

Cranial Nerves

Examination of the CNs is an important part of the neurologic examination, especially when disease of the brain is suspected. An abnormality of a CN constitutes evidence of a specific, localized area of disease not provided by postural reactions. The cranial nerve examination is not difficult, and the most commonly affected CNs can be evaluated quickly (Figure 1-23). The general outline of the cranial nerve examination was discussed under The Efficient Neurologic Examination at the beginning of this chapter.

Detection of any abnormalities on the screening examination may be followed by a more complete examination to define the abnormality further.

Olfactory Nerve (CN I)

The olfactory nerve is the sensory path for the conscious perception of smell.

Technique. A behavioral response to a pleasurable or a noxious odor, either inferred from the history or assessed by direct testing, may be used (Figure 1-24). Alcohol, cloves, xylol, benzol, or cat food containing fish appears to stimulate the olfactory nerves. Irritating substances such as ammonia or tobacco smoke cannot be used because they stimulate the endings of the trigeminal nerve in the nasal mucosa.

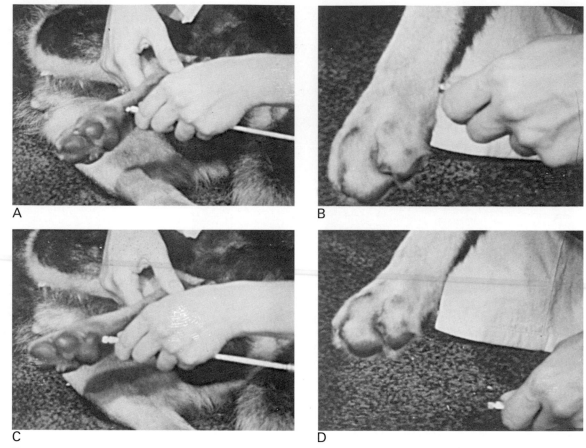

Figure 1-22 The extensor toe response (Babinski's reflex). **A** and **B,**The toes of the pelvic limbs are in the normal position. The instrument is moving down the metatarsus from the hock toward the digits. **C** and **D,** The digits extend and fan apart as the instrument completes the sweep. (Illustrations are frames from a motion picture.) (From Kneller SK, Oliver JE, Lewis RE: Differential diagnosis of progressive caudal paresis in an aged German Shepherd dog. *J Am Anim Hosp Assoc* 11:414-417, 1975.)

Anatomy and Physiology. Chemoreceptors in the nasal mucosa give rise to axons, which pass through the cribriform plate to synapse in the olfactory bulb. Axons from the olfactory bulb course through the olfactory tract to the ipsilateral olfactory cortex. Behavioral reactions to odors are controlled by connections to the limbic system.[7]

Assessment. Deficiencies in the sense of smell are difficult to evaluate. Rhinitis is the most common cause of *anosmia* (loss of olfaction). Tumors of the nasal passages and diseases of the cribriform plate also must be considered. Only rarely are structural lesions such as tumors of importance. Olfaction is also impaired by inflammatory diseases such as canine distemper and parainfluenza virus infection.[23]

Optic Nerve (CN II)

The optic nerve is the sensory path for vision and pupillary light reflexes (see Figures 11-1 and 11-2).

Technique. The optic nerve is tested in conjunction with the oculomotor nerve (CN III), which provides the motor pathway for the pupillary light reflex, and the facial nerve, which provides the motor pathway for the blink reflex. Vision can be assessed by observation of the animal's movements in unfamiliar surroundings, avoidance of obstacles, and following of moving objects. More objective evaluation requires three tests. The examiner elicits the menace reaction by making a threatening gesture with the hand at one eye. The normal response is a blink and, sometimes, an aversive movement of the head (Figure 1-25). The visual placing reaction (see the section on postural reactions) is an excellent method of assessing vision. The examiner induces the pupillary light reflex by shining a light in each eye and observing for pupillary constriction in both eyes.

Anatomy and Physiology. See Chapters 2 and 11.

Assessment. See Chapters 2 and 11.

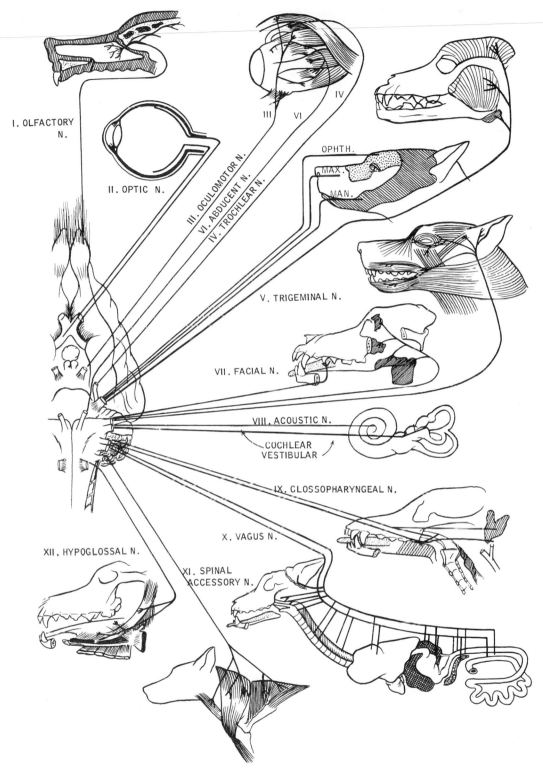

Figure 1-23 The origin and distribution of the cranial nerves in the dog. *N,* Nerve; *OPHTH,* ophthalmic nerve; *MAX,* maxillary nerve; *MAN,* mandibular nerve. (From Hoerlein BF: *Canine neurology,* 3rd ed. Philadelphia, 1978, WB Saunders.)

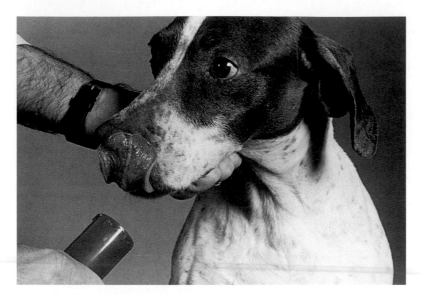

Figure 1-24 Noxious odors that are nonirritating cause an aversion or licking reaction.

Oculomotor Nerve (CN III)

The oculomotor nerve contains the parasympathetic motor fibers for pupillary constriction and innervates the following extraocular muscles: dorsal, medial, and ventral recti and ventral oblique. This nerve also innervates the levator palpebrae muscle of the upper lid (see Figure 11-4).

Technique. The examiner tests the pupillary light reflex by shining a light in the animal's eye and observing for pupillary constriction in both eyes. One can assess eye movement by observing the eyes as the animal looks in various directions voluntarily or in response to movements in the peripheral fields of vision. A more direct method is to elicit vestibular eye movements (normal nystagmus) by moving the head laterally (Figure 1-26). The fast beat of the nystagmus is in the direction of the head movement. The eyes should move in coordination with each other (conjugate movements). One can easily test the rectus muscles by this method.

A drooping upper lid (*ptosis*) is indicative of paresis of the levator palpebrae muscle. Lesions of the oculomotor nerve cause a fixed ventrolateral deviation (*strabismus*) of the eye and a dilated pupil. In cattle, the eye usually remains horizontal regardless of the head position. The function of each of the extraocular muscles can be assessed in the same manner if the examiner bears this difference in mind. The functions of the extraocular muscles of large animals have not been directly

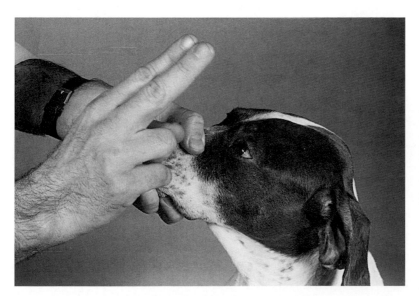

Figure 1-25 The menace reaction is elicited by making a threatening gesture at the eye, which should result in a blink. The examiner must avoid creating wind currents or touching the hairs around the eye, which will cause a palpebral reflex. The sensory pathway is in the optic nerve and the visual pathway. The motor pathway is in the facial nerve.

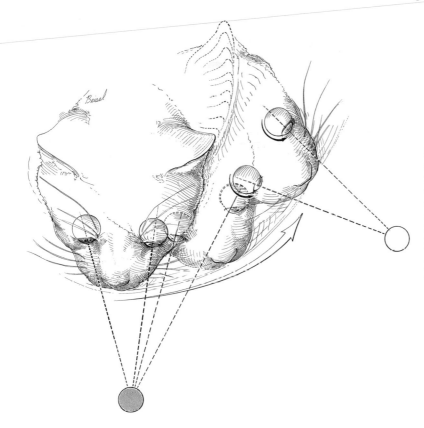

Figure 1-26 Vestibular eye movements are elicited by turning the animal's head from side to side. The eyes lag behind the head movement and then rotate to return to the center of the palpebral fissure. Both visual (oculokinetic or physiologic nystagmus) and vestibular pathways are active in this response, but vestibular pathways predominate and produce these movements in the absence of vision.

established, but presumably they are similar to the functions of the corresponding muscles in other species.

Anatomy and Physiology. See Chapters 2 and 11.

Assessment. See Chapters 2 and 11.

Trochlear Nerve (CN IV)

The trochlear nerve is the motor pathway to the dorsal oblique muscle of the eye.

Technique. The trochlear nerve is difficult to assess. Lesions may cause a lateral rotation of the eye, which can be seen most clearly in animals with a horizontal pupil (cow) or a vertical pupil (cat) or by ophthalmoscopic examination of the dorsal retinal vein (see Figure 11-4). A slight deficit is present in dorsomedial gaze.

Anatomy and Physiology. See Chapters 2 and 11.

Assessment. See Chapters 2 and 11.

Trigeminal Nerve (CN V)

The trigeminal nerve is the motor pathway to the muscles of mastication and the sensory pathway to the face.

Technique. The motor branch of the trigeminal nerve is in the mandibular nerve and innervates the masseter, temporal, rostral digastric, pterygoid, and mylohyoid muscles.[7] Bilateral paralysis produces a dropped jaw that cannot be closed voluntarily.

Unilateral lesions may cause decreased jaw tone. Atrophy of the temporal and masseter muscles is recognized by careful palpation approximately 1 week after the onset of paralysis. Sensation should be tested over the distribution of all three branches: ophthalmic, maxillary, and mandibular. A touch of the skin may be an adequate stimulus in some animals, whereas a gentle pinch with a forceps may be needed in others. The palpebral reflex is a blink response to a touch at the medial canthus of the eye that tests the ophthalmic branch (Figure 1-27). Touching the lateral canthus tests the maxillary branch. The blink response is dependent on innervation of the muscles by the facial nerve. Stimulation of the nasal mucosa tests the maxillary branch and should elicit a response even in depressed or stoic animals (Figure 1-28). Pinching the jaw tests the mandibular branch.

Anatomy and Physiology. See Chapters 2 and 9.

Assessment. See Chapters 2 and 9.

Abducent Nerve (CN VI)

The abducent nerve innervates the lateral rectus and the retractor bulbi muscles.

Technique. Eye movements are tested by the method described for the oculomotor nerve. The retractor bulbi muscles can be tested with a palpebral or a corneal reflex. Normally, the globe is

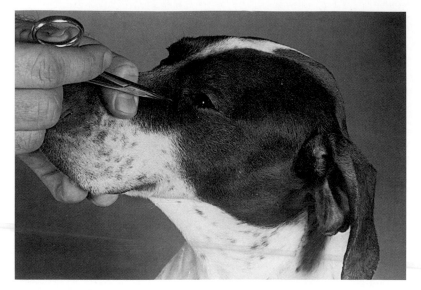

Figure 1-27 The palpebral reflex is checked by touching the eyelid and observing for a blink. The sensory pathway is in the trigeminal nerve; the motor pathway is in the facial nerve.

retracted, allowing extrusion of the third eyelid. Lesions of the abducent nerve cause a loss of lateral (abducted) gaze and medial strabismus combined with inability to retract the globe (see Figure 11-4). **Anatomy and Physiology.** See Chapters 2 and 11. **Assessment.** See Chapters 2 and 11.

Facial Nerve (CN VII)

The facial nerve is the motor pathway to the muscles of facial expression and the sensory pathway for taste to the palate and the rostral two thirds of the tongue. It also provides sensory innervation to the inner surface of the pinna.
Technique. Asymmetry is usually seen in cases of facial paralysis. The lips, eyelids, and ears may droop. The nose may be slightly deviated to the normal side, and the nostril may not flare on inhalation. The palpebral fissure may be slightly widened and fails to close when a palpebral or a corneal reflex is attempted (see Figure 1-27). Pinching the lip produces a behavioral response, but the lip may not retract. The examiner can test the animal's sense of taste by moistening a cotton-tipped applicator with atropine and touching it to the rostral part of the tongue. The affected side is tested first. Normal dogs react immediately to the bitter taste. Delayed reactions may occur as the atropine spreads to normal areas of the tongue.
Anatomy and Physiology. See Chapters 2 and 9.
Assessment. See Chapters 2 and 9.

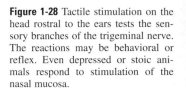
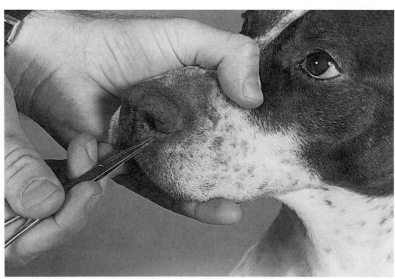

Figure 1-28 Tactile stimulation on the head rostral to the ears tests the sensory branches of the trigeminal nerve. The reactions may be behavioral or reflex. Even depressed or stoic animals respond to stimulation of the nasal mucosa.

Vestibulocochlear Nerve (CN VIII)

The vestibulocochlear nerve has two branches: the *cochlear division,* which mediates hearing, and the *vestibular division,* which provides information about the orientation of the head with respect to gravity.

Technique

Cochlear Division. Most tests for hearing are dependent on behavioral reactions to sound and therefore are subject to misinterpretation. No good test exists for unilateral deficits other than those involving electrophysiologic systems. Crude tests involve startling the animal with a loud noise (clap, whistle). Similar responses may be monitored by an electroencephalogram (EEG) or by observation or direct measurement of the respiratory cycle. Human audiometry equipment can also be adapted for animals. The most precise equipment involves a signal-averaging computer, which measures electrical activity of the brainstem in response to auditory stimuli (brainstem auditory-evoked response [BAER]). BAER not only detects auditory deficits but also may indicate the location of the lesion (see Chapter 4).

Vestibular Division. Abnormalities of the vestibular system produce several characteristic signs. Most vestibular lesions are unilateral except in congenital anomalies and occasionally in inflammatory diseases. Unilateral vestibular disease usually produces ataxia, nystagmus, and a head tilt to the side of the lesion.[6]

The head tilt should be apparent on observation (see Figure 1-5). The examiner can accentuate the head tilt by removing visual compensation or by removing tactile proprioception. Ataxia (an uncoordinated, staggering gait) usually is accompanied by a broad-based stance and a tendency to fall or to circle to the side of the lesion.

Nystagmus is involuntary rhythmic movement of the eyes. Two forms of nystagmus are recognized. *Jerk nystagmus* has a slow phase in one direction and a rapid recovery phase to return. *Pendular nystagmus* is small oscillations of the eyes with no slow or fast components. Pendular nystagmus is associated with visual defects and cerebellar diseases. Jerk nystagmus is associated with vestibular and brainstem diseases. See Chapter 11 for a more complete discussion of nystagmus. Nystagmus should be observed with the head held in varying positions. The direction of the fast component is noted (e.g., left horizontal nystagmus). Jerk nystagmus may be horizontal, vertical, or rotatory. Forced deviation of the globe (strabismus) also may be seen when the head is elevated or lowered. Typically, in small animals, the ipsilateral eye deviates ventrally when the head is elevated. Producing eye movements by moving the animal's head from side to side, physiologic nystagmus (see the section on CN III) also tests the vestibular system (see Figure 1-26). Vestibular lesions may alter the direction or may abolish the response. In some cases, the eyes do not move together (dysconjugate movement).

Lesions of the receptors or the vestibular nerve cause a horizontal or rotatory nystagmus that does not change with varying head positions. Lesions of the vestibular nuclei and associated structures may cause nystagmus in any direction that may change that direction with varying head positions. We have observed a few relatively rare instances of nystagmus that changes direction with confirmed peripheral disease and no evidence of central disease.

Postrotatory nystagmus may help to evaluate vestibular disease. As an animal is rotated rapidly, physiologic nystagmus is induced. When rotation is stopped, nystagmus (postrotatory) occurs in the opposite direction and is observed for a short time. The receptors opposite the direction of rotation are stimulated more than the ipsilateral receptors because they are farther from the axis of rotation. Unilateral lesions produce a difference in the rate and duration of postrotatory nystagmus when the animal is tested in both directions. The test is performed in the following manner: The animal is held by an assistant, who rapidly turns 360 degrees 10 times and then stops. The examiner counts the beats of nystagmus. After several minutes, the test is repeated in the opposite direction. Normal animals have three to four beats of nystagmus, with the fast phase opposite the direction of rotation. Peripheral lesions usually depress the response when the animal is rotated away from the side of the lesion. Central lesions may depress or prolong the response.

The caloric test is a specific test for vestibular function. This test has the advantage of assessing each side independently. It is difficult to perform in many animals, however, and may be unreliable if the patient is uncooperative. Negative responses occur in many normal animals. The examiner performs the test by holding the animal's head securely in one position, irrigating the ear canal with ice water, and observing for nystagmus. A rubber ear syringe should be used for the irrigation. Usually, 50 to 100 mL of cold water is adequate, and the infusion takes approximately 3 minutes. The test should not be performed if the tympanic membrane is ruptured or if the ear canal is plugged. Nystagmus is induced with the fast phase away from the side being tested. Warm water also produces the same effect, except that the nystagmus is in the opposite direction. Warm water is even less reliable. If the animal resists and shakes its head, the response usually is abolished. The test is helpful for the evaluation of brainstem function in comatose animals but has been replaced by the BAER test at most institutions.

Anatomy and Physiology. See Chapters 2 and 8.

Assessment. See Chapters 2 and 8.

Glossopharyngeal Nerve (CN IX) and Vagus Nerve (CN X)

Cranial nerves IX and X are considered together because of their common origin and intracranial pathway. The glossopharyngeal nerve innervates the muscles of the pharynx along with some fibers from the vagus nerve. The glossopharyngeal nerve also supplies parasympathetic motor fibers to the zygomatic and parotid salivary glands. It is sensory to the caudal one third of the tongue and the pharyngeal mucosa, including the sensation of taste. The vagus nerve innervates the pharynx, the larynx, and the palate and supplies parasympathetic motor fibers to the viscera of the body, except for the pelvic viscera, which are innervated by sacral parasympathetic nerves. Gastric abnormalities are common in vagus nerve problems in ruminants. The vagus nerve is the sensory pathway to the caudal pharynx, the larynx, and the viscera.

Technique. Taste can be evaluated by the method described for CN VII, although making an accurate assessment of the caudal part of the tongue is more difficult. The simplest test for function is to observe the palate and the larynx for asymmetry and to elicit a gag or a swallowing reflex by inserting a tongue depressor to the pharynx. Stertorous breathing may be observed with laryngeal paralysis. Endoscopic observation of the larynx is useful in the horse. The laryngeal adductor response (*slap test*) is performed during endoscopic observation. The skin caudal to the dorsal part of the scapula is slapped gently with the hand during expiration. The normal response is brief adduction of the contralateral arytenoid cartilage.[9]

Historical evidence of an inability to swallow may be suggestive of an abnormality in CNs IX and X. The clinician should be cautious when examining animals with swallowing problems because dysphagia is one of the signs of rabies.

Anatomy and Physiology. See Chapters 2 and 9.

Assessment. See Chapters 2 and 9.

Accessory Nerve

The accessory nerve is the motor pathway to the trapezius muscle and parts of the sternocephalicus and brachiocephalicus muscles.

Technique. The detection of an abnormality in an accessory nerve injury may be difficult, except by careful palpation for atrophy of the affected muscles. Passive movement of the head and the neck may demonstrate a loss of resistance to lateral movements in a contralateral direction.

Anatomy and Physiology. The accessory nerve arises from fibers in the ventral roots of C1-7 spinal cord segments and from the medulla. The fibers course cranially as the spinal root of the accessory nerve, which lies between the dorsal and the ventral spinal nerve roots. It emerges from the skull by way of the tympanooccipital fissure and then courses caudally in the neck to innervate the trapezius and portions of the sternocephalicus and brachiocephalicus muscles. These muscles elevate and advance the limb and fix the neck laterally.[7]

Assessment. Lesions of the accessory nerve are either rare or rarely recognized. An injury to the nerve in the vertebral canal or the cranium probably would be masked by other, more severe signs of paresis. The course of the nerve in the neck is well protected by muscle but could be damaged by deep penetrating wounds, injections, or contusions. Atrophy of the affected muscles would be the most obvious sign of injury. Electromyography (EMG) may be necessary for diagnosis. Lesions in the vertebral canal should produce other signs of spinal cord dysfunction.

Hypoglossal Nerve

The hypoglossal nerve is the motor pathway to the intrinsic and extrinsic muscles of the tongue and the geniohyoideus muscle.

Technique. The muscles of the tongue protrude and retract it. Each side is innervated independently. Protrusion is tested by wetting the animal's nose and observing the ability to extend its tongue forward (Figure 1-29). The strength of retraction can be tested by grasping the tongue with a gauze sponge. Atrophy can be observed if a lesion has been present for 5 to 7 days.

Anatomy and Physiology. See Chapters 2 and 9.

Assessment. See Chapters 2 and 9.

Sensation

The sensory examination provides information relative to the anatomic location and severity of the lesion. At this point in the neurologic examination, sensation has been tested by assessment of the cranial nerves, spinal reflexes, and proprioceptive positioning. Sensory modalities still to be tested include hyperesthesia, superficial pain, and deep pain from the limbs and the trunk.

Technique. Testing for pain perception is usually done last in the examination to avoid losing cooperation of the patient. The objective of the sensory examination is threefold: (1) map areas of increased sensation (*hyperesthesia*), (2) map any

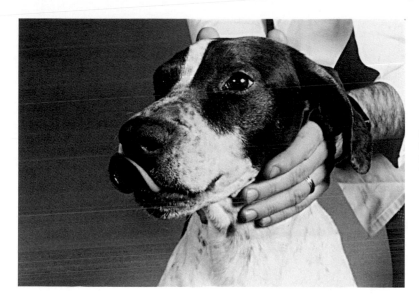

Figure 1-29 Most animals can be induced to lick if their noses are moistened. The tongue should be extended without forced deviation to the side.

areas of decreased sensation (*hypesthesia*), and (3) ensure that the animal can perceive a noxious stimulus. The first two are accomplished by testing for hyperesthesia and the ability to perceive superficial pain, respectively. The ability to perceive a noxious stimulus is tested if no reaction occurs to superficial stimuli. Always apply the minimum stimulus that elicits a reaction.

Hyperesthesia is an increased sensitivity to stimulation. For a comprehensive discussion of hyperesthesia and pain, see Chapter 14. Behavioral reactions to what should be a nonnoxious stimulus are interpreted as "pain." Testing should be done first from distal to proximal or caudal to cranial. *Lesions of the nervous system decrease sensation caudal or distal to the lesion, sometimes increase sensation at the lesion site, and leave sensation normal proximal to the lesion.* Therefore testing from distal to proximal or caudal to cranial goes from decreased sensation through increased sensation to normal sensation. The direction can be reversed to define more clearly the boundaries of abnormality. The pelvic limbs are palpated first, followed by the vertebral column. Beginning with L7 and progressing cranially, the examiner squeezes the transverse processes. Alternatively, one can press each spinous process firmly. The severity of the stimulus is increased from light touch to deep palpation. Proper palpation causes no reaction in normal areas and a behavioral reaction in areas that are painful. Animals that are in extreme pain may react regardless of where they are palpated. Localization of the source of pain may be more accurate if the animal is sedated before examination. Increased muscle tension may be noticed when the painful area is palpated, even under light

anesthesia. By placing one hand on the abdomen during palpation of the vertebral column, one can detect splinting of the abdominal muscles when pain is experienced (Figure 1-30). At the opposite extreme, some hounds may almost let you amputate a leg without flinching.

Sometimes the animal's reaction can be increased by mashing a toe until it reacts. One or two repetitions often overcome the animal's reluctance to protest, and they then react when you palpate the painful areas. During palpation of the animal, areas of increased sensitivity (hyperesthesia) are noted.

Testing for superficial pain or eliciting the cutaneous (panniculus) reflex is best done with a small hemostat. Gently grasp a fold of skin, then pinch (Figure 1-31). Needles may be applied, but they are less reliable and may cause injury. As in palpating, testing should be done from distal to proximal or caudal to cranial. The examiner tests the skin just lateral to the midline and then repeats on a line lateral to the site of the first evaluation. The opposite side is tested similarly. Three responses may be observed: a behavioral response, a reflex withdrawal of a limb, or a twitch of the skin (the cutaneous or panniculus reflex). A behavioral response such as a display of anxiety, an attempt to escape, a turning of the head, or a vocalization indicates perception of superficial pain. Withdrawal of a limb is a reflex and only indicates an intact reflex arc (see Flexor Reflexes). The cutaneous reflex is a contraction of the cutaneous trunci muscle causing a twitch of the skin along the dorsal and lateral areas of the trunk. A significant behavioral response at any step indicates the presence of sensation, and more severe stimuli are not needed once sensation has been established. If a

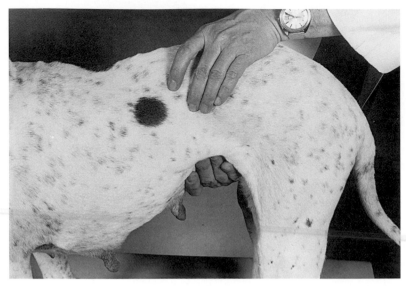

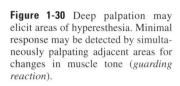

Figure 1-30 Deep palpation may elicit areas of hyperesthesia. Minimal response may be detected by simultaneously palpating adjacent areas for changes in muscle tone (*guarding reaction*).

dog turns and snaps when its toe is touched, one need not squeeze the toe with a hemostat.[24]

The caudal margins of normal superficial pain can be determined bilaterally. Spinal cord or nerve root lesions produce an area of hyperesthesia or a transition from decreased to normal sensation in a pattern conforming to the dermatomal distribution of the nerves (Figure 1-32). Testing of cutaneous sensation of the neck is unreliable for localizing cervical lesions. Manipulation of the head and the neck and deep palpation of the cervical vertebrae are more useful for localizing pain in this area.

A noxious stimulus that elicits any behavioral response is adequate for determining the presence of deep pain. When a response is difficult to elicit, a hemostat is used to squeeze a digit. *Withdrawal of the limb is not a behavioral response* (see the section on the flexor reflex in this chapter).

Anatomy and Physiology. Newer concepts emphasize the integration and interaction of all sensory systems and the effect of descending pathways that modify sensation. The concepts presented in this section are in general agreement with current research and are adequate for the clinical interpretation of sensory signs.[25-27]

Sensory fibers from the skin, the muscles, the joints, and the viscera enter the spinal cord at each segment by way of the dorsal nerve root. Fibers that innervate the skin are arranged in regular patterns called *dermatomes* (see Figure 1-32). A dermatome is the area of skin innervated by one spinal nerve root. Because of overlap, each

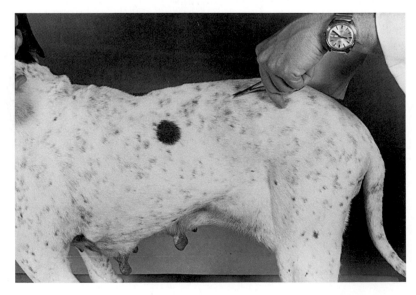

Figure 1-31 Gentle pricking or pinching of the skin can be used to outline the area of hyperesthesia more precisely. Both behavioral reactions and the cutaneous reflex may be elicited. The skin should be stimulated dorsally and laterally for the examiner to develop a map of abnormal reactions.

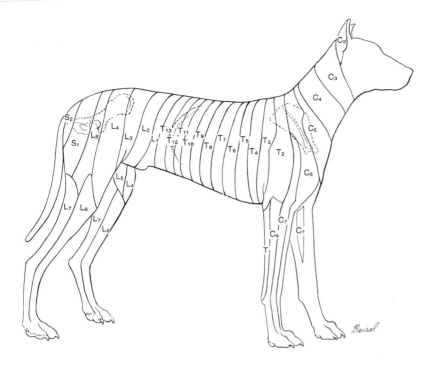

Figure 1-32 Dermatomes of the dog. This illustration represents the results of several studies. Dermatomes differ among individuals, and overlapping innervation of approximately three segments is present in most areas. The distribution to thoracic limbs is tentative. (From Oliver JE, Hoerlein BF, Mayhew IG: *Veterinary neurology.* Philadelphia, 1987, WB Saunders.)

strip of skin has some innervation from three segments.[28-32]

Proprioceptive fibers entering the spinal cord may ascend in the dorsal columns and the spinomedullothalamic tract to relay information to nuclei in the medulla (see Figure 1-8). Other fibers synapse on neurons in the dorsal horn of the gray matter. The neurons then send axons cranially along one of several named pathways, both ipsilaterally and contralaterally. The primary functions of these pathways include unconscious proprioception and sensitivity to touch, temperature, and superficial pain.

The deep pain pathway (spinoreticular and propriospinal tracts) is interrupted at three- to five-segment intervals to synapse on neurons in the spinal cord gray matter. These neurons give rise to axons, which rejoin the pathway on the same side or on the opposite side. The deep pain system is bilateral and multisynaptic and is composed of small-diameter fibers (Figure 1-33).[26]

The *cutaneous* or *panniculus reflex* is a twitch of the cutaneous muscle in response to a cutaneous stimulus. The sensory nerves from the skin enter by way of the dorsal root. The ascending pathway is probably the same as that for superficial pain. The synapse occurs bilaterally at the C8, T1 segments with motor neurons of the lateral thoracic nerve that innervates the cutaneous trunci muscle (Figure 1-34).[7]

Assessment. Alterations in a sensory modality are described as absent (0), decreased (+1), normal (+2), or increased (hyperesthesia, +3). Absent or decreased sensation indicates damage to a sensory nerve or a pathway. Increased sensitivity may indi-

cate irritation of a nerve or, more commonly, irritation of adjacent structures (e.g., disk herniation with irritation of meninges).

The cutaneous reflex is most prominent in the "saddle" area of the trunk. It cannot be elicited from stimulation over the sacrum or the neck. The response is absent caudal to the level of a lesion that disrupts the superficial pain pathway. For example, a severe compression of spinal cord segment L1 results in a normal panniculus response when stimulation is applied to the T13 dermatome but no response caudal to that point.

When alterations in touch, superficial pain, or hyperesthetic areas are found, the pattern of abnormality is carefully mapped. The pattern generally conforms to one of three possibilities:

1. Transverse spinal cord lesions cause an abnormality in all areas caudal to the lesion. The line of demarcation between normal and abnormal areas follows the pattern of a dermatome (see Figure 1-32).
2. Hyperesthesia, reflecting an irritation at a spinal cord segment or a nerve root, follows the distribution of one or more dermatomes but usually no more than three.
3. Lesions of a peripheral nerve produce a pattern of abnormality conforming to the distribution of that peripheral nerve (Figure 1-35).

One of these three patterns localizes the lesion to a peripheral nerve (e.g., sciatic nerve, radial nerve) or to a spinal cord segment accurate to within three segments (e.g., L1-3).

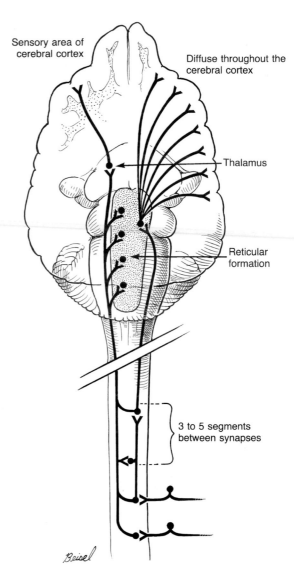

Sensory area of
cerebral cortex

Diffuse throughout the
cerebral cortex

Thalamus

Reticular
formation

3 to 5 segments
between synapses

Beisel

Figure 1-33 The pain pathway in animals is bilateral and multisynaptic (see also Figure 1-8). The deep pain pathway apparently has synapses every three to five segments, with projections continuing cranially on both sides of the spinal cord.

The presence or absence of sensation provides an important assessment of the extent of neural damage, especially in compressive lesions. When nerves are compressed, large nerve fibers are the first to lose function. With greater compression, small nerve fibers may be affected. In the spinal cord, loss of function develops in the following sequence: (1) loss of proprioception, (2) loss of voluntary motor function, (3) loss of superficial pain sensation, and (4) loss of deep pain sensation (see Figure 1-3). An animal with a spinal cord compression that has lost proprioception and voluntary motor function (paralyzed) but still has superficial and deep pain sensation therefore has less spinal cord damage than one that has lost all four functions. A loss of deep pain sensation indicates a severely damaged spinal cord and a poor prognosis.

Case Histories

The following case histories are presented for two purposes. First, they provide examples of the kinds of histories obtained in cases involving neurologic problems and demonstrate the processes used in evaluating this information. Second, they can be used to gauge one's understanding of the material in this chapter. After reading the history, but before reading about the neurologic examination, draw a sign-time graph and list the most probable categories of disease. Then read the results of the neurologic examination and decide what is normal and abnormal. Try to assess the findings in relation to the anatomic components of each test. Learning to assess the findings of the neurologic examination requires practice. Practice with immediate feedback from an experienced examiner is best but not always possible. The following cases are designed to illustrate the kinds of abnormalities that may be present in the various reactions and reflexes and to assist in making decisions

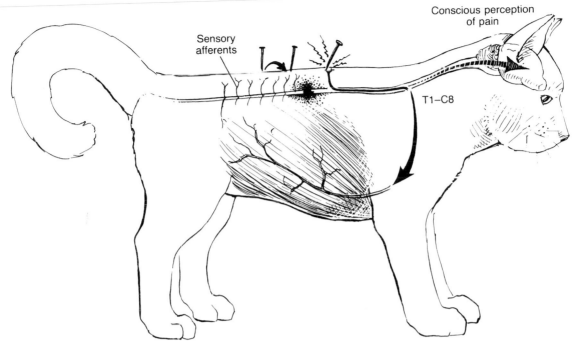

Figure 1-34 The cutaneous (panniculus) reflex is the contraction of cutaneous trunci muscle, producing a skin twitch from stimulation of cutaneous sensory fibers. (From Greene CE, Oliver JE: Neurologic examination. In Ettinger SJ, editor: *Textbook of veterinary internal medicine,* 2nd ed. Philadelphia, 1982, WB Saunders.)

regarding normality or abnormality. Later chapters include the complete findings in the cases and the final diagnoses. In this chapter, first make a sign-time graph and establish a list of disease categories (see Figure 1-1 and Table 1-4). Then evaluate the findings of the neurologic examination. Lesion localization for each case is presented at the conclusion of Chapter 2.

CASE HISTORY 1A

Signalment
Canine, West Highland white terrier, female, 6 years old.

History
The dog has had no significant previous medical problems, and vaccinations are current. She was found lying down in the fenced in backyard 4 days earlier. She was unable to walk, although some apparently voluntary movements were noticed in the left thoracic and pelvic limbs. The owners do not believe that conditions have changed since they first found the dog. They do not think the dog is in any pain. Appetite and eliminations are normal, and the dog seems alert and responsive.

Physical Examination
No abnormalities are found other than those detected on the neurologic examination.

Neurologic Examination
The dog is bright, alert, and responsive. She is unable to walk. When placed in a standing position, she falls to the right. Proprioceptive positioning is good in the left thoracic limb, slightly delayed in the left pelvic limb, and absent in the limbs on the right. The hopping reactions appear good in the left thoracic limb, with quick initiation of movement and accurate placement of the limb to support weight. The left pelvic limb

has a slow initiation of movement, but the limb is accurately placed. The right limbs do not initiate movement at all. The tactile and visual placing reactions are prompt and accurate in the left thoracic limb, somewhat delayed and inconsistent in the left pelvic limb, and absent in the right limbs. The quadriceps reflex is a single, brisk response, and withdrawal is present when the toes in the left pelvic limb are touched. The extensor carpi radialis reflex is decreased but present in the left thoracic limb. Attempts to elicit a triceps or a biceps reflex in the left thoracic limb are unsuccessful, but withdrawal is strong with a weak pinch of the digits. The quadriceps reflex is slightly more brisk in the right pelvic limb than in the left pelvic limb. Withdrawal is strong. The extensor carpi radialis reflex is present. Withdrawal is weak compared with the response of the left thoracic limb. The biceps and triceps reflexes cannot be elicited. The cranial nerves are normal. Sensation is present except pinching the skin of the right thoracic limb produces no reaction, and pinching a digit on this limb requires considerably more force to produce a behavioral response than does pinching a digit on the other limbs.

CASE HISTORY 1B

Signalment
Canine, German shepherd dog, female, 7 years old.

History
The dog has hip dysplasia, first diagnosed at 1 year of age. She has no other medical problems and vaccinations are current. The owners noticed the dog having difficulty with the pelvic limbs approximately 6 months ago. At first she just stumbled a bit on the steps or slipped on the kitchen floor. The problem has progressed slowly, and now she can no longer go up steps. Swaying of the caudal trunk occurs when she walks.

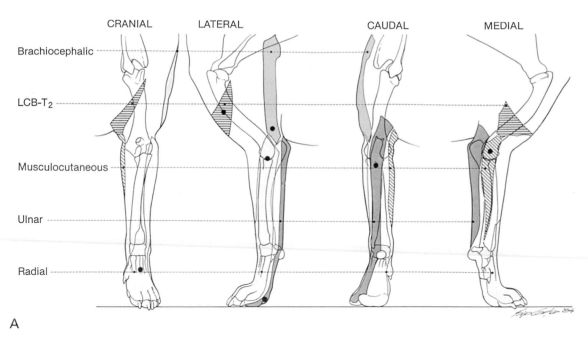

CRANIAL   LATERAL   CAUDAL   MEDIAL

Brachiocephalic

LCB-T$_2$

Musculocutaneous

Ulnar

Radial

A

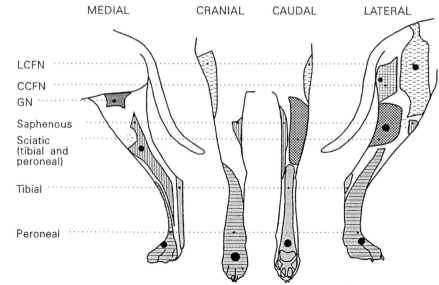

MEDIAL   CRANIAL   CAUDAL   LATERAL

LCFN
CCFN
GN
Saphenous
Sciatic
(tibial and
peroneal)
Tibial
Peroneal

B

Figure 1-35 A, Cutaneous innervation of the left thoracic limb of the dog. Autonomous zones, innervated by only one nerve, are shown along with recommended sites for testing of sensation *(dots)*. The median nerve does not have an autonomous zone. *LCB-T$_2$*, Lateral cutaneous branch of the second thoracic nerve. **B,** Cutaneous innervation of the right pelvic limb of the dog. Autonomous zones and testing sites are shown as in **A.** *LCFN,* Lateral cutaneous femoral nerve L3, L4 (L5); *CCFN,* caudal cutaneous femoral nerve (L7), S1-2; *GN,* genitofemoral nerve L(2), L3-4. (**A** is based on Kitchell RL, et al: Electrophysiological studies of cutaneous nerves of the thoracic limb of the dog. *Am J Vet Res* 41:61, 1980 and Bailey CS, Kitchell RL: Clinical evaluation of the cutaneous innervation of the canine thoracic limb. *J Am Anim Hosp Assoc* 20:939, 1984. **B** is based on Haghighi SS, et al: Electrophysiologic studies of cutaneous innervation of the pelvic limb of male dogs. *Am J Vet Res* 52:352, 1991 and Bailey CS, Kitchell RL: Cutaneous sensory testing in the dog. *J Vet Intern Med* 1:128, 1987.)

Occasionally she stumbles and falls, even on good footing. The owners are not aware of any pain. Appetite is normal, and neither urinary nor fecal incontinence has occurred.

Physical Examination
No significant physical abnormalities are evident other than neurologic dysfunction.

Neurologic Examination
The dog is alert and responsive. She has some difficulty getting up, especially on a slick surface. When she walks on the grass, she shows some swaying of the caudal trunk from side to side. Occasionally, she knuckles one of the pelvic limbs and stumbles but does not fall. The pelvic limbs cross at times, but

generally they are set wide apart. The thoracic limbs seem normal, but she carries much of her weight on them. The hopping and proprioceptive positioning reactions are good in the thoracic limbs. Hopping on the pelvic limbs is poor. When the dog's weight is shifted laterally, a long delay occurs before the limb is moved. When she shifts the limb, it is not moved far enough to support her weight adequately, so after approximately two hops, she falls over. When the digits are knuckled over, she stands in that position without attempting to replace them in a normal position. Both pelvic limbs have similar reactions.

The spinal reflexes are considered normal in the thoracic limbs. The quadriceps reflex is brisker in the left pelvic limb than in the right. The flexor reflexes are present in both pelvic limbs. The cranial nerves are normal. No areas of hyperesthesia are evident on deep palpation of the limb and trunk. The panniculus reflex is present, beginning at approximately L7. The dog immediately reacts to a pinching of the skin of the pelvic limbs in all areas.

CASE HISTORY 1C

Signalment
Feline, domestic shorthair, female, 3 months old.

History
The kitten has always seemed clumsier than the others in the litter. Of four kittens, one was born dead and the other two seem normal. This kitten had some difficulty nursing but has grown well and is alert and active. She has a peculiar prancing gait and trembles at times. The owners do not think the condition is getting worse. If anything, the kitten is able to get around somewhat better than when she first started walking.

Physical Examination
No abnormalities are found other than those detected on the neurologic examination.

Neurologic Examination
The kitten is alert and eager to play. The gait is characterized by jerky, exaggerated steps and a swaying of the body. The limbs are picked up rapidly and slapped on the floor. At times, she appears to stop the step before reaching the floor and lurches to one side. She tries to grab a piece of string with the thoracic limbs but is seldom successful. A head tremor is noticed at times. All postural reactions can be performed, but the movements are exaggerated. Initiation of hopping is slightly delayed, and the response is often too far or too short for proper support of weight. Proprioceptive positioning is present, but the foot is often placed more laterally than expected.

Myotatic reflexes are difficult to test because the kitten is so excited. Flexor reflexes are present in all four limbs.

The menace reaction is absent in both eyes, although the kitten can follow movements of objects such as a piece of string. At times her eyes show a slight side-to-side oscillation. No fast and slow components to the eye movements are apparent. The pupillary light reflexes and the palpebral reflex are normal.

No hyperesthesia is present, and the kitten feels a weak pinch of the skin on all four limbs. The panniculus reflex is present, starting at approximately S1.

CASE HISTORY 1D

Signalment
Feline, Siamese, male, 2 years old.

History
The right eye has seemed irritated for the past 2 months. Uveitis was diagnosed by another veterinarian, but treatment gave only temporary relief. The cat now seems to be lame in the left thoracic limb. The owners report a trembling of the head when the cat eats. In the last 2 days, the cat has seemed depressed and has refused to eat. He has had no other problems in the past and vaccinations are current.

Physical Examination
An ophthalmic examination confirms the diagnosis of anterior uveitis in the right eye. The cat is slightly depressed. No other abnormalities are found other than those detected on the neurologic examination.

Neurologic Examination
The cat is slightly depressed but responsive. The left thoracic limb knuckles over when he walks. A tremor of the head is evident when the cat is active, but it tends to resolve when he is at rest. Palpation reveals atrophy of the triceps and all the muscles ventral to the elbow of the left thoracic limb. The postural reactions are normal on the right side. The hopping reaction is poor (+1) in the left thoracic limb and absent (0) in the left pelvic limb. The proprioceptive positioning reaction is absent in both limbs on the left side. The extensor carpi radialis and flexor reflexes are absent in the left thoracic limb. The quadriceps reflex is exaggerated (+3) in the left pelvic limb compared with the right pelvic limb. The flexion reflex is present and of about the same strength in the left pelvic limb as in the right pelvic limb. Perineal reflexes are present. The cranial nerves are normal except for miosis of the left eye, which presumably is related to the uveitis. No areas show hyperesthesia, and sensation is intact, including superficial and deep pain sensation in the left thoracic limb.

CASE HISTORY 1E

Signalment
Canine, Yorkshire terrier, male, 8 months old.

History
The dog has been vaccinated in your clinic. Although he has had a reasonably good appetite, he has always been thin and small. Recently the dog had episodes of abnormal behavior. He paces continuously and resents being held. At times he stops and just stands and stares straight ahead. If someone tries to pick him up at these times, he appears startled. The episodes usually last for 2 to 3 hours, but on occasion he has seemed abnormal for an entire day. The owners cannot recall any day in the past 3 weeks when the dog did not have an "attack."

Physical Examination
The dog is very thin but otherwise normal.

Neurologic Examination
At the time of the initial examination, the dog is normal. Because of the history and the suspicion of metabolic disease, the dog is hospitalized for further evaluation. Food is withheld for 12 hours, blood and urine are collected for laboratory examination, and the dog is given a meal of cat food. Six hours later, the dog is reexamined. At this time he seems depressed. Although his gait seems relatively normal, he walks continually around the room. Limb movement is somewhat jerky, and he occasionally bumps into a chair or a table. Postural reactions are present, but they all appear somewhat slow in all limbs.

The dog becomes agitated during these reactions. If he is restrained on the table, he becomes quiet and almost goes to sleep. The spinal reflexes are normal. The menace response is present at times but is not consistent. Other cranial nerve responses are normal. The dog's reaction to painful stimuli is somewhat slow but present.

Construct a sign-time graph and a list of rule-outs (general categories of diseases) and interpret the neurologic examination before reviewing the assessments.

ASSESSMENT 1A

History. This dog's problem is tetraparesis with an acute onset and no progression. Two primary groups of diseases fit: trauma and vascular lesions. Inflammatory (infectious) diseases may have an acute onset but are usually progressive. Intervertebral disk problems may have a sudden onset but usually progress.

Rule-outs
1. Vascular lesion
2. Trauma
3. Inflammation (low probability)

Asking additional questions regarding possible sources of trauma proved unrewarding.

Neurologic Examination. The dog's mental status suggests that the cerebrum, the diencephalon, and the rostral brainstem are relatively normal. The dog cannot support weight and cannot move the right limbs voluntarily, indicating hemiparesis. Is the problem strictly unilateral? This question is answered by assessing postural reactions. The right side is obviously abnormal. The left thoracic limb has normal postural reactions, but some delay exists in initiating the hopping reaction in the left pelvic limb. Is that finding abnormal? The answer is maybe. If the hopping reaction is only slightly delayed, you should be cautious in calling it abnormal. Most dogs do not hop as well on the pelvic limbs as on the thoracic limbs. Placing reactions also are difficult to assess in the pelvic limbs. Proprioceptive positioning is more reliable, and this reaction is normal in the left pelvic limb. The extensor postural thrust reaction also can be helpful. In this dog, it appears to be somewhat slow in initiation. We assessed the postural reactions as absent on the right, normal in the left thoracic limb, and questionable in the left pelvic limb.

The quadriceps reflex in the left pelvic limb is brisk but not abnormal for this breed. Smaller dogs have relatively brisk reflexes. The significant finding is that the right quadriceps reflex is stronger than the left. Comparing the two sides gives the examiner a built-in control. We assessed the left quadriceps reflex as normal (+2) and the right as exaggerated (+3). Withdrawals (flexor reflex) are present and strong in both pelvic limbs. The extensor carpi radialis reflex is small but present and approximately equal in both thoracic limbs. This reflex is rarely strong and usually is abnormal if it is strong. The triceps and biceps reflexes are absent in both thoracic limbs. Is this finding abnormal? Not in our assessment. These reflexes are so difficult to elicit that we rarely use them. The flexor reflex is markedly weaker on the right than on the left. This is the most significant finding. Either the sensory or motor neurons (or both) of the reflex are damaged. The sensory examination is useful for deciding which neuron type is involved.

Sensation, both superficial and deep, is normal, except in the right thoracic limb. No response is obtained to pinching or to pinprick of the skin distal to the elbow. The cranial, caudal, medial, and lateral surfaces are similar. The dog does respond to a forceful pinch of the digits. The mapping of the distribution of sensory deficits is important for differentiating peripheral nerve lesions from spinal cord lesions.

The localization of the lesion in this case is discussed at the end of Chapter 2.

ASSESSMENT 1B

History. The dog's problems are pelvic limb paresis and ataxia with a chronic onset and a progressive course. A number of diseases can be chronic and progressive (see Figure 1-2). When the neurologic examination is performed, establishing whether the disease is focal or diffuse is important. With the information we have, we would include degenerative diseases, neoplasia, and inflammation as the primary rule-outs. Metabolic and nutritional diseases are more likely to affect the whole animal.

Rule-outs
1. Degenerative diseases
2. Neoplasia
3. Inflammation

Neurologic Examination. The gait can be described as pelvic limb ataxia and paresis. The swaying movements of the caudal trunk indicate some loss of function in paraspinal muscles. The hopping reactions are indicative of both sensory and motor deficits. The slow initiation of the reaction usually means that proprioception is poor. This finding is also confirmed by the complete absence of proprioceptive positioning. The inadequate movement of the limb as the weight is shifted indicates some paresis and loss of motor function. This dog also has some asymmetry in the quadriceps reflex, with the left slightly more brisk than the right. The dog's cranial nerves and sensation are considered normal.

The localization of the lesion in this case is discussed at the end of Chapter 2.

ASSESSMENT 1C

History. The history suggests that the problem is ataxia and tremors of the entire body with onset at birth and no progression. The onset suggests an anomaly or a birth injury. Either of these problems could be nonprogressive. Most of the other diseases affecting neonates, such as degenerative or inflammatory diseases, are progressive.

Rule-outs
1. Anomaly
2. Trauma

Neurologic Examination. The gait can be described as truncal ataxia with dysmetria of all four limbs. Paresis is not present at gait or on postural reactions. Dysmetria is caused by a loss of coordination between the initiation and the follow-through of a movement. The movement overshoots or undershoots its target. The head tremor was most apparent when the kitten initiated a movement and resolved at rest. This is an intention tremor. Postural reactions can be difficult to induce when an animal is uncoordinated, but determining the presence of any paresis is important. Spinal reflexes also may be difficult to elicit, especially in a young, excited animal. Flexor reflexes can always be tested. The absent menace reaction ordinarily indicates an abnormality in the visual pathways (afferent) or in the facial nerve (efferent). The animal can see and can follow moving objects, however, and the palpebral reflex is intact.

The localization of the lesion is discussed at the end of Chapter 2.

ASSESSMENT 1D

History. The cat has ocular disease, trembling of the head, lameness of the left thoracic limb, and depression. The disease is chronic and progressive. Chronic progressive diseases include degenerative, metabolic, neoplastic, inflammatory, and nutritional diseases. If the neurologic examination substantiates that the signs are multifocal in origin, as the history suggests, then metabolic and nutritional diseases would be much lower on the list.

Rule-outs
1. Inflammatory disease
2. Neoplastic disease
3. Degenerative disease

Neurologic Examination. The slight depression and the head tremor suggest that this cat has brain disease, although these findings may be merely manifestations of generalized disease. The lameness of the left thoracic limb suggests a more focal abnormality. The postural reactions confirm the diagnosis of an abnormality in this limb and in the left pelvic limb; therefore this is a hemiparesis. The spinal reflexes are absent in the left thoracic limb and present (flexion) to exaggerated (quadriceps reflex) in the left pelvic limb. Atrophy of the muscles of the left thoracic limb is also significant. You should immediately consider whether the atrophy is a result of disuse or denervation. The history does not give a clear indication of the duration of the lameness. (Disuse atrophy is slow, whereas denervation atrophy is rapid.) Note, however, that the triceps and the muscles ventral to the elbow are atrophied but that the flexors of the elbow and the scapular muscles are not. This finding is strongly indicative of denervation rather than disuse. The sensory examination indicates that the afferent nerves of the limb are intact. With a peripheral nerve lesion, one would expect both motor and sensory loss. Atrophy, loss of reflexes, and intact sensation indicate a lesion in the ventral spinal nerve roots or the motor neurons in the spinal cord. The postural reaction deficits in the pelvic limb on the same side indicate spinal cord disease.

Localization of the lesions is discussed at the end of Chapter 2.

ASSESSMENT 1E

History. The problem is primarily an abnormality in mental status. The neurologic examination is needed to determine whether other abnormalities are present. The onset is chronic and the course progressive, but the entire syndrome is episodic. Episodic disorders other than seizures are usually metabolic in origin. Toxicities can wax and wane with exposure, but this phenomenon is rare. Structural disorders such as degeneration, neoplasia, and inflammation may be accompanied by signs that wax and wane but are rarely associated with periods of normal activity.

Rule-outs
1. Metabolic disorder
2. Toxic disorder

Neurologic Examination. In addition to being depressed, the dog makes inappropriate responses. He becomes agitated during postural reaction testing but then dozes when restrained on the table. The menace reaction is not always present. A sharp tap on the eyelid (palpebral reflex) followed by a menacing gesture almost always elicits a response. Menacing gestures at other times may not produce a reaction. This finding is suggestive of inattention rather than loss of vision and may be seen in animals that are severely depressed, disoriented, or demented. The reaction to painful stimuli is interpreted similarly.

The localization of the lesion is discussed at the end of Chapter 2.

Further questioning regarding the timing of the episodes with feeding revealed that the dog was fed morning and evening. The usual diet was canned dog food. The episodes usually occurred 2 to 4 hours after feeding. This situation is typical of hepatic encephalopathy (see Chapter 12).

References

1. Weed LL: *Medical records, medical education and patient care.* Chicago, 1971, Year Book Medical Publishers.
2. Osborne CA, Low DG: The medical history redefined: idealism vs. realism. In *Proceedings of the American Animal Hospital Association,* Denver, 1976, AAHA, pp 207-213.
3. Oliver JE: Neurologic examinations: taking the history. *Vet Med Small Anim Clin* 67:433-434, 1972.
4. Oliver JE: Neurologic examinations: observations on mental status. *Vet Med Small Anim Clin* 67:654-659, 1972.
5. Oliver JE: Neurologic examinations: observations on posture. *Vet Med Small Anim Clin* 67:882-884, 1972.
6. Oliver JE: Neurologic examinations: observations on movement. *Vet Med Small Anim Clin* 67:1105-1106, 1972.
7. de Lahunta A: *Veterinary neuroanatomy and clinical neurology,* 2nd ed. Philadelphia, 1983, WB Saunders.
8. Oliver JE, Hoerlein BF, Mayhew IG: *Veterinary neurology.* Philadelphia, 1987, WB Saunders.
9. Mayhew IG: *Large animal neurology: a handbook for veterinary clinicians.* Philadelphia, 1983, Lea & Febiger.
10. Grillner S: Neurobiological bases of rhythmic motor acts in vertebrates. *Science* 228:143-149, 1985.
11. Grillner S: Locomotion in vertebrates: central mechanisms and reflex interaction. *Physiol Rev* 55:247-304, 1975.
12. Willis JB: On the interaction between spinal locomotor generators in quadripeds. *Brain Res Rev* 2:171-204, 1980.
13. Breazile JE, Blaugh BS, Nail N: Experimental study of canine distemper myoclonus. *Am J Vet Res* 27:1375-1379, 1966.
14. Oliver JE: Neurologic examinations: palpation and inspection. *Vet Med Small Anim Clin* 67:1327-1328, 1972.
15. Oliver JE: Neurologic examinations—sensation: proprioception and touch. *Vet Med Small Anim Clin* 67:295-298, 1972.
16. Holliday TA: The origins of the neurological examination: the postural and attitudinal, placing and righting reactions. In *Proceedings of the Seventh Annual Veterinary Medical Forum.* San Diego, 1989, American College of Veterinary Internal Medicine, pp 980-983.
17. Roberts TDM: *Neurophysiology of postural mechanisms.* New York, 1967, Plenum Press.
18. Thor KB, Morgan C, Nadelhaft I, et al: Organization of afferent and efferent pathways in the pudendal nerve of the female cat. *J Comp Neurol* 288:263-279, 1989.
19. Oliver JE: Neurologic examinations: flexion and crossed extension reflexes. *Vet Med Small Anim Clin* 68:383-385, 1973.

20. Oliver JE: Neurologic examinations—spinal reflexes: extensor thrust reflex. *Vet Med Small Anim Clin* 68:763, 1973.

21. Kneller S, Oliver J, Lewis R: Differential diagnosis of progressive caudal paresis in an aged German shepherd dog. *J Am Anim Hosp Assoc* 11:414-417, 1975.

22. Hoff H, Breckenridge C: Observations on the mammalian reflex prototype of the sign of Babinski. *Brain* 79:155-167, 1966.

23. Myers LJ, Nusbaum KE, Swango LJ, et al: Dysfunction of sense of smell caused by canine parainfluenza virus infection in dogs. *Am J Vet Res* 49:188-190, 1988.

24. Oliver JE: Neurologic examinations—sensation: pain. *Vet Med Small Anim Clin* 69:607-610, 1974.

25. Willis WD, Coggeshall RE: *Sensory mechanisms of the spinal cord,* 2nd ed. New York, 1991, Plenum Press.

26. Willis WD Jr: *The pain system: the neural basis of nociceptive transmission in the mammalian nervous system.* Basel, 1985, S Karger.

27. Willis W, Chung J: Central mechanisms of pain. *J Am Vet Med Assoc* 191:1200-1202, 1987.

28. Kirk E: The dermatomes of the sheep. *J Comp Neurol* 134:353-370, 1968.

29. Bailey C, Kitchell R, Haghighi S, Johnson R: Cutaneous innervation of the thorax and abdomen of the dog. *Am J Vet Res* 45:1689-1698, 1984.

30. Fletcher T, Kitchell R: The lumbar, sacral and coccygeal tactile dermatomes of the dog. *J Comp Neurol* 128:171-180, 1966.

31. Kirk E, Kitchell R, Johnson R: Neurophysiologic maps of cutaneous innervation of the hind limb of sheep. *Am J Vet Res* 48:1485-1492, 1987.

32. Hekmatpanah J: Organization of tactile dermatomes, C1 through L4, in cat. *J Neurophysiol* 24:129-140, 1961.

Localization of Lesions in the Nervous System

ANATOMIC AND FUNCTIONAL ORGANIZATION OF THE NERVOUS SYSTEM

Lesion localization is dependent on understanding basic concepts of neuroanatomy and neurophysiology and the terminology commonly used in clinical neurology. Although considerable debate exists over the amount of neuroanatomy that must be learned, for practitioners and students, it is much less than the total body of information currently available. The following sections present an overview of the organization and function of the nervous system.

CENTRAL NERVOUS SYSTEM

Anatomic Organization

The central nervous system (CNS) is composed of the brain and spinal cord. Embryologically, the CNS develops from ectoderm that forms the neural tube. The brain is divided into the cerebral hemispheres, brainstem, and cerebellum. The five major areas of the brain are the telencephalon (cerebrum), diencephalon, mesencephalon, metencephalon, and myelencephalon (Figure 2-1).

Telencephalon (Cerebrum)

This large area includes the lobes of the cerebral hemispheres, subcortical basal nuclei, olfactory bulbs (cranial nerve I [CN I]) and peduncles, pyriform lobes, and hippocampus. The following are the lobes of the cerebral cortex:

Frontal: This lobe includes the neurons responsible for voluntary motor functions, especially learned or skilled responses. The major motor pathways are the corticospinal tracts.
Parietal: This lobe largely functions for conscious perception of touch, pain, pressure, temperature, and noxious stimuli.

Temporal: This lobe functions for conscious perception of sound (hearing) and shares some functions with the parietal lobe.
Occipital: This lobe contains vision centers.

The following are the three types of axons *(fibers)* from cortical neurons:

Association fibers: axons that communicate with other neurons in the same cerebral hemisphere.
Projection fibers: axons that leave the cerebrum via the internal capsule to enter the brainstem (e.g., the corticospinal tracts). These fibers have important clinical application to lesion localization and will be described further under Motor Functions.
Commissural fibers: axons that cross from one cerebral hemisphere to the other.

Diencephalon

The diencephalon includes the thalamus and hypothalamus. The rostral ventral border is demarcated by the optic chiasm. The optic tracts lie on the lateral surfaces. The thalamus contains nuclei that receive sensory information from many areas. It serves as the major relay center for afferent *(sensory)* fibers projecting to the cerebral cortex. The hypothalamus lies ventral to the thalamus and has neuroendocrine and autonomic functions. It connects to the pituitary gland via the infundibular stalk.

Mesencephalon (Midbrain)

The mesencephalon contains the neurons for CN III *(oculomotor)* and CN IV *(trochlear),* which innervate extraocular muscles. The rostral and caudal colliculi are associated with visual and auditory reflexes and relay information to the cerebellum. The centers for pupillary light reflexes (parasympathetic–pupillary constriction) are located in the midbrain. Finally, centers for motor control (nucleus rubra/red nucleus) are located here.

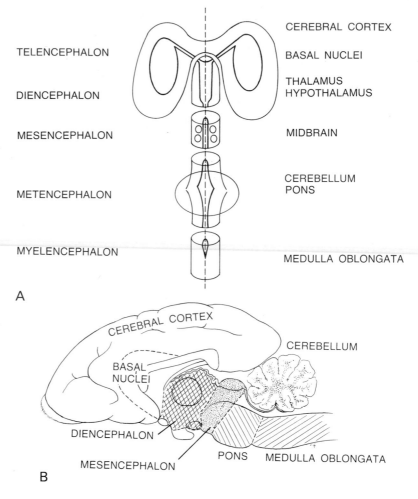

Figure 2-1 Segmental organization of the brain. Five major regions are significant clinically: the cerebrum, including the cerebral cortex, cerebral white matter, and the basal nuclei; the diencephalon, including the thalamus and the hypothalamus; the brainstem, including the midbrain, the pons, and the medulla oblongata; the vestibular system, including the labyrinth (peripheral) and the vestibular nuclei (central) in the rostral medulla; and the cerebellum. (From Hoerlein BF: *Canine neurology,* 3rd ed. Philadelphia, 1978, WB Saunders.)

Metencephalon

The metencephalon contains the pons and cerebellum. The pons contains neurons for CN V *(trigeminal),* whose axons innervate the muscles of mastication. It is also provides sensory innervation to the face and mandible. The pons contains motor pathways from the cerebrum that synapse in the cerebellum. The cerebellum composes the dorsal metencephalon. It coordinates motor activity and helps regulate muscle tone.

Myelencephalon (Medulla Oblongata)

The mylencephalon contains the neurons of CN VI through XII (see Figure 1-23) and central components of the vestibular system.

Forebrain: The forebrain contains the telencephalon and diencephalon. Lesions affecting these areas generally create contralateral clinical signs and generally are similar. Forebrain signs include blindness, depression, seizures, contralateral loss of postural reactions, and contralateral sensory deficits.

Midbrain: The midbrain has been described already (see Mesencephalon). Lesions in the midbrain produce depression, disorders of ocular movement *(strabismus),* constricted pupil(s), poor or absent pupillary light reflexes, gait deficits, and contralateral or ipsilateral postural deficits.

Hindbrain: The hindbrain includes the pons, medulla, and cerebellum. The pons and medulla contain neurons responsible for the generation of gait. Lesions in the pons and medulla cause ipsilateral motor and sensory deficits, vestibular syndromes, deficits in cranial nerve function (CN V-XII), and depression. Clinical signs of cerebellar disease include incoordination and spasticity. These three structures lie in the caudal fossa of the skull.

Brainstem: Anatomically, the brainstem contains the diencephalon, mesencephalon, metencephalon, and myelencephalon. Functionally, it includes all structures except the diencephalon. Clinically, most clinicians restrict *brainstem* to the pons and medulla. Clinical signs are those previously described for the midbrain and hindbrain.

Anatomic Organization of the Spinal Cord

The spinal cord comprises peripheral white matter composed of nerve tracts. The tracts are organized into specific motor (*efferent*) and sensory (*afferent*) pathways. Gray matter is located centrally and is composed of interneurons and motor neurons that innervate muscle. Specific structures are discussed in sections on functional organization of the CNS.

PERIPHERAL NERVOUS SYSTEM

The peripheral nervous system contains the axons of the spinal and cranial nerves and their receptors or effector organs. It includes both general and autonomic components. Peripheral nerves may contain fibers that are motor, sensory, or both. The anatomic distribution and function of spinal nerves are discussed later (see Lower Motor Neurons, or LMNs) and in Chapters 3 and 5. Cranial nerves are discussed in Chapters 1, 8, 9, and 11.

THE AUTONOMIC NERVOUS SYSTEM

The autonomic nervous system contains sympathetic and parasympathetic divisions. It is a multi-neuron system. Central neurons are located in the hypothalamus, midbrain, pons, and medulla. The hypothalamus is the primary center for integrating autonomic functions. Axons traverse the brainstem to affect LMNs located in the brainstem and spinal cord. Autonomic LMNs innervate the smooth muscle of blood vessels and visceral structures, glands, and cardiac muscle. Sensory fibers from body viscera are included in the peripheral component.

The LMNs of the sympathetic nervous system are distributed in the thoracolumbar spinal cord segments and generally use the spinal nerves for distribution to muscle and skin. Specific nerves control visceral function. The cranial sympathetic nerve has considerable importance to clinical neurologists in lesion localization (see Figure 11-3). The LMNs are located in spinal cord segments T1-3, and axons leave the spinal cord associated with roots of the brachial plexus. It traverses the thorax and the cervical region in association with the vagus nerve. It synapses on neurons in the cranial cervical ganglion. Axons from these neurons course near the middle ear and are distributed to the head via other cranial nerves. Axons innervate the dilator muscle of the pupil.

The LMNs of the parasympathetic nervous system are located in the brainstem (cranial nerves) and sacral spinal cord segments. The pupillary light reflex has been previously described (see Figure 11-2). The vagus nerve (CN X) is the major motor nerve for innervation of the muscles of the larynx, esophagus, and thoracic and abdominal viscera (see Chapter 9). The pelvic nerve innervates the detrusor muscle of the bladder (see Chapter 3).

FUNCTIONAL ORGANIZATION OF THE CENTRAL NERVOUS SYSTEM

Functionally, the CNS can be classified in several ways, but a simple scheme includes motor (efferent), sensory (afferent), and autonomic systems (efferent and afferent). The term *efferent* means conducting away from a center and usually indicates motor function. *Afferent* means conducting toward a center and usually indicates sensory function. Neuroanatomists may divide the major functions according to a scheme that relates function to embryologic development. That scheme is presented because the terms are still used in clinical literature.[1]

General Somatic Efferent System

The general somatic efferent (GSE) system includes motor neurons that innervate voluntary striated muscle of the head and skeleton. These neurons are found in CN III, IV, VI, and XII and all spinal nerves.

General Visceral Efferent System

The general visceral efferent (GVE) system includes motor neurons of the autonomic nervous system. It includes neurons in CN III, VII, IX, X, and XI and all spinal nerves. It includes sympathetic and parasympathetic divisions.

Special Visceral Efferent System

Neurons in the special visceral efferent (SVE) innervate striated muscle derived from brachial arch mesoderm. They are found in CN V, VII, IX, X, and XI.

General Somatic Afferent System

The general somatic afferent (GSA) system includes sensory neurons that have receptors in the surface of the head, body, and limbs. The neurons are located in CN V and all spinal nerves. It detects touch, temperature, and noxious stimuli.

Special Somatic Afferent System (SSA)

This system includes vision and hearing and neurons are associated with CN II and VIII.

General Visceral Afferent System (GVA)

This system includes sensory neurons from visceral structures of the head, body cavities, and blood vessels. Neurons are located in CN VII, IX, and X and spinal nerves.

Special Visceral Afferent (SVA)

This is the system for taste and smell. Taste receptors are associated with CN VII, IX, and X, and smell is associated with CN I.

General Proprioception (GP)

Proprioception is detection of changes in position of the trunk, limbs, and head. General proprioception neurons are associated with all spinal nerves and CN V.

Special Proprioception (SP)

This is the vestibular system, and neurons are associated with CN VIII.

Over the years, we have determined that this "classic" scheme is difficult for students and practitioners to remember. Therefore we use a scheme that describes function based on motor, GP, vestibular, general sensory (pain, touch, temperature, and pressure), special sensory (smell, taste, vision, and hearing), cerebellar, and cognitive systems. These major systems are described in subsequent sections.

MOTOR SYSTEMS

The motor system is composed of two divisions, the upper and lower motor neurons. Lesions of the motor system produce clinical signs called *paresis or paralysis*, depending on the severity or completeness of lesions.

Upper Motor Neurons

Upper motor neurons (UMN) are responsible for initiating voluntary motor functions. They are located in the cerebral cortex and brainstem and are found in both the somatic and autonomic systems. Their axons are organized into specific tracts, and they synapse in spinal cord gray matter on interneurons or directly on LMNs. The UMN system is divided into the pyramidal and extrapyramidal

systems (Figure 2-2; see also discussion under Gait in Chapter 1).

The pyramidal system allows animals to perform finely skilled movements but is not necessary for initiation of gait in animals. Neurons are located in the frontal lobe of the cerebral cortex and the axons are contained in the corticospinal tracts. Axons cross at the pyramids located in the caudal medulla and descend on the contralateral side. Axons synapse on LMNs in the spinal cord and cranial nerve LMNs in the brainstem. Lesions of the motor cortex or section of the pyramids produce little gait deficit but will cause postural reaction deficits in contralateral limbs.

The extrapyramidal system allows animals to gait and to initiate voluntary movement. Neurons are located in nuclei in all divisions of the brain. Some of the more clinically important motor pathways include the tectospinal, reticulospinal,

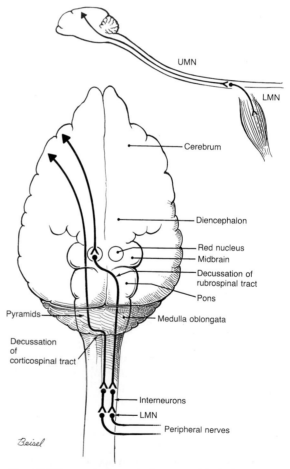

Figure 2-2 Neurons in the cerebral cortex and the brainstem send axons to the lower motor neurons (LMN) in the brainstem and the spinal cord. The upper motor neurons (UMN) provide voluntary control of movement. Two of the major voluntary motor pathways, the corticospinal (pyramidal) pathway and the corticorubrospinal pathway, are illustrated.

rubrospinal, and vestibulospinal tracts. Caudal to the midbrain, lesions generally produce signs in ipsilateral limbs and severe gait deficits. Lesions above the midbrain cause signs in contralateral limbs and less gait involvement.

Upper motor neurons may stimulate or inhibit motor actions. For instance, the UMN is necessary for voluntary motor action and at the same time exerts inhibitory action on other functions, such as spinal cord reflexes. Animals with UMN lesions caudal to the midbrain may have increased reflexes and increased muscle tone.

Signs of Upper Motor Neuron Lesions

Upper motor neuron lesions produce a characteristic set of clinical signs caudal to the level of the injury. These signs are summarized in Table 2-1 and are compared with signs of LMN lesions. The primary sign of motor dysfunction is *paresis*. With UMN disease, the paresis or paralysis is associated with normal or increased extensor tone and normal or exaggerated reflexes. Abnormal reflexes (e.g., a crossed extensor reflex) may be seen in some cases. Loss of descending inhibition on the LMN produces these findings. Disuse muscle atrophy may occur and is slow to appear, is not complete, and includes entire limbs in most cases. UMN signs are more common than LMN signs in clinical patients.

Because lesions at many different levels of the CNS may produce UMN signs, localization of a lesion to a specific segment usually is not possible when only UMN signs are considered. Proper interpretation of UMN signs and other associated signs, however, allows one to localize a lesion to a region. For example, UMN paresis of the pelvic limbs indicates a lesion cranial to L4. If the lesion were at L4-S2, LMN paresis would be present. If the thoracic limbs are normal, the lesion must be caudal to T2. Therefore pelvic limb paresis

(UMN) with normal thoracic limbs indicates a lesion between T3 and L3.

Lower Motor Neurons

The lower motor neurons (LMN) connect the CNS with muscles and glands. All motor activity of the nervous system ultimately is expressed through LMNs. The LMNs are located in all spinal cord segments in the intermediate and ventral horns of the gray matter and in cranial nerve nuclei (CN III-VII, IX-XII) in the brainstem. The axons extending from these cells form the peripheral spinal (Figure 2-3) and cranial nerves.

The nervous system is arranged in a segmental fashion. A spinal cord segment is demarcated by a pair of spinal nerves. Each spinal nerve has a dorsal *(sensory)* and a ventral *(motor)* root (see Figure 2-3). The muscle or group of muscles innervated by one spinal nerve is called a *myotome*. Myotomes are arranged segmentally in the paraspinal muscles but are more irregular in the limbs. Dysfunction of a specific muscle is localizing to a spinal nerve or a ventral root (Figures 2-4 and 2-5). The approximate relationship of spinal cord segments to vertebrae is illustrated in Figure 2-4.

Signs of LMN Lesions

Lesions of the LMN, whether of the cell body, the axon, or motor endplate, produce a characteristic group of clinical signs summarized in Table 2-1. Signs of LMN lesions are easily recognized on neurologic examination. Paralysis, loss of muscle tone, and loss of reflexes occur immediately after the neuron is damaged. Muscle atrophy is detectable within 1 week and becomes severe. Atrophy is limited to denervated muscles. Proper interpretation of LMN signs allows the clinician to localize accurately lesions to a peripheral nerve, a

Table 2-1 **Summary of Lower Motor Neuron (LMN) and Upper Motor Neuron (UMN) Signs**

	LMN: Segmental Signs	**UMN: Long-Tract Signs**
Motor function	Paresis to paralysis: loss of muscle power, flaccidity	Paresis to paralysis: loss of voluntary movements
Reflexes	Hyporeflexia to areflexia	Normal to hyperreflexia (especially myotatic reflexes)
Muscle atrophy	Early and severe: neurogenic; contracture after several weeks	Late and mild: disuse
Muscle tone	Decreased	Normal to increased
Electromyographic changes	Abnormal potentials (fibrillation, positive sharp waves) after 5 to 7 days	No changes
Associated sensory signs	Anesthesia of innervated area (dermatome); paresthesia or hyperesthesia of adjacent areas	Decreased proprioception, decreased perception of superficial and deep pain

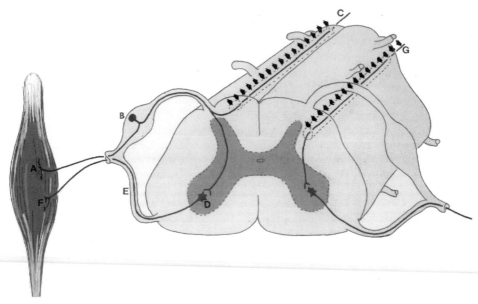

Figure 2-3 Components of the spinal reflex. **A,** Muscle spindle. **B,** Dorsal root ganglion. **C,** Ascending sensory pathway in the dorsal column. **D,** Ventral horn motor neuron (lower motor neuron). **E,** Ventral (motor) root. **F,** Neuromuscular junction. **G,** Descending motor pathway in the lateral column (upper motor neuron). The dorsal and ventral roots join to form the peripheral nerve. (From Oliver JE: Neurologic examination. *Vet Med Small Anim Clin* 68:151-154, 1973.)

nerve root, or a motor neuron within the brain or the spinal cord.

Most muscles are innervated by nerves that originate in more than one spinal cord segment. For example, the quadriceps muscle is innervated by neurons originating in segments L4-6. Loss of one segment or one root causes partial loss of the innervation of the muscle. The clinical sign is paresis, but not paralysis, of the affected muscles. The reflexes may be depressed. Lesions of peripheral nerves are more likely to cause severe loss of function, and all muscles innervated by the nerve are affected. The reflexes are usually absent in these lesions (see Figure 2-5).

Differentiating UMN and LMN signs is extremely important for localizing lesions in the spinal cord and brainstem. UMN signs localize lesions to spinal cord regions, whereas LMN signs help localize lesions to specific nerves, nerve roots, or spinal cord segments.

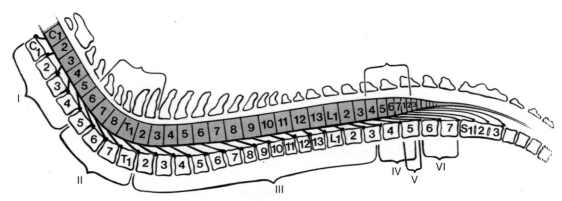

Figure 2-4 The spinal cord has a segmental arrangement; each segment has a pair of spinal nerves. The approximate relationship of spinal cord segments and vertebrae in the dog is illustrated here. Regions of the spinal cord that give rise to characteristic clinical signs when damaged are labeled. *I,* C1-5, Upper motor neuron (UMN) to all limbs; *II,* C6-T2, lower motor neuron (LMN) to thoracic, UMN to pelvic limbs; *III,* T3-L3, normal thoracic, UMN to pelvic limbs; *IV,* L4-S2, normal thoracic, LMN to pelvic limbs; *V,* S1-3, partial LMN to pelvic limbs, absent perineal reflex, atonic bladder; *VI,* caudal nerves, atonic tail.

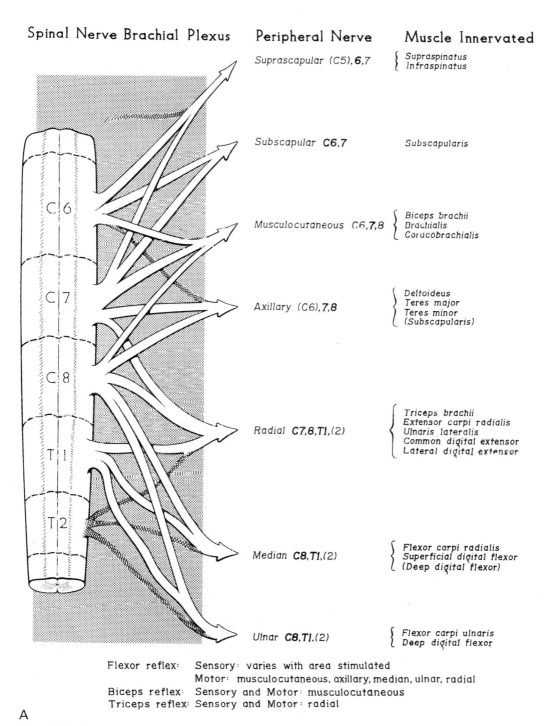

Spinal Nerve Brachial Plexus Peripheral Nerve Muscle Innervated

Suprascapular (C5),**6**,**7** { Supraspinatus / Infraspinatus

Subscapular **C6**,**7** Subscapularis

Musculocutaneous C6,**7,8** { Biceps brachii / Brachialis / Corucobrachialis

Axillary (C6),**7,8** { Deltoideus / Teres major / Teres minor / (Subscapularis)

Radial **C7,8,T1**,(2) { Triceps brachii / Extensor carpi radialis / Ulnaris lateralis / Common digital extensor / Lateral digital extensor

Median **C8,T1**,(2) { Flexor carpi radialis / Superficial digital flexor / (Deep digital flexor)

Ulnar **C8,T1**,(2) { Flexor carpi ulnaris / Deep digital flexor

Flexor reflex: Sensory: varies with area stimulated
Motor: musculocutaneous, axillary, median, ulnar, radial
Biceps reflex: Sensory and Motor: musculocutaneous
Triceps reflex: Sensory and Motor: radial

A

Figure 2-5 A, Segmental innervation from cervical intumescence of thoracic limb muscles in the dog.

Continued

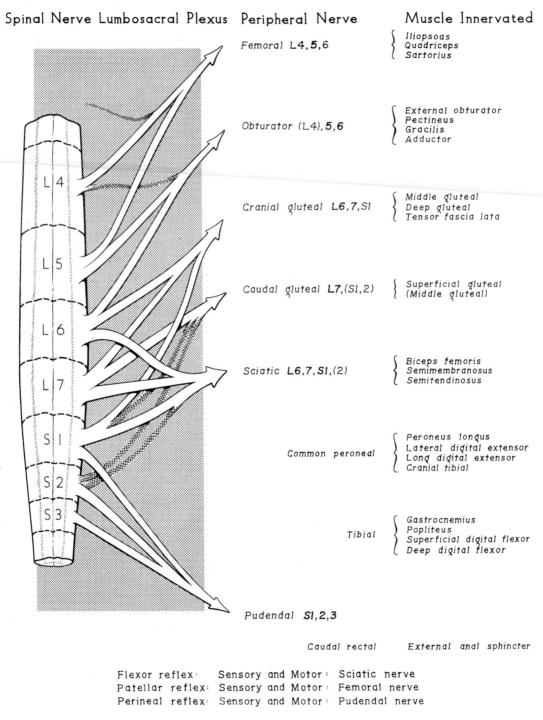

Spinal Nerve   Lumbosacral Plexus   Peripheral Nerve   Muscle Innervated

Femoral L4,**5**,6
{ Iliopsoas
  Quadriceps
  Sartorius

Obturator (L4),**5,6**
{ External obturator
  Pectineus
  Gracilis
  Adductor

Cranial gluteal L6,7,Sl
{ Middle gluteal
  Deep gluteal
  Tensor fascia lata

Caudal gluteal **L7**,(Sl,2)
{ Superficial gluteal
  (Middle gluteal)

Sciatic L6,7,**Sl**,(2)
{ Biceps femoris
  Semimembranosus
  Semitendinosus

Common peroneal
{ Peroneus longus
  Lateral digital extensor
  Long digital extensor
  Cranial tibial

Tibial
{ Gastrocnemius
  Popliteus
  Superficial digital flexor
  Deep digital flexor

Pudendal **Sl,2,3**

Caudal rectal   External anal sphincter

Flexor reflex: Sensory and Motor: Sciatic nerve
Patellar reflex: Sensory and Motor: Femoral nerve
Perineal reflex: Sensory and Motor: Pudendal nerve

B

Figure 2-5 Cont'd. B, Segmental innervation from lumbosacral intumescence of pelvic limb muscles in the dog. (From de Lahunta A: *Veterinary neuroanatomy and clinical neurology*. Philadelphia, 1977, WB Saunders.)

SENSORY SYSTEMS

In our organizational scheme, sensory systems are divided into general proprioception, general sensory (segmental and long tract), and special sensory systems.

Segmental Sensory Neurons

Sensory neurons are located in the ganglia of the dorsal roots along the spinal cord (see Figure 2-3) and in the ganglia of CN V. The receptors for pain, temperature, pressure, touch, and noxious stimuli are located on or near body surfaces. Axons are located in peripheral nerves and enter the spinal cord via the dorsal roots (see Figure 2-3). After entering the spinal cord, axons synapse on interneurons that stimulate limb flexion and inhibit limb extension in the ipsilateral limb and facilitate extension and inhibit flexion in the contralateral limb. This is the sensory component of withdrawal and crossed extensor reflexes (see Figure 1-19). Fibers are also projected to the brain for conscious perception of sensory information (see Figure 1-33).

The area of skin innervated by one spinal nerve is called a *dermatome*. Dermatomes also are arranged in regular segmental fashion, except for some variation in the limbs (see Figure 1-32). Alterations in the sensation of a dermatome can be used to localize a lesion to a spinal nerve or a dorsal root. The area of skin innervated by the sensory neurons of a named peripheral nerve has a different distribution (see Figure 1-35), allowing localization of lesions of peripheral nerves.

Cranial nerve V is the major nerve for facial sensation (see Figure 1-23). Sensory fibers project to the contralateral cerebral cortex.

Signs of Segmental Sensory Neuron Lesions

Lesions of the sensory neurons also produce characteristic clinical signs. Segmental sensory signs include (1) anesthesia (complete lesion), (2) hypesthesia (decreased sensation, partial lesion), (3) hyperesthesia (increased sensation of pain, irritative lesion), and (4) loss of reflexes. Increased or decreased sensation of a dermatome can be mapped by pinching the skin. Mapping the distribution of sensory loss is accurate to within three spinal cord segments (see Chapter 1). Similarly, the alteration of sensitivity in the distribution of a named peripheral nerve localizes the lesion accurately.

Long-tract Sensory Pathways

Sensory pathways of clinical significance include those responsible for proprioception (position sense) and pain. In animals, two types of pain fibers traverse the spinal cord. Based on the location of receptors, these are called *superficial* and *deep-pain pathways*. Superficial pain pathways (for perception of discrete pain in the skin [e.g., a pinprick]) are located primarily in the ventrolateral (primate) or dorsolateral (cat) portion of the spinal cord, with a relay in the thalamus.[2] The pathway primarily projects to the contralateral cerebral cortex for conscious recognition of pain. The deep-pain pathway (for perception of severe pain in the bones, the joints, or the viscera [e.g., a crushing pain]) is a bilateral, multisynaptic system that projects to the reticular formation, the thalamus, and the cerebral cortex.[3,4] In general, damage must be bilateral and severe to block conscious perception of pain distal to lesions.

General Proprioception

Proprioception means "sense of position." The clinical sign of proprioception dysfunction is ataxia *(incoordination)*. *General proprioception* describes the position of muscles, joints, and tendons because proprioceptors are located in neuromuscular spindles and Golgi tendon organs. Axons ascend within peripheral nerves and enter the spinal cord via dorsal roots. Neurons are located in the dorsal root ganglion. On entering the spinal cord, axons may (1) synapse directly on alpha motor neurons for initiation of extensor reflexes such as the patellar or knee jerk reflex (see Figure 1-13), (2) synapse on interneurons to indirectly influence alpha motor neurons, or (3) synapse on interneurons and then send afferent fibers via the spinal cord to the brainstem, cerebellum, and cerebrum (see Figure 1-8).

Proprioception is transmitted to the cerebellum via spinocerebellar tracts. This information is used by the cerebellum to regulate muscle tone, posture, locomotion, and equilibrium. Lesions involving these tracts have a profound effect on gait and may create clinical signs similar to cerebellar dysfunction (i.e., truncal swaying, hypermetria). Spinocerebellar tracts activate Purkinje neurons in the cerebellum that inhibit protraction *(flexion)* of limbs. This facilitates limb extension for weight bearing. Lesions in spinocerebellar tracts result in overflexion of limbs, known as *hypermetria*. Clinical signs are ipsilateral to lesions.

Conscious proprioception is carried to the medulla via the dorsal columns (fasciculus gracilis and cuneatus), whose fibers first synapse in medullary nuclei. Axons from these nuclei traverse the brainstem and cross to the opposite side in the region of the midbrain and diencephalon (medial lemniscus). Fibers are projected to the contralateral parietal lobe of the cerebral cortex. Lesions of this pathway are associated with delayed responses in the initiation of postural reactions (hopping, knuckling-paw placement) and less profound gait abnormalities. Lesions above and below the midbrain create deficits in contralateral and ipsilateral limbs, respectively.

Signs of Long-tract Sensory Lesions

The signs of sensory long-tract lesions are valuable for the formulation of a prognosis of CNS disorders and for localization. Spinal cord lesions frequently cause decreased sensation caudal to the level of the lesion. Proprioceptive deficits usually are the first signs observed with compressive lesions of the spinal cord. Abnormal positioning of the feet and ataxia may be present before any significant loss of voluntary motor activity occurs. Superficial pain sensation (the conscious perception of a pinprick) and voluntary motor activity are often lost at the same time. Deep pain sensation (perception of a strong pinch of a bone or a joint) is the last neurologic function to be lost during spinal cord compression.[5] The level of a spinal cord lesion can be determined if a level of hypesthesia or anesthesia can be detected (see Figure 1-34).

Special Sensory: Vision

The retina serves the function of a digital scanner. It contains photosensitive cells (rods and cones), bipolar neurons, and ganglion cells. Axons from ganglion cells form the optic nerve. Just rostral to the ventral diencephalon, the optic nerves join at the optic chiasm. The percentage of optic nerve axons that cross to the opposite varies in animal species: dog, 75%; cat, 65%; horse and ox, 85% to 90%. All fibers from the medial (nasal) half of the retina and about 25% from the lateral (temporal) half cross. Post chiasm, fibers continue in bilateral optic tracts located on the caudodorsolateral surface of the diencephalon. Most optic-tract fibers synapse in the lateral geniculate nucleus of the thalamus; however, about 20% to 25% of fibers pass over the geniculate nucleus and terminate in the pretectal area of the midbrain and participate in pupillary light reflexes. Visual fibers project from the lateral geniculate nucleus to the contralateral occipital cortex, where the image is perceived (see Figure 11-2).

Pupillary Light Reflexes

Axons that pass over the lateral geniculate body enter the midbrain and synapse on parasympathetic nuclei in the pretectal area. A second neuron then synapses on the parasympathetic motor nucleus of CN III. This is a bilateral pathway that influences both nuclei. Parasympathetic axons follow CN III and synapse in the ciliary ganglion. The short ciliary nerve synapses on the iris sphincter muscle, resulting in both direct and consensual pupillary light reflexes (see Figure 11-2).

Disorders of vision (blindness), pupil size (anisocoria), ocular movement (nystagmus), and ocular position (strabismus) are discussed in Chapter 11.

Special Sensory: Hearing

The cochlea is the receptor organ for hearing and is located in the inner ear. Movement of special hair cells in the cochlea activates fibers in the cochlear nerve. The cochlear nerve joins the vestibular nerve to form CN VIII, the vestibulocochlear nerve, which enters the rostral medulla. The cochlear nerve neurons are located in nuclei just inside the medulla. Numerous pathways and synapses are available for reflex activity and conscious perception of sound. Conscious perception of sound is bilateral and resides in the temporal lobes of the cerebral cortex. These pathways provide little help in localizing lesions within the brain. Deafness is discussed in Chapter 9.

Vestibular System

This is a special proprioception system that maintains an animal's orientation relative to gravity and position in face of linear or rotatory acceleration or tilting of the head. It maintains proper position of the eyes, trunk, and limbs relative to head position or movement. Neurons are located in brainstem nuclei and connect to receptors in the inner ear via CN VIII. The receptors for balance are located in the semicircular canals. To maintain proper posture and coordinated (conjugate) eye movements, vestibular stimuli are projected from vestibular nuclei to the cerebellum and rostrally via the medial longitudinal fasciculus (MLF) to nuclei of CN III, IV, and VI. Motor fibers from vestibular nuclei project to all levels of the spinal cord via vestibulospinal tracts and synapse on interneurons in ventral gray matter. The net effect is facilitation of ipsilateral *(same side)* extensor muscles and inhibition of ipsilateral flexor muscles. This is important for maintenance of extensor tone and facilitation of the stretch reflex mechanism. Both are important components of the animal's antigravity system.

Vestibular syndromes are characterized by ataxia, head tilt, circling, nystagmus, and falling toward the side of the lesion. Vestibular syndromes are classified as peripheral (inner ear, vestibular nerve) or central (medulla) and are discussed in Chapter 8.

Cerebellum

The cerebellum functions as a coordinator of movements that originate in the UMN system. It also functions to help maintain equilibrium, posture, body support against gravity, and eye movements.

The cerebellum receives sensory information and compares or measures where body parts are in relationship to the action required to perform coordinated movements. It contains both efferent and afferent pathways, which enter or leave the cerebellum via three pairs of peduncles that connect the brainstem to the cerebellum. For the cerebellum to function, it must receive sensory information related to position of the head, trunk, and limbs. The most important sensory pathways are the spinocerebellar tracts (general proprioception from the limbs, trunk, and neck), vestibulocerebellar tracts (special proprioception for head position), and visual and auditory sensation via the colliculi and tectocerebellar processes. Extrapyramidal motor information is projected to the cerebellum via the olivary nuclei located in the caudal medulla. Axons from all areas of the cerebral cortex project fibers to the cerebellum via the pontine nuclei. Finally, the cerebellum receives motor information from the red nucleus (midbrain) and reticular formation. No efferent cerebellar axons project into the spinal cord and directly influence the LMNs. The cerebellum exerts its regulatory functions via efferent fibers that influence UMNs in the brainstem.

In general, cerebellar disease causes severe ataxia, dysmetria (both hypermetria and hypometria), tremors (both generalized and intention), and rarely vestibular signs. Because the cerebellum does not initiate motor action, paresis and paralysis are not signs of cerebellar disease. Postural reactions and gait can be initiated, and muscle tone is normal or increased. Movements may be spastic or uncoordinated but not paretic. Cerebellar syndromes are discussed in Chapters 8 and 10.

Cerebrum: Cognitive Function

Sensory and motor functions that involve specific areas of the cerebral cortex have been previously described. The cerebrum contains areas for cognitive (thought, thinking) function, learned responses, and behavior. Generalized disease of the cerebrum may cause alterations of mental status (depression, stupor, coma), loss of learned responses such as house training, and aimless pacing or walking. Seizures can be a sign of cerebral disease.

LOCALIZATION OF LESIONS
Localization to a Region of the Spinal Cord or the Brain
Upper and Lower Motor Neuron Signs

Examination of the motor system should allow the clinician to localize the lesion to one of five levels of the spinal cord or to the brain (Figure 2-6). Gait

and postural reactions detect paresis or paralysis; spinal reflexes detect LMN abnormality. The thoracic and pelvic limbs should be classified as normal or as exhibiting LMN or UMN signs (see Table 2-1). Briefly, LMN signs are paresis, a loss of reflexes, and a loss of muscle tone. UMN signs are a loss of voluntary motor activity *(paresis),* an increase in tone, and normal or exaggerated reflexes. Note that in both cases, paresis *(paralysis)* is the primary finding. The status of the reflexes distinguishes between the two.

The examiner can localize a lesion to a region of the spinal cord or the brain by using these findings and the material presented in Figure 2-6, which is an algorithm that explains the logic of the diagnosis. For example, paresis in the pelvic limbs with normal thoracic limbs indicates that the brain and spinal cord as far caudal as T2 are functioning. Therefore, a lesion is caudal to T2. To determine whether the lesion is in the T3-L3 or L4-S2 segments, the reflexes of the pelvic limb must be evaluated. If they are normal or exaggerated, the L4-S2 segments must be functioning and the lesion is between T3 and L3. If the reflexes are decreased or absent, the lesion is in the L4-S2 segments. Paresis or paralysis of all four limbs indicates a lesion cranial to T3. Reflexes are tested in all four limbs. Normal or exaggerated reflexes of all limbs indicate a lesion cranial to C6. Other findings are used to localize the lesion further. With a lesion cranial to C6, one should examine the cranial nerves to rule out brainstem disease. The sensory examination is reviewed for possible signs related to the neck (i.e., C1-5).

Using only the information related to LMN and UMN signs of the limbs, the examiner can localize the lesion to one of the following regions: (1) the brain, (2) C1-5, (3) C6-T2–brachial plexus (thoracic limb), (4) T3-L3, (5) L4-S2–lumbosacral plexus (pelvic limb), or (6) S3-Cd5. Case histories at the end of the chapter can be used to test the reader's understanding of this concept.

Localization to a Segmental Level of the Spinal Cord
Lower Motor Neuron Signs

If LMN signs are present in the limbs, the examiner can localize the lesion further by identifying the affected muscles. Table 2-2 lists spinal cord segments (roots) and peripheral nerves for the most commonly tested reflexes. The examiner can localize within two to four segments or to a peripheral nerve if LMN signs are present. Spinal cord segments do not correlate directly with vertebral levels. When the examiner has determined the spinal cord

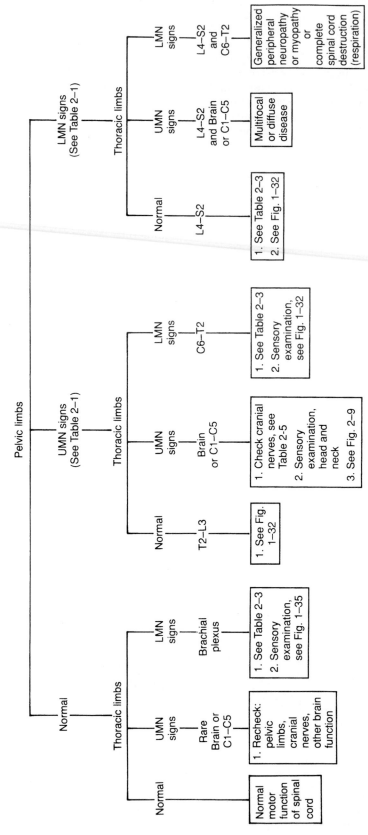

Figure 2-6 Localization of lesions based on motor function. *UMN*, Upper motor neuron; *C*, cervical; *T*, thoracic; *L*, lumbar; *S*, sacral spinal cord segments. (From Hoerlein BF: *Canine neurology*, 3rd ed. Philadelphia, 1978, WB Saunders.)

level, Figure 2-4 can be referred to for an estimation of the vertebral level. As a general rule, the sacral segments overlie L5. This can be remembered because S (for sacral) resembles the number 5.

Peripheral nerve lesions usually cause monoparesis (paresis of one limb) because the most common lesions are the result of injury to a limb. Localization of lesions in monoparesis is reviewed in Chapter 5. The primary exception is generalized peripheral neuropathies, which affect all of the limbs. These conditions are discussed in Chapter 7.

Pain

Hyperesthesia (increased sensitivity) is a useful localizing sign and may be present with little or no motor deficit. The animal's limbs and trunk, especially the vertebral column, are palpated and manipulated while the examiner observes for signs of pain. Obvious reactions may include resistance to movement and tensing of the muscles. If the clinician places one hand on the animal's abdomen while squeezing each vertebral segment with the other hand, increased tension of the abdominal muscles may be felt as painful areas are palpated. The skin is pinched with a hemostat after palpation is completed. A fold of skin is grasped gently with the hemostat, and the skin is pinched lightly so that no significant behavioral reaction is elicited from normal areas. Pinching areas of hyperesthesia elicits an exaggerated skin twitch or a behavioral response.

The superficial pain examination should be performed in a caudal to cranial direction because areas caudal to a lesion usually have decreased skin sensation. A level of normal or increased sensation can be ascertained by this method. If a spinal lesion is present, the sensory level should have the conformation of a dermatome (see Figure 1-32). Peripheral nerves have a different pattern of sensory distribution (see Figure 1-35).

The cutaneous (panniculus) reflex is elicited with a hemostat in the same manner as that just described for detecting hyperesthesia. Cutaneous sensation enters the spinal cord at each segment (dermatomes) and ascends to the brachial plexus (C8-T1) to the *lateral thoracic* nerve, which innervates the cutaneous trunci (panniculus carnosus) muscle. Contraction of the cutaneous muscle causes a skin twitch. A segmental lesion blocks the ascending afferent stimulus, abolishing the reflex. Pinching the skin in a caudal to cranial direction identifies the first level at which the reflex can be elicited. This segment is normal, and the lesion is one segment caudal to this level. The superficial pain pathways must be blocked to abolish the reflex. Normally the cutaneous reflex is most apparent in the thoracolumbar (saddle) area. A minimal response is obtained from a stimulus applied to the sacral or caudal regions, and no response is obtained from a stimulus applied to the cervical region. Cervical pain is assessed by manipulation of the neck and deep palpation of the vertebrae. Although defining the location of the pain precisely may be difficult, determining whether it is in the cranial, middle, or caudal cervical segments is usually possible by performing palpation carefully and gently.

Hypesthesia (decreased sensation) and *anesthesia* (no sensation) also are good localizing signs. Single nerve-root lesions usually do not produce a clinically detectable area of decreased sensation because of the overlapping pattern of cutaneous innervation (see Figure 1-32). Multiple nerve roots may be involved in some lesions, especially in the area of the cauda equina. Lesions of the spinal cord may result in decreased perception of pain caudal to the lesion. Determining the level of decreased sensation was discussed earlier, and the prognostic implications of the loss of sensation are discussed later. The motor examination localizes the lesion to

Table 2-2 **Spinal Reflexes**

Reflex	Muscle(s)	Peripheral Nerve	Segments*
Myotatic (stretch)	Biceps brachii	Musculocutaneous	(C6), C7-8, (T1)
	Triceps brachii	Radial	C7-8, T1, (T2)
	Extensor carpi radialis	Radial	C7-8, T1, (T2)
	Quadriceps	Femoral	(L3), L4-5, (L6)
	Cranial tibial	Peroneal (sciatic)	L6-7, S1
	Gastrocnemius	Tibial (sciatic)	L6-7, S1
Flexor (withdrawal)	Thoracic limb	Radial, ulnar, median, musculocutaneous	C6-T2
	Pelvic limb	Sciatic	L6-S1, (S2)
Perineal	Anal sphincter	Pudendal	S1-S2, (S3)

*Parentheses indicate segments that sometimes contribute to a nerve.
Modified with permission from Oliver JE Jr: Localization of lesions in the nervous system. In Hoerlein BF, editor: *Canine neurology*, 3rd ed. Philadelphia, 1978, WB Saunders.

Table 2-3 **Signs of Lesions in the Spinal Cord**

Site of Lesion	Sign
Cd1-5	LMN–tail
S1-3	UMN–tail
Pelvic plexus	LMN–anal sphincter, bladder
Pudendal nerve	
L4-S2	UMN–tail
Lumbosacral plexus	LMN–hindlimbs
	UMN or LMN–bladder, sphincter
T3-L3	UMN–hindlimbs, bladder, sphincter
	LMN–segmental spinal muscles
C6-T2	UMN–hindlimbs, bladder
Brachial plexus	LMN–forelimbs
C1-5 or brainstem	UMN–all four limbs, bladder

LMN, Lower motor neuron; *UMN*, upper motor neuron.

one of six regions of the spinal cord or to the brain (Table 2-3). A carefully performed sensory examination localizes the lesion to within three segments of the spinal cord or to a peripheral nerve. For additional details on pain, see Chapter 14.

Localization in the Brain

If the lesion has been localized to the brain, the next step is to determine what part of the brain is involved. Localization to one of five regions of the brain or to the peripheral vestibular apparatus

(labyrinth) is made on the basis of clinical signs (Table 2-4).

BRAINSTEM

For our purposes, the functional brainstem includes the midbrain, pons, and medulla oblongata. Lesions of the brainstem produce UMN signs in all four limbs (tetraparesis) or in the thoracic and pelvic limbs on one side *(hemiparesis)*. The paresis or paralysis produced by brainstem lesions is obvious both in the gait and in postural reactions.

Table 2-4 **Signs of Lesions in the Brain and Peripheral Vestibular System**

Lesion Site	Mental Status	Posture	Movement	Postural Reactions	Cranial Nerves
Cerebral cortex	Abnormal behavior, depression, seizures	Normal	Gait normal to slight hemiparesis (contralateral)	Deficits (contralateral)	Normal (vision may be impaired on contralateral side)
Diencephalon (thalamus and hypothalamus)	Abnormal behavior, depression, endocrine and autonomic dysfunction	Normal	Gait normal to hemiparesis or tetraparesis	Deficits (contralateral)	CN II
Brainstem (midbrain, pons, medulla)	Depression, stupor, coma	Normal, turning, falling	Hemiparesis to tetraparesis, ataxia	Deficits (ipsilateral or contralateral)	CN III-XII
Vestibular, central (medulla)	Depression (may be normal in focal lesions)	Head tilt, falling (usually toward affected side)	Hemiparesis, (usually ipsilateral), ataxia	Deficits (usually ipsilateral, rarely contralateral)	CN VIII, may also affect CN V and VII; nystagmus
Vestibular, peripheral (labyrinth)	Normal	Head tilt, circling, falling, rolling	Normal to ataxia	Normal, although may be awkward	CN VIII, sometimes CN VII; Horner's syndrome, nystagmus
Cerebellum	Normal	Normal unless paradoxical vestibular disease is present	No paresis; dysmetria, ataxia, and tremors are common	Normal to dysmetria	Normal, may see menace reaction deficit or nystagmus

Cerebral lesions affect postural reactions with minimal change in gait, although compulsive walking and circling may be seen. Abnormal posture resulting from vestibular involvement may also be seen.

Cranial nerve signs (CN III–XII) are present in larger brainstem lesions and provide important localizing signs (LMN or sensory) (Figure 2-7). The evaluation of cranial nerves is outlined in Table 2-5 (see Chapters 1, 9, 10, and 11).

Cranial nerve signs are ipsilateral to the lesion, whereas motor signs may be ipsilateral or contralateral, depending on the level and the pathways involved. The animal's mental status may be altered, especially in lesions of the midbrain and the pons, which disrupt the reticular activating system. Signs vary from depression to coma (see Chapter 12).

Diencephalon

Diencephalic lesions (lesions of the thalamus or hypothalamus) may produce UMN signs in all four limbs *(tetraparesis)* or in the thoracic and pelvic limbs on one side *(hemiparesis),* depending on the extent of the lesion. The gait is not severely affected (similar to cerebral lesions), but postural reaction deficits are obvious. CN II (optic) may be affected in diencephalic lesions. Space-occupying lesions (e.g., tumors, abscesses) of the diencephalon also may affect CN III, IV, and VI (see Table 2-5). Cranial nerve signs are *ipsilateral* to the lesion, whereas postural reaction deficits are *contralateral* to the lesion.

The most characteristic signs of diencephalic lesions are related to abnormal function of the hypothalamus and its connections with the pituitary gland. The hypothalamus is the control center for the autonomic nervous system and most of the endocrine system. If the hypothalamus is not affected, distinguishing diencephalic from cerebral lesions is difficult.

All sensory pathways of the body, with the exception of those serving olfaction, relay in the diencephalon en route to the cerebral cortex. Clinical signs of lesions in these systems in the diencephalon usually are not localizing. A rare generalized hyperesthesia has been described as a result of an abnormality in the relay nuclei of the pain pathways. Large lesions in the diencephalon may produce alterations in the level of consciousness (stupor, coma) because of interference with the reticular activating system (see Chapter 12).

Vestibular System

Vestibular signs may be the result of central (brainstem) or peripheral (labyrinth) disease.

Distinguishing central disease from peripheral disease is important because of the differences in treatment and prognosis. Signs of vestibular disease include falling, rolling, head tilting, circling, nystagmus, positional strabismus (deviation of one eye in certain positions of the head), and asymmetric ataxia (Figures 2-8 and 2-9).

Peripheral lesions involve the labyrinth in the petrosal bone. Middle-ear lesions (bulla ossea) usually produce a head tilt with no other signs, presumably through pressure changes on the windows of the inner ear. Horizontal or rotatory nystagmus may be seen occasionally. Inner-ear disease, which actually involves the receptors and the vestibular nerve, usually produces one or more of the signs listed earlier in addition to the head tilt. In either case, the head tilt is ipsilateral to the lesion. Horners syndrome (miosis, ptosis, enophthalmos) of the ipsilateral eye may be present with either middle- or inner-ear disease in the dog and cat because the sympathetic nerves pass through the middle ear in proximity to the petrosal bone. CN VII (facial) may be affected in inner-ear disease as it courses through the petrosal bone in contact with the vestibulocochlear nerve (CN VIII). The primary characteristics of peripheral vestibular disease are an asymmetric ataxia without deficits in postural reactions and a horizontal, or rotatory, nystagmus that does not change direction with different head positions. The quick phase of the nystagmus is away from the side of the lesion.

Any signs of brainstem disease in association with vestibular signs indicate that central involvement is present. The most important differentiating feature is a deficit in postural reactions. Peripheral vestibular disease does not cause paresis or loss of proprioception, whereas central disease frequently does. Postural reactions must be evaluated critically because an animal with peripheral vestibular disease has deficits in equilibrium, which make the performance of tests such as hopping awkward. An evaluation of proprioceptive positioning is an excellent method for discrimination. Alterations in mental status or deficits in CN V and CN VI also are indicative of central disease (see Figure 2-8); however, some polyneuropathies may affect the cranial nerves, including CN V, VI, and VIII.

Lesions near the caudal cerebellar peduncle may produce what has been called a *paradoxic vestibular syndrome.* The signs are usually similar to those of central vestibular disease except that the direction of the head tilt is contralateral to the side of the lesion.[6] Additional signs of cerebellar disease, such as dysmetria and ataxia, may be seen.

Bilateral vestibular disease, which is usually peripheral, produces a more symmetric ataxia. The animal walks with the limbs flexed and spread

Text continued on p. 64.

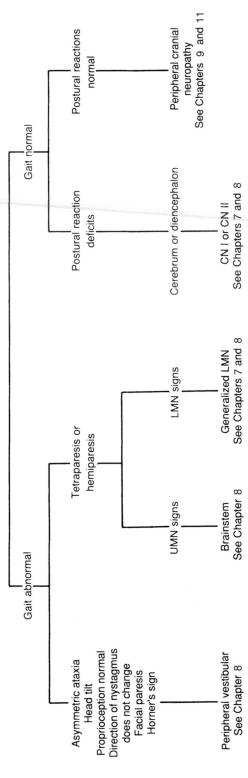

Figure 2-7 Localization of lesions causing cranial nerve signs.

Table 2-5 Cranial Nerves

Number and Name	Origin or Termination in Brain	Course	Function	Test	Normal Response	Abnormal Response	Occurrence
CN I olfactory	Pyriform cortex	Nasal mucosa, cribriform plate, olfactory bulbs, olfactory tract, olfactory stria, pyriform cortex	Sense of smell	Smelling of nonirritating volatile substances (alcohol, food)	Behavioral reaction; aversion or interest	No reaction	Rare: nasal tumors and infections (evaluation difficult)
CN II optic	Lateral geniculate nucleus (vision), pretectal nucleus (pupillary reflex)	Retina, optic nerve, optic tract, lateral geniculate nucleus, optic radiation, visual cortex, optic tract, pretectal nucleus, parasympathetic nucleus of CN III, oculomotor nerve	Vision pupillary light reflexes	Menace reaction, obstacle test and behavior, placing reaction, following movement, pupillary light reflex, ophthalmoscopy	Blinks, avoids obstacles and responds to visual cues, placing good, follows objects, pupillary light reflexes present, retina normal	No blink, poor avoidance of obstacles, no visual placing, direct pupillary light reflex absent, retina or optic disk may be abnormal	Optic neuritis, neoplasia, orbital trauma, orbital abscess
CN III oculomotor	Midbrain, tegmentum (level of rostral colliculus)	Nucleus ventral to mesencephalic aqueduct, exits ventral to midbrain between cerebral peduncles, courses through tentorial notch, runs in cavernous sinus with CN IV and CN VI, exits orbital fissure	Constriction of pupil: ciliary muscle for accommodation reaction of lens; extraocular muscles: dorsal, ventral, and medial rectus, ventral oblique	Pupillary size, pupillary light reflex, eye position, eye movements	Pupils symmetric, pupils constrict to light, eyes centered in palpebral fissure, eyes move in all directions	Mydriasis, ipsilateral, no direct pupil response, ventrolateral strabismus, no movement except laterally (CN VI)	Orbital lesions, tentorial herniation, midbrain lesion
CN IV trochlear	Midbrain, tegmentum (level of caudal colliculus)	Nucleus ventral to mesencephalic aqueduct, exits dorsal to tectum, caudal to caudal colliculus, contralateral to origin, courses along ridge of petrosal bone, follows course of CN III	Dorsal oblique muscle, rotates dorsal portion of eye medioventrally	Eye position, eye movements	Eye centered in palpebral fissure, eyes move in all directions	Normal; rotation may be detected in animal with elliptical pupil or by position of vessels ophthalmoscopically	Rare, difficult to evaluate; reported in polioencephalomalacia of cattle, but eyes move

Continued

Table 2-5　Cranial Nerves—Continued

Number and Name	Origin or Termination in Brain	Course	Function	Test	Normal Response	Abnormal Response	Occurrence
CN V trigeminal ophthalmic, maxillary and mandibular nerves	*Motor nucleus:* Pons *Sensory nucleus:* Pons, medulla, C1 spinal cord segment	*Motor:* Pons, exits at cerebellopontine angle, trigeminal canal of petrosal bone, oval foramen, mandibular nerve *Sensory:* Same except trigeminal ganglion in trigeminal canal; ophthalmic, maxillary, and mandibular nerves	*Motor:* Muscles of mastication *Sensory:* Face rostral to ears	*Motor:* Ability To close mouth, jaw tone *Sensory:* Palpebral reflex, pinch face, touch nasal mucosa	Closed mouth, good jaw tone; no atrophy of temporal or masseter muscles; palpebral reflex present; behavioral response to noxious stimulus	Jaw hangs open (bilateral), poor jaw tone, atrophy, loss of palpebral reflex or behavioral response to noxious stimulus (check all three branches)	Idiopathic mandibular paralysis, trigeminal neuritis, cerebellopontine angle tumors, rabies, trauma
CN VI abducent	Medulla (rostral and dorsal)	Medulla, lateral to pyramid, courses ventral to brainstem to join CN III And IV	Lateral rectus and retractor muscles; lateral movement of eye, retraction of globe	Eye position, eye movements	Eye centered in palpebral fissure, eye moves laterally and retracts	Medial strabismus, lack of lateral eye movements or retraction	Orbital trauma, orbital abscess, brainstem disease
CN VII facial	Medulla (rostral and ventrolateral)	*Motor:* Axons leave nucleus, loop around abducent nucleus, and exit ventrolateral medulla ventral to CN VIII to internal acoustic meatus, facial canal in petrosal bone, and stylomastoid foramen to muscles of face *Taste:* Solitary nucleus and tract, medulla follows course of trigeminal nerve *Sensory:* Geniculate ganglion and branches from vagus nerve	Muscles of facial expression and taste, rostral two thirds of tongue, and cutaneous sensation of inner surface of pinna	Facial symmetry, palpebral reflex, ear movements *Taste:* Atropine applied to rostral two thirds of tongue with cotton swabs *Sensory:* Touch inner surface of pinna	Face symmetric; normal movements of lips, ears, eyelids; palpebral reflex present; ears move in response to stimulation *Taste:* Aversive reaction immediately *Sensory:* Behavioral and ear twitch response	Asymmetry of face, ptosis, lip drops, deviation of nasal philtrum, palpebral reflex absent (check CN V), ears do not move *Taste:* No reaction until mouth is closed and material reaches caudal portion of tongue *Sensory:* No behavioral or ear twitch response	Idiopathic facial paralysis, polyneuropathies, inner ear infections, brainstem lesions

Cranial nerve	Location (nuclei)	Anatomy	Function	Test	Normal response	Abnormal signs	Causes
CN VIII vestibulocochlear	Vestibular nuclei medulla; cochlear nuclei medulla	Inner ear, petrosal bone, internal acoustic meatus, cerebellomedullary angle, medulla	Equilibrium, hearing	*Vestibular:* Posture and gait, eye movements, rotatory and caloric tests. *Hearing:* Startle response, electrophysiology (EEG alerting, brainstem evoked response)	*Vestibular:* Normal posture and gait, oculocephalic responses normal, brief postrotatory nystagmus and caloric-induced nystagmus. *Hearing:* Startled reaction to handclap, evoked response present	*Vestibular:* Head tilt, head twist, circling, spontaneous nystagmus, prolonged or absent postrotatory nystagmus, abnormal or absent caloric response. *Hearing:* Poor startle reaction, no evoked response	Otitis media and otitis interna, idiopathic vestibular disease, polyneuropathy, brainstem disease
CN IX glossopharyngeal	Medulla (caudal)	*Sensory:* Solitary tract and nucleus. *Motor:* Parasympathetic, ambiguus nucleus, exit together along lateral surface of medulla, exit through jugular foramen	Sensory and motor to pharynx and palate, parasympathetic to zygomatic and parotid salivary glands (in CN V); sensory to carotid body and sinus	Gag reflex	Swallowing	Poor gag reflex, dysphagia	Rare; common in rabies!
CN X vagus	Medulla (caudal)	Same as CN IX	Sensory and motor to pharynx and larynx, thoracic and abdominal viscera	Gag reflex, laryngeal reflex, slap test, oculocardiac reflex	Swallowing, coughing, bradycardia	Poor gag reflex, dysphagia, inspiratory dyspnea, no retraction of laryngeal folds, regurgitation	Rare, except in laryngeal paralysis (idiopathic); polyneuropathy
CN XI accessory	Medulla (caudal) and cervical spinal cord	Ambiguus nucleus of medulla and cervical gray matter, axons run rostrally from cervical cord to join cranial roots, exit jugular foramen	Trapezius and parts of sternocephalicus and brachiocephalicus muscles	Palpate for atrophy of muscles; EMG	Normal muscles	Atrophied muscles, denervation	Rare
CN XII hypoglossal	Medulla (caudal)	Axons exit medulla lateral to pyramid, hypoglossal canal to tongue	Movements of tongue	Protrusion of tongue (wet nose), retraction of tongue	Tongue protrudes symmetrically and can lick in both directions, strong withdrawal of tongue	Tongue deviates to side of lesion, atrophy, weak withdrawal	Brainstem disease, polyneuropathy

CN, Cranial nerve; *EEG*, electroencephalography; *EMG*, electromyography.

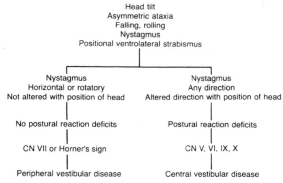

Head tilt
Asymmetric ataxia
Falling, rolling
Nystagmus
Positional ventrolateral strabismus

Nystagmus Horizontal or rotatory Not altered with position of head	Nystagmus Any direction Altered direction with position of head
No postural reaction deficits	Postural reaction deficits
CN VII or Horner's sign	CN V, VI, IX, X
Peripheral vestibular disease	Central vestibular disease

Figure 2-8 Algorithm for differentiating central and peripheral vestibular diseases.

apart to maintain balance. The head often sways from side to side. No nystagmus is present, and vestibular eye movements are usually absent.[7]

CEREBELLUM

The cerebellum coordinates movements. It controls the rate and range of movements without actually initiating motor activity. Cerebellar lesions may be unilateral or bilateral, depending on cause. Characteristic signs include ataxia, wide-based stance, dysmetria, and intention tremor with little weakness. Involvement of the head differentiates cerebellar lesions from spinal tract lesions, which may produce similar signs in the limbs. For example, dysmetria usually is recognized as a severe head drop when the head is elevated and suddenly released. The animal may stick its nose too far into its water dish when drinking or may even hit the edge of the dish. Intention tremors are uncoordinated movements that become much worse as the animal initiates an activity such as eating or drinking (see Figure 2-9).[8]

Nystagmus may occur in cerebellar disease but is usually more of a tremor of the globe than the slow-quick (*jerk*) movements associated with vestibular disease. Cerebellar nystagmus is most pronounced as the animal shifts its gaze and fixates on a new field (*an intention tremor*).

Acute injury to the cerebellum causes a different clinical picture, typically extensor hypertonus in the thoracic limbs, flexion in the pelvic limbs, and opisthotonos.[6] Isolated cerebellar trauma is unusual because of the protected location of the cerebellum. These signs are most pronounced when combined with brainstem lesions at the level of the midbrain or the pons.

Lesions of the flocculonodular lobes of the cerebellum produce signs similar to those of vestibular disease, including loss of equilibrium, nystagmus, and tendency to fall (see Chapter 8).

Diffuse cerebellar lesions may cause the menace reaction to be absent even if vision is normal.

CEREBRUM

Cerebral lesions (including the cerebral hemispheres and basal nuclei) usually cause alterations in behavior or mental status, seizures, loss of vision with intact pupils, contralateral decrease in facial sensation, and mild hemiparesis with deficits in postural reactions.[9] Only one or two of these signs may be present because the cerebrum is a relatively large structure with well-localized functional areas. Signs are generally contralateral to the lesion.

Behavioral changes usually reflect a lesion of the limbic system or the frontal or temporal lobes of the cortex. Frontal-lobe lesions often cause a disinhibition that results in excessive pacing. Compulsive pacing may continue until the animal walks into a corner and stands with its head pressed against the obstruction. If the lesion is unilateral or asymmetric, the animal may circle. Circling in an animal with a cerebral lesion is usually to the same side as the lesion. The animal's movement tends to be in large circles. The gait is reasonably normal, although obstacles may not be perceived. Circling is not a localizing sign because it can be caused by lesions in the forebrain, brainstem, and vestibular system.

Depression, stupor, and coma represent decreasing levels of consciousness caused by a separation of the cerebral cortex from the reticular activating system of the brainstem. Severe depression usually is caused by brainstem lesions (see Chapter 12). Conscious visual perception requires intact visual pathways to the occipital lobes of the cerebral cortex. Occipital cortical lesions cause blindness with intact pupillary reflexes (see Chapter 11).

The sensorimotor cortex is important for voluntary motor activity but is not necessary for relatively normal gait and posture. Animals with lesions in this area can stand, walk, and run with minimal deficits. The animal's ability for fine discrimination is lost, however, and it is unable to avoid obstacles smoothly or to perform fine maneuvers, such as walking on the steps of a ladder. Markedly abnormal postural reactions are found.

Localization to one of the five regions of the brain is usually adequate for a clinical diagnosis. Cranial nerve signs provide positive evidence for precise localization within the brainstem. Clinical signs referable to several parts of the nervous system indicate diffuse or multifocal disease, such as infection, metabolic disorder, or malignant neoplasia (see Chapter 15).

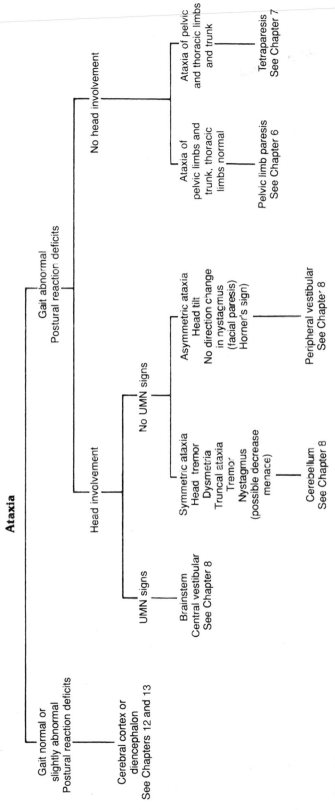

Figure 2-9 Algorithm for the diagnosis of ataxia based on gait, head involvement, and motor function of the limbs.

Case Histories

You now should be able to localize the lesion in the cases presented in Chapter 1. The signalment and pertinent neurologic abnormalities are repeated. Make your assessment before reading ours.

CASE HISTORY 2A

Signalment
Canine, West Highland white terrier, female, 6 years old.

History
The dog was found lying down in the backyard 4 days earlier. The owners describe some voluntary movements in the left thoracic and pelvic limbs. The condition has not changed since its onset. The animal is not in pain. Appetite, urination, and defecation are normal (see Case History 1A, Chapter 1).

Physical Examination
Nothing significant was found on the physical examination other than the neurologic deficits.

Neurologic Examination[*]
(See Case History 1A, Chapter 1.)

A. Observation
   1. Mental status: Alert
   2. Posture: Recumbent; falls to right when placed on feet
   3. Gait: None
B. Palpation: No abnormalities
C. Postural reactions

Left	Reactions	Right
	Proprioceptive positioning	
+1	PL	0
+2	TL	0
NE	Wheelbarrowing	NE
	Hopping	
+1	PL	0
+2	TL	0
NE	Extensor postural thrust	NE
NE	Hemistand–hemiwalk	NE
NE	Tonic neck	NE
	Placing, tactile	
+1	PL	0
+2	TL	0
	Placing, visual	
+1	PL	0
+2	TL	0

D. Spinal reflexes

Left	Reflex, Spinal Segment	Right
+2	Quadriceps L4-6	+3
+2	Extensor carpi radialis C7-T1	+2
NE	Triceps C7-T1	NE
+2	Flexion–PL L5-S1	+2
+2	Flexion–TL C6-T1	+1
0	Crossed extensor	0
+2	Perineal S1-2	+2

E. Cranial nerves: All normal
F. Sensation: Location
   Hyperesthesia: None
   Superficial pain: Decreased in right thoracic limb
   Deep pain: Decreased in right thoracic limb
   Complete sections G and H before reviewing case summary.
G. Assessment (anatomic diagnosis and estimation of prognosis)
H. Plan (diagnostic)

   Rule-outs
   1.
   2.
   3.
   4.

CASE HISTORY 2B

Signalment
Canine, German shepherd, female, 7 years old.

History
The animal has had hip dysplasia since 1 year of age. Stumbling on the pelvic limbs started 6 months ago and progressed slowly. The dog cannot go up steps and falls even with good footing. No evidence of pain is present (see Case History 1B, Chapter 1).

Physical Examination
Nothing significant was found on the physical examination other than neurologic deficits.

Neurologic Examination[*]
(See Case History 1B, Chapter 1.)

---

[*]*0,* Absent; *+1,* decreased; *+2,* normal; *+3,* exaggerated; *+4,* very exaggerated or clonus; *PL,* pelvic limb; *TL,* thoracic limb; *NE,* not evaluated.

[*]*0,* Absent; *+1,* decreased; *+2,* normal; *+3,* exaggerated; *+4,* very exaggerated or clonus; *PL,* pelvic limb; *TL,* thoracic limb; *NE,* not evaluated.

A. Observation
1. Mental status: Alert
2. Posture: Difficulty getting up; wide-based stance
3. Gait: Truncal ataxia, stumbles; crosses pelvic limbs, knuckles toes of pelvic limbs
B. Palpation: Normal
C. Postural reactions

Left	Reactions	Right
	Proprioceptive positioning	
0	PL	0
+2	TL	+2
NE	Wheelbarrowing	NE
	Hopping	
+1	PL	+1
+2	TL	+2
NE	Extensor postural thrust	NE
NE	Hemistand–hemiwalk	NE
NE	Tonic neck	NE
	Placing, tactile	
NE	PL	NE
NE	TL	NE
	Placing, visual	
NE	PL	NE
NE	TL	NE

D. Spinal reflexes

Left	Reflex, Spinal Segment	Right
	Quadriceps L4-6	
+3		+2
	Extensor carpi radialis C7-T1	
+2		+2
	Triceps C7-T1	
NE		NE
	Flexion-PL L5-S1	
+2		+2
	Flexion-TL C6-T1	
+2		+2
0	Crossed extensor	0
	Perineal, S1-2	
+2		+2

E. Cranial nerves: All normal
F. Sensation: Location
Hyperesthesia: No
Superficial pain: +2
Deep pain: +2
Complete sections G and H before reviewing case summary.
G. Assessment (anatomic diagnosis and estimation of prognosis)
H. Plan (diagnostic)

Rule-outs
1.
2.
3.
4.

CASE HISTORY 2C

Signalment
Feline, domestic shorthair, female, 3 months old.

History
The kitten has been clumsy since birth. It was one of four in the litter: one was born dead, and the other two are normal. The kitten has a peculiar prancing gait and tremors at times. It seems to be getting around better now (see Case History 1C, Chapter 1).

Physical Examination
Nothing significant was found on the physical examination other than neurologic deficits.

Neurologic Examination[*]
(See Case History 1C, Chapter 1.)

A. Observation
1. Mental status: Alert
2. Posture: Slightly wide-based stance; head tremor that resolves at rest
3. Gait: Ataxia, dysmetria of all four limbs
B. Palpation: Normal
C. Postural reactions

Left	Reactions	Right
	Proprioceptive positioning	
+2	PL	+2
+2	TL	+2
NE	Wheelbarrowing	NE
	Hopping	
+3	PL	+3
+3	TL	+3

Initiation is normal, but movements are hypermetric.

---

[*]*0,* Absent; *+1,* decreased; *+2,* normal; *+3,* exaggerated; *+4,* very exaggerated or clonus; *PL,* pelvic limb; *TL,* thoracic limb; *NE,* not evaluated.

NE	Extensor postural thrust	NE
NE	Hemistand-hemiwalk	NE
NE	Tonic neck	NE

	Placing, tactile	
NE	PL	NE
NE	TL	NE

	Placing, visual	
NE	PL	NE
NE	TL	NE

D. Spinal reflexes: All normal
E. Cranial nerves

Left	Nerve Function (Response/Test)	Right
	CN II–vision	
0	(Menace)	0

	CN II, III	
Pupil size: Normal and equal		

	PLRs	
+2	(Stimulate left eye)	+2
+2	(Stimulate right eye)	+2

	CN II–fundus	
No abnormalities detected.		

	CN III, IV, VI	
Strabismus: None		
Nystagmus: Pendular noted in both eyes		

+2	CN V–sensation	+2
+2	CN V–mastication	+2

+2	CN VII–facial muscles	+2
+2	(Palpebral)	+2

+2	CN IX, X–swallowing	+2
+2	CN XII–tongue	+2

F. Sensation: Location
   Hyperesthesia: No
   Superficial pain: +2
   Deep pain: +2
   Complete sections G and H before reviewing case summary.
G. Assessment (anatomic diagnosis and estimation of prognosis)
H. Plan (diagnostic)

   Rule-outs
   1.
   2.
   3.
   4.

CASE HISTORY 2D

Signalment
Feline, Siamese, male, 2 years old.

History
Uveitis has been present in the right eye for 2 months. The cat is lame in the left thoracic limb and its head tremors when the cat eats. The animal has been depressed for 2 days (see Case History 1D, Chapter 1).

Physical Examination
Physical examination reveals anterior uveitis in the right eye. The remaining findings are normal except for those pertaining to neurologic status.

Neurologic Examination*
(See Case History 1D, Chapter 1.)

A. Observation
   1. Mental status: Depressed
   2. Posture: Head tremor that resolves when the animal is at rest
   3. Gait: Knuckles left thoracic limb
B. Palpation: Atrophy of triceps and muscles distal to elbow in left thoracic limb
C. Postural reactions

Left	Reactions	Right
	Proprioceptive positioning	
0	PL	+2
0	TL	+2

NE	Wheelbarrowing	NE

	Hopping	
0	PL	+2
+1	TL	+2

0	Extensor postural thrust	+2

NE	Hemistand–hemiwalk	NE

NE	Tonic neck	NE

	Placing, tactile	
NE	PL	NE
NE	TL	NE

	Placing, visual	
NE	PL	NE
NE	TL	NE

D. Spinal reflexes

Left	Reflex, Spinal Segment	Right
	Quadriceps	
+3	L4-6	+2

*0, Absent; +1, decreased; +2, normal; +3, exaggerated; +4, very exaggerated or clonus; PL, pelvic limb; TL, thoracic limb; NE, not evaluated.

0	Extensor carpi radialis C7-T1	+2
NE	Triceps C7-T1	NE
+2	Flexion–PL L5-S1	+2
0	Flexion–TL, C6-T1	+2
0	Crossed extensor	0
+2	Perineal, S1-2	+2

E. Cranial nerves

Left	Nerve–Function (Response/Test)	Right
+2	CN II–vision (Menace)	+2
+2 +2	CN II, III–pupil size: miosis present in right eye PLRs (Stimulate left eye) (Stimulate right eye)	+2 +2
	CN II–fundus No abnormalities detected in retina. Uveitis in right eye.	
	CN III, IV, VI Strabismus: None Nystagmus: None Conjugate eye movements: Normal	
+2	CN V–sensation	+2
+2	CN V–mastication	+2
+2 +2	CN VII–facial muscles (Palpebral)	+2 +2
+2	CN IX, X–swallowing	+2
+2	CN XII–tongue	+2

F. Sensation: Location
   Hyperesthesia: No
   Superficial pain: +2
   Deep pain: +2
   Complete sections G and H before reviewing case summary.
G. Assessment (anatomic diagnosis and estimation of prognosis)
H. Plan (diagnostic)

   Rule-outs
   1.
   2.

3.
4.

CASE HISTORY 2E

Signalment
Canine, Yorkshire terrier, male, 8 months old.

History
The animal has always been small and thin. Episodes of abnormal behavior have occurred recently. The dog paces, is restless, and resents being held. These episodes typically last 2 to 3 hours, occasionally for a whole day, and have occurred every day for the past 3 weeks (see Case History 1E, Chapter 1).

Physical Examination
On physical examination the dog appears thin. Other findings are normal except for those pertaining to neurologic status.

Neurologic Examination*
A. Observation
   1. Mental status: Mildly depressed. At times acts confused and agitated.
   2. Posture: Normal
   3. Gait: Paces, sometimes bumps into objects
B. Palpation
C. Postural reactions

Left	Reactions	Right
+1 +1	Proprioceptive positioning PL TL	+1 +1
+1	Wheelbarrowing	+1
+1 +1	Hopping PL TL	+1 +1
+1	Extensor postural thrust	+1
NE	Hemistand–hemiwalk	NE
+1 +1	Placing, tactile PL TL	+1 +1
+1 +1	Placing, visual PL TL	+1 +1

D. Spinal reflexes: All normal
E. Cranial nerves: All normal
F. Sensation: Location
   Hyperesthesia: No

---

*0, Absent; +1, decreased; +2, normal; +3, exaggerated; +4, very exaggerated or clonus; *PL*, pelvic limb; *TL*, thoracic limb; *NE*, not evaluated.

Superficial pain: +2
Deep pain: +2
Complete sections G and H before reviewing case summary.
G. Assessment (anatomic diagnosis and estimation of prognosis)
H. Plan (diagnostic)

Rule-outs
1.
2.
3.
4.

The following abbreviated cases are presented to give you additional practice in localizing lesions. Use Table 2-2 or 2-5 or Figure 2-7 if necessary. The findings on the neurologic examination are all that are needed to localize the lesion.

CASE HISTORY 2F

Signalment
Canine, dachshund, male, 2 years old.

Neurologic Examination*
A. Observation
 1. Mental status: Normal
 2. Posture: Cannot stand
 3. Gait: Moves thoracic limbs but not pelvic limbs (paraparesis)
B. Palpation: Normal
C. Postural reactions

Left	Reactions	Right
	Proprioceptive positioning	
0	PL	0
+2	TL	+2
+2	Wheelbarrowing	+2
	Hopping	
0	PL	0
+2	TL	+2
0	Extensor postural thrust	0
NE	Hemistand–hemiwalk	NE
NE	Tonic neck	NE
	Placing, tactile	
0	PL	0
+2	TL	+2
	Placing, visual	
0	PL	0
+2	TL	+2

D. Spinal reflexes

Left	Reflex, Spinal Segment	Right
0	Quadriceps L4-6	0
+2	Extensor carpi radialis C7-T1	+2
+2	Triceps C7-T1	+2
0	Flexion–PL L5-S1	0
+2	Flexion–TL C6-T1	+2
0	Crossed extensor	0
0	Perineal S1-2	0

E. Cranial nerves: All normal
F. Sensation: Location
 Hyperesthesia: No
 Superficial pain: NE
 Deep pain: NE
 Complete section G before reviewing case summary.
G. Assessment (anatomic diagnosis and estimation of prognosis)

CASE HISTORY 2G

Signalment
Feline, domestic, male, 6 years old.

Neurologic Examination*
A. Observation
 1. Mental status: Normal
 2. Posture: Recumbent
 3. Gait: The cat has slight voluntary movements of limbs but cannot walk (severe tetraparesis)
B. Palpation: Normal
C. Postural reactions

Left	Reactions	Right
	Proprioceptive positioning	
0	PL	0
0	TL	0
0	Wheelbarrowing	0
	Hopping	
0	PL	0
0	TL	0

---

*0, Absent; +1, decreased; +2, normal; +3, exaggerated; +4, very exaggerated or clonus; *PL*, pelvic limb; *TL*, thoracic limb; *NE*, not evaluated.

*0, Absent; +1, decreased; +2, normal; +3, exaggerated; +4, very exaggerated or clonus; *PL*, pelvic limb; *TL*, thoracic limb; *NE*, not evaluated.

0	Extensor postural thrust	0
0	Hemistand–hemiwalk	0
0	Tonic neck	0
0 0	Placing, tactile PL TL	0 0
0 0	Placing, visual PL TL	0 0

D. Spinal reflexes

Left	Reflex, Spinal Segment	Right
+3	Quadriceps, L4-6	I3
+2	Extensor carpi radialis C7-T1	+2
+2	Triceps C7-T1	+2
+2	Flexion–PL L5-S1	+2
+2	Flexion–TL C6-T1	+2 +2
0	Crossed extensor	0
+2	Perineal S1-2	+2

E. Cranial nerves: All normal
F. Sensation: Location
   Hyperesthesia: No
   Superficial pain: +2
   Deep pain: +2
   Complete section G before reviewing case summary.
G. Assessment (anatomic diagnosis and estimation of prognosis)

CASE HISTORY 2H

Signalment
Equine, quarter horse, male, 2 years old.

Neurologic Examination*
A. Observation
   1. Mental status: Alert

---

2. Posture: Normal
3. Gait: Knuckles pelvic limbs, sways trunk; difficulty in backing, will fall
B. Palpation: Normal
C. Postural reactions

Left	Reactions	Right
+1 +2	Proprioceptive positioning PL TL	+1 +2
+1 +2	Hopping PL TL	+1 +2
0 +2	Placing, tactile (curb) PL TL	0 +2

D. Spinal reflexes

Left	Reflex, Spinal Segment	Right
+3	Quadriceps L4-6	+3
+2	Extensor carpi radialis C7-T1	+2
NE	Triceps C7-T1	NE
+2	Flexion–PL L5-S1	+2
+2	Flexion–TL C6-T1	+2
0	Crossed extensor	0
+2	Perineal S1-2	+2

E. Cranial nerves: All normal
F. Sensation: Location
   Hyperesthesia: No
   Superficial pain: +2
   Deep pain: +2
   Complete section G before reviewing case summary.
G. Assessment (anatomic diagnosis and estimation of prognosis)

CASE HISTORY 2I

Signalment
Canine, cocker spaniel, female, 8 years old.

Neurologic Examination*

A. Observation
   1. Mental status: Normal
   2. Posture: Head tilt to right
   3. Gait: Tends to circle to the right; disoriented when picked up for assessment of postural reactions
B. Palpation: Normal
C. Postural reactions: All normal
D. Spinal reflexes: All normal
E. Cranial nerves

Left	Nerve Function (Response/Test)	Right
	CN II–vision (Menace)	
+2		0
	CN II, III–pupil size Normal and equal	
+2	(Stimulate left eye)	+2
+2	(Stimulate right eye)	+2
+2	CN II–fundus	+2
	CN III, IV, VI	
Strabismus:	None	
Nystagmus: Horizontal, fast (jerk) phase to left.		
+2	CN V–sensation	+2
+2	CN V–mastication	+2
	CN VII–facial muscles	
Drooping of right lip.		
+2	(Palpebral)	0
+2	CN IX, X–swallowing	+2
+2	CN XII–tongue	+2

F. Sensation: Location
   Hyperesthesia: No
   Superficial pain: +2
   Deep pain: +2
   Complete section G before reviewing case summary.
G. Assessment (anatomic diagnosis and estimation of prognosis)

CASE HISTORY 2J

Signalment
Bovine, Jersey, female, 6 months old.

Neurologic Examination*

A. Observation
   1. Mental status: Coma
   2. Posture: Recumbent, increased extensor tone in all four limbs
   3. Gait: None

B. Palpation: Normal
C. Postural reactions: Recumbent, none possible
D. Spinal reflexes

Left	Reflex, Spinal Segment	Right
+3	Quadriceps L4-6	+3
+3	Extensor carpi radialis C7-T1	+3
Slow; extensor hypertonus	Flexion–PL L5-S1	Slow; extensor hypertonus
Slow; extensor hypertonus	Flexion–TL, C6-T1	Slow; extensor hypertonus
0	Crossed extensor	0
+2	Perineal S1-2	+2

E. Cranial nerves

Left	Nerve–Function (Response/Test)	Right
	CN II–vision (Menace)	
0		0
	CN II, III	
Pupil size: midposition and equal		
	PLRs	
0	(Stimulate left eye)	0
0	(Stimulate right eye)	0
	CN II–fundus	
No abnormalities noted		
	CN III, IV, VI	
No eye movements noted		
0	CN V–sensation	0
+2	CN V–mastication	+2
	CN VII–facial muscles	
+2	(Palpebral)	+2
+1	CN IX, X–swallowing	+1
+2	CN XII–tongue	+2

F. Sensation: Location
   Hyperesthesia: No
   Superficial pain: 0
   Deep pain: 0
   Complete section G before reviewing case summary.
G. Assessment (anatomic diagnosis and estimation of prognosis)

*0, Absent; +1, decreased; +2, normal; +3, exaggerated; +4, very exaggerated or clonus; *PL*, pelvic limb; *TL*, thoracic limb; *NE*, not evaluated.

ASSESSMENT 2A

Postural reactions are abnormal in both limbs on the right side and are possibly decreased in the left pelvic limb. This finding is not characteristic of peripheral nerve lesions, which ordinarily are restricted to one limb or affect all four limbs (generalized polyneuropathy). Because both pelvic and thoracic limbs are affected, the lesion must be cranial to T2. The right pelvic limb has an exaggerated quadriceps reflex, a UMN sign. Would the interpretation be different if the reflex was normal? No, this would not matter. Reflexes may be normal or exaggerated with UMN disease. The weak or absent myotatic reflexes in the thoracic limbs should not be considered diagnostic. They are frequently difficult to elicit. If a good response occurred on one side and none on the other, you might be more confident in diagnosing an abnormality. The weak flexion reflex in the right thoracic limb is abnormal, however. This finding is a sign of sensory or motor deficit at the segmental level, a LMN sign. From this observation, you should assess the lesion as between C6 and T2 on the right side. There is decreased sensation in the right thoracic limb. Can the lesion be in the peripheral nerves of the brachial plexus? No, not unless more than one lesion exists. Remember the abnormalities of the right pelvic limb. One lesion in the C6-T2 spinal cord segments could account for both thoracic and pelvic limb abnormalities. A gray matter lesion affecting sensory and motor neurons to the brachial plexus and a white matter lesion affecting the proprioceptive and UMN pathways to the pelvic limb account for all the signs. Why is pain sensation still present in the pelvic limbs? The pain pathways are bilateral, and this lesion is unilateral. If the lesion were bilateral, both pelvic limbs would have severe postural reaction deficits. The slow initiation of hopping in the left pelvic limb may be caused by a partial loss of the proprioceptive pathways to that side. This hypothesis cannot be substantiated by proprioceptive positioning tests. Is the spinal cord lesion the only lesion? The animal's mental status and cranial nerves are normal, and no other signs are present that cannot be explained by the lesion. Always assume that one lesion is present unless evidence exists to the contrary.

Localization
Spinal cord, C6-T2, right side.

Rule-outs
1. Vascular lesion
2. Trauma
3. Inflammation (low probability)

The plan for a definitive diagnosis is discussed at the end of Chapter 4.

ASSESSMENT 2B

Pelvic limb ataxia and paresis suggest a lesion caudal to T2. The postural reactions and the spinal reflexes confirm that the thoracic limbs are not affected. The spinal reflexes are normal or exaggerated in the pelvic limbs, indicating that the lesion is cranial to L4. Therefore, the lesion should be between T3 and L3. The sensory examination does not provide any definitive evidence for a more specific localization. The animal's mental status and the reactions of the cranial nerves and the thoracic limbs do not suggest that more than one lesion exists.

Localization
Spinal cord, T3-L3, symmetric.

Rule-outs
1. Degenerative disease
2. Neoplasia
3. Inflammation

The plan for a definitive diagnosis is discussed at the end of Chapter 4.

ASSESSMENT 2C

Ataxia, dysmetria, and tremor are signs of cerebellar disease. Paresis is not associated with cerebellar disease, and so ensuring that no loss of voluntary movement exists is important. Brainstem or spinal cord disease may mimic some of the signs of cerebellar dysfunction. In this case the head is affected; the cat shows a head tremor, an absent menace reaction, and pendular nystagmus, indicating brain disease. Neither paresis nor proprioceptive deficits are present, although the postural reactions are not normal. The abnormality in hopping is dysmetria. The absence of the menace reaction with an intact palpebral reflex (CN V and VII) and good vision is indicative of cerebellar disease. The nystagmus, which does not have a fast and slow component, is similar in origin to the intention tremor of the head. All these signs are compatible with cerebellar disease, and no signs exist that cannot be explained by the presence of this lesion.

Localization
Cerebellum.

Rule-outs (see Chapter 1)

Rule-outs
1. Anomaly
2. Trauma

The plan for a definitive diagnosis is discussed at the end of Chapter 4.

ASSESSMENT 2D

The clinical findings cannot be explained by one lesion. The animal's altered mental status and head tremor should immediately signal brain disease. Depression can be caused by a lesion in almost any part of the brain except the cerebellum, or it could be merely a manifestation of systemic illness. The head tremor suggests cerebellar involvement. If the depression is caused by a brain lesion, more than one lesion exists. The postural reactions indicate a left hemiparesis. Hemiparesis is caused by brain disease more often than by spinal cord disease, but spinal reflexes are absent in the left thoracic limb, indicating either C6-T2 spinal cord disease or peripheral nerve lesions.

Absent reflexes with intact sensation are unusual with peripheral nerve disease (with the exception of polyneuropathies); so the lesion is more likely in the ventral roots or the spinal cord gray matter. The left pelvic limb has an UMN paresis, further indicating spinal cord or brainstem involvement. Miosis of the left pupil is most likely caused by the uveitis, but a lesion involving the left cranial sympathetic nerve cannot be totally excluded, especially with the presence of a C6-T2 spinal cord lesion. In summary, this cat has multifocal lesions affecting the left C6-T2 spinal cord, the cerebellum, and, possibly, other brain structures (depression).

Localization

Multifocal or systemic disease, left C6-T2 spinal cord, cerebellum; cerebrum or brainstem.

Rule-outs
1. Inflammation
2. Neoplasia
3. Degenerative disease

The plan for a definitive diagnosis is discussed at the end of Chapter 4.

ASSESSMENT 2E

The primary abnormality is altered mental status. The dog's mood fluctuates between depression and agitation. He does not always make appropriate responses. The slowness of the postural reactions must be interpreted cautiously in view of the dog's mental status. Severely depressed animals may not be cooperative when postural reaction tests are performed. Compulsive walking is usually a sign of prefrontal cerebral cortex (forebrain) disease. In severe forms of the disease, the animal walks until it bumps into a wall and stands pressing its head against the wall. The dog's neurologic signs suggest cerebral (forebrain) disease.

Localization

Forebrain (cerebrum).

Rule-outs (see Chapter 1)

Rule-outs
1. Metabolic disease
2. Toxic disease

ASSESSMENT 2F

Normal thoracic limbs, LMN signs in the pelvic limbs.

Localization

L4-S3.

ASSESSMENT 2G

UMN signs in all four limbs; normal brain.

Localization

C1-5.

ASSESSMENT 2H

Normal thoracic limbs, UMN signs in the pelvic limbs.

Localization

T3-L3.

ASSESSMENT 2I

The head tilt and the nystagmus indicate an abnormality of the vestibular system. The lack of paresis or proprioceptive deficits is diagnostic of a peripheral vestibular lesion. The dog has right-sided peripheral vestibular disease.

The drooping lip, negative palpebral reflex, and normal facial sensation indicate involvement of the facial nerve (CN VII). CN VII and CN VIII are both affected by disease in the right labyrinth.

ASSESSMENT 2J

Coma, decerebrate posture, tetraparesis, and cranial nerve signs indicate involvement of the brainstem. The menace reaction is absent because of the coma and disconnection of the cortex from CN VII.

The pupils indicate a loss of both sympathetic and parasympathetic input and involvement of the midbrain. The absence of eye movements indicates involvement of the core brainstem (medial longitudinal fasciculus). The lesion is in the midbrain (see Chapter 11). Localization to the brainstem is adequate for the formulation of a clinical diagnosis.

References

1. De Lahunta A: *Veterinary neuroanatomy and clinical neurology.* Philadelphia, 1977, WB Saunders, pp 3-6.
2. Willis W, Chung J: Central mechanisms of pain. *J Am Vet Med Assoc* 191:1200-1202, 1987.
3. Breazile JE, Kitchell RL: A study of fiber systems within the spinal cord of the domestic pig that subserve pain. *J Comp Neurol* 133:373-382, 1968.
4. Kennard MA: The course of ascending fibers in the spinal cord of the cat essential to the recognition of painful stimuli. *J Comp Neurol* 100:511-524, 1954.
5. Tarlov IM: *Spinal cord compression: mechanism of paralysis and treatment.* Springfield, Ill, 1957, Charles C Thomas.
6. Holliday T: Clinical signs of acute and chronic experimental lesions of the cerebellum. *Vet Res Commun* 3:259-278, 1980.
7. Holliday TA: Clinical signs caused by experimental lesions in the vestibular system. In *Proceedings of the Eighth Annual Veterinary Medical Forum.* Washington, DC, 1990, pp 1025-1028.
8. Kornegay JN: Ataxia of the head and limbs: cerebellar diseases in dogs and cats. *Prog Vet Neurol* 1:255-274, 1990.
9. Oliver JE: Localization of lesions in the nervous system. In Hoerlein BF, editor: *Canine neurology,* 3rd ed. Philadelphia, 1978, WB Saunders, pp 71-102.

Disorders of Micturition

Abnormal visceral function may reflect a pathologic change in the nervous system; however, the importance of nervous control of the viscera is often overlooked.

The classic view of the autonomic nervous system as one with discrete boundaries is giving way to a concept of a more integrated system with no limits. For example, conventional theory held that the autonomic system controlled functions that the individual could not modify voluntarily; however, the fact that one can regulate blood pressure, heart rate, micturition, and many other autonomic activities has been proven. In conventional theory, the sympathetic *(adrenergic)* system functions as an antagonist to the parasympathetic *(cholinergic)* system. This simplistic view, which separates the autonomic system from the somatic system, does not explain well-defined somatovisceral and viscerosomatic reflexes.

Problems associated with micturition are common in neurologic disorders. Other forms of visceral dysfunction traditionally have been the concern of cardiologists and internists, and these are discussed in books on cardiology and internal medicine. This chapter reviews the anatomy, physiology, and clinical syndromes of micturition.

ANATOMY AND PHYSIOLOGY OF MICTURITION

Micturition is the reaction that ultimately occurs if a bladder is gradually distended, leading to the coordinated expulsion of its contents.[1] The micturition reflex is a complex integration of parasympathetic, sympathetic, and somatic pathways extending from the sacral segments of the spinal cord to the cerebral cortex. The components of the micturition reflex are discussed in functional groups before a complete description of the micturition reflex is discussed.

Detrusor Reflex

The primary component of micturition is the detrusor (the muscle of the urinary bladder) reflex. As the bladder fills with urine, a slight increase in bladder pressure occurs with each increase in volume until the limit of elasticity of the smooth muscle is reached. The sensory nerve endings in the bladder wall are tension recorders and are arranged in series with the muscle fibers. As the bladder nears its capacity, these nerves begin to discharge. The sensory fibers from the bladder are located in the pelvic nerve and originate from the sacral segments of the spinal cord (Figure 3-1).[2,3] The sensory discharge ascends in the spinal cord to the pontine reticular formation in the brainstem. Integration occurs at this level, eventually giving rise to a motor discharge down the spinal cord to the preganglionic parasympathetic neurons in the intermediate horn of the sacral segments.

The preganglionic parasympathetic neurons are located in segments S1-3 in the cat and the dog.[2,3] They have not been located precisely in other species, but gross dissections indicate that they are in the sacral segments. The preganglionic neurons discharge and activate postganglionic neurons, which are located in the pelvic ganglia, along the course of the pelvic nerves, and in the wall of the bladder. Some integration of activity apparently takes place in the ganglia. Ultimately, the postganglionic neurons synapse on detrusor muscle fibers and cause a contraction—the detrusor reflex (Figure 3-2, *A*).

Integration in the brainstem is necessary for the detrusor reflex to be coordinated and sustained long enough for bladder evacuation. Complete lesions of any portion of this pathway abolish the detrusor reflex.

Voluntary Control of the Detrusor Reflex

The sensory pathway to the brainstem that signals distention of the bladder also sends collaterals to the cerebral cortex (see Figure 3-1). Integration at the cortical level allows voluntary initiation (e.g., in territorial marking) or inhibition (e.g., in house training) of micturition. The precise location of the control center of the cerebral cortex is not clear. Stimulation and evoked-response studies indicate that several areas of the cortex influence the detrusor reflex.[4]

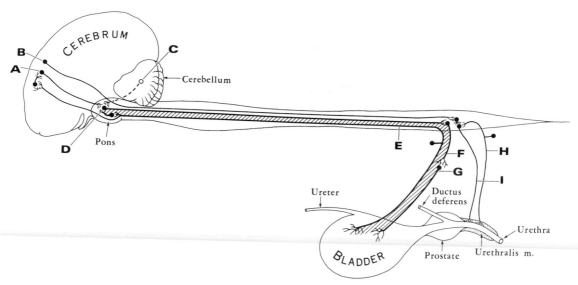

Figure 3-1 Anatomic organization of micturition. **A,** Cortical neurons for voluntary control of micturition. **B,** Cortical neurons for voluntary control of sphincters. **C,** Cerebellar neurons that have an inhibitory influence on micturition. **D,** Pontine reticular neurons that are necessary for the detrusor reflex. **E,** Afferent (sensory) pathway for the detrusor reflex. **F,** Preganglionic pelvic (parasympathetic) neuron to the detrusor. **G,** Postganglionic pelvic (parasympathetic) neuron to the detrusor. **H,** Afferent (sensory) neuron from the urethral spincter, pudendal nerve. **I,** Efferent (motor) neuron to the urethral sphincter, pudendal nerve. (From Oliver JE Jr, Osborne CA: Neurogenic urinary incontinence. In Kirk RW, editor: *Current veterinary therapy,* VII. Philadelphia, 1980, WB Saunders, pp 1122-1127.)

Lesions of the cerebral cortex may cause a loss of voluntary control of micturition and may reduce the capacity of the bladder.[5] For example, animals with cerebral tumors may start voiding in the house for no apparent reason.

Cerebellar Inhibition of the Detrusor Reflex

The cerebellum can inhibit the detrusor reflex (see Figure 3-1). Stimulation of the fastigial nucleus abolishes detrusor reflex contraction.[6] Lesions of

Figure 3-2 Schematic representation of sequential pressure and neural changes during micturition (not drawn to scale). **A,** Intravesical pressure. **B,** Urethral pressure. **C,** Pelvic nerve. **D,** Hypogastric nerve. **E,** Pudendal nerve. **F,** Bladder volume. (Modified from Jonas U, Tanagho EA: Studies on vesicourethral reflexes. *Invest Urol* 12:357-373, 1975; and Bradley WE, Teague CT: Hypogastric and pelvic nerve activity during the micturition reflex. *J Urol* 101:438-440, 1969.)

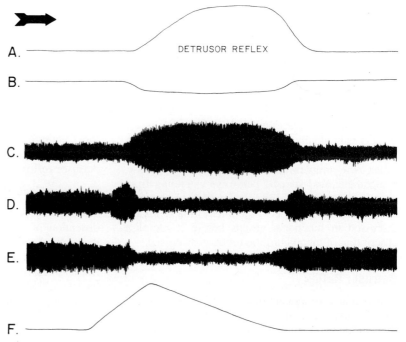

the cerebellum, such as cerebellar hypoplasia, may produce increased frequency of voiding with a reduced bladder capacity.[1]

Urethral Sphincter

The muscle surrounding the urethra contains spindles that discharge in response to stretch, as do other skeletal muscles. Sensory discharges ascend in the pudendal nerves to the sacral segments. The pudendal urethral motor neurons are located in segments L7-S3 in the dog and the cat, although they are found primarily in S1 and S2 in both species.[2,7] Monosynaptic activation of the motor neurons is transmitted back down the pudendal nerve to the muscle (see Figure 3-1). Afferent discharge through the pelvic nerves also activates the pudendal nerve. These pathways produce urethral contraction in response to a sudden stretch, maintaining continence during a cough, a sneeze, and so forth. Voluntary control of the urethral sphincter is provided by cortical pathways to the sacral segments (see Figure 3-1).

Lesions of the sacral segments or the pudendal nerve cause a hypotonic paralysis of the sphincter. Cortical or spinal lesions may abolish voluntary control of the sphincter and may produce increased sphincter tone, which increases outflow resistance.[8] Typically, T3-L3 lesions of the spinal cord abolish the long-routed detrusor reflex and cause increased tone in the sphincter.

Sympathetic Innervation

The detrusor reflex is mediated through the parasympathetic nervous system *(sacral spinal cord segments)*. The skeletal muscle in the urethral sphincter is innervated by somatic nerves. Sympathetic nerves found in the pelvic plexus, the pelvic ganglia, and the urinary bladder serve to enhance the storage function of micturition.

The preganglionic sympathetic neurons to the bladder are located in the lumbar spinal cord (L2-5 in the cat, L1-4 in the dog).[2,3] The fibers course through the caudal mesenteric ganglion and the hypogastric nerve to the bladder and the pelvic plexus. Both alpha- and beta-adrenergic (sympathetic postganglionic) synapses have been found on neurons in the pelvic ganglia, in the bladder wall, and on the detrusor muscle, especially in the area of the trigone.[9]

Pharmacologic studies have demonstrated that alpha-adrenergic receptors are located primarily in the region of the trigone, the bladder neck, and the proximal urethra, causing contraction of the smooth muscle. Beta-adrenergic receptors are found in all parts of the bladder and cause relaxation of smooth muscle. The presence of adrenergic synapses on cholinergic ganglion cells suggests that the sympathetic pathways can also modulate the activity of the parasympathetic pathway, but this effect has not been demonstrated in naturally occurring sympathetic firing.[8] Adrenergic innervation of the bladder neck and the trigone has been demonstrated to have major significance in the prevention of retrograde ejaculation.

Lesions of the sympathetic pathways apparently do not have a major effect on micturition; however, acceptance of the theory that the sympathetic pathways play an important role in animals and in humans with lesions of the parasympathetic pathways is increasing.[9-11] Patients with neurogenic bladder dysfunction complicated by a narrowing of the bladder neck or spasms of the urethra may be helped by alpha-adrenergic blockade.[9]

Sensory Pathways from the Bladder

Sensory fibers originating in the bladder run in both the pelvic and the hypogastric nerves. Stretch receptors in the bladder wall give rise to fibers that run through the pelvic nerve into the sacral spinal cord (S1-3 in the cat and the dog) and ascend to the pontine reticular formation to initiate the detrusor reflex. Sensory fibers in the hypogastric nerve reach the spinal cord at the lumbar segments (L2-5 in the cat, L1-4 in the dog).[2,3] Afferent fibers from both pelvic and hypogastric nerves reach the cerebral cortex in the cat, whereas only hypogastric neural activity is relayed to the cortex in the dog.[12] The hypogastric fibers respond to overdistention of the bladder. Activation of these fibers is perceived as pain.[13] A lesion of the caudal lumbar or sacral spinal cord could abolish micturition, although the animal would still perceive overdistention of the bladder as a painful sensation mediated through the hypogastric nerve.

Motor Innervation of the Detrusor Muscle

Each motor nerve in the bladder wall innervates many muscle cells, although not all muscle cells have direct innervation. The neuromuscular junction is characterized by a varicosity of the axon-containing synaptic vesicles, a thinning of the Schwann cell layer, and a close apposition to specialized areas of the detrusor muscle fibers. Excitation of the innervated muscle cell (pacemaker cell) initiates a spread of excitation and contraction through adjacent cells by means of "tight junctions."[8] The spread of excitation has also been hypothesized to occur by diffusion of a neurotransmitter in the extracellular space to adjacent detrusor muscle fibers.

Disruption of tight junctions between muscle fibers may occur when the bladder is overdistended (e.g., obstruction of the urethra). If tight junctions are disrupted, the wave of excitation cannot spread and a flaccid bladder results. Reconnection of the junction occurs in 1 to 2 weeks if the distention is relieved early. If the bladder remains distended too long or if infection is present, fibrosis develops between the cells, preventing restoration of function.

Reflex Integration

The micturition reflex involves a coordinated and sustained contraction of the detrusor muscle and relaxation of the urethra. Pelvic-nerve sensory neurons that produce the detrusor reflex also send collaterals to inhibitory interneurons in the sacral spinal cord.[13] The inhibitory interneurons synapse on the pudendal motor neurons, which are also in the sacral segments, to reduce motor activity in the pudendal nerves and the periurethral striated muscle (see Figure 3-2, *B* and *E*). As the detrusor contracts, the urethra relaxes, allowing urine to pass. If the long pathways are intact, voluntary activation of the pudendal neurons by the corticospinal pathways can override this effect and block micturition. Lesions of the long tracts or at the segmental level may interfere with reflex integration. Detrusor contraction without urethral relaxation is called *reflex dyssynergia.*[14]

Reflex connections between the pelvic (parasympathetic) nerve afferents and the lumbar (sympathetic) motor neurons also have been demonstrated.[13] The effect seems similar to that observed in the pudendal (somatic) nerve—that is, as the pelvic motor neuron begins to fire to initiate a detrusor contraction, the hypogastric nerve becomes silent (see Figure 3-2, *C* and *D*). When the pelvic nerve stops firing as the bladder is emptied, the hypogastric nerve discharges once more. Presumably, the effect of the hypogastric nerve is on bladder relaxation and urethral contraction.

Micturition Reflex

Integration of filling, storage, and contraction of the bladder with contraction and then relaxation of the sphincters is the *micturition reflex.* The following discussion presents each of the components for a more complete picture.

Urine is transported from the kidneys to the bladder through the ureters. Peristaltic waves move the urine into the bladder in spurts. Vesicoureteral reflux is prevented by the oblique course of the ureter through the bladder wall, resulting in the formation of a flap valve. The detrusor muscle spirals around the ureter, assisting in the maintenance of the valve effect.

The bladder fills without a significant increase in pressure as the smooth muscle stretches (see Figure 3-2, *A* and *F*). The sympathetic *(adrenergic)* pathways may assist by inhibiting parasympathetic *(cholinergic)* neurons or by direct relaxation of smooth muscle. If the bladder fills beyond the normal elasticity of the smooth muscle, pressure increases linearly with the increase in volume.

In the intact animal, as the limits of stretch of the smooth muscle are approached, stretch receptors in the bladder wall are excited and send sensory discharges through the pelvic nerves to the sacral spinal cord. These discharges are relayed up the spinal cord to the reticular formation in the pons. The activation of neuronal pools in the pons results in a motor discharge down the spinal cord to the sacral segments. Preganglionic parasympathetic motor neurons in the intermediate horn of the sacral gray matter are activated. The motor discharge passes down the pelvic nerves to activate postganglionic neurons in the pelvic ganglia and in the wall of the bladder, which in turn activate the bladder smooth muscle *(detrusor).* The sustained discharge of neurons through these pathways produces a coordinated, sustained contraction of the detrusor muscle (see Figure 3-2, *A* and *C*).

The fibers of the detrusor muscle spiral into the neck of the bladder and help to maintain continence in the relaxed state. As the fibers contract, the bladder neck is pulled open into a funnel shape. Simultaneously, sensory discharges from the pelvic nerves are relayed to the lumbar segments (inhibiting the output of the sympathetic pathway) and to the pudendal motor neurons in the ventral horn of the sacral segments (inhibiting the tonic output in the nerves to the skeletal sphincter) (see Figure 3-2, *C* to *E*).

The result is a coordinated contraction of the bladder and a relaxation of the sphincter, which is maintained until voiding is complete (see Figure 3-2, *A* and *B*). Sustaining the contraction also is enhanced by sensory fibers in the urethra, which respond to the flow of urine.

When the bladder is empty, sensory discharges in the pelvic nerve stop. Motor discharges in the pelvic nerve cease and activity in the sympathetic and pudendal nerves returns. The bladder relaxes, and the sphincter closes.

DISORDERS OF MICTURITION

The neurogenic disorders of micturition are caused by abnormal detrusor or sphincter function or both (Table 3-1). Detrusor or sphincter activity may be decreased, increased, or normal. Typical syndromes

Table 3-1 **Effect of Lesions of the Neuromuscular System on Micturition**

Location of Lesion	Normal Function	Bladder					Sphincter			
		Voluntary Control	Sustained Detrusor Reflex	Tone	Volume	Residual Urine	Voluntary Control	Perineal Reflex	Tone	Synergy with Detrusor
Forebrain	Voluntary control	Absent	N	N	↑, N, ↓	None	Absent	N to ↑	N to ↑	N
Cerebellum	Inhibition of detrusor reflex	Normal, ↑ frequency	May be hyperreflexic	N	↓	None	N	N	N	N
Brainstem to sacral spinal cord	Sustained detrusor reflex	Absent	None early; small unsynchronized contractions late	Atonic early, may be ↑ late	↑	↑	Absent	N to ↑	N to ↑	Absent
Partial lesions; brainstem to sacral spinal cord (reflex dyssynergia)	Coordination of detrusor and sphincter	May be present	May be present	N to ↓	↑	↑ to ↓	May be present	N	N to ↑	Absent
Sacral spinal cord or roots	LMN to detrusor and sphincter	Absent	Absent	↓	↑	↑	Absent	Absent	↓	Absent
Detrusor muscle (tight junctions)	Spread of excitation in detrusor	Absent	Absent	↓	↑	↑	N	N	N	N (impossible to evaluate)

Modified from Oliver JE Jr, Osborne CA: Neurogenic urinary incontinence. In Kirk RW, editor: *Current veterinary therapy, VI.* Philadelphia, 1977, WB Saunders.
↑, Increased; ↓, decreased; *N*, normal; *LMN*, lower motor neuron.

include inappropriate voiding; inadequate voiding with an overflow of urine; increased frequency, reduced capacity, or both; and incomplete voiding when normal voiding reactions are interrupted by abrupt contractions of the urethral sphincter.[8]

Clinical Signs

The clinical signs of abnormal micturition are summarized in Table 3-2.

Detrusor Areflexia with Sphincter Hypertonus

The most frequently recognized disorder of micturition is a loss of the detrusor reflex with increased tone in the urethral sphincter. Lesions from the pontine reticular formation to the L7 spinal cord segments may cause these complications. The most common cause is compression of the spinal cord such as from a herniated disk, which disrupts the long pathways that are responsible for the detrusor

reflex and the upper motor neuron (UMN) pathways to the skeletal muscle of the urethral sphincter. Loss of micturition occurs at about the same time that voluntary function of the limbs is lost and recovers similarly. The animal is unable to void and the bladder becomes greatly distended, and expressing the bladder manually is difficult or impossible. The perineal reflex is intact.

Detrusor Areflexia with Normal Sphincter Tone

Lesions of the spinal cord or the brainstem may produce detrusor areflexia without causing increased tone in the urethral sphincter. Traumatic injuries of the pelvis may damage the pelvic plexus without damage to the pudendal nerve. The animal is unable to void, but manual expression can be accomplished. Females have a short skeletal sphincter so that even with UMN lesions, sphincter tone may not be excessive. Perineal reflexes are intact.

Table 3-2   Signs of Abnormal Micturition

Problem	Voiding	Attempts to Void	Expression of Bladder	Residual Urine	Perineal Reflex	Probable Lesion
Detrusor areflexia, sphincter hypertonus	Absent	No	Difficult	Large amount	Present	Brainstem to L7 spinal cord
Detrusor areflexia, normal sphincter tone	Absent	No	Possible, some resistance	Large amount	Present	Brainstem to L7 spinal cord
Detrusor areflexia, sphincter areflexia	Absent	No	Easy, often leaks urine	Large to moderate amounts	Absent	Sacral spinal cord or nerve roots
Detrusor areflexia (overdistention)	Absent	Yes	Possible, some resistance	Large amount	Present	Detrusor muscle
Detrusor hyper-reflexia	Frequent, small quantity	Yes	Possible, some resistance	None	Present	Brainstem to L7, partial, or cerebellum; also inflammation of bladder
Reflex dyssynergia	Frequent, spurting, unsustained	Yes	Difficult	Small to large amount	Present	Brainstem to L7, partial lesions
Normal detrusor reflex, incompetent sphincter	Normal, but with leakage of urine with stress or full bladder	Yes	Easy	None	May or may not be present	Pudendal nerves, sympathetic nerves, hormone deficiency

Detrusor Areflexia with Sphincter Areflexia

Lesions of the sacral spinal cord or the nerve roots, such as fractures of the L6 or L7 vertebrae, cause a loss of the detrusor reflexes and urethral sphincter reflexes and tone. The bladder is easily expressed and may leak urine continuously. Perineal reflexes are diminished or absent.

Detrusor Areflexia from Overdistention

Loss of excitation–contraction coupling in the detrusor muscle may occur as a result of severe overdistention of the bladder. Manual expression of the bladder may be difficult because the sphincter is normal. The animal may empty the bladder partially by abdominal contraction. Attempts to void indicate that sensory pathways are intact and suggest a primary detrusor muscle abnormality. The most frequent cause is obstruction of the outflow tract (e.g., calculi).

Detrusor Hyperreflexia

Frequent voiding of small quantities of urine, often without warning, may be caused by partial lesions of the long pathways or of the cerebellum. Inflammation of the bladder *(cystitis)* may produce similar signs. Little or no residual urine is present, the capacity of the bladder is reduced, and perineal reflexes are intact.

The so-called upper motor neuron bladder as seen in chronic paraplegic human beings is rare in animals. In animals, complete chronic spinal cord lesions cause detrusor areflexia, not hyperreflexia. The bladder may have small uncoordinated contractions, but these are inadequate to empty the bladder. Animals with partial lesions, especially in the recovery phase, may have increasing amplitude of the detrusor contractions as they approach normal.

Reflex Dyssynergia

Normal initiation of voiding is followed by interruption of the stream through an involuntary contraction of the urethral sphincter. The stream of urine is normal at first, followed by short spurts and then by a complete cessation of the flow. Frequently the animal continues to strain with no success. Reflex dyssynergia is seen primarily in male dogs. The pathogenesis is not certain but is presumed to be the result of a partial UMN lesion causing a loss of the normal inhibition of the pudendal nerves during the detrusor reflex. The detrusor reflex is present, and the perineal reflex is often hyperactive. Increased sensory input from abnormal structures innervated by the sacral nerves may also play a role. Examples include prostatic disease, perineal trauma, and surgical wounds in this area. Sympathetic innervation may also play a role in some cases of dyssynergia. We have observed an abnormality clinically similar to reflex dyssynergia in a male dog recovering from tetanus.

Normal Detrusor Reflex with Decreased Sphincter Tone

Loss of normal urethral resistance with a normal detrusor reflex causes leaking of urine when voiding is delayed. The animal can empty the bladder, but as soon as a small amount of urine accumulates, leakage occurs. The leakage may occur during an abdominal press (barking, coughing) or during complete rest. The most frequent cause is the lack of sex hormones in a neutered animal. Hormone-responsive incontinence has been well documented in ovariectomized bitches[15] and less frequently in neutered male dogs. Both are responsive to hormone replacement therapy with or without supplementation with adrenergic agents. A similar clinical picture may be seen in some animals that are not responsive to hormone therapy. The lesion may be a structural abnormality of the urethra, a loss of pudendal innervation, or a loss of sympathetic innervation to the urethra.[15]

Diagnosis

The minimum database recommended for the evaluation of an animal with a problem associated with micturition is presented in Table 3-3. The minimum database is designed to reveal any additional problems as well as to provide the information necessary to make a diagnosis and to formulate a prognosis. Figure 3-3 outlines the process of establishing a diagnosis. Specific steps in the process are discussed in the following sections.

Table 3-3   Minimum Database for Diagnosis of Disorders of Micturition

History
Physical examination
  Includes: Observation of voiding and measurement of residual urine
Neurologic examination
  Includes: Sphincter reflexes
Clinical pathology
  Includes: Complete blood cell count, urinalysis, blood urea nitrogen or creatinine determinations
Radiologic examination
  Includes: Survey of abdomen and pelvis, contrast cystography and urethrography, intravenous pyelogram.

Modified from Oliver JE Jr, Osborne CA: Neurogenic urinary incontinence. In Kirk RW, editor: *Current veterinary therapy, VI*. Philadelphia, 1977, WB Saunders.

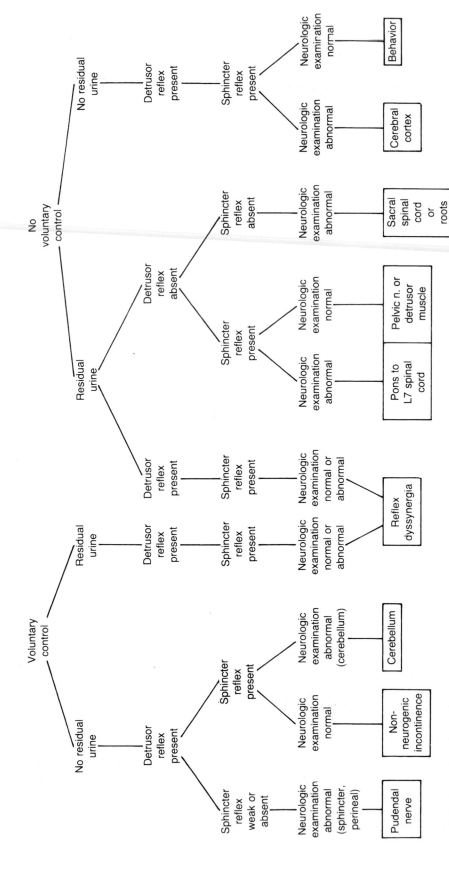

Figure 3-3 Algorithm for diagnosis of disorders of micturition. (From Oliver JE Jr, Osborne CA: Neurogenic urinary incontinence. In Kirk RW, editor: *Current veterinary therapy*, VII. Philadelphia, 1980, WB Saunders, pp 1122-1127.)

History

In addition to the usual items in the history, the examiner should obtain some specific information pertinent to micturition.

Previous History. The clinician should determine the animal's pattern of micturition habits from as early an age as possible. Age when house trained, frequency of micturition at various ages, and changes in habits may provide insight into the onset of a problem before the owner's recognition of its significance.

Signs of abnormality in the nervous system or the urinary tract and previous trauma are important. Previous operative procedures, especially neurologic, abdominal, or pelvic (e.g., ovariohysterectomy), should be analyzed in relation to the time of onset of the problem.

History of the Problem. Information regarding the onset and the chronologic course of the problem allows the examiner to construct a sign-time graph, which is useful for determining the cause of the disease (see Chapter 1).

Voluntary control of micturition is often best established by the owner's perceptions, which are supplemented and confirmed by direct observations of the animal in natural surroundings (e.g., outside on the grass). If the animal can volitionally initiate voiding, the detrusor reflex is probably present. Voluntary control also implies that micturition can be withheld for a reasonable length of time (house training) and can be interrupted if necessary. Interruption of micturition is difficult to evaluate. A dog that is lead-trained can be interrupted by a pull on the lead and a command to "come." Individual interpretation of interruption is quite subjective.

Reflex dyssynergia begins with a normal initiation of voiding followed by a narrowing of the stream and a sudden interruption of the flow. The animal often strains and may continue voiding in brief spurts. Dyssynergia must be differentiated from *partial obstruction* (e.g., that caused by urethral calculi), which can be demonstrated by catheterization and urethral contrast-enhanced radiography.

Various types of incontinence may be described by the owner. Precipitate voiding *(detrusor hyperreflexia),* in which the animal voids suddenly in inappropriate places without apparent warning, is characteristic of cerebellar lesions and some partial spinal cord or brainstem lesions (see Table 3-2). Differentiation between precipitate voiding and loss of normal voluntary control, as in cortical lesions or behavioral changes, may be difficult on the basis of the history alone. Dribbling of urine may result from loss of urethral resistance or overflow from an areflexic bladder (see Table 3-2).

Physical Examination

Observation of the animal may confirm the characteristics of micturition as described in the history. The differences in the various abnormalities of micturition may be subtle; therefore the problem described by the owner must be verified by the examiner.

The presence of a detrusor reflex can be assumed if voiding is sustained (see Figure 3-3); however, bladder contractions with incomplete voiding are common in neurologic disorders. Such contractions are not the result of a true detrusor reflex. The residual urine must therefore be measured in every animal with a problem associated with micturition. After the animal has voided, preferably outside in natural surroundings, the bladder is catheterized and the residual urine is measured. Residual urine should be less than 10% of the normal volume. Most animals have less than 10 ml remaining (0.2 to 0.4 ml/kg).[9]

Except for urethral flaps, which are rare, obstructions in the urethra can be detected when a catheter is passed. A flap can be demonstrated only by excretory urethrography.[16]

Palpation of the bladder before and after the animal voids provides some information regarding bladder tone. The tone of the detrusor muscle is intrinsic and is not directly related to innervation; however, a normal bladder contracts to accommodate the volume of urine present. An overdistended bladder with rupture of the tight junctions does not contract. A chronically infected bladder is often small and has thickened, fibrotic walls. A small, contracted bladder with infection may not be the primary problem because bladder infection is a common sequela of urine retention from neurogenic disorders. Some of the nonneurogenic causes of incontinence, such as tumors or calculi, may be identified by palpation.

Manual expression of the bladder provides some information regarding urethral sphincter tone. Normally, expression of the bladder is more difficult in the male than in the female. Urethral sphincter tone is decreased in lesions of the sacral spinal cord, the sacral roots, or the pudendal nerve (lower motor neuron [LMN]) and is increased in lesions between the L7 spinal cord segment and the brainstem (see Table 3-2). The sacral spinal cord segments lie within the body of the fifth lumbar vertebra in the dog so that lesions of the vertebrae from L5-6 caudad can affect the sacral roots. In large animals, lesions at the level of the midsacrum affect the sacral segments and nerve roots.

Neurologic Examination

The complete neurologic examination is described in Chapter 1. Reflexes related to the sacral spinal cord segments are especially important in evaluating micturition disorders.

The anal and urethral sphincters are innervated by the pudendal nerve, primarily from sacral segments 1 and 2 but occasionally with fibers from S3. Anal sphincter function is easy to observe or to palpate, whereas the urethral sphincter is evaluated best by electrodiagnostic procedures.

Tone of the anal sphincter can be observed, or the sphincter can be palpated with a gloved digit. Two sacral reflexes also can be evaluated. The *bulbocavernosus reflex* is a sharp contraction of the sphincter in response to a squeeze of the bulb of the penis or the clitoris. The *perineal reflex* is a contraction of the sphincter in response to a pinch or pinprick of the perineal region. The perineal reflex also is used to test sensory distribution in the perineal region. Unilateral lesions are detected in this manner.

Lesions of the sacral spinal cord, sacral roots, or pudendal nerves abolish these reflexes, and the anal sphincter is atonic.

The history, physical examination, and neurologic examination provide sufficient data to differentiate neurogenic from nonneurogenic bladder disorders and to localize the lesion in the nervous system if a neurogenic disorder is present (see Tables 3-1 and 3-2). Additional data are necessary for the formulation of diagnosis and prognosis.

Clinical Pathology

The minimum database includes a complete blood cell count, urinalysis, and biochemical profile. Each is essential to the formulation of a prognosis of urinary tract dysfunction, and each may assist in the diagnosis of nonneurogenic problems of micturition.

All animals with neurogenic bladder disorders are likely to have urinary tract infections. Constant surveillance and appropriate treatment, when indicated, are imperative if a favorable outcome is to be expected. Ureteral reflux is also a frequent complication of neurogenic bladder dysfunction. Reflux of infected urine may lead to chronic pyelonephritis and renal failure.

Radiologic Examination

Radiography is important for the identification of nonneurogenic problems, for the evaluation of the extent of urinary tract disease (which may be a complication of neurogenic disorders), and for the assessment of the primary neurologic problem.

Contrast-enhanced cystourethrography, especially when performed in conjunction with cystometry, augments assessment of the functional morphology of the lower urinary tract.[16]

Electrophysiologic Examination

Electrophysiologic tests were not included in the minimum database described in Chapter 1 because they currently are not widely available. In some cases, however, electrophysiologic tests are needed to make a definitive diagnosis.

The cystometrogram (CMG) measures intravesical pressure during a detrusor reflex (Figure 3-4).[16-20] A sustained detrusor reflex is difficult to document clinically in most cases. Additionally, the CMG provides data on threshold volume and pressure, capacity, ability of the bladder to fill at a normal pressure (a measure of elasticity of the bladder wall), and presence of uninhibited bladder contractions (a sign of denervation). Normal data from the CMG of the dog and horse are presented in Table 3-4.

Simultaneous measurement of the CMG and urinary flow allows more complete assessment of the function of the bladder and urethra, especially in disorders of coordination of bladder contraction and urethral relaxation.[21,22] An electromagnetic flow transducer records the flow of urine collected in a funnel. Intravesical pressure is measured simultaneously. The major disadvantage of this technique is the necessity of placing two catheters through the abdominal wall into the bladder. Normal dogs have minimal problems, but we have had leakage from cystocentesis with 22-gauge needles in animals with neurogenic bladders. This procedure must therefore be used with caution.[23]

Electromyography (EMG) of the skeletal muscles of the anal and urethral sphincters and other muscles in the pelvic diaphragm provides direct

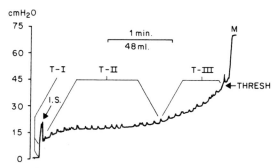

Figure 3-4 Cystometrogram of a dog showing segments of the tonus limb. *T-I*, Resting pressure; *T-II*, bladder filling pressure change (smooth muscle elasticity); *T-III*, bladder filling pressure change after capacity is reached. Scale indicates time and volume. *THRESH*, Threshold of detrusor reflex; *M*, maximal contraction; *I.S.*, initial spike, an artifact.

$$\text{T-II} = \frac{(\text{Pressure at inflection} - \text{Resting pressure}) \times 100}{\text{Volume}}$$

(From Oliver JE Jr, Young WO: Air cystometry in dogs under xylazine-induced restraint. *Am J Vet Res* 34:1433, 1973.)

Table 3-4 **Normal Values for Cystometrograms (CMG) Using Xylazine for Restraint***

Measurement	Values of CMG	
	Dog	Horse
Tonus limb I	9.7 ± 4.3	1.9 ± 1.6
Tonus limb II	12.6 ± 12.2	1.0 ± 0.7
Threshold pressure	24.4 ± 10.0	22.0 ± 7.5
Threshold pressure minus tonus limb I	14.4 ± 8.7	14.4 ± 10.6
Threshold volume	206.6 ± 184.4	2,554 ± 1,087
Maximal contraction pressure	77.6 ± 33.8	100.1 ± 5.9

Data from Oliver JE Jr, Young WO: Air cystometry in dogs under xylazine-induced restraint. *Am J Vet Res* 34:1433-1435, 1973; and Clark ES et al: Cystometrography and urethral pressure profiles in healthy horse and pony mares. *Am J Vet Res* 48:552-555, 1987.

*All values are means ± SD and are given in centimeters of H₂O except for threshold volume, which is given in milliliters of air (see Figure 3-4).

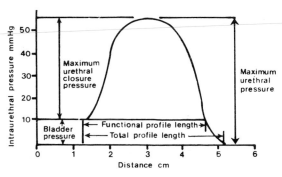

Figure 3-5 Schematic representation of the urethral closure pressure profile. (From Rosin A, Rosin E, Oliver JE Jr: Canine urethral pressure profile. *Am J Vet Res* 41:1113-1116, 1980.)

evidence of the status of innervation. The perineal or bulbocavernosus reflex also can be tested while a recording is being taken directly from these muscles in cases in which clinical evaluation is equivocal.

An EMG recorded from the anal sphincter while the urethra or the bladder is stimulated with a catheter electrode is termed an *electromyelograph* (EMyG).[23] Urethral stimulation evokes a response similar to the bulbocavernosus reflex. Stimulation of the bladder wall evokes a comparable response, except that the sensory pathway is in the pelvic nerves. The evoked bladder response is difficult to record in most animals. An EMyG from bladder stimulation provides evidence of the integrity of the pelvic nerves. The main advantages of the electrical tests are the following: (1) the response is objective, (2) the response can be measured accurately, and (3) the latencies are recorded that provide information about partial denervation.

The urethral pressure profile measures the pressure along the length of the urethra.[19,20,24-26] An EMG of the striated urethral sphincter can be recorded simultaneously. The maximum urethral closure pressure and the functional profile length are the most important parameters (Figure 3-5). Normal values are listed in Table 3-5.

Averaged somatosensory-evoked responses can be recorded from the scalp (cortex) or the spinal cord during stimulation of the bladder or the urethra (see the section on the somatosensory-evoked response in Chapter 4). The cortical-evoked response is a method of evaluating the sensory

pathways. Results of these tests are useful for lesion localization. Table 3-6 summarizes data provided by physical examination findings and electrophysiologic tests.

The final diagnosis should include (1) location of the lesion in the nervous system, (2) cause of the lesion, (3) functional central nervous system (CNS) deficit, and (4) functional deficit related to micturition.

Treatment

Management of a case depends on the final diagnosis. The treatment of primary CNS disease is described throughout this text. Functional deficits of micturition secondary to CNS disease may be temporary or permanent, depending on the reversibility of the CNS lesion and the maintenance of the integrity of the urinary system. If the bladder is severely infected and secondary fibrosis of the bladder wall occurs, normal function cannot be restored even if the CNS lesion is corrected. This section presents management of the urinary tract based on the functional disorder of micturition. Table 3-7 lists the most common drugs used in the pharmacologic management of disorders of micturition.

Medical therapy includes control of the urinary tract infection and management of the functional abnormality of the bladder and urethra. Treatment of urinary tract infections is described in detail in most general veterinary medical books.

Detrusor Areflexia with Sphincter Hypertonus

Lesions from the pons to the L7 spinal cord segments may abolish the detrusor reflex and may produce a UMN-type sphincter characterized by hyperreflexia and increased tone (see Table 3-2). The animal is unable to void, and the bladder is difficult if not impossible to express manually.

The primary consideration in all neurogenic bladder disorders is to evacuate the bladder

Table 3-5   **Normal Values for Urethral Pressure Profiles***

Study Animal (Condition)	Maximal Urethral Pressure (cm H$_2$O)	Maximal Urethral Closure Pressure (cm H$_2$O)	Functional (cm) Profile Length
Female dogs (xylazine)	35.2 ± 16.2	31.0 ± 15.3	7.2 ± 1.9
Male dogs (xylazine)	42.5 ± 5.3	36.79 ± 5.2	28.3 ± 3.9
Female dogs (no sedation)	90.18 ± 4.48	79.72 ± 4.61	8.68 ± 0.57
Male dogs (no sedation)	109.77 ± 11.52	99.77 ± 11.71	24.00 ± 0.9
Female cats, intact (xylazine)	76.6 ± 26.7	71.4 ± 25	4.4 ± 1.5
Female cats, ovariohysterectomized (xylazine)	81.3 ± 31.7	77.5 ± 31.3	5.78 ± 0.9
Male cats (xylazine)	163.2 ± 47.5	161.6 ± 47.1	10.53 ± 0.5
Female horse (xylazine)		43.4 ± 21.6	3.7 ± 1.4
Female horse (no sedation)		49.1 ± 19.4	5.0 ± 1.8

Data sources: Female and male dogs (xylazine)—Rosin A, Rosin E, Oliver JE Jr: Canine urethral pressure profile. *Am J Vet Res* 41:1113-1116, 1980 (values converted from mm Hg). Female and male dogs, no sedation—Richter KP, Ling GV: Effects of xylazine on the urethral pressure profile of healthy dogs. *Am J Vet Res* 46:1881-1886, 1985. Female cats, intact versus ovariohysterectomized (xylazine)—Gregory CR, Willits NH: Electromyographic and urethral pressure evaluations: assessment of urethral function in female and ovariohysterectomized female cats. *Am J Vet Res* 47:1472-1475, 1986. Male cats (xylazine)—Gregory CR et al: Electromyographic and urethral pressure profilometry: assessment of urethral function before and after perineal urethrostomy in cats. *Am J Vet Res* 45:2062-2065, 1984. Female horse, xylazine or no sedation—Clark ES et al: Cystometrography and urethral pressure profiles in healthy horse and pony mares. *Am J Vet Res* 48:552-555, 1987.
*Values are means ± SD.

completely at least three times daily. When tone in the urethra is exaggerated, manual expression is not only ineffective but also dangerous. Aseptic catheterization is required. Indwelling catheters are associated with a high risk of infection, and their use should be avoided if possible. Female dogs become infected even with closed systems using Foley catheters. Detrusor areflexia from overdistention (described later) requires an indwelling catheter.

Urethral tone may be reduced pharmacologically, making management easier. Phenoxybenzamine, an alpha-adrenergic blocking agent, is sometimes effective in a dosage of 0.5 mg per kilogram of body weight daily divided into two doses (small animals). Hypotension is the most common side effect. Diazepam is used for relaxation of the striated sphincter. Bethanechol, a cholinergic agent, can be given to stimulate bladder contraction. We have not found it effective if the bladder is areflexic, however. If bladder contractions are present but are inadequate for good voiding, bethanechol in doses of 2.5 to 10 mg given subcutaneously three times daily may be beneficial. Side effects include increased motility of the gastrointestinal tract. Oral doses of up to 50 mg also may be

Table 3-6   **Diagnostic Tests of Micturition**

Test	Detrusor Reflex	Detrusor Tone and Capacity	Complete Voiding	Sensation to Bladder	Urethral Resistance/ Obstruction	Synchrony of Bladder and Urethra
Cystometrogram	+	+		+		
Urethral pressure profile					+	
Flow	+	+			+	+
Evoked potentials				+		
Observation of voiding	+	+	+	+		+
Palpate bladder		+				
Measure residual urine			+			
Resistance to expression and catheterization					+	

+, Test evaluates this function or this anatomic component.

Table 3-7 **Drugs Used in Treating Disorders of Micturition**

Drug Action	Drug	Dosage	Side Effects
Increase detrusor contractility	Bethanechol (Urecholine)	2.5-15 mg PO q8h (dog) 1.25-5 mg PO q8h (cat)	Cholinergic: GI hypermotility, hypotension
Decrease detrusor contractility	Propantheline (Pro-Banthine)	0.25-0.5 mg/kg PO q8-12h	Anticholinergic: decreased GI motility, decreased salivation, tachycardia
	Oxybutynin (Ditropan)	0.5 mg PO q8-12h	
Increase urethral resistance	Phenylpropanolamine	1.5 mg/kg PO q8-12h (dog and cat)	Sympathomimetic: Urine retention, hypertension
	Diethylstilbestrol (in female)	0.1-1.0 mg/day PO for 3-5 days, then 1 mg/wk (dog)	Estrus, bone marrow toxicity
	Testosterone cypionate (male)	2 mg/kg IM at intervals of weeks to months	Caution in animals with prostatic hyperplasia, perineal hernia, perianal adenoma
Decrease urethral resistance	Phenoxybenzamine (Dibenzyline)	0.25-0.5 mg/kg PO q12h	Sympatholytic: hypotension
	Diazepam (Valium)	0.2 mg/kg PO q8h	Tranquilizer and skeletal muscle relaxant: sedation
	Baclofen (Lioresal)	1-2 mg/kg PO q8h (dog)	Skeletal muscle relaxant: weakness

Modified from Oliver JE, Hoerlein BF, Mayhew IG: *Veterinary neurology.* Philadelphia, 1987, WB Saunders.
GI, gastrointestinal; PO, orally; q8h, every 8 hours.

effective. The combination of bethanechol and phenoxybenzamine may be necessary to reduce urethral resistance.[11,27,28]

Urinalysis is performed weekly or anytime the urine appears abnormal. At the first sign of infection, urine is obtained for quantitative culture and sensitivity tests.[16] Appropriate antibiotic therapy should be continued until the urinalysis verifies correction of the problem. Animals receiving antiinflammatory drugs such as corticosteroids are at increased risk of urinary tract infection. In addition, corticosteroids can suppress the inflammatory response to infection. Asymptomatic infection may go undetected unless urine is cultured repeatedly for microorganisms.

If the detrusor reflex returns with good voiding of urine, the bladder is catheterized periodically to ensure that no residual urine is present. Voiding is often incomplete in the early stages, and residual urine in quantities of 10 to 20 ml or more can result in a urinary tract infection.

Detrusor Areflexia with Normal Sphincter Tone

Some lesions of the spinal cord and brainstem may abolish the detrusor reflex without producing hypertonus of the urethral sphincter. The bladder can be expressed manually in many of these cases. The urethra of the female dog is short and has less resistance than observed with male dogs. Manual expression may be effective even in the context of sphincter hypertonus. Manual expression, if adequate, is less likely to produce infection than is repeated catheterization. Other aspects of management are the same as when sphincter tone is increased.

Detrusor Areflexia with Sphincter Areflexia

Lesions of the sacral spinal cord or nerve roots produce a deficit of LMN of both bladder and sphincter. Management of the bladder is the same as that described previously.

Constant leakage of urine through an incompetent sphincter leads to soiling of the skin, irritation, and ulceration. Frequent evacuation of the bladder reduces the problem but does not eliminate it. Frequent hydrotherapy and protective emollients are useful adjuncts.

Long-term management of the patient with paralysis of the sphincter is problematic. Surgical reconstruction of the bladder neck and the urethra is sometimes successful. Prosthetic urethral sphincters have been successfully used in people, but the cost of these devices currently limits their applicability in animals.

Detrusor Areflexia from Overdistention

Severe overdistention of the bladder can separate the tight junctions between the detrusor muscle fibers, which prevents excitation–contraction coupling. Neural elements may be normal.

Complete evacuation of the bladder must be accomplished early and maintained for 1 to 2 weeks. Manual expression is not recommended because of the increased stress on the detrusor muscle. Intermittent aseptic catheterization can be performed at least three times a day, but to prevent iatrogenic urinary tract infection, closed-system indwelling catheterization is recommended. The system should be used for several days, followed by intermittent catheterization, if needed. Function should return in 1 to 2 weeks. Bethanechol may be of benefit, especially if partial contractions are present.

Antibiotics or urinary antiseptics are administered throughout the treatment period. Frequent urinalysis, with cultures when indicated, is mandatory. Infection in the overdistended bladder leads to fibrosis of the detrusor muscle, and adequate function cannot be restored in this case.

Detrusor Hyperreflexia

Frequent voiding of small volumes of urine, often without much warning and with little or no residual urine, is characteristic of detrusor hyperreflexia.[29] Partial long-tract lesions or abnormalities of the cerebellum may produce these signs. The condition is not usually detrimental to the patient, but it may be an early sign of a progressive disease of the nervous system. Additionally, it is socially unacceptable in the house pet. The condition must be differentiated from the small, contracted, irritable bladder associated with chronic cystitis.

Anticholinergic medication may be of benefit. Propantheline (Pro-Banthine) is used in dosages of 0.25 to 0.5 mg per kilogram of body weight every 8 to 12 hours. The lowest dose should be tried first, and the dose should be increased in small increments until a response is obtained. Oxybutynin may be more effective than propantheline in some cases. Overdosage may result in urine retention in addition to the other side effects characteristic of this group of drugs.[29]

Reflex Dyssynergia

Initiation of a detrusor reflex with voiding followed by an uncontrolled reflex contraction of the urethral sphincter is termed *reflex dyssynergia*. Partial lesions of the long tracts are presumed to be responsible, although the condition has been seen in a dog with a cauda equina lesion.[14]

The problem may be related to uninhibited reflexes of the external urethral sphincter (skeletal muscle) or to increased tone in the smooth muscle related to adrenergic innervation. Limited reports in humans and dogs have not yet provided a definitive therapeutic regimen. Skeletal muscle

reflexes may be reduced with diazepam or dantrolene. Sympathetic (adrenergic) activity can be reduced with an alpha-blocking agent such as phenoxybenzamine.

Normal Detrusor Reflex with Decreased Sphincter Tone

If hormone therapy is ineffective in an animal with normal voiding but leakage, an alpha-adrenergic stimulating drug, such as phenylpropanolamine, may be effective. The dosage is 1.5 mg per kilogram of body weight administered orally every 8 to 12 hours. Side effects include restlessness and irritability. Surgical management may be of benefit.[15]

Case Histories

For the following cases, the reader should concentrate on the problem related to micturition, even though it may be only a part of the total deficit. Using Table 3-2, decide the location of the lesion causing the problem.

CASE HISTORY 3A

Signalment
Canine, dachshund, male, 5 years old.

History
The dog became paralyzed in the pelvic limbs last night. The dog was alone in a fenced-in backyard when the owners found him.

Physical Examination
The bladder is large and easily palpated. It cannot be expressed, even with considerable pressure. The dog makes no attempt to initiate urination.

Neurologic Examination
The dog is alert and paraplegic. The postural reactions are normal in the thoracic limbs and absent in the pelvic limbs. The spinal reflexes are normal in the thoracic limbs. In the pelvic limbs the quadriceps reflexes are exaggerated (+3) bilaterally, and the flexion reflexes are normal (+2). The perineal and bulbocavernosus reflexes are present. The anal sphincter has good tone. Hyperesthesia is evident on palpation of the T13-L2 area. The panniculus reflex is absent caudal to L1. Deep pain sensation is present in the pelvic limbs.

CASE HISTORY 3B

Signalment
Canine, pekingese, female, 6 years old.

History
The dog suddenly became paralyzed in the pelvic limbs while playing with the owners' children. When first seen by the referring veterinarian 4 hours later, the dog was paraplegic with increased muscle tone in the pelvic limbs, had exaggerated quadriceps reflexes but decreased flexion reflexes bilaterally, and no sensation caudal to L4 vertebra. The dog was referred to you.

Physical Examination
The dog is seen 12 hours after the onset of paralysis. Urine has leaked during the trip to the clinic, and the dog is

obviously in pain. The bladder is large and is easily expressed on palpation.

Neurologic Examination

The dog is alert and anxious. The thoracic limbs are normal. The postural reactions and the spinal reflexes are absent in the pelvic limbs. The perineal reflex is absent, and the anal sphincter is dilated. No sensation exists caudal to T13.

CASE HISTORY 3C

Signalment

Canine, chihuahua, male, 3 years old.

History

The dog has had generalized seizures at least three times in the past 2 weeks. The previous medical history is noncontributory. The dog started urinating in the house within the past 3 months, although he was well house-trained since a puppy. The dog has not been taking medication.

Physical Examination

The skull is dome shaped, and the fontanelle is 1.5 cm in diameter. The bladder is empty.

Neurologic Examination

The postural reactions are judged to be a bit slow, but the rest of the examination is normal.

ASSESSMENT 3A

The neurologic examination indicates a UMN paralysis of the pelvic limbs. The sensory examination localizes the lesion to T13-L2. The bladder problem can be characterized as detrusor areflexia with sphincter hypertonia, which is typical of a lesion cranial to L7. Cystometry confirms detrusor areflexia. Management of the bladder should include a closed indwelling urinary catheter system. The dog has a herniated intervertebral disk, which is decompressed by hemilaminectomy. Seven days after surgery, voluntary movements of the pelvic limbs are seen, and voiding begins with minimal pressure of the abdomen. Voiding returns to normal in 10 days.

ASSESSMENT 3B

The dog has LMN paralysis of the pelvic limbs and the sphincters. This finding indicates a lesion from L4 through S3. Initially the lesion spared the L4-6 segments because the quadriceps reflex was intact and extension of the limb occurred. The loss of sensation has progressed from L4 to T13 in 8 hours, and the quadriceps reflex has disappeared, indicating a progressive lesion. Detrusor areflexia and sphincter areflexia are present, consistent with a lesion of the sacral segments of the spinal cord. The dog has a herniated disk with hemorrhagic myelomalacia (see Chapter 6). The prognosis is so poor that no other tests are performed. Cystometry would confirm the detrusor areflexia. The urethral pressure profile would be expected to show pressures below normal. EMG would demonstrate no voluntary or reflex activity, but fibrillation potentials would not be present this early. If management were attempted, manual evacuation of the bladder probably would be effective.

ASSESSMENT 3C

The seizures indicate abnormality of the cerebrum or diencephalon or a metabolic problem. The change in urinary habits also could be either cerebral or metabolic (polyuria). A laboratory evaluation is indicated to rule out metabolic diseases. The evaluation was performed, and all tests were normal.

Rule-outs
1. Hydrocephalus
2. Encephalitis
3. Tumor (unlikely)
4. Idiopathic epilepsy

The cystometrogram was normal and showed adequate capacity and a good detrusor reflex. An electroencephalogram showed high-voltage slow waves in all leads. This finding is typical of hydrocephalus. Computed tomography confirmed the diagnosis. The dog was treated with corticosteroids, and complete remission of the signs resulted (see Chapter 12 for a discussion of hydrocephalus). The voiding behavior was related to cerebral dysfunction.

References

1. Oliver JE, Selcer RR: Neurogenic causes of abnormal micturition in the dog and cat. *Vet Clin North Am* 4:517-524, 1974.
2. Purinton PT, Oliver JE: Spinal cord origin of innervation to the bladder and urethra of the dog. *Exp Neurol* 65:422-434, 1979.
3. Oliver JE Jr, Bradley WE, Fletcher TF: Spinal cord representation of the micturition reflex. *J Comp Neurol* 137:329-346, 1969.
4. Gjone R, Setekleiv J: Excitatory and inhibitory bladder responses to stimulation of the cerebral cortex in the cat. *Acta Physiol Scand* 59:337-348, 1963.
5. Langworthy OR, Hesser FH: An experimental study of micturition released from cerebral control. *Am J Physiol* 115:694-700, 1936.
6. Bradley WE, Teague CT: Cerebellar influence on the micturition reflex. *Exp Neurol* 23:399-411, 1969.
7. Oliver JE, Bradley WE, Fletcher TF: Spinal cord distribution of the somatic innervation of the external urethral sphincter in the cat. *J Neurol Sci* 10:11-23, 1970.
8. Oliver JE: Disorders of micturition. In Hoerlein BF, editor: *Canine neurology*, 3rd ed. Philadelphia, 1978, WB Saunders, pp 461-469.
9. Moreau PM: Neurogenic disorders of micturition in the dog and cat. *Compend Cont Educ Pract Vet* 4:12-22, 1982.
10. O'Brien D: Neurogenic disorders of micturition. *Vet Clin North Am* 18:529-544, 1988.
11. O'Brien D: Disorders of the urogenital system. *Semin Vet Med Surg* 5:57-66, 1990.
12. Purinton PT, Oliver JE, Bradley WE: Differences in routing of pelvic visceral afferent fibers in the dog and cat. *Exp Neurol* 73:725-731, 1981.
13. DeGroat WC: Nervous control of the urinary bladder of the cat. *Brain Res* 87:201-211, 1975.
14. Oliver JE: Dysuria caused by reflex dyssynergia. In Kirk RW, editor: *Current veterinary therapy, VIII*. Philadelphia, 1983, WB Saunders, p 1088.
15. Holt PE: Urinary incontinence in the bitch due to sphincter mechanism incompetence: prevalence in referred dogs and retrospective analysis of sixty cases. *J Small Anim Pract* 26:181-190, 1985.
16. Barsanti JA: Diagnostic procedures in urology. *Vet Clin North Am* 14:3-14, 1984.
17. Oliver JE, Young WO: Air cystometry in dog under xylazine-induced restraint. *Am J Vet Res* 34:1433-1435, 1973.

18. Johnson CA, Beemsterboer JM, Gray PR, et al: Effects of various sedatives on air cystometry in dogs. *Am J Vet Res* 49:1525-1528, 1988.

19. Barsanti J, Finco D, Brown J: Effect of atropine on cystometry and urethral pressure profilometry in the dog. *Am J Vet Res* 49:112-114, 1988.

20. Clark E, Semrad S, Bichsel P, et al: Cystometrography and urethral pressure profiles in healthy horse and pony mares. *Am J Vet Res* 48:552-555, 1987.

21. Moreau PM, Lees GE, Gross DR: Simultaneous cystometry and uroflowmetry (micturition study) for evaluation of the caudal part of the urinary tract in dogs: studies of the technique. *Am J Vet Res* 44:1769-1773, 1983.

22. Moreau PM, Lees GE, Gross DR: Simultaneous cystometry and uroflowmetry (micturition study) for evaluation of the caudal part of the urinary tract in dogs: reference values for healthy animals sedated with xylazine. *Am J Vet Res* 44:1774-1781, 1983.

23. Oliver JE: Urodynamic assessment. In Oliver JE, Hoerlein BF, Mayhew IG, editors: *Veterinary neurology*. Philadelphia, 1987, WB Saunders, pp 180-184.

24. Kay AD, Lavoie J-P: Urethral pressure profilometry in mares. *J Am Vet Med Assoc* 191:212-216, 1987.

25. Gregory C, Willits N: Electromyographic and urethral pressure evaluations: assessment of urethral function in female and ovariohysterectomized female cats. *Am J Vet Res* 47:1472-1475, 1986.

26. Richter KP, Ling GV: Effects of xylazine on the urethral pressure profile of healthy dogs. *Am J Vet Res* 46:1881-1886, 1985.

27. Moreau PM, Lappin MR: Pharmacologic management of urinary incontinence. In Kirk RW, editor: *Current veterinary therapy, X: small animal practice*. Philadelphia, 1989, WB Saunders, pp 1214-1222.

28. Moreau PM: Management of micturition disorders in the dog and cat. In *Proceedings of the Eighth Annual Veterinary Medical Forum*. Washington, DC, 1990, American College of Veterinary Internal Medicine, pp 369-374.

29. Lappin MR, Barsanti JA: Urinary incontinence secondary to idiopathic detrusor instability: cystometrographic diagnosis and pharmacologic management in two dogs and a cat. *J Am Vet Med Assoc* 191:1439-1442, 1987.

Chapter
4

Confirming a Diagnosis

After the history has been taken and the physical and neurologic examinations have been completed, a list of problems is made. For each problem, an initial plan is formulated that contains a list of the most likely diseases, which are ruled in or out by appropriate diagnostic tests. Chapters 1 through 3 provide the information necessary for identifying neurologic problems and for making an anatomic diagnosis. Chapters 5 through 15 elaborate on each problem in terms of arriving at a differential diagnosis through appropriate diagnostic tests. This chapter discusses the tests available; indicates the feasibility of performing them; suggests references for further reading on techniques and interpretation; and outlines the indications, contraindications, and limitations of the tests. The most useful tests for each major category of disease are listed in Table 4-1.

CLINICAL LABORATORY STUDIES
Hematology, Blood Chemistry Analysis, and Urinalysis
Availability

All clinical practices have access to routine hematology studies, chemistry analysis, and urinalysis.

Indications

A laboratory database is required for all sick animals so that common diseases are not overlooked and the general status of the animal can be assessed. Clinical laboratory studies are especially important in evaluating animals with brain disorders, seizures, signs of multisystem disease, and where general anesthesia is required for diagnostic procedures or surgery.

Cerebrospinal Fluid Analysis
Availability

Cerebrospinal fluid (CSF) analysis can be performed in any practice. The CSF sample is collected routinely by cerebellomedullary cisternal puncture. CSF can also be obtained, with somewhat greater difficulty, from the lumbar cistern at L5-6 or L6-7 in dogs and at the lumbosacral interspace in cats and large animals.[1,2] The examiner should perform the procedures often enough to maintain confidence and accuracy. Lumbar CSF is more likely to provide positive information in animals with thoracolumbar spinal cord disease.[3]

To avoid movement of the animal during needle placement, CSF is collected using general anesthesia in dogs and cats. In food animals and horses, lumbar puncture can be accomplished with sedation and the animal standing. The hair is clipped and the skin is prepared for an aseptic procedure. The needle (a 22-gauge, 1.5-inch disposable spinal needle with a stylet for most small animals; a 20-gauge, 3.5-inch needle for most large animals) should be handled with sterile gloves. For cerebellomedullary puncture, the landmarks for the midline are the occipital protuberance and the spinous process of the axis (C2) (Figure 4-1). The needle is inserted on the midline near the cranial border of the wings of the atlas (C1). A slight loss of resistance is felt as the needle penetrates the dorsal atlantooccipital membrane and enters the subarachnoid space. The stylet is withdrawn, and fluid is allowed to flow from the hub of the needle into sterile tubes. The CSF sample should be divided into three aliquots collected in separate tubes. The initial collection may contain red blood cells (RBCs) from trauma, but subsequent collections may be devoid of this contamination. In horses, three or four 2-ml samples should be collected in separate tubes and analyzed. Total protein concentration and red cell contamination are significantly lower in samples 2, 3, and 4, and sample 1 may not be suitable for serologic or cytologic examinations.[4]

The syringe is not attached to the needle because aspiration is likely to worsen hemorrhage. If CSF pressure is to be measured, a three-way valve is attached before any fluid is collected.[5] Fluid is allowed to rise in a spinal manometer attached to the valve. The reading is taken at the

Table 4-1 **Selection of Diagnostic Tests**

Site	Disease Category	Diagnostic Tests	
		Useful	*Usually Diagnostic*
Brain	Degenerative	EEG, CSF	Biopsy
	Anomalous	Examination	Radiography
	Neoplastic	EEG, radiography	CT or MR imaging
Spinal cord	Degenerative	Myelography, CSF	None
	Anomalous	Radiography	Myelography
	Neoplastic	CSF, radiography	Myelography
Vertebrae	Degenerative	CSF	Radiography, myelography
	Anomalous	Examination	Radiography
	Neoplastic	CSF	Radiography, myelography
	Inflammation	CSF	Radiography, myelography
Peripheral nerve, muscle	Demyelinating	EMG, EDT	Biopsy
	Inflammation	EMG, EDT, CK	Biopsy
	Neoplastic	EMG, EDT	Biopsy
	Traumatic	EMG, EDT	Biopsy
	Toxic	EMG, EDT	Biopsy
Systemic or any site	Metabolic	History	Clinical laboratory profile
	Nutritional	History	Radiography
	Inflammation	History, examination	CSF, serology
	Traumatic	History, examination	Radiography
	Toxic	History	Clinical laboratory profile

EEG, Electroencephalography; *CSF,* cerebrospinal fluid; *CT,* computed tomography; *MR,* magnetic resonance; *EMG,* electromyography; *EDT,* electrodiagnostic testing; *CK,* creatine kinase.

bottom of the meniscus. Pulsations of the fluid indicate that the needle is patent. Increased CSF pressure occurs nonspecifically with a variety of CNS diseases. Because of this lack of specificity and the fact that additional manipulation of the needle increases the frequency of blood contamination, we rarely measure CSF pressure.

Total and differential white blood cell (WBC) counts are the most important parts of a CSF analysis. Unless a preservative is added, cell counts must be determined within 30 minutes of collection because WBCs deteriorate rapidly. Total cell counts can be done with a hemacytometer. Several methods exist for determining the differential count, including sedimentation and centrifugation techniques that can be done in practice. Techniques for RBC and WBC counts and differentials are described in the references.[2,6,7] Techniques for using a preservative and a filtration method of obtaining cell counts have been described by Roszel.[8] Not all laboratories are prepared to use this method. The addition of cell-free autologous serum protects cellular morphology for up to 48 hours when samples are stored at 4° C.[9] To make an 11% serum concentration, 30 µl of serum is added to 250 µl of CSF. The disadvantage of this technique is that undiluted CSF must be submitted for protein determination. Referral institutions may also perform electron microscopy on the sample to identify microorganisms.

The examiner should observe the appearance of the CSF. Hemorrhage caused by the puncture produces a red tinge to the fluid that decreases as the fluid continues to flow. WBC counts may be corrected for hemorrhage by subtracting approximately 1 WBC for each 500 RBCs; however, the validity of correction formulas has been questioned.[10] High CSF nucleated cell counts and protein concentrations correlate with the presence of neurologic disease, even when samples contain moderate amounts of blood contamination.[11] Centrifugation should leave a clear, colorless fluid. A yellowish tinge to the CSF is called *xanthochromia* and is caused by free bilirubin. Previous subarachnoid hemorrhage is the usual cause, although prolonged icterus can produce xanthochromia. Turbidity is caused by an increase in the cell content of the fluid to more than 500 cells/mm^3. Shaking the sample produces foam if the protein content is markedly elevated. Fibrin clots may be seen if the elevated protein includes fibrinogen.

Measurement of CSF protein levels is necessary for a complete examination. Simple qualitative studies such as the Pandy test are adequate, although quantitative methods are preferred. The Pandy test can be performed in the practice; it qualitatively estimates globulin concentrations. Quantitative analysis also can be done in the practice, or the sample can be sent to a reference laboratory. Electrophoresis is used

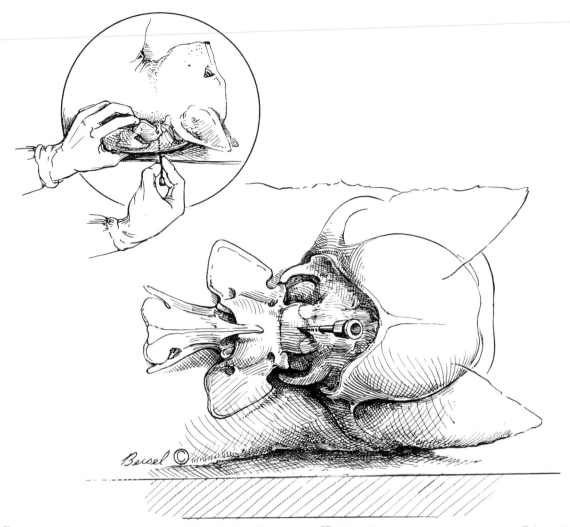

Figure 4-1 Landmarks for cerebrospinal fluid collection. (From Greene CE, Oliver JE Jr: Neurologic examination. In Ettinger SJ, editor. *Textbook of veterinary internal medicine,* 2nd ed. Philadelphia, 1982, WB Saunders.)

to determine quantitatively the levels of protein fractions or immunoglobulins in CSF. Increased albumin indicates a disturbance of the blood-brain barrier, whereas significant increased immunoglobulin indicates synthesis intrathecally.[12-16]

Other chemical values, including glucose, creatine kinase (CK), and lactic dehydrogenase (LDH), may be determined. The quantities of CSF necessary for these tests are difficult to obtain from small animals, and the usefulness of these studies has not been demonstrated clearly.[17-20] CSF glucose levels may be decreased in bacterial infections, but the increase in cells and protein is more significant. Increased CK concentrations do not provide useful diagnostic information. Concentrations of LDH reportedly increase with CNS lymphosarcoma.

If bacterial infection is strongly suspected based on clinical findings or if neutrophils are increased in the CSF, culture and sensitivity testing should be done. Fluid should be obtained in two sterile syringes, one for laboratory analysis and one for culture.

Titers to agents such as viruses,[21,22] fungi,[23] and protozoa[24,25] also may be indicated when encephalitis is suspected. The CSF titer is compared with the serum titer because serum antibodies may cross the blood-brain barrier in inflammatory diseases. Indirect fluorescent antibody testing for canine distemper virus may be positive in 60% to 82% of dogs with noninflammatory and inflammatory distemper, respectively.[26]

Indications

Increased WBC counts and protein levels are expected with active CNS inflammatory diseases and in any disease process that disrupts the blood-brain barrier. In general, the WBCs are predominantly polymorphonuclear leukocytes in bacterial diseases and predominantly lymphocytes in viral diseases. Fungal and protozoal diseases may produce mixed populations of leukocytes. An eosinophilic pleocytosis is found in some protozoal, parasitic, or idiopathic diseases such as granulomatous or eosinophilic meningoencephalomyelitis.[27,28] Mixed populations of neutrophils, lymphocytes, and monocytes (pyogranulomatous pleocytosis) are characteristic of granulomatous meningoencephalomyelitis of dogs and the neurologic form of feline infectious peritonitis. The CSF may be completely normal in animals with inflammatory diseases.[22,24,26]

Primary degenerative or demyelinating diseases, neoplasia, infarction, or CNS compression may produce an increase in CSF protein with little or no increase in cells (*albuminocytologic dissociation*) (Table 4-2).

Free blood or xanthochromia may be seen after subarachnoid hemorrhage. Hemorrhage may be caused by trauma, primary vascular disease, or vascular lesions secondary to inflammation or neoplasia. Blood contamination may also occur at the time of CSF collection.

Contraindications

The animal should be anesthetized when CSF is collected; therefore, if anesthesia is contraindicated, CSF should not be obtained. When the animal is positioned for cerebellomedullary cisternal puncture, the anesthetist should be certain that the airway is patent and pulmonary ventilation is adequate.

Cerebrospinal fluid should not be collected if increased intracranial pressure is suspected. Removal of CSF from the cerebellomedullary or lumbar cistern causes a pressure gradient, and the cerebrum or cerebellum may be displaced caudally. Herniation of the cerebellum through the foramen magnum may lead to apnea and death because of compression of the medullary respiratory centers or pathways (see Chapter 12). The temporal cortex may herniate through the tentorial notch and compress the midbrain, with resultant pupillary dilation. Either foramen magnum or transtentorial herniation may also lead to tetraplegia and stupor or coma because of involvement of the descending pathways and the reticular activating system, respectively. Increased pressure from generalized brain inflammation, tumors, large abscesses, or intracranial trauma also predisposes the animal to brain herniation. The information obtained from the CSF analysis may not be worth the risk to the animal in these cases. Pressure shifts may occur with either cerebellomedullary or lumbar puncture. Herniation of the cerebellum, however, compromises the cerebellomedullary cistern. For this reason, if CSF

aspiration is deemed necessary in animals with the potential for herniation, we prefer the lumbar site. Steps should be taken to reduce CSF pressure before collecting fluid (see Chapter 12).

Radiography

Radiography is the most frequently employed and the most helpful diagnostic tool in neurology (Table 4-3).

Availability

Most veterinary practices have radiographic capabilities adequate for the formulation of a neurologic diagnosis in small animals. Before taking radiographs, the neurologic examination should be reviewed so that the underlying lesions can be accurately localized. Special attention is given to these areas during the radiographic examination. Meticulous technique is essential to detection of subtle changes that are often the key to a diagnosis.[30] Proper positioning of the animal and correct film exposure and development are imperative. Beyond these parameters, the only limitation is the interpretive skill of the veterinarian. Interpretive skill is developed through practice.

An approach to the interpretation of radiographs is as follows:

1. Scan the entire radiograph for quality of exposure, positioning, and the presence of artifacts or motion. Recognize the limitations imposed by these factors.
2. Scan the structures on the radiograph that are not of primary interest, such as the soft tissue, abdomen, and chest.
3. Systematically evaluate the area of primary interest.

Vertebral Column and Spinal Cord

1. Scan the entire vertebral column for contour: the ventral surface of the vertebral bodies, the floor of the vertebral canal, and the lamina, articulations, and spinous processes (Table 4-4).
2. Scan the entire vertebral column for changes in bone density, such as lytic or proliferative changes (see Table 4-4).
3. Scan the vertebral canal for changes in density, especially at the intervertebral foramina and the disk spaces.
4. Compare the size of adjacent intervertebral disk spaces and foramina and the joint spaces of facets. A narrowing of one or more of these spaces is suggestive of disk herniation.
5. Stand back and scan the vertebral column again. Changes in contour or spacing are sometimes more apparent from a distance.

Table 4-2 Cerebrospinal Fluid

Disease	Appearance	Pressure (mm H₂o)	White Blood Cells* per mm³	Cell Type	Protein (mg/dl)	Other
Normal dog	Clear	<140	<5	Mononuclear	<25†	Glucose: 60%–70% of blood glucose
Normal cat	Clear	<100	<5	Mononuclear	<25	Same as dog
Normal horse	Clear	<500	<6	Mononuclear	<100	Same as dog
Normal cow	Clear	<200	<10	Mononuclear	<40	Same as dog
Normal pig	Clear		<30	Mononuclear	<40	Same as dog
Normal sheep	Clear		<10	Mononuclear	<40	Same as dog
Inflammatory						
Bacterial	Clear to turbid	Slight increase	Increased, usually >100	Mostly neutrophils	Increased, usually >100	Glucose decreased
Viral	Clear	Slight increase	Increased, usually <100	Mostly mononuclear‡	Increased, usually <100	Electron microscopy: viral particles
Fungal	Turbid	Increased	Increased, usually >100	Mixed	Increased, usually >100	Organisms may be seen, especially *Cryptococcus*
Protozoal	Clear	Increased	Increased, may be >100	Mononuclear, sometimes neutrophils	Increased, usually >100	
Parasitic	Clear to xanthochromic	Increased	Increased, variable	Mixed, sometimes eosinophils	Increased, usually >100	
Degenerative, including compression	Clear	Normal	Normal to slight increase	Mononuclear	Increased, usually <100	
Neoplastic	Clear	Increased	Normal to increased	Mononuclear	Increased, usually <100	Tumor cells may be seen if tumor adjacent to subarachnoid space; usually contraindicated in suspected brain tumors
Traumatic	Xanthochromic	Increased	Normal to increased	RBCs, WBCs	Increased, variable	Usually contraindicated
Vascular	Xanthochromic	Increased	Normal to Increased	RBCs, WBCs	Increased, variable	

* White blood cell counts may be normal in animals with encephalitis; this is particularly true of some viral and protozoal infections.
† Protein is normally higher in lumbar versus cerebellomedullary CSF and may exceed 25 mg/dL.
‡ Neutrophils may predominate in some viral diseases; e.g., feline infectious peritonitis and eastern equine encephalomyelitis.

Data from Hoerlein BF: *Canine neurology: diagnosis and treatment,* 3rd ed. Philadelphia, WB Saunders, 1978; Kornegay JN: Cerebrospinal fluid collection, examination, and interpretation in dogs and cats. *Compendium Continuing Educ Pract Vet* 3:85–92, 1981; deLahunta A: *Veterinary neuroanatomy and clinical neurology,* 2rd ed. Philadelphia, WB Saunders, 1983; Mayhew IG, Whitlock RH, Tasker JB: Equine cerebrospinal fluid: Reference values of normal horses. *Am J Vet Res* 38:1271–1274, 1977; Simpson ST, Reed RB: Manometric values for normal cerebrospinal fluid pressure in dogs. *J Am Anim Hosp Assoc* 23:629–632, 1987; Bailey CS, Higgins RJ: Comparison of total white blood cell count and total protein content of lumbar and cisternal cerebrospinal fluid of healthy dogs. *Am J Vet Res* 46:1162–1165, 1985.

Table 4-3 **Radiography**

Test	Indications	Possible Usefulness	Contraindications	Availability
Spinal radiography	Degenerative disease (vertebral)	High	Anesthesia usually required	Practice
	Anomaly	High		
	Neoplasia	Moderate		
	Inflammatory disease (vertebral)	High		
	Trauma	High		
Myelography	Degenerative disease	High	Anesthesia required; not done if active inflammation is present or if intracranial pressure is increased	Specialty practice
	Anomaly	High		
	Neoplasia	High		
	Inflammatory disease (vertebral)	Low		
	Trauma	High		
Epidurography (primarily for evaluation of caudal lumbar and sacral area)	Degenerative disease	High	Anesthesia required	Specialty practice
	Anomaly	Variable		
	Neoplasia	High		
	Inflammatory disease (vertebral)	Variable		
	Trauma	Low		
Vertebral sinus venography	Same as those for epidurography	Low	Anesthesia required	Specialty practice
Diskography	L7-S1 disk protrusion	Moderate	Anesthesia required	Specialty practice
Skull radiography	Anomaly	High	Anesthesia required	Practice
	Neoplasia	Low		
	Inflammatory disease (especially otitis media)	Low (except otitis media)		
	Trauma	High		
Ventriculography	Anomaly (hydrocephalus)	High	Anesthesia required	Specialty practice
	Neoplasia	Low		
Ultrasonography	Hydrocephalus, with persistent fontanelles	High	None	Specialty practice
Cavernous sinus venography	Neoplasia (floor of skull)	Moderate	Anesthesia required	Specialty practice
Cranial thecography	Neoplasia (floor of skull)	Moderate	Anesthesia required	Specialty practice
Cerebral arteriography	Neoplasia	Moderate	Anesthesia required	Specialty practice
Radioisotope scans	Neoplasia	Moderate	Anesthesia required	Institutions
Computed tomography and magnetic resonance imaging	Degenerative disease	Moderate	Anesthesia required; expensive	Institutions; local imaging centers
	Anomaly	High		
	Neoplasia	High		
	Trauma	High		

96

Table 4-4 **Radiographic Findings and Interpretation**

Radiographic Change	Possible Causes
Vertebrae Proliferation	*Degenerative:* Spondylosis, dural ossification (linear density in vertebral canal) *Neoplastic:* Primary or metastatic vertebral tumor *Nutritional:* Ankylosing spondylosis, hypervitaminosis A *Inflammatory:* Osteomyelitis involving disk space, diskospondylitis (osteomyelitis usually is proliferative and lytic) *Traumatic:* Healing fracture
Lysis	*Neoplastic:* Primary or metastatic vertebral tumor, widening of vertebral canal (spinal cord tumor), widening of intervertebral foramen (nerve root tumor) *Nutritional:* Generalized loss of density, hypocalcemia, hyperparathyroidism *Inflammatory:* Osteomyelitis involving disk space, diskospondylitis (osteomyelitis usually is proliferative and lytic)
Abnormal shape of vertebrae	*Degenerative:* Cervical instability *Anomalous:* Hemivertebrae, spina bifida, fused vertebrae *Traumatic:* Compression fractures
Displacement	*Degenerative:* Cervical spondylopathy (Wobbler syndrome), lumbosacral spondylopathy, intervertebral disk herniation (narrowing of interspace, foramen, and facet space) *Anomalous:* Hemivertebrae, agenesis of dens (atlantoaxial luxation) *Neoplastic:* Pathologic fractures *Nutritional:* Pathologic fractures *Inflammatory:* Pathologic fractures *Traumatic:* Fractures, luxations
Skull	
Proliferation	*Degenerative:* Hypertrophic osteopathy of the mandible and skull (possibly inflammatory) *Neoplastic:* Primary or metastatic tumor *Inflammatory:* Osteomyelitis, otitis media, otitis interna
Lysis	*Anomalous:* Loss of digital markings, persistent fontanelles or suture lines, loss of osseous tentorium (may be caused by chronic hydrocephalus) *Neoplastic:* Primary or metastatic tumor *Nutritional:* Generalized loss of density, hypocalcemia, hyperparathyroidism *Inflammatory:* Osteomyelitis, otitis media, otitis interna
Abnormal shape	*Anomalous:* Hydrocephalus, rarely otocephaly, hydranencephaly, other cranial malformations *Traumatic:* Fractures
Alterations in shape of foramina	*Anomalous:* Occipital dysplasia, hydrocephalus *Neoplastic:* Tumor of a cranial nerve

Skull

1. Ventrodorsal and frontal (craniocaudal) views are especially useful because the two sides can be compared.
2. Scan the periphery of the calvaria for asymmetry, cracks, deviations, or abnormal shape (see Table 4-4).
3. Compare the nasal passages, the frontal sinuses, and the bullae of the middle ears for similarity in density.
4. Survey the calvaria for changes in density (proliferative or lytic), normal digital impressions, the presence of persistent suture lines or fontanelles, or linear fractures.
5. Evaluate the structures inside the calvaria-osseous tentorium cerebelli, foramina, and petrous temporal bone.

Contrast-enhanced procedures, especially *myelography* (radiographs made after the injection of contrast material into the subarachnoid space), are within the capabilities of most practices. As with most procedures, however, they must be performed often enough that the veterinarian maintains confidence in both technique and interpretation. Table 4-3 lists the special imaging techniques available in specialty practice. Arteriography and ventriculography are rarely performed with the advent of radioisotope brain scans, computed tomography (CT), and magnetic resonance (MRI). Most institutions have one or more of these techniques available.[31-33] Practicing veterinarians often can have CT or MRI done at a local hospital or imaging center. In animals likely to have brain tumors, one of these imaging methods should be performed after the minimum database has been obtained and, ideally, in advance of CSF collection.[33-36]

Indications

Nervous tissue has essentially the same radiographic density as other soft tissues. Radiographs of the head and the vertebral column reveal changes in the skull and the vertebrae. Lesions of nervous tissue such as hemorrhage, tumor, or degeneration are detected only rarely when calcification of the lesion or lytic change in adjacent bone is present. The most common radiographic changes and their causes are listed in Table 4-4. Examples of radiographic changes associated with specific disease processes are included in the discussion of each disease (see Chapters 5 through 15).

Imaging with CT or MR is used to confirm a suspected lesion that cannot be identified definitively on survey radiographs or to identify the extent or location of a lesion more precisely.

Myelography is the most frequently employed contrast-enhanced imaging procedure.[37-41] The development of nonionic, water-soluble contrast media has dramatically reduced the complications of myelography. Iohexol (Omnipaque; 240 mg of iodine per ml, 0.3 to 0.5 ml/kg of body weight) is used most commonly. Injections may be made in either the lumbar area at L5-6 or L6-7 or at the cerebellomedullary cistern. In our experience, compressive lesions are better defined when the contrast medium is injected into the lumbar area. The injection pressure attained there forces the medium past lesions. Medium injected from the cerebellomedullary cistern may be blocked by compressive lesions and may flow cranially into the skull. Seizures are the most common complication of myelography. Factors that predisposed animals to seizures in one study included body weight $\geq$ 29 kg, multiple injections, and injections made at the cerebellomedullary cistern.[41]

Masses that occupy space in the vertebral canal (e.g., tumors, abscesses, disks) cause alterations in the myelographic contrast column. The epidural, intradural-extramedullary, or intramedullary location can be determined by the type of distortion occurring in the contrast column (Figure 4-2).[42] Evaluating both the lateral and ventrodorsal views is critical. As an example, asymmetric extradural lesions cause a pattern typical of intradural-extramedullary masses on lateral radiographs. Similarly, midline extradural lesions appear intramedullary on ventrodorsal radiographs. Focal atrophy causes narrowing of the spinal cord with widening of the contrast column. Severe malacia may allow the contrast media to pool in the cord substance (Figure 4-3). The central canal may be outlined by the contrast medium in some cases, without

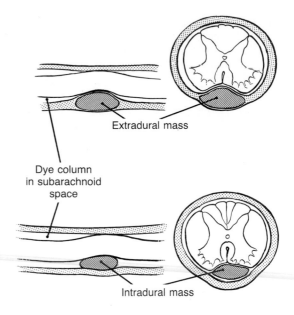

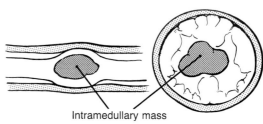

Extradural mass

Dye column in subarachnoid space

Intradural mass

Intramedullary mass

Figure 4-2 Effect of a mass lesion on a myelogram. *Top:* An extradural mass causes thinning or complete obliteration of the contrast column. *Middle:* An intradural-extramedullary mass deviates the spinal cord and obstructs the contrast column. The cranial and caudal borders of the mass may have a cup-shaped outline of contrast material. *Bottom:* An intramedullary mass expands the spinal cord, causing thinning or obliteration of the contrast column on all sides.

apparent clinical consequences, particularly when injections are made cranial to L5 in small dogs.[43]

Myelography for the diagnosis of lumbosacral lesions is limited by the fact that the spinal cord terminates cranial to this site in some dogs. This varies among breeds. In one study, the spinal cord extended further caudally in dachshunds than in German shepherd dogs.[44] *Epidurography* (radiographs made after injection of contrast material into the epidural space of the vertebral canal) is indicated in animals in which the lumbosacral region cannot be defined with myelography.[45-47] The toxic effects of the procedure are minimized with the use of water-soluble contrast agents, and the technique is simple. Considerable experience with normal variations is required for proper interpretation of the radiographs.

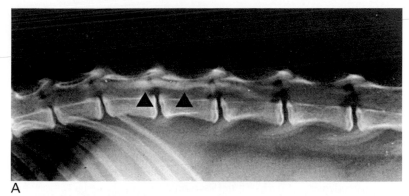

A

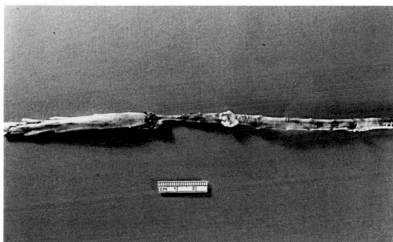

B

Figure 4-3 A, Myelogram of a cat with malacia in the spinal cord caused by an infarct. Note the contrast media pooled in the area of the malacia *(arrowheads).* **B,** Spinal cord showing the area of malacia.

Vertebral sinus venography requires filling the venous sinuses on the floor of the vertebral canal with contrast material. This procedure has limited value, because false-positive results are common.

Diskography involves injection of the contrast medium into the intervertebral disk and has been used primarily to define disk protrusions at L7-S1. In one study, a 20- or 22-gauge spinal needle was passed into the L7-S1 disk space and 0.2 to 0.3 ml of 20% iopamidol was injected.[48] Injection was facilitated considerably by fluoroscopy. Contrast material remained confined to the disk space in normal dogs but outlined the protruded disk in those affected.

Ventriculography is delineation of the cerebral ventricular system with air or a positive contrast agent.[30] Ventriculography can be employed to establish a diagnosis of hydrocephalus; CSF can also be obtained. The needle is placed about midway between the lateral canthus of the eye and the external occipital protuberance, 0.5 to 1.0 cm from the midline, to enter the lateral ventricle.[49] Ultrasonography, CT, and MRI are less invasive and are preferred for a diagnosis of hydrocephalus.

Ultrasonography can be used when the fontanelle is persistent or during either brain or spinal surgery.[50-54] Precise localization of masses is best accomplished using CT or MRI. Ultrasonography, however, can be helpful in delineating lesions at surgery. Masses tend to be hyperechoic and cause shifts in the ventricular system.[53] Hydrocephalus can be diagnosed in dogs with persistent fontanelles.[51,52]

Cavernous sinus venography is relatively simple to perform. Contrast material is injected into the angularis oculi vein.[55] The medium flows through the orbit into the cavernous sinuses on the floor of the cranial vault. Compression or occlusion of the sinus from masses in the area of the pituitary gland can be demonstrated.

Intracranial thecography entails injection of a water-soluble contrast agent into the subarachnoid space of the brain. The head is tilted down, and radiographs are taken in the dorsoventral projection. The floor of the cranial vault is outlined. The pituitary gland, optic nerves, and any mass lesion of this area may be seen. The procedure is safe and within the capability of most practices.[56, 57]

Cerebral arteriography is performed by injecting contrast material into the internal carotid or vertebral arteries.[30] Arteriography is rarely used because CT and MRI are noninvasive and provide more information about mass lesions. Primary arterial disease, a possible indication, is rare in animals.

Computed tomography and *MRI* are preferred for assessment of mass lesions (Figures 4-4 and 4-5).[31-36] CT is a special radiographic technique that generates transverse images. Images are done before and after intravenous injection of contrast medium (iodine, 600 to 900 mg/kg). Lesions identified on precontrast images are either hypodense, isodense, or hyperdense relative to surrounding brain. Greater cellularity, hemorrhage, and mineralization increase brain density. Edema is the main cause of decreased density. Masses change brain density and shift brain structures. Contrast medium is excluded from the normal brain by the blood-brain barrier but accumulates in most tumors. Myelography may be combined with CT to increase the diagnostic sensitivity for spinal cord disease.[58,59]

Magnetic resonance images are generated through a computer-assisted technique that depends on the magnetic properties of atomic nuclei in tissue.[33] Two principal forms of images, termed T_1- and T_2-weighted, are produced. The CSF appears dark (signal hypointense) in T_1-weighted images and bright (signal hyperintense) on T_2-weighted images. The magnetic properties of edema and most tumors are similar to those of CSF.[33, 60] Lesions can

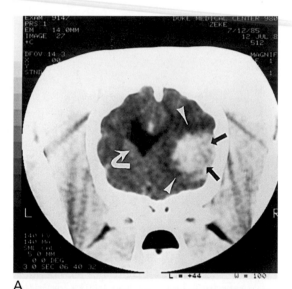

A

Figure 4-4 Iodine-enhanced, transverse computed tomography (CT) images at the level of the thalamus and caudal pole of the caudate nucleus from an 11-year-old male boxer with a 2-week history of decreased visual acuity, circling to the right, and left hemiparesis. The CT window level (L) and width (W) have been manipulated so that greater brain detail is appreciated in **A** (soft tissue or narrow window; L 44; W 100), whereas bony detail of the calvaria is better seen in **B** (bone or wide window; L 283; W 2000). Note that a somewhat irregular, heterogeneously enhancing mass (arrows in **A**) is present at the level of the right temporal cortex. The mass is poorly seen in **B**, but it is identified with arrows to provide a point of reference. This mass and the resultant peritumoral edema (decreased opacity surrounding the tumor [arrowheads]) compresses the right lateral ventricle. The caudal pole of the caudate nucleus is seen in **A** (curved arrow). The calvaria adjacent to the lesion is well delineated in **B** and does not seem involved. The lesion was partially resected surgically; a diagnosis of meningeal sarcoma was made. (From Kornegay JN: Imaging brain neoplasms: computed tomography and magnetic resonance imaging, *Vet Med Rep* 2:372-390, 1990.)

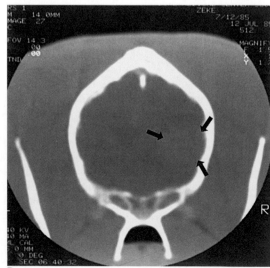

B

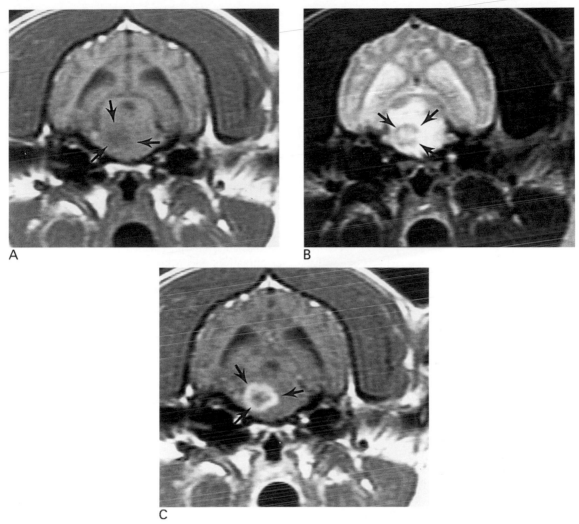

Figure 4-5 Transverse magnetic resonance images at the level of the midbrain from a 9-year-old female mixed-breed dog with a 1-week history of circling to the left and right and disorientation. Images **A** and **C** are T1 weighted, and image **B** is T2 weighted. Gadolinium diethylenetriamine pentaacetic acid (Gd-DTPA) has been given in **C.** A relatively distinct lesion is seen in the midbrain (arrows) in all three images. In the precontrast T1-weighted image **(A),** the lesion is hypointense, whereas it has a ring pattern of enhancement after Gd-DTPA **(C).** With T2 weighting, the lesion contains a central area of hyperintensity (presumably corresponding to tumor), a surrounding zone of hypointensity, and adjacent hyperintensity, probably representing edema **(B).** This apparent edema appears hypointense in **A** and is not distinguished from the central tumor. A relatively high-grade glioma was suspected. Irradiation was initiated; however, the dog died during treatment. Necropsy was not allowed. Spin echo in all three: TR, 0.5 seconds in **A** and **C** and 2.0 seconds in **B;** TE, 20 msec in **A** and C and 70 msec in **B.** (From Kornegay JN: Imaging brain neoplasms: computed tomography and magnetic resonance imaging, *Vet Med Report* 2:372-390, 1990.)

be further characterized using a paramagnetic contrast medium such as gadolinium diethylenetriamine pentaacetic acid (Gd DTPA) (0.1 mmol/kg). Most animals with probable brain tumors should be referred to a facility with CT or MRI capabilities.

Contraindications

Anesthesia is required for good-quality radiographs of the nervous system. Many patients with CNS disease are poor risks for anesthesia. The veterinarian must make a decision by weighing the risks of the procedure against the risk of doing nothing. For example, vertebral fractures usually require early decompression if spinal cord function is to be preserved. These patients may be in shock or have other injuries. The issue of risk versus benefit must be resolved on an individual basis.

Increased intracranial pressure is a contraindication to spinal puncture; hence, myelography should not be performed in such cases. Because contrast media are irritating, myelography is usually not done in the presence of meningitis. When the puncture is made for myelography, a CSF cell count is determined. If the count indicates active inflammation, myelography is not performed unless it is considered essential to diagnosis and treatment (e.g., with strong suspicion of an abscess). The CSF analysis must be performed *before* myelography because contrast agents cause inflammation.

In an animal with increased intracranial pressure, a ventricular tap not only is diagnostic but also may be therapeutic. Excessive removal of fluid, however, can cause collapse of the cerebral cortex and subdural hematoma.

Electrophysiology

Availability

Electrophysiologic techniques require expensive equipment and extensive training and experience for valid interpretation of results. These factors generally limit electrophysiologic studies to specialty practices and institutional settings. Electroencephalography (EEG), electromyography (EMG), and evoked potentials are the most widely used techniques and are available in a number of specialty practices. The other techniques are in varying stages of development for clinical application and are available primarily at research institutions (Table 4-5).

Indications

Electroencephalography, the graphic recording of the electrical activity of the brain, is helpful in the evaluation of cerebral disease.[61, 62] As with most diagnostic tools, the EEG often does not provide a specific diagnosis but supports determination of a category of disease. The EEG varies with the level of consciousness. Low voltage and fast activity are seen in the alert animal. Higher voltage and slower activity occur during drowsiness and sleep. Drugs such as sedatives, tranquilizers, and anesthetics produce higher voltage and slower activity similar to sleep patterns. Results of the EEG usually can indicate that cerebral disease is present and whether it is focal or diffuse, acute or chronic, and inflammatory or degenerative.

The following general principles of EEG changes have been listed by Klemm and Hall[63]:

1. Low voltage, fast activity (LVFA) and spikes (very fast activity) indicate irritation from any cause (usually inflammatory disease).
2. High voltage, slow activity (HVSA) suggests neuronal death or compression.
3. Neither change is diagnostic of a disease but rather reflects the kind of process occurring (e.g., inflammation or degeneration).

4. A focal EEG abnormality indicates a focal cortical lesion.
5. A generalized EEG abnormality indicates a diffuse cortical disease or a subcortical abnormality that alters the activity of the majority of the cerebral cortex.
6. The EEG can change with time, suggesting progression or resolution of the disease process.

Quantitative electroencephalography provides more objective data on the spectral frequency content and amplitudes of the EEG recording.[64]

Electromyography, the measurement of the electrical activity of muscle, and the measurement of *nerve-conduction velocity* (NCV) are performed on the same equipment, usually during the same examination. Electromyography and NCV are the best diagnostic tools for the evaluation of neuropathies and myopathies.[65] The information provided by these procedures regarding the location and the extent of the abnormality may support a diagnosis.

The EMG examination includes evaluation of the electrical activity of the muscle at the following times: (1) during insertion or movement of the electrode (insertion activity), (2) when the muscle is resting (resting activity), (3) during muscle contraction (voluntary or reflex), and (4) in response to electrical stimulation of a motor nerve (also called *electrodiagnostic testing*). Mechanical distortion of the muscle membrane by the needle electrode causes the membrane to depolarize, producing a brief burst of electrical activity (i.e., insertion activity). Resting muscle is electrically silent.

Loss of nerve supply to a muscle causes an increase in the excitability of the muscle membrane within 7 to 10 days. Insertion activity is greatly prolonged. Small, abnormal potentials (called *fibrillation potentials* and *positive sharp waves*) are produced spontaneously while the muscle is at rest. Contraction of the muscle voluntarily, by activation of a reflex or by direct stimulation of a nerve, usually is reduced because of denervation.

Myopathies may be associated with EMG changes similar to those of neuropathies, except that muscle action potentials are smaller and muscle activation is possible and may even be hyperactive. In addition, many myopathies are characterized by prolonged complex repetitive discharges that sound like dive bombers or motorcycles on the speaker of the EMG unit.

Localization to a spinal cord segment, nerve root, or peripheral nerve is determined on the basis of the distribution of abnormal findings. Lesions of spinal cord segments and roots typically cause partial denervation of several muscle groups, whereas

Table 4-5 **Electrophysiology**

Test	Indications	Probable Usefulness	Contraindications	Availability
Electroencephalography	Degenerative disease	Moderate	None	Specialty practice
	Anomaly	High		
	Metabolic disease	Moderate		
	Neoplasia	Moderate		
	Inflammatory disease	High		
	Trauma	Low		
	Toxic disease	Moderate		
Electromyography, nerve conduction, and nerve stimulation	Lower motor neuron diseases	High	None	Specialty practice
	Peripheral neuropathies	High		
	Myopathies	High		
Electroretinography	Retinal disease	High	None	Specialty practice
Evoked response (cortical, brain-stem, and spinal)	Localization of lesions in pathways	Insufficient data in most areas	None	Specialty practice
Visual-evoked response	Cortical function	Moderate		
Auditory-evoked response	Test of hearing, location of brain stem lesions	High		
Somatosensory-evoked response	Spinal cord, plexus lesions	Moderate		
Urodynamics (cystometrogram, urethral pressure, sphincter reflexes)	Neurogenic bladder disorders	(See Ch. 3)		
Tympanometry	Otitis media, otitis interna, hearing disorders	Moderate	None	Institutions (few)

peripheral nerve lesions are more likely to cause complete denervation in the distribution of that nerve. Spinal cord segment lesions are more likely to be bilateral.

Either *motor-nerve-conduction velocity* (MNCV) or *sensory-nerve-conduction velocity* (SNCV) may be evaluated. For SNCV, the nerve to be tested is stimulated and a potential is recorded directly from the nerve proximal to the site of stimulation.[66] The distance between the recording and stimulation sites is divided by the latency of the potential to give a conduction velocity in m/s. For MNCV, the nerve to be evaluated is stimulated at two sites to factor out the time required for transmission across the neuromuscular junction (Figure 4-6). The length of the nerve segment between the two stimulation sites is divided by the difference in latency between

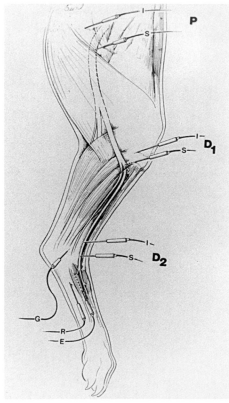

Figure 4-6 Drawing illustrating proximal (P) and distal (D$_1$ and D$_2$) stimulation sites for measuring motor-nerve conduction velocity in proximal and distal segments of the peroneal nerve in a dog. I and S illustrate indifferent (reference) (I) and stimulating (S) electrodes. In this method, potentials are recorded from the extensor digitorum brevis muscle using ground (G), reference (R), and exploring (recording) (E) electrodes. The interelectrode distance is divided by the difference in onset latency values to give motor nerve conduction velocity. (From Tuler SM, Bowen JM: Measurement of conduction velocity of the peroneal nerve based on recording from extensor digitorum brevis muscle, *J Am Anim Hosp Assoc* 26:164-168, 1990.)

the compound muscle action potentials to give a conduction velocity in m/s.[67] The primary *compound muscle action potential* or *M-wave* used in calculating MNCV occurs because of orthodromic stimulation of motor fibers. Nerve stimulation also elicits smaller, more delayed secondary action potentials in muscle.[68] Orthodromic stimulation of sensory fibers produces the *H-wave* or *reflex,* whereas antidromic stimulation of motor fibers produces the *F-wave.* Evaluation of these secondary waves provides information about the nerve roots and the integrity of reflex arcs.

Decrement of the compound muscle action potential subsequent to *repetitive motor nerve stimulation* at rates of less than 5 per second is suggestive of myasthenia gravis.[69] *Single-fiber electromyography* (SFEMG) also is used to evaluate neuromuscular transmission. Delayed neuromuscular conduction, as with myasthenia gravis, causes latency variability termed *jitter.*[70]

Electroretinography (ERG) is the electrical recording of the retinal response to light. Simple strip-chart recorders can be used, but a cathode ray oscilloscope is necessary to obtain better results. Signal-averaging computers provide even better resolution and allow recording in nonsedated animals.[71] The ERG is helpful for differentiating retinal from central blindness.

The *visual-evoked response* (VER) is the cortical electrical activity that occurs in response to a light stimulus administered to the eye. A signal-averaging computer is needed to record this response. The response provides an objective evaluation of central visual pathways.[72,73] Pattern stimuli, light-emitting diode goggles, or a red filter has made this technique more useful.[74,75]

The *brainstem auditory-evoked response* (BAER) entails the recording of brainstem potentials in response to a click stimulus in the ear canal. A signal-averaging computer is necessary to record this response.[76-79] The peripheral auditory system can be evaluated rapidly and accurately with this system. Partial hearing loss requires pure tone stimuli, which present more difficult technical problems. Brainstem function also can be evaluated. The recording consists of a series of waves that represent electrical activity at successive levels of the brainstem. A lesion at one level of the brainstem blocks the responses at that level and at all succeeding levels. The BAER has been used most commonly to diagnose inherited unilateral or bilateral deafness in susceptible breeds such as the dalmatian.[80,81] Brainstem lesions also cause BAER abnormalities.[82] BAER can confirm a diagnosis of complete loss of brainstem function in brain death.

Impedance audiometry (IA) is a method of assessing the integrity of the middle ear system.[83,84]

Impedance audiometry measures the compliance of the tympanic membrane at rest, with changes in pressure, and in response to auditory stimuli. Middle-ear effusion, occlusion of the auditory (eustachian) tube, conduction alterations in the ossicles, retrocochlear hearing loss, and facial motor nerve function (through the stapedial reflex) can be identified through IA.

Somatosensory-evoked potentials (SEPs) are the potentials recorded from the spinal cord, brainstem, or brain in response to a stimulus administered to a peripheral nerve.[85,86] A signal-averaging computer is required. The SEP is used to determine the functional capacity of sensory pathways, as with a paraplegic animal with questionable sensory function on neurologic examination.[87] Adequate information is not yet available to determine the clinical value of this test. The fastest potentials recorded are those of the faster pathways (e.g., the dorsal columns). More trials are needed to determine whether the slower-conducting pain pathways can be evaluated in clinical patients.[88] Similar *motor-evoked potentials* (MEPs) can be recorded from either muscle or the spinal cord in response to either magnetic or electrical stimulation of the motor cortex.[89-91] These waveforms may have more clinical significance because they involve motor pathways necessary for walking.

Urodynamics includes cystometrography, urethral pressure profiles, and electrophysiologic testing of bladder and sphincter reflexes (see Chapter 3 for details).

Contraindications

No significant contraindications exist to any of the electrophysiologic tests unless anesthesia or tranquilization is necessary and is contraindicated.

Biopsy

Availability

Biopsy of neural or muscular tissue can be performed by any veterinary surgeon; however, the difficulties in obtaining good diagnostic samples generally limit this procedure to specialty practices and institutions. Histopathologic evaluation requires a trained pathologist.

Indications

Brain biopsy is used to confirm a diagnosis of a diffuse encephalopathy such as viral inflammation or storage disease.[92] Samples of the cerebral cortex or cerebellum can be obtained. Many of the diseases cannot be definitively diagnosed antemortem with other procedures. Because of the invasive nature of the procedure, it is not generally recommended;

however, biopsy is useful for establishing the diagnosis in a potential animal model of neurologic disease or when the owner of the animal wants a definitive diagnosis of a potentially untreatable disease. Minimal deficits in neurologic function are produced by removal of small samples of the cerebral or cerebellar cortex. Biopsy of focal lesions identified with CT or MRI also is indicated.

Fine-needle aspiration of spinal cord masses can be accomplished with fluoroscopy.[93] Lymphosarcoma is readily identified. We have obtained histologic diagnosis for parenchymal tumors as well.

Biopsy of a peripheral nerve is indicated in neuropathies. Excision of a few fascicles of a mixed nerve is preferred if a motor neuropathy is suspected, but small sensory nerves may be sampled in many disorders.[94,95] A muscle biopsy usually is performed simultaneously with a peripheral nerve biopsy to differentiate neuropathies from myopathies. Multiple muscles should ideally be sampled because pathologic changes may differ widely among muscles. Tissues must be handled properly for satisfactory histopathologic evaluation. The nerve or muscle specimen must be maintained straight, without excess tension, during fixation. This positioning usually is attained by suspending the nerve with a weight on the end, tying or pinning the ends of the nerve to a tongue depressor, or using double clamps on the muscle.[94] The histochemical staining necessary to diagnose or better characterize most muscle diseases must be done on unfixed muscle. The pathologist should be consulted regarding the proper handling of the tissues.

Contraindications

The invasive nature of these procedures must be weighed against the benefits of the information to be gained. A brain biopsy usually is reserved for animals with serious, usually untreatable, encephalopathies. The brain biopsy has gained favor as a procedure for the diagnosis of certain human viral encephalitides, such as herpes encephalitis. Deficits produced by the biopsy are minimal. A spinal cord biopsy is generally contraindicated because the procedure may seriously compromise spinal cord function; however, fine-needle aspiration of mass lesions in the vertebral canal is useful and produces little damage. Peripheral nerve and muscle biopsies are performed more commonly and do not produce serious deficits if care is exercised in the selection of the peripheral nerve.

Case Histories

The case studies presented in Chapters 1 and 2 involve the history (Chapter 1), which was used to develop a sign time graph and a list of probable categories of disease (rule-outs); neurologic examination (Chapter 1); and, from it, localization of the lesion (Chapter 2). At this point in each case, an anatomic diagnosis and a list of rule-outs have been established. The next step is to perform appropriate diagnostic tests to confirm or exclude the possible causes of the problem and, in some cases, to pinpoint the location of the lesion. The signalment, localization, and list of rule-outs are repeated. The reader should decide which diagnostic tests are appropriate in each case before reading the diagnostic plan.

CASE HISTORY 4A

Signalment
Canine, West Highland white terrier, female, 6 years old.

Problems
Right hemiparesis, slight paresis in the left pelvic limb.

Localization
(See Chapter 2.) Spinal cord, C6-T2, primarily the right side.

Rule-outs:
(See Chapter 1.)
1. Vascular lesion
2. Trauma
3. Inflammation

CASE HISTORY 4B

Signalment
Canine, German shepherd dog, female, 7 years old.

Problems
Pelvic limb ataxia and paresis.

Localization
(See Chapter 2.) Spinal cord, T3-L3, symmetric.

Rule-outs:
(See Chapter 1.)
1. Degenerative disease
2. Neoplasia
3. Inflammation

CASE HISTORY 4C

Signalment
Feline, domestic shorthair, female, 3 months old.

Problems
Ataxia and dysmetria, nystagmus, and menase deficit.

Localization
(See Chapter 2.) Cerebellum.

Rule-outs:
(See Chapter 1.)
1. Anomaly
2. Trauma

CASE HISTORY 4D

Signalment
Feline, Siamese, male, 2 years old.

Problems
1. Depression
2. Head tremor

3. Left hemiparesis
4. Uveitis in left eye

Localization
(See Chapter 2.)

1. Left C6-T2 spinal cord
2. Cerebellum
3. Possibly cerebrum or brainstem

Rule-outs:
(See Chapter 1.)
1. Inflammation
2. Neoplasia
3. Degenerative disease

CASE HISTORY 4E

Signalment
Canine, Yorkshire terrier, male, 8 months old.

Problems
1. Mental status: Episodic depression and agitation
2. Compulsive walking with slight dysmetria and mild postural reaction deficits

Localization
(See Chapter 2.) Cerebrum, diffuse.

Rule-outs:
(See Chapter 1.)
1. Metabolic disease
2. Toxic disease

ASSESSMENTS

Diagnostic Plan 4A
Radiography: Rule out trauma (vertebral fracture or luxation). Survey radiographs are normal.

Cerebrospinal fluid (CSF) analysis: Rule out inflammation. Possible evidence of hemorrhage. The protein level is 50 mg/dl, with 1 WBC per mm^3 in the CSF.

Myelography: Rule out compression from trauma. Check for possible swelling of the spinal cord, which may be seen with a vascular lesion. The myelogram is normal, lessening the likelihood of trauma.

The probable diagnosis is spinal cord infarction. Infarcts usually are diagnosed by exclusion, as in this case. The CSF may have a slight increase in protein and, more rarely, may be xanthochromic. See Chapter 6 for a discussion of spinal cord infarction.

Diagnostic Plan 4B
Radiography: Rule out vertebral inflammation (diskospondylitis) or vertebral neoplasia.

CSF analysis: Rule out inflammation.

Myelography: Rule out degenerative disk disease and spinal cord tumor.

Primary degenerative diseases of the spinal cord or the brain are diagnosed by exclusion because the lesion is microscopic. Tumors and herniated intervertebral disks also may cause these signs, so they must be ruled out. This dog had a protruding disk that was evident on the myelogram and was resected surgically. For a discussion of these diseases, see Chapter 6.

Diagnostic Plan 4C

This kitten has been abnormal since birth: a congenital lesion. Trauma is a possible diagnosis if we consider the possibility of a birth injury. The problem has been present for at least 6 to 8 weeks (from the time of significant motor activity) and probably since birth (poor nursing). The lack of progression and the severity of the signs suggest a static lesion, which is not likely to be treatable. This syndrome is typical of cerebellar malformations associated with in utero infection with panleukopenia virus. In contrast, degenerative conditions such as the lysosomal storage diseases and inflammatory diseases typically cause progressive, multifocal involvement. Diagnostic tests other than a cerebellar biopsy or MRI or CT scans are not likely to be rewarding. Sometimes the client should be advised not to spend additional money on diagnostic procedures. The cat can live a reasonably normal life if it stays in the house. See Chapter 8 for a discussion of this syndrome.

Diagnostic Plan 4D

Funduscopic Examination: Characterize the eye lesion.

Hematology and Blood Chemistry Analysis: Rule out systemic disease.

CSF analysis: Rule out inflammation and neoplasia.

Serum titers: Rule out feline infectious peritonitis (FIP) and feline leukemia virus. Remember that the benign enteric coronavirus may cross-react with the FIP virus.

Radiography and myelography are performed if these tests are negative. Rule out neoplasia. The funduscopic examination is an integral part of the neurologic examination. Inflammatory diseases may cause uveitis and retinal lesions. Neoplasia can lead to cerebral edema and optic disk swelling. Hematology and blood chemistry analyses should be performed for any animal with neurologic disease (see the section on the minimum database in Chapter 1), but they are not likely to provide positive information in this case. The chronic progressive history and the multifocal signs are most likely caused by an infectious agent or a degenerative disease. Ocular involvement is more compatible with an inflammatory condition. Feline infectious peritonitis, systemic fungal disease, toxoplasmosis, and feline leukemia virus (FeLV) are the most likely causes of this syndrome. Specific immunologic tests for these diseases are available and should be used if the results are questionable. Radiographs are unlikely to be needed. This cat had an increased plasma protein (9.2 g/dl), primarily in the globulin fraction (6.2 g/dl). A granulomatous uveitis and retinitis were seen on ophthalmoscopic examination. The CSF protein level was 400 mg/dl, with 300 WBCs per mm^3, which were 80% neutrophils and 20% lymphocytes. These findings are typical of FIP. The FeLV test was positive, and the FIP titer was high. For a discussion of these diseases, see Chapter 15.

Diagnostic Plan 4E

Consider the results of the minimum database (see Chapter 1) before proceeding. The history and clinical findings are typical of hepatic encephalopathy. Affected animals generally have signs of forebrain disease. Any suggestion of liver disease in the minimum database indicates the need for specific tests. Levels of serum enzymes that indicate acute liver disease may be normal. Decreased values of blood urea nitrogen and serum albumin are significant. Specific tests include sulfobromophthalein sodium excretion (BSP), serum bile acid levels, blood ammonia levels, and the ammonia tolerance test. For a discussion of hepatic encephalopathy, see Chapter 15.

References

1. Mayhew I: Collection of cerebrospinal fluid from the horse, *Cornell Vet* 65:500-511, 1975.
2. Kornegay JN: Cerebrospinal fluid collection, examination, and interpretation in dogs and cats, *Compendium Continuing Educ Pract Vet* 3:85-94, 1981.
3. Thomson CE, Kornegay JN, Stevens JB: Analysis of cerebrospinal fluid from the cerebellomedullary and lumbar cisterns of dogs with focal neurologic disease: 145 cases (1985-1987), *J Am Vet Med Assoc* 196:1841-1844, 1990.
4. Sweeney CR, Russell GE: Differences in total protein concentration, nucleated cell count, and red blood cell count among sequential samples of cerebrospinal fluid from horses, *J Am Vet Med Assoc* 217:54-57, 2000.
5. Simpson ST, Reed RB: Manometric values for normal cerebrospinal fluid pressure in dogs, *J Am Anim Hosp Assoc* 23:629-632, 1987.
6. Duncan JR, Oliver JE, Mayhew IG: Laboratory examinations. In Oliver JE, Hoerlein BF, Mayhew IG, editors: *Veterinary neurology.* Philadelphia, 1987, WB Saunders.
7. Jamison EM, Lumsden JH: Cerebrospinal fluid analysis in the dog: methodology and interpretation, *Semin Vet Med Surg* 3:122-132, 1988.
8. Roszel J: Membrane filtration of canine and feline cerebrospinal fluid for cytologic evaluation, *J Am Vet Med Assoc* 160:720-725, 1972.
9. Bienzle D, McDonnell JJ, Stanton JB: Analysis of cerebrospinal fluid from dogs and cats after 24 and 48 hours of storage, *J Am Vet Med Assoc* 216:1761-1764, 2000.
10. Wilson JW, Stevens JB: Effects of blood contamination on cerebrospinal fluid analysis, *J Am Vet Med Assoc* 171:256-258, 1977.
11. Hurtt AE, Smith MO: Effects of iatrogenic blood contamination on results of cerebrospinal fluid analysis in clinically normal dogs and dogs with neurologic disease, *J Am Vet Med Assoc* 211:866-867, 1997.
12. Bichsel P, Vandevelde M, Vandevelde E, et al: Immunoelectrophoretic determination of albumin and IgG in serum and cerebrospinal fluid in dogs with neurological diseases, *Res Vet Sci* 37:101-107, 1984.
13. Sorjonen DC, Warren JN, Schultz RD: Qualitative and quantitative determination of albumin, IgG, IgM and IgA in normal cerebrospinal fluid in dogs, *J Am Anim Hosp Assoc* 17:833-839, 1981.
14. Sorjonen D: Total protein, albumin quota, and electrophoretic patterns in cerebrospinal fluid of dogs with central nervous system disorders, *Am J Vet Res* 48:301-305, 1987.
15. Kristensen F, Firth EC: Analysis of serum proteins and cerebrospinal fluid in clinically normal horses, using agarose electrophoresis, *Am J Vet Res* 38:1089-1092, 1977.
16. Rand JS, Parent J, Jacobs R, et al: Reference intervals for feline cerebrospinal fluid: biochemical and serologic variables, IgG concentration, and electrophoretic fractionation, *Am J Vet Res* 51:1049-1054, 1990.
17. Wright JA: Cerebrospinal fluid enzyme estimation in the diagnosis of central nervous damage in the dog, *Vet Rec* 106:54-57, 1980.
18. Wilson JW: Clinical application of cerebrospinal fluid creatine phosphokinase determination, *J Am Vet Med Assoc* 171:200-202, 1977.

19. Indrieri RJ, Holliday TA, Keen CL: Critical evaluation of creatine phosphokinase in cerebrospinal fluid of dogs with neurologic disease, *Am J Vet Res* 41:1299-1303, 1980.

20. Jackson C, de Lahunta A, Divers T, Ainsworth D: The diagnostic utility of cerebrospinal fluid creatine kinase activity in the horse, *J Vet Intern Med* 10:246-251, 1996.

21. Vandevelde M, Zurbriggen A, Steck A, Bichsel P: Studies on the intrathecal humoral immune response in canine distemper encephalitis, *J Neuroimmunol* 11:41-51, 1986.

22. Thomas WB, Sorjonen DC, Steiss JE: A retrospective evaluation of 38 cases of canine distemper encephalomyelitis, *J Am Anim Hosp Assoc* 29:129-133, 1993.

23. Berthelin CF, Legendre AM, Bailey CS, et al: Cryptococcosis of the nervous system in dogs, part 2: diagnosis, treatment, monitoring, and prognosis, *Prog Vet Neurol* 5:136-146, 1994.

24. Dunigan CE, Oglesbee MJ, Podell M, et al: Seizure activity associated with equine protozoal myeloencephalitis, *Prog Vet Neurol* 6:50-54, 1995.

25. Munana KR, Lappin MR, Powell CC, et al: Sequential measurement of *Toxoplasma gondii* specific antibodies in the cerebrospinal fluid of cats with experimentally induced toxoplasmosis, *Prog Vet Neurol* 6:27-31, 1995.

26. Tipold A: Diagnosis of inflammatory and infectious diseases of the central nervous system in dogs: a retrospective study, *J Vet Intern Med* 9:304-314, 1995.

27. Smith-Maxie LL, Parent JP, Rand J, et al: Cerebrospinal fluid analysis and clinical outcome of eight dogs with eosinophilic meningoencephalomyelitis, *J Vet Intern Med* 3:167-174, 1989.

28. Sorjonen DC: Clinical and histopathological features of granulomatous meningoencephalomyelitis in dogs, *J Am Anim Hosp Assoc* 26:141-147, 1990.

29. Tipold A, Vandevelde M, Jaggy A: Neurological manifestations of canine distemper virus infection, *J Small Anim Pract* 33:466-470, 1992.

30. Barber DL, Oliver JE, Mayhew IG: Neuroradiography. In Oliver JE, Hoerlein BF, Mayhew IG, editors: *Veterinary neurology*. Philadelphia, 1987, WB Saunders.

31. Fike JR, LeCouteur RA, Cann CE: Anatomy of the canine brain using high resolution computed tomography, *Vet Radiol* 22:236-243, 1981.

32. LeCouteur RA, Fike JR, Cann CE, et al: X-ray computed tomography of brain tumors in cats, *J Am Vet Med Assoc* 183:301-305, 1983.

33. Kornegay JN: Imaging brain neoplasms: computed tomography and magnetic resonance imaging, *Vet Med Report* 2:372-390, 1990.

34. Turrel J, Fike J, LeCouteur RA, et al: Computed tomographic characteristics of primary brain tumors in 50 dogs, *J Am Vet Med Assoc* 188:851-856, 1986.

35. LeCouteur RA, Fike JR, Cann CE, et al: Computed tomography of brain tumors in the caudal fossa of the dog, *Vet Radiol* 22:244-251, 1981.

36. Fike JR, LeCouteur RA, Cann CE, et al: Computerized tomography of brain tumors of the rostral and middle fossas in the dog, *Am J Vet Res* 42:275-281, 1981.

37. Cox F, Jakovljevic S: The use of iopamidol for myelography in dogs: a study of twenty-seven cases, *J Small Anim Pract* 27:159-165, 1986.

38. May S, Wyn-Jones G, Church S: Iopamidol myelography in the horse, *Equine Vet J* 18:199-202, 1986.

39. Wheeler SJ, Davies JV: Iohexol myelography in the dog and cat: a series of one hundred cases, and a comparison with metrizamide and iopamidol, *J Small Anim Pract* 26:247-256, 1985.

40. Wood AK: Iohexol and iopamidol: new nonionic contrast media for myelography in dogs, *Compendium Continuing Educ Pract Vet* 10:31-36, 1988.

41. Lewis DD, Hosgood G: Complications associated with the use of iohexol for myelography of the cervical vertebral column in dogs: 66 cases (1988-1990), *J Am Vet Med Assoc* 200:1381-1384, 1992.

42. Suter PF, Morgan JP, Holliday TA, et al: Myelography in the dog: diagnosis of tumors of the spinal cord and vertebrae, *J Vet Radiol Soc* 12:29-44, 1971.

43. Kirberger RM, Wrigley RH: Myelography in the dog: review of patients with contrast medium in the central canal, *Vet Radiol Ultrasound* 34:253-258, 1993.

44. Morgan JP, Atilola M, Bailey CS: Vertebral canal and spinal cord mensuration: a comparative study of its effect on lumbosacral myelography in the Dachshund and German Shepherd Dog, *J Am Vet Med Assoc* 191:951-957, 1987.

45. Selcer BA, Chambers JN, Schwensen K, et al: Epidurography as a diagnostic aid in canine lumbosacral compressive disease: 47 cases (1981-1986), *Vet Comp Orthop Trauma* 2:97-103, 1988.

46. Feeney DA, Wise M: Epidurography in the normal dog: technic and radiographic findings, *Vet Radiol* 22:35-39, 1981.

47. Klide AM, Steinberg SA, Pond MJ: Epiduralograms in the dog: the uses and advantages of the diagnostic procedure, *J Vet Radiol Soc* 8:39-44, 1967.

48. Sisson AF, LeCouteur RA, Ingram JT, et al: Diagnosis of cauda equina abnormalities by using electromyography, discography, and epidurography in dogs, *J Vet Intern Med* 6:253-263, 1992.

49. Savell CM: Cerebral ventricular tap: an aid to diagnosis and treatment of hydrocephalus in the dog, *J Am Anim Hosp Assoc* 10:500-501, 1974.

50. Hudson JA, Cartee RE, Simpson ST, et al: Ultrasonographic anatomy of the canine brain, *Radiology* 30:13-21, 1989.

51. Spaulding KA, Sharp NJH: Ultrasonographic imaging of the lateral cerebral ventricles in the dog, *Vet Radiol* 31:59-64, 1990.

52. Rivers WJ, Walter PA: Hydrocephalus in the dog: utility of ultrasonography as an alternate diagnostic imaging technique, *J Am Anim Hosp Assoc* 28:333-343, 1992.

53. Gallagher JG, Pennick D, Boudrieau RJ, et al: Ultrasonography of the brain and vertebral canal in dogs and cats: 15 cases, *J Am Vet Med Assoc* 207:1320-1324, 1995.

54. Finn-Bodner ST, Hudson JA, Coates JR, et al: Ultrasonographic anatomy of the normal canine spinal cord and correlation with histopathology after induced spinal cord trauma, Vet *Radiol Ultrasound* 36:39-48, 1995.

55. Oliver JE: Cranial sinus venography in the dog, *J Am Vet Radiol Soc* 10:66-71, 1969.

56. LeCouteur RA, Scagliotti RH, Beck KA, et al: Indirect imaging of the optic nerve, using metrizamide (optic thecography), *Am J Vet Res* 43:1424-1428, 1982.

57. Voorhout G, Rijnberk A: Cisternography combined with linear tomography for visualization of pituitary lesions in dogs with pituitary dependent hyperadrenocorticism, *J Vet Radiol* 31:74-78, 1990.

58. Sharp NJH Cofone M, Robertson ID, et al: Computed tomography in the evaluation of caudal cervical spondylopathy of the Doberman pinscher, *Vet Radiol Ultrasound* 36:100-108, 1995.

59. Drost WT, Love NE, Berry CR: Comparison of radiography, myelography and computed tomography for the evaluation of canine vertebral and spinal cord tumors in sixteen dogs, *Vet Radiol Ultrasound* 37:28-33, 1996.

60. Thomas WB, Wheeler SJ, Kramer R, Kornegay JN: Magnetic resonance imaging features of primary brain tumors in dogs, *Vet Radiol Ultrasound* 37:2027, 1996.

61. Redding RW, Knecht CE: *Atlas of electroencephalography in the dog and cat.* New York, 1984, Praeger.

62. Redding RW: Electroencephalography, *Prog Vet Neurol* 1:181-188, 1990.

63. Klemm WR, Hall CL: Current status and trends in veterinary electroencephalography, *J Am Vet Med Assoc* 164:529-532, 1974.

64. Moore MP, Greene SA, Keegan RD, et al: Quantitative electroencephalography in dogs anesthetized with 2.0% end-tidal concentration of isoflurane anesthesia, *Am J Vet Res* 52:551-560, 1991.

65. Bowen JM: Electromyography. In Oliver JE, Hoerlein BF, Mayhew IG, editors: *Veterinary neurology.* Philadelphia, 1987, WB Saunders.

66. Redding RW, Ingram JT: Sensory nerve conduction velocity of cutaneous afferents of the radial, ulnar, peroneal, and tibial nerves of the cat: reference values, *Am J Vet Res* 45:1042-1045, 1984.

67. Tuler SM, Bowen JM: Measurement of conduction velocity of the peroneal nerve based on recordings from extensor digitorum brevis muscle, *J Am Anim Hosp Assoc* 26:164-168, 1990.

68. Knecht CD, Redding RW: Monosynaptic reflex (H wave) in clinically normal and abnormal dogs, *Am J Vet Res* 42:1586-1589, 1981.

69. Sims MH, McLean RA: Use of repetitive nerve stimulation to assess neuromuscular function in dogs: a test for suspected myasthenia gravis, *Prog Vet Neurol* 1:311-318, 1990.

70. Hopkins AL, Howard JF, Wheeler SJ, Kornegay JN: Single fibre electromyography in normal dogs, *J Small Anim Pract* 34:271-276, 1993.

71. Acland GM: Diagnosis and differentiation of retinal diseases in small animals by electroretinography, *Semin Vet Med Surg* 3:15-27, 1988.

72. Sims MH, Laratta LJ, Bubb WJ, et al: Waveform analysis and reproducibility of visual-evoked potentials in dogs, *Am J Vet Res* 50:1823-1828, 1989.

73. Strain GM, Claxton MS, Olcott BM, et al: Visual-evoked potentials and electroretinograms in ruminants with thiamine-responsive polioencephalomalacia or suspected listeriosis, *J Am Vet Med Assoc* 51:1513-1517, 1990.

74. Sims MH, Laratta LJ: Visual-evoked potentials in cats, using a light-emitting diode stimulator, *Am J Vet Res* 49:1876-1881, 1988.

75. Bichsel P, Oliver JE, Coulter DB, et al: Recording of visual-evoked potentials in dogs with scalp electrodes, *J Vet Intern Med* 2:145-149, 1988.

76. Rolf SL, Reed SM, Melnick W, et al: Auditory brain stem response testing in anesthetized horses, *Am J Vet Res* 48:910-914, 1987.

77. Sims MH, Moore RE: Auditory-evoked response in the clinically normal dog: early latency components, *Am J Vet Res* 45:2019-2027, 1984.

78. Holliday TA, Te Selle ME: Brain stem auditory-evoked potentials of dogs: wave forms and effects of recording electrode positions, *Am J Vet Res* 46:845-851, 1985.

79. Strain GM, Olcott BM, Thompson DR, et al: Brainstem auditory-evoked potentials in Holstein cows, *J Vet Intern Med* 3:144-148, 1989.

80. Holliday TA, Nelson HJ, Williams DC, Willits N: Unilateral and bilateral brainstem auditory-evoked response abnormalities in 900 Dalmatian dogs, *J Vet Intern Med* 6:166-174, 1992.

81. Strain GM, Kearney MT, Gignac IJ, et al: Brainstem auditory-evoked potential assessment of congenital deafness in Dalmatians: associations with phenotypic markers, *J Vet Intern Med* 6:175-182, 1992.

82. Steiss JE, Cox NR, Hathcock JT: Brain stem auditory-evoked response abnormalities in 14 dogs with confirmed central nervous system lesions, *J Vet Intern Med* 8:293-298, 1994.

83. Penrod JP, Coulter DB: The diagnostic uses of impedance audiometry in the dog, *J Am Anim Hosp Assoc* 16:941-948, 1980.

84. Sims M, Weigel J, Moore R: Effects of tenotomy of the tensor tympani muscle on the acoustic reflex in dogs, *Am J Vet Res* 47:1022-1032, 1986.

85. Oliver JE, Purinton PT, Brown J: Somatosensory evoked potentials from stimulation of thoracic limb nerves of the dog, *Prog Vet Neurol* 1:433-443, 1990.

86. Strain GM, Taylor DS, Graham MC, et al: Cortical somatosensory-evoked potentials in the horse, *Am J Vet Res* 49:1869-1872, 1988.

87. Shores A, Redding RW, Knecht CD: Spinal-evoked potentials in dogs with acute compressive thoracolumbar spinal cord disease, *Am J Vet Res* 48:1525-1530, 1987.

88. Holliday T, Ealand B, Weldon N: Ascending pathways of average evoked spinal cord potentials of dogs. In *Proceedings of the American College of Veterinary Internal Medicine,* Seattle, 1979, ACVIM, p 104.

89. Cook JR, Konrad PE, Tacker WA: Amplitude and latency characteristics of spinal cord motor-evoked potentials in dogs, *Am J Vet Res* 51:1340-1344, 1990.

90. Sylvestre AM, Cockshutt JR, Parent JM, et al: Magnetic motor evoked potentials for assessing spinal cord integrity in dogs with intervertebral disc disease, *Vet Surg* 22:5-10, 1993.

91. Van Ham LML, Mattheeuws DRG, Vanderstraeten GGW: Transcranial magnetic motor evoked potentials in anesthetized dogs, *Prog Vet Neurol* 6:5-12, 1995.

92. Swaim SF, Vandevelde M, Faircloth JC: Evaluation of brain biopsy techniques in the dog, *J Am Anim Hosp Assoc* 15:627-633, 1979.

93. Irving G, McMillan MC: Fluoroscopically guided percutaneous fine-needle aspiration biopsy of thoracolumbar spinal lesions in cats, *Prog Vet Neurol* 1:473-475, 1990.

94. Braund KG: Nerve and muscle biopsy techniques, *Prog Vet Neurol* 2:35-56, 1991.

95. Braund K, Walker T, Vandevelde M: Fascicular nerve biopsy in the dog, *Am J Vet Res* 40:1025-1030, 1979.

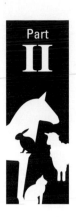

Clinical Problems: Signs and Symptoms

Chapter 5

Paresis of One Limb

The term *monoparesis,* or *monoplegia,* denotes partial or complete loss of voluntary motor function in one limb resulting from a neurologic lesion. Monoparesis must be distinguished from lameness that is due to musculoskeletal involvement. Severe neural lesions cause characteristic sensory and motor deficits (see Lesion Localization). Peripheral nerve and nerve root compression and neoplastic involvement, however, often initially cause lameness and pain *(nerve root signature)* suggestive of musculoskeletal disease (Figure 5-1). Results of the neurologic examination must be reviewed critically in these animals to identify typical deficits. Electrodiagnostic testing may be particularly helpful in localizing lesions to the peripheral nerve or nerve root in such cases (see Chapter 4).

Peripheral or spinal nerves may be injured owing to skeletal fractures or luxations. Thus both systems must be critically evaluated in animals with monoparesis after trauma. In general, the prognosis for recovery is better with skeletal than with neurologic injuries.

LESION LOCALIZATION

The basic anatomic and physiologic principles that enable a clinician to localize lesions based on motor or sensory deficits are presented in Chapter 2.

Concepts related to the localization of lesions producing monoparesis or monoplegia are reviewed here (Figure 5-2).

Monoparesis usually is caused by disease or injury to the lower motor neurons (LMNs) innervating the affected limb. Thus, dysfunction of the neuron (motor nerve cell body), axon (ventral root, spinal nerves, peripheral nerves), or neuromuscular end plate results in motor dysfunction and denervation atrophy. Monoparesis most commonly occurs because of involvement of axons of either peripheral or spinal nerves but less frequently results from lesions affecting neuronal cell bodies in the ventral gray matter of the spinal cord. In most cases, unilateral spinal cord lesions cranial to T3

cause hemiparesis and bilateral lesions cause tetraparesis. Unilateral spinal cord lesions caudal to T2 produce paresis or paralysis of the ipsilateral pelvic limb, whereas bilateral lesions produce paraparesis or paraplegia. Thus, in animals with thoracic limb monoparesis and no involvement of the other limbs, primary consideration is given to the brachial plexus or the peripheral nerves (Table 5-1). Spinal cord lesions at C6-T2 confined entirely to the ventral gray matter could cause thoracic limb monoparesis but more commonly these lesions also involve upper motor neurons (UMNs) to the ipsilateral pelvic limb. Pelvic limb monoparesis may occur because of unilateral spinal cord lesions between the T3-S1 segments or more commonly because of involvement of spinal or peripheral nerves of the pelvic plexus. Unilateral T3-L3 spinal cord lesions cause UMN signs in the ipsilateral limb, whereas lesions at L4-S2 or in the spinal or peripheral nerves cause LMN signs.

Disease of the spinal or peripheral nerves results in both sensory and motor dysfunction distal to the lesion. In contrast, lesions confined to the ventral gray matter of the spinal cord produce only motor dysfunction. Unilateral T3-L3 spinal cord lesions do not cause anesthesia of the affected limb because deep pain sensation is transmitted over bilateral, multisynaptic pathways (see Chapter 1). Anesthesia in the affected limb therefore suggests peripheral or spinal nerve involvement. If sensory loss cannot be detected in the affected limb, lesions in the spinal cord gray matter or the ventral spinal roots should be considered. Figure 5-2 outlines the localization of lesions that produce monoparesis of the thoracic and pelvic limbs.

The distribution of sensory loss in an affected limb has great localizing value because lesions can be pinpointed to a particular nerve or within two to three spinal cord segments (see Figure 1-35).[1,2] The total area innervated by a particular cutaneous nerve is termed its *cutaneous area.*[3] The cutaneous area includes a peripheral *overlap zone* innervated by other cutaneous nerves and a central *autonomous zone* innervated solely by that nerve.

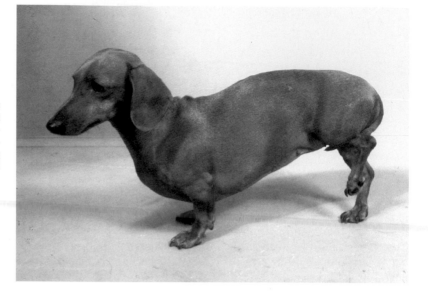

Figure 5-1 Dachshund with "nerve root signature" involving the left pelvic limb resulting from compression of the left L5 nerve root by a laterally extruded disk at L5-6. The dog held the limb off the floor and had pain when the limb was manipulated.

These zones can be detected clinically using a method termed the "two-step pinch technique." Using a mosquito hemostat, a small fold of skin is lifted and gently grasped, activating mechanoreceptors in adjacent cutaneous areas. After the animal is quiet, the small fold of skin is pinched, stimulating only the autonomous zone of the particular nerve. Either a conscious response or reflex withdrawal indicates functional integrity of the particular nerve. The degree of sensory loss also influences the prognosis for functional recovery.

The pattern of denervation atrophy (Figure 5-3) facilitates localization of lesions to a particular nerve or nerve group. Tables 5-1 and 5-2 outline the motor and sensory distribution of the brachial and lumbosacral plexus and the neurologic signs associated with lesions in each major nerve. Animals with peripheral nerve disease or injury also may mutilate the area normally innervated by the affected nerves.[4] This behavior apparently occurs because of *dysesthesia (paresthesia)* caused by ectopic excitation of axonal sprouts in the neuroma or sensory neurons in the dorsal root ganglion of the injured nerve. Self-mutilation can become particularly problematic and necessitate amputation of the involved digits, limb, or tail.

Lesions in the gray matter of the spinal cord at T1-T3 or in the roots of the brachial plexus may injure the LMNs of the sympathetic nerve fibers that form the cranial sympathetic trunk. Loss of sympathetic stimulation to the ipsilateral eye produces signs of miosis, enophthalmos with extrusion of the third eyelid, and ptosis (Horner's syndrome). In the horse, miosis is not as obvious and sweating is seen on the face and neck to the level of C2 on the side of the lesion.[5] Horner's syndrome commonly is associated with traumatic injuries of the brachial plexus. Similarly, lesions of the C8-T1 gray matter or spinal nerves affect the lateral thoracic nerve, which is the motor component of the cutaneous (panniculus) reflex. Therefore, lesions of the brachial plexus may cause LMN paresis of the limb, Horner's syndrome, and loss of the cutaneous reflex on the same side.

Mononeuropathy refers to a disease or an injury of a specific peripheral nerve or its nerve roots. If a large nerve such as the sciatic or radial nerve is injured, severe monoparesis may occur. In most cases, mononeuropathies result from physical injury secondary to compression, laceration, or contusion or from intramuscular injection of drugs. In addition to motor dysfunction and atrophy, variable degrees of sensory loss are encountered because peripheral nerves innervating the limbs contain both motor and sensory fibers.

Polyneuropathy refers to a disease or an injury of several peripheral nerves or their nerve roots. The term is generally used to indicate systemic involvement of many nerves. Those diseases are described in Chapter 7.

In regard to monoparesis, polyneuropathy suggests an injury or a disease of the brachial plexus, the lumbosacral plexus, or the cauda equina. As for mononeuropathies, physical injury is the most common cause of polyneuropathy and subsequent monoparesis. Occasionally, monoparesis occurs because of neoplastic involvement of a specific peripheral nerve, nerve root, or nerve

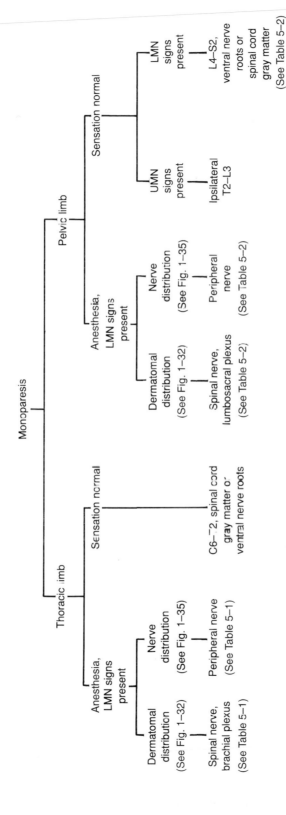

Figure 5-2 An algorithm for localization of lesions that produce monoparesis.

Table 5-1 **Nerves of the Brachial Plexus**

Nerve	Spinal Cord Segments*	Motor Function	Cutaneous Sensory Distribution	Signs of Dysfunction
Suprascapular	*C6*, C7	Extension and lateral support of the shoulder	None	Little gait abnormality, pronounced atrophy of supraspinatus and infraspinatus muscles (sweeney)
Brachiocephalicus	*C6*, C7	Advance limb	Cranial surface of brachium	Little gait abnormality, anesthesia of cranial brachium
Musculocutaneous	C6, *C7*, C8	Flexion of the elbow	Medial antebrachium	Little gait abnormality, weakened flexion of the elbow; anesthesia of medial antebrachium
Axillary	C6, C7, C8	Flexion of the shoulder	Dorsolateral brachium	Little gait abnormality, decreased shoulder flexor reflex; anesthesia of lateral side of brachium
Radial	*C7*, C8, T1, T2	Extension of the elbow, the carpus, and the digits	Dorsal surface of the foot and dorsal and lateral parts of the antebrachium	Loss of weight bearing, knuckling of pes, decreased extensor carpi radialis and triceps reflexes, anesthesia of dorsal surface distal to elbow
Median and ulnar	*C8*, T1, T2	Flexion of the carpus and the digits	Palmar surface of the foot; caudal antebrachium	Little gait abnormality, slight sinking of the carpus; loss of carpal flexion on withdrawal reflex; partial loss of sensation of the palmar surface of the foot and caudal antebrachium
Lateral thoracic	*C8*, T1	Cutaneous muscle of the trunk	None	Absent ipsilateral cutaneous reflex, normal sensation
Sympathetic†	T1, T2, T3	Dilation of the pupil	None	Miosis, ptosis, enophthalmos and protrusion of third eyelid

*The major spinal cord segments that form the peripheral nerves are italicized.
†The sympathetic nerve is not considered part of the brachial plexus; however, its nerve fibers travel along the roots of the brachial plexus as they exit the vertebral column.

plexus. Resulting clinical signs progress insidiously, in contrast to the acute, nonprogressive course typical of physical injuries. Specific diseases that cause monoparesis are discussed in greater detail next.

MONOPARESIS OF THE PELVIC LIMBS
Peripheral Nerve Injuries

Traumatic peripheral nerve injuries are classified into three categories based on the degree of injury. *Neurapraxia* refers to transient interruption of nerve function and conduction, sometimes associated with a lesion of the myelin but without evidence of wallerian degeneration. Neurapraxia is usually caused by a loss of blood supply, such as that produced by application of a tourniquet or by pressure from the weight of the animal during anesthesia. The condition can last for days to months. Demyelination has probably occurred if signs persist for more than a few days. A period of 3 to 4 weeks is required for remyelination.

Axonotmesis denotes separation of the axon from the neuronal cell body with subsequent degeneration of the distal axon (wallerian degeneration) and loss of conduction in 3 to 5 days. The endoneurium and the Schwann sheath supporting

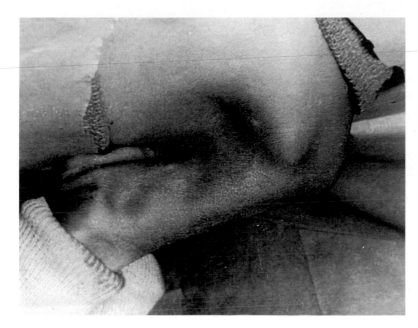

Figure 5-3 Right thoracic limb of a 6-year-old mixed-breed dog with lameness ("nerve root signature") that progressed to monoparesis with associated hyporeflexia and neurogenic muscle atrophy. Atrophy of the triceps muscle group is shown here. On exploration of the brachial plexus, multiple nerves were infiltrated by a nerve sheath tumor. The limb was amputated.

Table 5-2 **Nerves of the Lumbosacral Plexus**

Nerve	Spinal Cord Segments[*]	Motor Function	Cutaneous Sensory Distribution	Signs of Dysfunction
Obturator	L4, *L5, L6*	Adduction of pelvic limb	None	Little gait abnormality, abduction on slick surface
Femoral	L3, *L4, L5*, L6	Extension of stifle, flexion of hip	Saphenous branch supplies medial surface of limb and medial digit	Severe gait dysfunction, no weight bearing, decreased or absent knee jerk reflex, loss of sensation in medial limb and medial digit
Sciatic	*L6, L7, S1, S2*	Extension of hip, extension and flexion of stifle (see tibial and peroneal branches)	Caudal and lateral surfaces of limb distal to stifle (see tibial and peroneal branches)	Severe gait dysfunction; paw is knuckled, but weight bearing occurs; hip cannot be extended, hock cannot be flexed or extended (in more central lesions, hip is flexed and drawn toward the midline); loss of cutaneous sensation distal to stifle (except for areas supplied by saphenous nerve); absent withdrawal reflex
Peroneal	*L6, L7*, S1,S2	Flexion of hock, extension of digits	Cranial surface of limb distal to stifle	Hock is straightened and foot tends to knuckle; loss of sensation on cranial surface to limb distal to stifle, poor hock flexion on withdrawal reflex[†]
Tibial	L6, *L7, S1*, S2	Extension of hock, flexion of digits	Caudal surface of limb distal to stifle	Hock is dropped, loss of sensation on caudal surface of limb distal to stifle[†]

[*]The major spinal cord segments that form the peripheral nerves are italicized.
[†]Peroneal and tibial nerve paralysis commonly occurs in association with each other. Signs of peroneal nerve damage tend to predominate.

structures remain intact. Regeneration of the axon usually begins in about 1 week and progresses at a rate of approximately 1 mm per day (1 inch per month).

Neurotmesis refers to complete severance of the nerve. Regeneration may occur, but neuroma formation is likely. The degree of nerve injury dictates the relative likelihood of regeneration, with restoration of function being most likely with neurapraxia and least likely with neurotmesis.

Electromyography (EMG) and nerve conduction studies are useful for confirming a diagnosis of nerve injury, determining the distribution, and estimating the prognosis. Changes on EMG appear about 1 week after injury (see Chapter 4 for details).

The presence of motor-unit action potentials indicates an incomplete injury. The EMG also can be used to monitor the progress of recovery.

Sciatic Nerve Injury

The sciatic nerve is a mixed nerve that arises from spinal cord segments L6-S2 (see Table 5-2). Because caudal lumbar and sacral spinal cord segments lie cranial to the corresponding vertebrae, nerve fibers that become the sciatic nerve must course caudally before exiting from the vertebral canal. As a result, these nerve fibers are particularly subject to injury from lumbosacral fractures and subluxations, lumbosacral stenosis, and pelvic fractures. Traumatic injuries of the lumbosacral area rarely result in a true mononeuropathy because fibers forming the pudendal, pelvic, and caudal nerves are also injured. In degenerative lumbosacral stenosis, however, the L7 root may be entrapped in the L7-S1 foramen, causing lameness or monoparesis. Sciatic nerve paralysis is a common calving injury in cattle. Damage to the fibers within the vertebral canal usually results in bilateral injury and paraparesis. Occasionally the injury is asymmetric, involving only the fibers of one sciatic nerve.

After giving off branches within the pelvis, the major portion of the sciatic nerve exits at the greater ischiatic foramen and courses caudally to the coxofemoral joint, between and deep to the tuber ischii and the greater trochanter of the femur. The nerve then continues distally between the semimembranosus and biceps femoris muscles. Branches of the sciatic nerve supply muscles that extend the hip and flex the stifle. Between the hip and the stifle, the sciatic nerve bifurcates to form the peroneal and tibial nerves, which supply all muscles distal to the stifle and provide sensation to all areas of the foot except the medial digit, which is innervated by the saphenous branch of the femoral nerve.

Injuries below the distal third of the femur cause signs of peroneal and/or tibial nerve dysfunction. These injuries are described later. Damage to the proximal sciatic nerve results in severe monoparesis because the extensor muscles of the stifle (innervated by the femoral nerve) are the only group that remains functional. Although the animal can bear weight, the stifle does not flex. The hock and the digits do not flex or extend because of tibial and peroneal nerve involvement. The animal stands "knuckled over," and the hock usually is dropped. Sensation distal to the stifle is severely compromised laterally (peroneal), caudally (tibial), and cranially (peroneal), but it is preserved medially if the saphenous branch of the femoral nerve is intact (see Figure 1-35). The dorsal surface of the foot frequently is ulcerated if the animal drags or walks on the affected paw (Figure 5-4).

The sciatic nerve is the major nerve contributing to the pelvic limb flexor reflex. In proximal sciatic nerve injuries, the digits, hock, and stifle do not flex when the toes are stimulated. Stimulation of the medial digit or the medial aspect of the distal limb elicits a pain response and flexion of the hip, but the remainder of the joints of the affected limb do not flex. Atrophy of the caudal thigh muscles and the muscles distal to the stifle may be severe. Dogs with nerve entrapment may have severe pain. Self-mutilation also may occur. Clinical deficits usually are acute but may be delayed if fibrosis leads to nerve entrapment.

The proximal portion of the sciatic nerve is most frequently damaged by fractures of the shaft of the ilium, acetabulum, and proximal femur; after retrograde placement of intramedullary pins in the femur; and during calving injuries in cattle.[6-11] Less common causes include severe hip dysplasia and

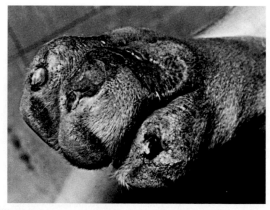

Figure 5-4 Ulcerated digits of the pelvic limb in a dog with peroneal nerve paralysis.

surgical procedures involving the coxofemoral joint.[12-14] The prognosis is poor if sciatic injuries are complete. Partial deficits may be temporary.

Surgical relief of compression injuries may be rewarding. Clinical outcome was studied in one series of 34 dogs with nerve injury subsequent to pelvic fractures and dislocations. Nerve entrapment was noted at surgery in 13 dogs.[11] Limb function was considered good or excellent 2 to 16 weeks after surgery in 11 dogs in which the nerve was decompressed and internal fixation was applied. Function was also good to excellent 2 to 12 weeks after injury in 10 of 12 dogs that did not undergo surgery. Clinical features of dogs managed surgically and conservatively were not well characterized. Many in both groups had decreased cutaneous sensation. The workers suggested that surgery is indicated in dogs with severe pain or "signs of moderate to severe peripheral nerve injury." Markedly blunted or absent pain sensation suggests severe involvement.

The sciatic nerve, or the peroneal or tibial nerves along the caudal aspect of the femur, can be injured by injections or femoral fractures. Injected materials intended for the biceps femoris or semimembranosus muscles may go instead into the fascial plane between these muscles.[15] Injury can occur from direct laceration of the nerve by the needle, from the agent being injected directly into the nerve, or from secondary scarring around the nerve. Injection injuries may be prevented by using another site for intramuscular injections, such as the quadriceps or lumbar muscles. The diagnosis is based on the history and the lack of another explanation for the deficits. Establishing a direct cause-and-effect relationship is usually difficult but may be important from a medicolegal standpoint.

Prognosis and management depend on the severity of the injury. Careful assessment of motor and sensory function determines whether both peroneal and tibial components are affected. Functionally, tibial paralysis is accommodated better. If both components are affected, sensory evaluation is important to determine whether the lesion is complete. If function remains, especially in the peroneal distribution, conservative treatment is recommended and a fairly good prognosis is given. Many of these injuries are due to neurapraxia, and function is recovered. If the lesion is complete, more aggressive treatment is indicated. Conservative treatment includes protecting the foot from injury by using a boot or splint and physical therapy to maintain muscle mass and range of motion. Boots for dogs are available from several sources, usually advertised in hunting magazines. Surgical exploration of the nerve with debridement of surrounding tissues, neurolysis, resection of neuromas, and anastomosis of the nerve segments is indicated with severe injuries.

Peroneal Nerve Injury

The peroneal nerve supplies the muscles that flex the hock and extend the digits. It provides cutaneous sensory innervation to the dorsal aspect of the foot and the cranial surface of the hock and the tibia. This nerve is subject to injury where it crosses the lateral aspect of the stifle joint. In large animals, prolonged recumbency may injure the nerve at this site. In small animals and calves, injuries usually result from intramuscular injection of drugs into or near the nerve.

The foot tends to "knuckle over," and the hock may be overextended. The cranial tibial muscle and the digital extensor muscles are atrophied in small animals. Loss of sensation occurs on the dorsal areas of the foot and the cranial surface of the hock and the tibia. The flexor reflex is severely depressed when the dorsal aspects of the foot or the digits are stimulated. Pinching the plantar surface of the digits or the foot elicits a definite pain response, and the flexor reflex is present, but the animal may not actively flex the hock joint. The examiner must exercise care in evaluating the flexor reflex because some passive flexion of the hock may occur as the stifle actively flexes. Although the foot tends to knuckle over, the dorsal surface usually does not become so severely abraded or ulcerated as it does in more proximal sciatic nerve lesions (see Figure 5-4). Dogs soon learn to place the foot by greater flexion of the hip and extension of the stifle. Transfer of tendons of muscles that are not denervated to affected muscles may be beneficial.[16] Horses reportedly have minimal gait deficits 3 months after injury.[5]

Tibial Nerve Injury

The tibial nerve supplies the muscles that extend the hock and flex the digits. It provides cutaneous sensory innervation to the plantar surface of the foot and the caudal surface of the limb. In a pure tibial nerve injury, the hock joint is dropped when the animal walks or supports weight (Figure 5-5). The gastrocnemius muscle is atrophied. Loss of sensation occurs from the plantar aspect of the foot. Large so-called trophic ulcers may develop in the digital pads of small animals because of decreased circulation over bony prominences.[17] Affected animals apparently do not move their limbs to the degree necessary to relieve soft tissue compression. The flexor reflex is severely depressed when the plantar surface of the foot is stimulated. Pinching the dorsal surface of the foot elicits a definite pain response, and the flexor reflex is present even though the toes are not flexed. Isolated tibial nerve

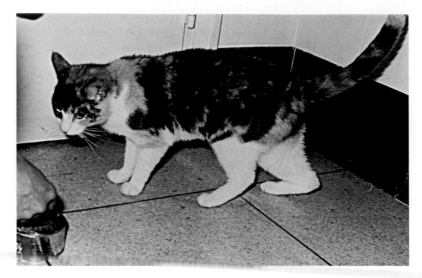

Figure 5-5 Tibial nerve paralysis in a cat resulting from an injection injury. Note the dropped hock of the right pelvic limb, a result of paralysis of the gastrocnemius muscle.

injury may follow injections into the thigh muscles. In most animals tibial nerve lesions occur in association with peroneal nerve injuries, and a mixture of neurologic signs occurs.

Femoral Nerve Injury

The femoral nerve arises from the L3-6 spinal cord segments and supplies the extensor muscles of the stifle. The major motor component is from L5.[18] The saphenous branch of the femoral nerve is the sensory pathway from the skin on the medial surface of the foot, limb, stifle, and thigh. Peripheral injuries to this nerve are not common because it is well protected. Rarely, unilateral damage restricted to the ventral gray matter of the L3-6 segments results in a neuronopathy involving the femoral nerve. Bilateral femoral nerve injury has been seen in dogs after extreme extension of the hips. With femoral nerve lesions, the stifle cannot be fixed (extended) for weight bearing. The affected animal usually carries the affected limb. Lesions involving the peripheral femoral nerve cause anesthesia in areas innervated by the saphenous nerve. Selective lesions involving the gray matter of the spinal cord produce motor dysfunction only. The knee jerk (patellar) reflex is absent or diminished; however, the flexor reflex is normal, except for decreased flexion of the hip. The hopping reaction is greatly decreased in the affected limb because weight bearing is inhibited.

In large animals, femoral nerve paralysis results in severe monoparesis. The affected limb is poorly advanced and collapses during weight bearing. In calves and foals, femoral nerve paralysis results from trauma during parturition. Forced extraction from the "hip-lock" position may hyperextend the hip and overstretches the nerve where it enters the quadriceps muscle. Incidence is increased in the heavily muscled cattle breeds.

Obturator Nerve Injury

Injuries to the obturator nerve in dogs or cats do not cause monoparesis, although the affected limb may slide laterally when the animal stands on a smooth surface. Obturator paralysis occurs most commonly during parturition in cows. The obturator nerve innervates the adductor muscles of the limb. Injuries cause marked pelvic limb ataxia, especially on slippery surfaces. The limbs may be placed in a wide-based stance that is exaggerated as the animal runs. The gait abnormality is less pronounced with unilateral lesions. Most calving injuries also damage branches of the sciatic nerve.[7]

Spinal Cord Diseases

Unilateral spinal cord lesions caudal to the T2 segment result in monoparesis. Lesions at L4-S2 cause LMN deficits, whereas those at T3-L3 cause UMN signs. Sensory deficits usually also occur. In most cases, several spinal cord segments are involved, and dysfunction affects multiple nerves (*polyneuropathy*). The most common cause is infarction caused by fibrocartilaginous embolism and other vascular-based diseases. Occasionally, spinal cord trauma, neoplasia, or, more rarely, inflammation has a unilateral distribution and produces monoparesis. Pertinent disorders that produce unilateral spinal cord lesions are discussed in the chapters on pelvic limb paresis (see Chapter 6) and tetraparesis (see Chapter 7).

MONOPARESIS OF THE THORACIC LIMBS

Peripheral Nerve Injuries

The nerves that innervate the muscles of the thoracic limbs and the clinical signs associated with injuries of these nerves are listed in Table 5-1. Proximal radial nerve injuries cause paralysis of the triceps brachii and carpal and digital extensors. Because the animal is unable to extend the elbow and carpus, it cannot bear weight or properly place the foot. The elbow also is dropped. Injury to the musculocutaneous nerve causes biceps brachii and brachialis muscle paralysis. Animals cannot flex the elbow. Paralysis of carpal flexors as a result of median and ulnar nerve injury is more subtle, causing overextension of the carpus during weight bearing.

Reflexes help to identify which muscle groups are functional. The flexor reflex is useful in assessing muscle strength and identifying partial lesions. Sensory evaluation is essential to mapping the area of decreased sensation (see Chapter 1). This section discusses injuries to the brachial plexus and radial and suprascapular nerves because injuries to these nerves are more common in clinical practice.

Avulsion of the Brachial Plexus

The nerves of the brachial plexus originate from the C6-T2 spinal cord segments (see Table 5-1). In addition, the sympathetic nerves that innervate the eye originate from neurons in the first three thoracic segments and travel along the roots of the brachial plexus as they exit the vertebral canal. Trauma that abducts and caudally displaces the thoracic limb may avulse the dorsal and ventral roots of the brachial plexus.[19-24]

Typically, the avulsion occurs intradurally at the point where the nerve roots arise from the spinal cord. Injuries of avulsion that place severe traction on the spinal cord also may damage spinal pathways. Rarely, the plexus is damaged by a direct blow to the shoulder, thus causing contusion or hemorrhage. This lesion is usually not complete.

The myotomal distribution of the ventral spinal nerve roots varies to some extent from one dog to the next so that the degree of dysfunction induced by any single root injury cannot be fully predicted. Avulsions have been broadly categorized as complete, cranial, and caudal, depending on the extent of nerve root avulsion.[20,21] Complete avulsions involve the entire plexus. In Griffiths' original classification, caudal avulsions involve the C8 and T1 nerve roots, whereas cranial avulsions involve the C6 and C7 roots.[20,21] Complete and caudal avulsions cause paralysis of the triceps brachii muscle so that affected dogs cannot extend the elbow or bear weight on the limb. Postural reactions and the flexor, extensor carpi radialis, and triceps brachii reflexes are weak or absent. The paw is knuckled over and dragged on the ground (Figure 5-6), potentially causing severe abrasion and ulceration of the dorsal surface. Dogs with caudal avulsions walk with the elbow and shoulder flexed and retain the flexor reflex. Elbow extensors are spared with cranial avulsions so that the dog can still bear weight on the limb but cannot flex the elbow or protract the limb. The supraspinatus and infraspinatus muscles are atrophied. With each form of avulsion, neurogenic muscle atrophy begins in the distribution of the denervation in about 1 week.

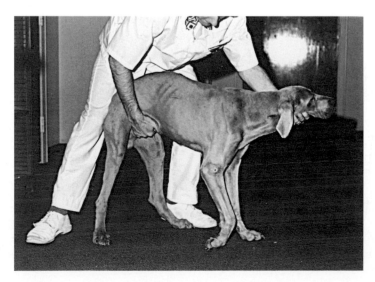

Figure 5-6 Right brachial plexus injury in a dog, a result of a car accident. Note the knuckled paw and the inability to support weight on the limb. Atrophy is present in the scapular and triceps muscles.

The pattern of sensory loss allows more critical clinical definition of the nature of the avulsion[21,22] (Figure 5-7). With complete avulsions, sensation is essentially lost distal to the elbow. Bailey[22] has provided a detailed description of sensory deficits in selected incomplete lesions. A cranial avulsion involving the C6-8 roots caused a loss of cutaneous sensation over the cranial antebrachium distal to the elbow (radial nerve), the lateral and cranial brachium overlying the humerus (axillary and brachiocephalicus nerves), and an area over the cranial aspect of the dorsal spine of the scapula (dorsal cutaneous branch of C6). Sensation over the caudal antebrachium, provided through cutaneous branches of the ulnar nerve, and a portion of the median antebrachium (musculocutaneous nerve) were spared. A caudal avulsion involving the C8 and T1 roots and the T2 communicating branch to T1 caused loss of sensation cranially and caudally over both the lateral and medial antebrachia (radial and ulnar nerves). Although pain sensation was lost over the lateral antebrachium, a sizeable medial portion retained sensation (musculocutaneous nerve). Areas innervated by cutaneous branches of the axillary and brachiocephalicus nerves over the cranial and lateral brachium also were spared.

Avulsion of the T1 ventral spinal nerve root injures preganglionic sympathetic nerve fibers, resulting in miosis of the ipsilateral pupil (partial Horner's syndrome).[20] Other features of Horner's syndrome, such as ptosis, enophthalmos, and protrusion of the membrana nictitans, occur rarely. Another feature of brachial plexus avulsion is loss of the panniculus reflex ipsilateral to the lesion. This loss occurs with either complete or caudal avulsions resulting from injury to the C8 and T1 ventral spinal nerve roots, thus interrupting lateral thoracic nerve innervation of the cutaneous trunci (panniculus carnosus) muscle. The reflex is present on the side of the body contralateral to the lesion. Avulsion injuries that place severe traction on the spinal cord also may cause damage to ascending/descending spinal pathways. This damage causes pelvic limb deficits, particularly on the ipsilateral side.

Some function may return relatively quickly when intact axons recover from temporary conduction block. The prognosis for recovery of function, however, is generally poor, particularly when elbow extensors are denervated. Corrective orthopedic procedures such as carpal arthrodesis or tendon transplantation are not indicated in these cases but may be helpful in selected cases in which the proximal branches of the radial and the musculocutaneous nerves are spared. If such surgery is contemplated, EMG should be done to ensure that the elbow extensors and muscles to be transplanted are not denervated. Affected animals often develop severe contractures and excoriations and may mutilate the limb, necessitating amputation.

Bilateral brachial plexus avulsion occurs in some animals, particularly when they have fallen from great heights and landed in a sternal position, severely abducting both thoracic limbs. Bilateral avulsion of the C5-7 nerve roots may cause diaphragmatic paralysis due to phrenic nerve involvement. Affected animals have dyspnea in addition to bilateral thoracic limb paralysis.

Suprascapular Nerve Injury

Suprascapular paralysis occurs most frequently in large animals secondary to trauma or fracture of the scapula. Severe supraspinatus and infraspinatus muscle atrophy occurs, resulting in a condition termed *sweeney*. Weight bearing is usually unaffected; however, the stride may be shortened and the shoulder may luxate laterally when weight is borne on the limb. Cattle may be injured in malfunctioning chutes or from striking the head gate

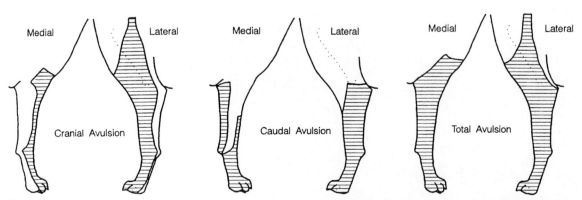

Figure 5-7 Maps of sensory loss in cranial, caudal, and total brachial plexus avulsions. (Data from Bailey CS: Patterns of cutaneous anesthesia associated with brachial plexus avulsions in the dog, *J Am Vet Med Assoc* 185:889, 1984.)

with the shoulders. Work horses may be injured from poorly fitting collars. EMG is useful to ensure that other nerves are not affected. Surgical decompression of the nerve as it passes around the cranial surface of the scapula is recommended if spontaneous improvement does not occur. Recommendations vary with early versus delayed surgery.[5] Results are probably best with exploration after about 1 month. Waiting for 3 months to ensure that spontaneous recovery does not occur is an alternative.

Contracture of the infraspinatus muscle occurs in dogs and results in thoracic limb lameness. The elbow and the antebrachium are abducted as the dog runs. The forward stride of the limb may be slightly shortened. Characteristically, the foot is moved laterally as the limb is advanced. The cause is presumed to be trauma to the muscle and possibly to the vasculature or the suprascapular nerve supplying the muscle.[25] Cutting the insertion of the infraspinatus muscle is beneficial.

Radial Nerve Injury

The entire radial nerve may be injured by fractures of the first rib. Fractures of the humerus may injure the nerve distal to the branches that supply the triceps muscle. In large animals, radial nerve injuries occur most commonly during anesthetic procedures or when the animal is in lateral recumbency on a hard surface for extended periods. Distal radial nerve injuries produce less severe gait abnormalities than do brachial plexus injuries. The elbow can be extended; however, the foot tends to knuckle over when the animal walks because the extensors of the carpus and the digits are paralyzed. Sensation is lost from the dorsal and cranial aspects of the limb distal to the elbow. Surgical exploration of the injured nerve with neurolysis or anastomosis is indicated, especially in distal radial nerve injuries. Carpal arthrodesis or transposition of a flexor tendon may be helpful. Paresthesia may lead to self-mutilation, however.

Spinal Cord Diseases

Unilateral spinal cord lesions restricted to the gray matter at C6-T2 may destroy the motor neurons of the brachial plexus, resulting in LMN monoparesis while sparing sensation, depending on the degree of involvement of the dorsal horn sensory relay neurons. Lesions at this level usually involve the motor and proprioceptive pathways to and from the ipsilateral pelvic limb, causing hemiparesis with UMN signs in the ipsilateral pelvic limb. The most common cause is infarction resulting from fibrocartilaginous embolism and other vascular-based diseases. Trauma, neoplasia, and inflammation also may cause focal spinal cord disease. Avulsion of the brachial plexus may be associated with paresis or paralysis of the ipsilateral pelvic limb if the spinal cord is compressed, contused, or otherwise damaged at the time of trauma. Spinal cord diseases are discussed in the chapters on pelvic limb paresis and tetraparesis.

PROGNOSIS

The prognosis of peripheral nerve injuries depends on the type of damage and the severity of neurologic dysfunction. Nerve fibers that have been contused, compressed, or stretched may regain function slowly. Nerves that have been lacerated or avulsed from their spinal cord attachments, however, seldom regain function. Unfortunately, in routine practice, establishing which of these situations has occurred is sometimes difficult at the initial examination. For nerve fibers to regenerate, the nerve sheath must remain intact. Compressive lesions may cause demyelination without disrupting the axon. Recovery begins in about 3 to 4 weeks and continues for 1 to 2 months. Axonal regeneration occurs slowly, at a rate of approximately 1 inch a month; however, the nerve sheath must be intact to guide the axon to the denervated muscle. The affected muscles may be reinnervated by axonal sprouting from adjacent intact neurons. Regardless of the repair process involved, return to function may take several months and may never be complete. As a general rule, reinnervation must occur in 12 months or less to be effective. Regeneration for distances greater than 12 inches is therefore unlikely.

In general, the prognosis for functional recovery of animals with severe motor dysfunction and complete anesthesia is poor. These lesions are usually severe and may involve complete disruption of nerve fibers. Some animals regain function; however, the outcome is often unsatisfactory. The prognosis is better for animals with partial loss of motor or sensory function because damage to the axons may be transitory and reinnervation from adjacent, intact nerve fibers is more predictable. In addition, animals with partial dysfunction may learn to compensate by using other, uninvolved muscle groups. In most cases, the distribution and the severity of sensory loss are the most important factors in establishing a prognosis.

If available, an EMG examination that includes nerve conduction and evoked potentials is useful for formulating a prognosis and assessing the recovery of peripheral nerve injuries. This technique helps the clinician establish the severity and distribution of nerve injury. A total lack of voluntary motor potentials, an absence of response to nerve stimulation, and evidence of diffuse denervation are highly correlated with a poor prognosis. The presence of some motor unit activity and patchy denervation suggests that the lesion is not complete and that a better chance for nerve regeneration exists. The EMG examination can be repeated periodically over several months to determine whether reinnervation is occurring. If tendon transplant surgery is contemplated, the muscle to be transplanted should be examined with EMG to ensure that denervation potentials are absent.

TREATMENT

Animals with peripheral nerve injury should be treated with glucocorticoids to relieve inflammation. The limb is immobilized to prevent further trauma. Nerve decompression or anastomosis is indicated if the site of injury is surgically accessible. Long-term management includes physical therapy to help prevent muscle atrophy and trauma to the foot. Tendon transplantation and joint arthrodesis are performed primarily for distal radial nerve and peroneal injuries in small animals.[16] The most important aspect of long-term management is probably prevention of trauma to the distal extremity. Commercially available boots that help protect the foot are easily applied by the owner and are well tolerated by the dog. Owners frequently request amputation of the affected limb because of distal extremity trauma. Generally, amputation of the limb should be delayed for 6 months unless traumatic complications cannot be prevented. This period is sufficient to determine whether nerve regeneration will occur. The owner should be warned that recovery is slow and that amputation is an irreversible solution to the problem.

Many peripheral nerve injuries can be avoided by proper management of large animals placed in lateral recumbency. Adequate padding must be provided at all times, and recumbent animals should be turned at least three times daily. Excessive traction on limbs should be avoided during anesthesia, animal movement, or fetal extraction. Injured limbs should be protected by bandages, splints, or casts. Cattle with obturator paralysis must be kept on a good surface. Hobbles on the pelvic limbs may be helpful. Recumbent animals should be supported with slings whenever possible.

PERIPHERAL NERVE TUMORS

Pathophysiology

Peripheral nerves may be affected primarily or secondarily by neoplasia. Primary nerve sheath tumors arise from Schwann's cells (schwannoma) or connective tissue surrounding the nerves (neurofibroma,

neurofibrosarcoma). These two tumors are distinguished in part because the schwannoma is encapsulated and distinct from the nerve, whereas the neurofibroma is not encapsulated and indistinct from the nerve. They are considered collectively under the term *nerve sheath tumor*.[26] Most nerve sheath tumors occur in the caudal cervical area, originating peripherally and then extending proximally to involve the spinal cord (Figure 5-8).[26,27] Tumors in the thoracolumbar area more commonly arise intradurally and compress the spinal cord initially.[27] Many tumors may secondarily involve peripheral nerves and nerve roots. Meningiomas originating at the outfoldings of meninges around the nerve roots may compress or invade the root. Bony and soft tissue tumors also may compress nerve roots or peripheral nerves. Lymphosarcoma, particularly in cats, may involve peripheral nerves and roots, especially at the brachial intumescence.[28]

Clinical Signs

Some nerve sheath tumors affect peripheral nerves in the skin and cause only disfigurement, particularly true in cattle.[29] Other tumors can involve major peripheral nerves or roots and cause monoparesis.

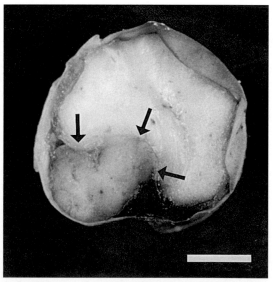

Figure 5-8 Transverse section of cervical spinal cord from a 9-year-old male Labrador retriever with progressive paraparesis and eventual cervical hyperesthesia. A compressive lesion was identified with myelography at C5-6 and a laminectomy was performed. The dog was euthanized when tumor extending to the subarachnoid space was noted. A distinct, roughly round mass is seen within the subarachnoid space ventrolateral to the C6 spinal cord segment on the left side (arrows). Schwannoma was diagnosed on histologic evaluation. Bar = 0.3 cm. (From Bagley RS, et al: Central nervous system neoplasia. In Slatter DH, editor: *Textbook of small animal surgery.* Philadelphia, 1993, WB Saunders.)

Those originating in the cervical area typically cause initial thoracic limb lameness *(nerve root signature).* Dogs are reluctant to bear weight on the involved limb and show pain when palpated. Eventually, neurologic deficits such as neurogenic muscle atrophy become more pronounced. Tumors generally are not palpable, but large masses can be identified in the axillary space in some dogs.[24] Tumors involving the brachial plexus often extend proximally to compress the spinal cord and cause deficits in the opposite limb and pelvic limbs. Cervical nerve root involvement causes loss of the ipsilateral panniculus reflex and Horner's syndrome.

Diagnosis

Nerve root neoplasia should be suspected in animals with chronic progressive monoparesis associated with neurogenic muscle atrophy and signs of nerve root signature. EMG evidence of denervation suggests neural involvement in animals with subtle neurologic deficits that otherwise might be thought to have musculoskeletal disease. Tumors that reach the vertebral canal may cause bone atrophy and enlargement of the intervertebral foramen on survey radiographs. Compression of the spinal cord causes a characteristic intradural-extramedullary pattern on myelography (also see Chapter 4).[27] The contrast material in the subarachnoid space splits at the tumor, resulting in a so-called golf-tee pattern in which the tumor is the golf ball and the dividing contrast columns are the tee. Tumors affecting the brachial plexus and paravertebral area may be detected by computed tomography.[30]

Treatment

Focal nerve sheath tumors can be resected.[31] Tumors often are invasive, however, and cannot be resected without injuring or removing portions of the involved nerve. In many cases, tumors arising in the brachial plexus have extended to other nerves by the time the diagnosis is made. Resection of tumors in the animals cannot be done without causing substantial neurologic dysfunction. Amputation is often the best option. Tumors that extend to the vertebral canal must be resected. Despite aggressive treatment, recurrence is common. Radiation and chemotherapy have no definite benefit in animals.

Case Histories

CASE HISTORY 5A

Signalment

Canine, weimaraner, male, 6 years old.

History

The dog was hit by a car 20 days ago. Since that day, he has been unable to use the right thoracic limb. He has been dragging the foot and is unable to advance the limb or bear weight. Open sores have developed on the dorsum of the foot.

Physical Examination

No abnormalities were found other than the neurologic problems described in the next section.

Neurologic Examination*

A. Observation
  1. Mental status: Alert
  2. Posture: Normal, see "Gait"
  3. Gait: Severe paresis of the right thoracic limb; drags the limb and the foot; the paw knuckles over, and the dog can bear little weight on the limb
B. Palpation: Atrophy of the triceps, supraspinatus, infraspinatus, biceps, and flexor carpi radialis muscles of the right thoracic limb
C. Postural reactions

Left	Reactions	Right
	Proprioceptive positioning	
+2	PL	+2
+2	TL	0
+2	Wheelbarrowing	0
	Hopping	
+2	PL	+2
+2	TL	0
+2	Extensor postural thrust	+2
+2	Hemistand-hemiwalk	0
	Placing, tactile	
+2	PL	+2
+2	TL	0
	Placing, visual	
+2	TL	0

D. Spinal reflexes

Left	Reflex	Right
	Spinal Segment	
	Quadriceps (L4-6)	
+2		+2
	Extensor carpi radialis (C7-T1)	
+2		0
	Triceps (C7-T1)	
+2		0

---

*0, Absent; +1, decreased; +2, normal; +3, exaggerated; +4, very exaggerated or clonus; *PL*, pelvic limb; *TL*, thoracic limb.

+2	Flexion, PL (L5-S1)	+2
+2	Flexion, TL (C6-T1)	0
0	Crossed extensor	0
+2	Perineal (S1-2)	+2

E. Cranial nerves (CN)

Left	Nerve—Function (Response/Test)	Right
+2	CN II—vision (menace)	+2
Normal +2 +2	CN II, III—pupil size (Stimulus, left eye) (Stimulus, right eye)	Constricted +2 +2
Normal	CN II—fundus	Normal
0 0	CN III, IV, VI (Strabismus) (Nystagmus)	0 0
+2	CN V—sensation	+2
Normal	CN V—mastication	Normal
Normal +2	CN VII—facial muscles (Palpebral)	Normal +2
Normal	CN IX, X—swallowing	Normal
Normal	CN XII—tongue	Normal

F. Sensation: Location
   Hyperesthesia: None
   Superficial pain: 0 right TL
   Cutaneous reflex: Absent on right
   Deep pain: 0 to +1 right TL

Complete sections G and H before reviewing the case summary.

G. Assessment (anatomic diagnosis and estimation of prognosis)
H. Plan (diagnostic)

Rule-outs	Procedure
1.	
2.	
3.	
4.	

CASE HISTORY 5B

Signalment
Canine, boxer, male, 1 year old.

History
The dog was hit by a car 10 months ago and was treated for shock and multiple pelvic fractures. He was referred 2 days after the initial injury because of severe dyspnea. Massive pleural effusion was treated with chest drains. The examination disclosed moderate paresis in the right pelvic limb and hypalgesia distal to the stifle. No treatment was given, and the dog was discharged 4 days later. He returned 10 months after the initial injury for follow-up examination, at which time no improvement in the right pelvic limb was noted.

Physical Examination
Negative except for the neurologic problems.

Neurologic Examination*

A. Observation
   1. Mental status: Alert
   2. Posture: Normal
   3. Gait: Moderate paresis of the right pelvic limb, with hyperflexion of the stifle; the paw knuckles over and the hock sinks during weight bearing; all other limbs are normal
B. Palpation: Atrophy of the cranial tibial muscle and flexors and extensors of the hock and digits; deep ulcers in the plantar surfaces of the middle two digital pads; these toes are swollen
C. Postural reactions

Left	Reactions	Right
+2 +2	Proprioceptive positioning PL TL	0 +2
+2	Wheelbarrowing	+2
+2 +2	Hopping PL TL	0 +2
+2	Extensor postural thrust	0
+2	Hemistand-hemiwalk	0
+2 +2	Placing, tactile PL TL	0 to +1 +2
+2	Placing, visual TL	+2

D. Spinal reflexes

Left	Reflex (Spinal segment)	Right
+2	Quadriceps (L4-6)	+2
+2	Extensor carpi radialis (C7-T1)	+2
+2	Triceps (C7-T1)	+2

*0, Absent; +1, decreased; +2, normal; +3, exaggerated; +4, very exaggerated or clonus; PL, pelvic limb; TL, thoracic limb.

	Reflex	
+2	Flexion, PL (L5-S1)	Flexes hip and stifle— 0 distal to stifle
+2	Flexion, TL (C6-T1)	+2
0	Crossed extensor	0
+2	Perineal (S1-2)	+2

E. Cranial nerves: Normal
F. Sensation: Location
   Hyperesthesia: None.
   Superficial pain: Blunted distal to stifle in right PL
   Deep pain: 0 from middle two digits in right Pl

Complete sections G and H before reviewing the case summary

G. Assessment (anatomic diagnosis and estimation of prognosis)
H. Plan (diagnostic)

Rule-outs	Procedure
1.	
2.	
3.	
4.	

CASE HISTORY 5C

Signalment
Feline, domestic, female, 7 years old.

History
Mild lameness was noted in the right thoracic limb 6 to 8 weeks ago. The condition has slowly worsened, and the cat now cannot bear weight on the limb. She holds the limb extended with the paw flexed and is knuckling occasionally on the right pelvic limb.

Physical Examination
Negative except for the neurologic problems.

Neurologic Examination*

A. Observation
   1. Mental status: Alert
   2. Posture: Normal
   3. Gait: Severe paresis of the right thoracic limb; the cat occasionally drags and knuckles the right pelvic paw
B. Palpation: Mild atrophy in the right scapular muscles
C. Postural reactions

Left	Reactions	Right
	Proprioceptive positioning	
+2	PL	+1
+2	TL	0

+2	Wheelbarrowing	0
	Hopping	
+2	PL	+1
+2	TL	0
+2	Extensor postural thrust	+1
+2	Hemistand-hemiwalk	0
	Placing, tactile	
+2	PL	+1
+2	TL	0
	Placing, visual	
+2	TL	0

D. Spinal reflexes

Left	Reflex (Spinal segment)	Right
+2	Quadriceps (L4-6)	+3
+2	Extensor carpi radialis (C7-T1)	0 to +1
+2	Triceps (C7-I1)	0 to +1
+2	Flexion, PL (L5-S1)	+2
+2	Flexion, TL (C6-T1)	0
0	Crossed extensor	0
+2	Perineal (S1-2)	+2

E. Cranial nerves

Left	Nerve—Function (Response/Test)	Right
+2	CN II—vision (Menace)	+2
Normal	CN II, III—pupil size	Constricted
+2	(Stimulus, left eye)	+2
+2	(Stimulus, right eye)	+2
Normal	CN II—fundus	Normal
0	CN III, IV, VI (Strabismus)	0
0	(Nystagmus)	0
Normal	CN V—sensation	Normal
Normal	CN V—mastication	Normal
Normal	CN VII—facial muscles	Normal
+2	(Palpebral)	+2

*0, Absent; +1, decreased; +2, normal; +3, exaggerated; +4, very exaggerated or clonus; *PL*, pelvic limb; *TL*, thoracic limb.

Normal	CN IX, X—swallowing	Normal
Normal	CN XII—tongue	Normal

F. Sensation: Location
    Hyperesthesia: Present in right axillary space
    Superficial pain: Normal
    Cutaneous reflex: Absent on right side
    Deep pain: Normal

Complete sections G and H before reviewing the case summary

G. Assessment (anatomic diagnosis and estimation of prognosis)
H. Plan (diagnostic)

Rule-outs	Procedure
1.	
2.	
3.	
4.	

ASSESSMENT 5A

Anatomic Diagnosis

The dog has monoparesis affecting the right thoracic limb and partial Horner's syndrome of the right eye. Lower motor neuron signs with sensory deficits in several nerves suggest a lesion of the right brachial plexus. A C6-T2 spinal cord lesion is discounted because the right pelvic limb is normal.

1. A brachial plexus injury
2. An injury to the roots of the right sympathetic nerve has caused Horner's syndrome

Diagnostic Plan (Rule-outs)

1. Caudal cervical trauma—Radiography (negative)
2. Brachial plexus injury—EMG (fibrillation potentials and positive sharp waves in several muscle groups)

Therapeutic Plan

1. Protect the foot with a boot.
2. Perform physical therapy.

Client Education

The prognosis is very poor for functional use of the limb because the nerve roots have been severely injured. Amputation may be needed in the future.

Case Summary

1. Diagnosis: Brachial plexus injury is present.
2. Result: The dog regained partial use of the limb in 6 months; however, he must wear a boot continually to protect the foot. Persistent mild pupil constriction is present in the right eye.

ASSESSMENT 5B

Anatomic Diagnosis

The dog has monoparesis of the right pelvic limb. The presence of LMN signs with sensory deficits distal to the stifle localizes the lesion to the distal sciatic nerve. A distal sciatic nerve (peroneal and tibial nerves) injury was diagnosed.

Diagnostic Plan (Rule-outs)

1. Pelvic fracture—Pelvic radiography (multiple pelvic fractures that are now healed but are displaced)
2. Injection injury—EMG (diffuse denervation distal to the stifle; few fibrillation potentials and positive sharp waves in the gastrocnemius, the semitendinosus, and the semimembranosus muscles; evidence of reinnervation in some muscles)

Therapeutic Plan

1. Physical therapy should be performed.
2. The middle two digits are infected and require antibiotic therapy.
3. A boot should be fitted on the dog to prevent further trauma.

Client Education

Because the sciatic nerve injury is partial and evidence of reinnervation is present, the dog may regain functional use of the limb.

Case Summary

One must debate the cause of the nerve injury, that is, a pelvic fracture versus a needle (injection) injury. The neurologic examination is more consistent with the diagnosis of a needle (injection) injury because nerve damage usually occurs at the origin of the peroneal and the tibial nerves in the area caudal to the femur. The EMG, however, provides evidence that the lesion is more proximal. Denervation of the semitendinosus and semimembranosus muscles probably is a result of the pelvic fractures because these muscles are rarely affected by injections in the thigh muscles.

Final Diagnosis

Sciatic nerve injury from a pelvic fracture.

Result

The dog regained good use of the limb, and the boot eventually was removed.

ASSESSMENT 5C

Anatomic Diagnosis

Lower motor neuron signs are present in the right thoracic limb, and UMN signs are present in the right pelvic limb. In addition, mild Horner's syndrome is present in the right eye. A unilateral right C6-T3 spinal cord lesion would explain these signs. The history suggests that the lesion may have begun in the brachial plexus and moved proximally.

Diagnostic Plan (Rule-outs)

1. Neoplasia—Radiology (survey films negative), myelography (intradural-extramedullary mass at the right side of the cord at the C7-T1 intervertebral space)
2. Inflammation—Cerebrospinal fluid (CSF) tap (0 cells, 20 mg/dl protein)

Therapeutic Plan

Administer dexamethasone to help relieve spinal cord edema. Surgical removal may be possible but probably will cause denervation of the limb, requiring amputation.

Case Summary

A nerve sheath tumor of the right brachial plexus is the most likely diagnosis causing spinal cord compression of C6, C7, C8, and T1. The history is typical for a primary nerve sheath tumor or secondary tumor such as lymphosarcoma involving the brachial plexus.

【F:

References

1. Bailey CS, Kitchell RL: Clinical evaluation of the cutaneous innervation of the canine thoracic limb, *J Am Anim Hosp Assoc* 20:939-950, 1984.
2. Haghighi SS, Kitchell RL, Johnson RD, et al: Electrophysiologic studies of the cutaneous innervation of the pelvic limb of male dogs, *Am J Vet Res* 52:352-362, 1991.
3. Bailey CS, Kitchell RL: Cutaneous sensory testing in the dog, *J Vet Intern Med* 1:128-135, 1987.
4. Bennett GJ: An animal model of neuropathic pain: A review, *Muscle Nerve* 16:1040-1048, 1993.
5. Mayhew IG: *Large animal neurology: A handbook for veterinary clinicians.* Philadelphia, 1989, Lea & Febiger.
6. Chambers J, Hardie E: Localization and management of sciatic nerve injury due to ischial or acetabular fracture, *J Am Anim Hosp Assoc* 22:539-544, 1986.
7. Cox V, Breazile J, Hoover T: Surgical and anatomic study of calving paralysis, *Am J Vet Res* 36:427-430, 1975.
8. Walker T: Ischiadic nerve entrapment, *J Am Vet Med Assoc* 178:1284-1288, 1981.
9. Palmer RH, Aron DN, Purinton PT: Relationship of femoral intramedullary pins to the sciatic nerve and gluteal muscles after retrograde and normograde insertion, *Vet Surg* 17:65-70, 1988.
10. Fanton J, Blass C, Withrow S: Sciatic nerve injury as a complication of intramedullary pin fixation of femoral fractures, *J Am Anim Hosp Assoc* 19:687-694, 1983.
11. Jacobson A, Schrader SC: Peripheral nerve injury associated with fracture-dislocation of the pelvis in dogs and cats: 34 cases (1979-1982), *J Am Vet Med Assoc* 190:569-572, 1987.
12. Stanton ME, Weigel JP, Henry RE: Ischiatic nerve paralysis associated with the biceps femoris sling: Case report and anatomical study, *J Am Anim Hosp Assoc* 24:429-432, 1988.
13. Sorjonen DC, et al: Hip dysplasia with bilateral ischiatic nerve entrapment in a dog, *J Am Vet Med Assoc* 197:495-497, 1990.
14. Cockshutt JR, Smith-Maxie LL: Delayed onset sciatic impairment following triple pelvic osteotomy, *Prog Vet Neurol* 4:60-63, 1993.
15. Autefage A, Fayolle P, Toutain P-L: Distribution of material injected intramuscularly in dogs, *Am J Vet Res* 51:901-904, 1990.
16. Bennett D, Vaughan LC: The use of muscle relocation techniques in the treatment of peripheral nerve injuries in dogs and cats, *J Small Anim Pract* 17:99-108, 1976.
17. Read RA: Probable trophic pad ulceration following traumatic denervation: Report of two cases in dogs, *Vet Surg* 15:40-44, 1986.
18. Wilson J: Relationship of the patellar tendon reflex to the ventral branch of the fifth lumbar spinal nerve in the dog, *Am J Vet Res* 39:1774-1777, 1978.
19. Griffiths IR: Avulsion of the brachial plexus, 1: Neuropathology of the spinal cord and peripheral nerves, *J Small Anim Pract* 15:165-176, 1974.
20. Griffiths IR, Duncan ID, Lawson DD: Avulsion of the brachial plexus, 2: Clinical aspects, *J Small Anim Pract* 15:177-182, 1974.
21. Griffiths IR: Avulsion of the brachial plexus in the dog, In Kirk RW, editor: *Current veterinary therapy, vol VI: Small animal practice,* Philadelphia, 1977, WB Saunders.
22. Bailey C: Patterns of cutaneous anesthesia associated with brachial plexus avulsions in the dog, *J Am Vet Med Assoc* 185:889-899, 1984.
23. Steinberg HS: Brachial plexus injuries and dysfunctions, *Vet Clin North Am* 18:565-580, 1988.
24. Wheeler S, Jones C, Wright J: The diagnosis of brachial plexus disorders in dogs: A review of twenty-two cases, *J Small Anim Pract* 27:147-157, 1986.
25. Bennett R: Contracture of the infraspinatus muscle in dogs: A review of 12 cases, *J Am Anim Hosp Assoc* 22:481-487, 1986.
26. Braund KG: Neoplasia. In Oliver JE, Hoerlein BF, Mayhew IG, editors: *Veterinary neurology,* Philadelphia, 1987, WB Saunders.
27. Bradley RL, Withrow SJ, Snyder SP: Nerve sheath tumors in the dog, *J Am Anim Hosp Assoc* 18:915-921, 1982.
28. Lane SB, et al: Feline spinal lymphosarcoma: A retrospective evaluation of 24 cases, *J Vet Intern Med* 8:99-104, 1994.
29. de Lahunta A: *Veterinary neuroanatomy and clinical neurology,* ed 2. Philadelphia, 1983, WB Saunders.
30. McCarthy RJ, Feeney DA, Lipowitz AJ: Preoperative diagnosis of tumors of the brachial plexus by computed tomography in three dogs, *J Am Vet Med Assoc* 202:291-294, 1993.
31. Bailey CS: Long-term survival after surgical excision of a schwannoma of the sixth cervical spinal nerve in a dog, *J Am Vet Med Assoc* 196:754-756, 1990.

Pelvic Limb Paresis, Paralysis, or Ataxia

Bilateral motor dysfunction of the pelvic limbs is termed *paraparesis* or *paraplegia*, depending on the severity of the motor loss. Loss of proprioception from the pelvic limbs results in sensory ataxia. In addition, loss of pain perception from the pelvic limbs may accompany the motor dysfunction. Lesion localization has been discussed in Chapter 2 and is summarized in Figure 6-1. A brief review follows.

LESION LOCALIZATION

Animals with pure pelvic limb paresis and ataxia have neurologic disease caudal to the second thoracic spinal cord segment. Lesions in the region of T3-L3 produce paraparesis of the upper motor neuron (UMN) type. The pelvic limb lower motor neurons (LMNs), located in segments L4-S2, remain intact and are capable of reflex motor activity; however, voluntary motor control from the brain is lost because the motor pathways in the spinal cord are damaged. The spinal reflexes are normal or exaggerated. Exaggerated reflexes result when UMN inhibitory influence on the LMNs is lost. Similarly, extensor hypertonus also may develop. Ataxia results from damage to the spinal cord proprioceptive pathways, which transmit position sense signals from receptors in the pelvic limbs to the brain. Hypalgesia or analgesia distal to the lesion results from disruption of pain pathways from the pelvic limbs to the brain. Deep pain sensation is lost only if the lesions are bilateral and severe. Voluntary visceral functions (see Chapter 3) such as micturition may be lost when motor or sensory pathways in the spinal cord are damaged. Muscle atrophy from disuse may develop with time.

In summary, spinal cord lesions in the region of T3-L3 result in paresis, ataxia, decreased or absent postural reactions, normal reflexes or hyperreflexia, impaired micturition, and variable degrees of sensory loss caudal to the lesion. Examination of the thoracolumbar dermatomes may be helpful in the localization of lesions to spinal segments within this spinal cord region (see Chapter 2).

Lesions in the area of L4-S2 or those that involve the cauda equina produce pelvic limb paresis of the LMN type. Lesions involving spinal cord segments of L4-S2 injure the motor neurons that form the lumbosacral plexus. Abnormalities related to femoral, sciatic, pudendal, and pelvic nerves are encountered in these patients. Pelvic limb reflexes are depressed or absent, and the muscles may be hypotonic. Neurogenic muscle atrophy develops. Sensory dysfunction (ataxia, hypalgesia, analgesia) results from an injury to the sensory neurons and the nerve fibers located in this region of the spinal cord. Abnormalities of visceral function result from an injury to the motor and sensory neurons that innervate the bladder and the anus. Lesions involving the caudal segments of the spinal cord and the cauda equina damage nerve fibers that form the sciatic, pudendal, pelvic, and caudal nerves. Because the femoral nerve is spared, the animal is able to support weight on the pelvic limbs. The knee-jerk reflex is normal, and pain is perceived from the medial digit and the thigh. The clinical signs are related to motor and sensory dysfunction of the involved nerves. Figure 6-2 summarizes lesion localization for the problem of pelvic limb paresis based on motor signs.

DISEASES

The disorders or diseases that affect the spinal cord segments T3-L3 are classified in Tables 6-1 through 6-3. Disorders that affect spinal cord segments L4-S2 and the cauda equina are presented in Tables 6-4 through 6-6. These tables are organized according to the logic used in the formulation of a neurologic diagnosis, discussed in Chapter 1. After the lesion has been localized to a region or segment of the spinal cord or nerve root, consideration is given to the possible etiologic categories that could produce the lesion. The etiologic categories are

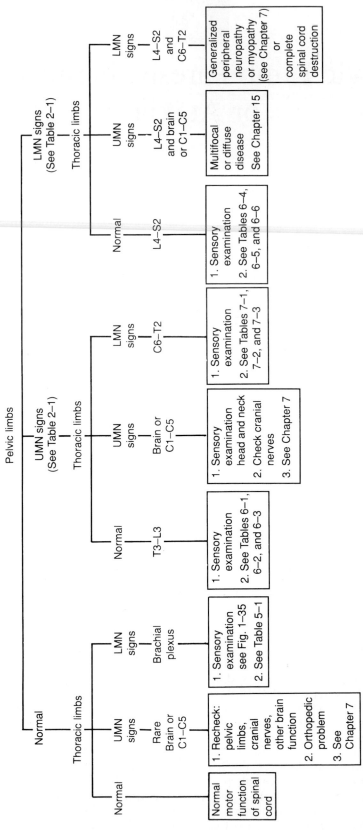

Figure 6-1 Localization of lesions based on motor function. *UMN,* Upper motor neuron; *LMN,* lower motor neuron; *C,* cervical; *T,* thoracic; *L,* lumbar; *S,* sacral. (From Hoerlein BF: *Canine neurology: diagnosis and treatment,* ed 3. Philadelphia, 1978, WB Saunders.)

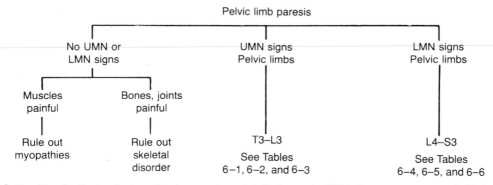

Figure 6-2 Algorithm for the localization of lesions causing pelvic limb paresis. *UMN,* Upper motor neuron; *LMN,* lower motor neuron.

Table 6-1 **Small Animal Thoracolumbar Spinal Cord Diseases: Differential Diagnosis of T3-L3 Spinal Cord Disease Based on Clinical Course and Etiologic Categories***

Etiologic Category	Acute Nonprogressive	Acute Progressive	Chronic Progressive
Degenerative	None	Type I disk disease (6) Hemorrhagic myelomalacia (6)	Type II disk disease (6) Degenerative myelopathy (6) Spondylosis deformans (6) Afghan Hound myelopathy (6) Demyelinating diseases (7) Neuronopathies (7)
Anomalous	None	None	Spinal dysraphism (6) Vertebral anomalies (6)
Metabolic	None	None	Endocrine neuropathies (8)
Neoplastic (6)	None	Metastatic Primary Skeletal Lymphoreticular	Primary Lymphoreticular Skeletal Metastatic
Nutritional	None	None	Hypervitaminosis A (cats) (15)
Inflammatory	None	Distemper myelitis (15) Bacterial myelitis (15) Diskospondylitis (6) Protozoal myelitis (15) Mycotic myelitis (15)	Feline infectious peritonitis (15) Distemper myelitis (15) Granulomatous meningoencephalomyelitis (15) Immune meningoencephalomyelitis (15)
Toxic	None	None	Various neuropathies (7,15)
Traumatic	Fractures (6) Luxations (6) Contusions (6) Intervertebral disk rupture (6)	Hemorrhagic myelomalacia (6) Intervertebral disk rupture (6)	None
Vascular	Fibrocartilaginous embolism (6) Aortic thromboem- bolism (6)	None	None

*Numbers in parentheses refer to chapters in which the entities are discussed.

Table 6-2   **Equine Thoracolumbar Spinal Cord Diseases: Differential Diagnosis of T3-L3 Spinal Cord Disease Based on Clinical Course and Etiologic Categories***

Etiologic Category	Acute Nonprogressive	Acute Progressive	Chronic Progressive
Degenerative	None	Degenerative myeloencephalopathy (7)	Spondylosis deformans (6) Neuronopathies (7) Demyelinating diseases (7) Axonopathies (7)
Anomalous	None	None	Vertebral anomalies (6) Spinal dysraphism (6)
Neoplastic (6)	None	Metastatic Primary Skeletal Lymphoreticular	Primary Skeletal Lymphoreticular
Inflammatory	None	Herpesvirus 1 (6) Protozoal myelitis (6) Verminous migration (6) Vertebral osteomyelitis (6) Mycotic myelitis (6)	See acute progressive
Toxic	None	None	Various neuropathies (7, 15)
Traumatic	Fractures (6) Luxations (6)	None	None
Vascular	Embolic myelopathy (6) Fibrocartilaginous emboli (6) Post-anesthetic myelopathy	None	None

*Numbers in parentheses refer to chapters in which the entities are discussed.

listed in the left-hand column of these tables and follow the DAMNIT scheme described in Table 1-4. The diseases are further divided into acute progressive, acute nonprogressive, and chronic progressive categories based on historical information or on the clinical course of the illness. Most diseases have been included in the tables. The most important disorders are described in subsequent sections of this chapter. They are reviewed briefly with an emphasis on diagnosis and treatment. Some diseases are discussed in other chapters, as noted in the tables.

Acute Progressive Diseases, T3-L3

Thoracolumbar Intervertebral Disk Disease

Intervertebral disk disease is one of the most common disorders that produces paraparesis in the dog. Disk disease occurs in about 2% of canine patients seen at teaching hospitals.[1] It is rarely a problem in cats, horses, or food animals. Degenerative changes within the disk can cause protrusion or herniation of the nucleus pulposus into the vertebral canal. Basically, two types of disk degeneration that result in different clinical syndromes have been described (Figure 6-3). Hansen type I disk

degeneration occurs primarily in the chondrodystrophoid (hypochondroplastic) breeds (small poodle, dachshund, beagle, cocker spaniel, Pekingese, or mixed chondrodystrophoid breeds). Type I degeneration develops when the animal is young (i.e., 2 to 9 months of age); clinical signs are present by the time the animal is 3 to 6 years of age.[2] The disk degeneration is basically a chondroid metaplasia of the nucleus pulposus with degeneration and weakening of the annulus fibrosus.

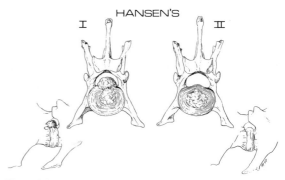

Figure 6-3 Drawings of Hansen type I and type II disk protrusions. (From Hoerlein BF: *Canine neurology: diagnosis and treatment,* ed 3. Philadelphia, 1978, WB Saunders.)

Table 6-3 **Food Animal Thoracolumbar Spinal Cord Diseases: Differential Diagnosis of T3-L3 Spinal Cord Disease Based on Clinical Course and Etiologic Categories**[*]

Etiologic Category	Acute Nonprogressive	Acute Progressive	Chronic Progressive
Degenerative	None	None	Progressive ataxia of Charolais cattle—B (7) Degenerative myeloencephalopathy—B (7) Spondylosis deformans—All (6) Arthrogryposis—All (7) Demyelinating diseases—B (7) Neuronopathies—O (7)
Anomalous	None	None	Spinal dysraphism—All (6) Vertebral anomalies—All (6)
Neoplastic (6)	None	Metastatic Primary Skeletal Lymphoreticular	Primary Lymphoreticular Skeletal Metastatic
Nutritional	None	None	Enzootic ataxia, copper deficiency—C, O (15)
Inflammatory	None	Caprine arthritis-encephalomyelitis—C (6) Bacterial myelitis—All (15) Vertebral osteomyelitis—All (6) Protozoal myelitis (15) Mycotic myelitis (15)	Visna-Maedi—O (15) Verminous migration—All (6)
Toxic	None	None	Various neuropathies (7, 15)
Traumatic	Fractures (6) Luxations (6) Contusions (6)	None	None
Vascular	Fibrocartilaginous embolism—B (6) Aortic thromboembolism—B (6)	None	None

[*]Numbers in parentheses refer to chapters in which the entities are discussed.
B, Bovine; *C,* caprine; *O,* ovine; *P,* porcine.

Calcification of the degenerative disk commonly occurs and is radiographically apparent in affected dachshunds at 6 to 18 months of age.[2] The weakened annulus cannot restrain the degenerative nucleus, and normal movements of the vertebral column are sufficient to initiate acute disk prolapse. These extrusions of disk material result primarily in an acute focal compressive myelopathy. In some cases a severe progressive myelopathy, known as *ascending-descending myelomalacia,* follows acute "blowouts" of the nuclear material.[3]

Hansen type II disk degeneration occurs in nonchondrodystrophoid breeds, such as German shepherd dogs and Labrador retrievers.[1] Type II degeneration develops at a slower rate, and clinical signs occur when the animal is 5 to 12 years of age. The disk degeneration is basically a fibroid metaplasia that can result in the gradual protrusion of disk material contained within an intact, but degenerate, annulus. True extrusion of free nuclear material into the epidural space does not occur. Compression from this protrusion results in a slowly progressive focal myelopathy. This syndrome is discussed in the section on chronic progressive spinal cord disorders.

Compressive myelopathy has been attributed primarily to the mechanical derangement of nerve tissue and hypoxic changes resulting from pressure on the vascular system in the spinal cord. Vascular factors that result in ischemia and edema undoubtedly play a role in the development of more severe spinal cord degeneration and the syndrome of ascending-descending myelomalacia. The severity of the spinal cord lesion is influenced by the magnitude of the protrusion and its rate of development. The inflammatory reaction induced by the

Table 6-4   **Small Animal Lumbosacral and Cauda Equina Diseases: Differential Diagnosis of L4-S3 and Caudal Spinal Cord Disease Based on Clinical Courses and Etiologic Categories**[*]

Etiologic Category	Acute Nonprogressive	Acute Progressive	Chronic Progressive
Degenerative	None	Type I disk disease (6) Hemorrhagic myelomalacia (6)	Type II disk disease (6) Degenerative myelopathy (6) Degenerative lumbosacral stenosis (6) Spondylosis deformans (6) Neuronopathies (7)
Anomalous	None	None	Spinal dysraphism (6) Vertebral anomalies (6)
Metabolic	None	None	Endocrine neuropathies (7)
Neoplastic (6)	None	Metastatic Primary Skeletal Lymphoreticular	Primary Lymphoreticular Skeletal Metastatic
Inflammatory	None	Distemper myelitis (15) Bacterial myelitis (15) Diskospondylitis (6) Protozoal myelitis (15) Mycotic myelitis (15)	Feline infectious peritonitis (15) Distemper myelitis (15) Granulomatous meningoencephalomyelitis (15) Immune meningoencephalomyelitis (15) Postvaccinal rabies
Toxic	None	None	Various neuropathies (7, 15)
Traumatic	Fractures (6) Luxations (6) Contusions (6) Intervertebral disk rupture (6)	Hemorrhagic myelomalacia (6) Intervertebral disk rupture (6)	None
Vascular	Fibrocartilaginous embolism (6) Aortic thromboembolism (6)	None	None

[*]Numbers in parentheses refer to chapters in which the entities are discussed.

extruded material and the diameter of the vertebral canal are also related to the severity of the clinical signs. Acute protrusions produce more severe spinal cord lesions than do chronic progressive protrusions. Less severe lesions occur in areas where the vertebral canal is large (e.g., the cervical area). Changes progress from edema, demyelination, and necrosis of myelin and axons to myelomalacia.

Ascending-descending myelomalacia has an unknown pathogenesis, but vascular lesions leading to severe ischemia probably are important. This syndrome follows severe acute spinal cord trauma of any cause and results in nearly complete nervous tissue destruction. The clinical signs result from necrosis of the motor neurons and the sensory fibers. LMN signs develop in the muscles supplied by the affected spinal cord segments. Analgesia develops caudal to the cranial edge of the lesion. This syndrome should be suspected in all animals that develop ascending or descending signs of LMN dysfunction and ascending analgesia after spinal trauma and severe compression. Affected animals usually die of respiratory failure 2 to 4 days after the onset of clinical signs. The lesion is irreparable, and euthanasia should be performed on affected animals to prevent needless suffering.

Clinical Signs. In addition to the signs of paresis or paralysis that characterize spinal cord lesions, the extruded material irritates the nerve roots and the meninges, resulting in severe pain and hyperesthesia when the vertebral column is manipulated. An animal may arch its back and tense its abdominal muscles/motions that are suggestive of acute abdominal disorders such as pancreatitis. Sensory examinations, such as pinching the skin and palpating the vertebrae, are important because they allow the clinician to localize the lesion to two or three spinal cord segments. Lesions that affect

Table 6-5   **Equine Lumbosacral and Cauda Equina Diseases: Differential Diagnosis of L4-S2 and Caudal Disease Based on Clinical Course and Etiologic Categories***

Etiologic Category	Acute Nonprogressive	Acute Progressive	Chronic Progressive
Degenerative	None	None	Spondylosis deformans (6) Neuronopathies (7) Demyelinating diseases (7) Axonopathies (7)
Anomalous	None	None	Vertebral anomalies (6) Spinal dysraphism (6)
Neoplastic (6)	None	Metastatic Primary Skeletal Lymphoreticular	Primary Skeletal Lymphoreticular
Inflammatory	None	Herpesvirus 1 (6) Protozoal myelitis (6) Verminous migration (6) Vertebral osteomyelitis (6) Mycotic myelitis (6)	Neuritis of the cauda equina (6) (see also acute progressive)
Toxic	None	None	Various neuropathies (7, 15) Sorghum cystitis (6)
Traumatic	Fractures (6) Luxations (6) Postfoaling paralyses (5)	None	None
Vascular	Embolic myelopathy (6) Fibrocartilaginous emboli (6) Post-anesthetic myelopathy	None	None

*Numbers in parentheses refer to chapters in which the entities are discussed.

the superficial pain pathways abolish the panniculus reflex caudal to the lesion. This reflex is normally most apparent when the skin over the thoracolumbar junction is stimulated. Students incorrectly believe that this apparent exaggeration of the skin twitch represents hyperesthesia and thus correlates with lesion location. Hyperesthesia is an exaggerated cerebral response to painful stimuli. Cooperative animals that cry out or try to bite when an area is palpated or pinched may be experiencing hyperesthesia, and the lesion is usually one or two segments cranial to the point at which the response was induced. In animals that are analgesic in the pelvic limbs, the point of analgesia along the spine should be found. The lesion is usually one or two segments cranial to the point at which the animal first feels painful stimuli.

Thoracolumbar disk disease may develop at intervertebral disk spaces T9-10 to L7-S1. The intercapital ligament usually prevents protrusion of the cranial and midthoracic disks. More than 65% of disk protrusions occur at sites T11-12, T12-13, T13-L1, and L1-2. These areas should be evaluated carefully in animals with suspected thoracolumbar disk disease. Less frequently, disk protrusions occur in sites caudal to L3-4. Protrusions at these

sites produce LMN signs in the pelvic limbs because the compressive myelopathy affects the motor neurons that form the lumbosacral plexus. These cases can be differentiated from those of descending myelomalacia as the result of a more cranial lesion by the location of hyperesthesia or the cranial level of decreased sensation.

Animals that develop progressive myelomalacia have ascending or descending signs of progressive LMN dysfunction and ascending levels of analgesia. Typically, affected dogs develop hypotonic abdominal muscles and hypotonic, areflexic pelvic limbs. The anus may be dilated, and the perineal reflex is weak or absent. The bladder is usually distended and easily expressed because of poor tone in the urethral sphincter.

Ascending signs of LMN paralysis include a loss of intercostal respirations and an inability to remain sternal because of paralysis of the paraspinal muscles. The thoracic limbs may be rigidly extended, and hyperesthesia may develop in the feet a few hours before the necrosis affects the lower cervical cord. Animals die of respiratory failure when the necrosis ascends to the level of the fifth and sixth cervical cord segments and thus destroys the neurons of the phrenic nerves. This

Table 6-6   **Food Animal Lumbosacral and Cauda Equina Diseases: Differential Diagnosis of L4-S3 and Caudal Disease Based on Clinical Course and Etiologic Categories**[*]

Etiologic Category	Acute Nonprogressive	Acute Progressive	Chronic Progressive
Degenerative	None	None	Spondylosis deformans—All (6)
			Arthrogryposis—All (7)
			Neuronopathies—0 (7)
Anomalous	None	None	Spinal dysraphism—All (6)
			Vertebral anomalies—All (6)
Neoplastic (6)	None	Metastatic	Primary
		Primary	Lymphoreticular
		Skeletal	Skeletal
		Lymphoreticular	Metastatic
Nutritional	None	None	Enzootic ataxia, copper deficiency—C, O (15)
Inflammatory	None	Bacterial myelitis—All (15)	Verminous migration—All (6)
		Vertebral osteomyelitis—All (7)	
		Protozoal myelitis—All (15)	
		Mycotic myelitis—All (15)	
Toxic	None	None	Various neuropathies (7, 15)
Traumatic	Fractures (6)	None	None
	Luxations (6)		
	Contusions (6)		
	Postcalving paralyses—B (5)		
Vascular	Fibrocartilaginous embolism—B (6)	None	None
	Aortic thromboembolism—B (6)		

[*]Numbers in parentheses refer to chapters in which the entities are discussed.
B, Bovine; C, caprine; O, ovine; P, porcine.

syndrome apparently occurs with greatest frequency in dogs that develop acute paralysis and sensory loss. Owners should be warned of this possibility, particularly in cases in which surgical therapy is contemplated.

Diagnosis. A tentative diagnosis of thoracolumbar disk disease is based on assessment of the clinical signs, knowledge of the typical breed involvement, and results of the neurologic evaluation. For example, an animal with asymmetric paresis and little hyperesthesia is more likely to have an infarct than a compressive lesion from a disk. The diagnosis can be confirmed by a conventional radiographic examination, but myelographic examination of the spine is usually required for surgical intervention. Figures 6-4 through 6-6 demonstrate diagnostic lesions observed on survey radiographs of the spine. General anesthesia is required for making diagnostic spinal radiographs. In our hospitals, radiographs are taken when the animal is treated surgically.

For cases treated by conservative medical procedures, radiographs are not routinely made unless another disease, such as diskospondylitis, is to be excluded. The expense and risk of anesthesia in a dog that probably has this disease are difficult to justify if medical therapy is contemplated. Survey radiographic changes include a narrowing of the intervertebral disk space, a narrowing of the articular space, and a smaller intervertebral foramen with some increase in density in the foramen as compared with adjacent spaces. Myelography is required to determine the site of the compression, particularly if the survey radiographs suggest several potential sites. Myelographic changes are consistent with an extradural compression, although if significant spinal cord swelling is present, the column of contrast agent may be absent for some distance. Surgeons should require myelography for all disk problems to be certain of the lesion site, to increase the probability of identifying the side of the protrusion, and to rule out other diseases. In some hospitals, magnetic resonance imaging (MRI) and computed tomography (CT) may be useful to document more obscure disk herniations.

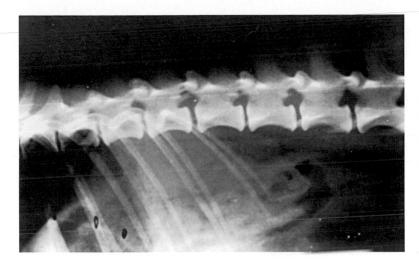

Figure 6-4 Lateral thoracolumbar radiograph showing narrowing of the intervertebral space, intervertebral foramen, and articular space between the facets at L1-2, a common radiographic lesion in type I intervertebral disk disease.

Treatment. Many dogs with intervertebral disk disease respond at least temporarily to attentive nursing care that promotes the spontaneous healing processes. Because of this finding, citing clear-cut evidence of the superiority of one therapy over another is extremely difficult. The major treatment controversy centers on the benefit of surgery versus conservative medical management. In addition, the relative benefits of the various surgical procedures are still being debated. In comparing any treatment protocols, the severity and duration of the problem must be recognized as critical factors in recovery, regardless of treatment.[1] When those factors are constant, the literature is reasonably clear on appropriate treatment. Table 6-7 summarizes the indications for treatment and the forms of management currently recommended.

Medical Therapy. Medical therapy is indicated for animals that experience an initial episode of mild neurologic dysfunction or pain or for those that have other medical problems precluding surgery. Therapy should support the normal healing processes but not totally relieve pain or totally inhibit the beneficial inflammatory process induced by the extruded disk material. Analgesics and antiinflammatory drugs can be used but only if strict confinement is possible. Total relief of pain may allow overactivity of the animal, which could result in further disk extrusion and rapidly worsening clinical signs. The most important aspect of therapy is enforced cage rest, preferably under direct veterinary supervision.

Animals should not be confined in baby cribs or playpens because to do so encourages the animal to jump in attempt to get out. Confinement at home should be in a small pet crate placed in a quiet room where the animal will not be disturbed. The animal should be exercised twice a day on a leash,

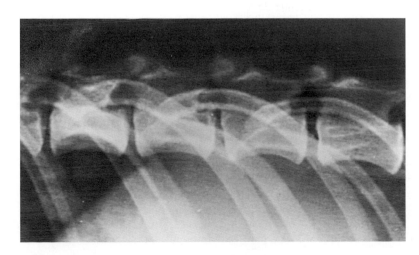

Figure 6-5 Lateral thoracolumbar radiograph showing wedging of the intervertebral space at T12-13. This is another radiographic lesion indicative of disk protrusion.

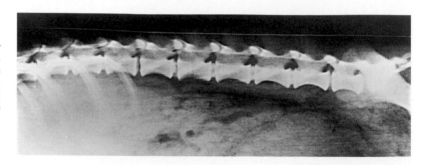

Figure 6-6 Lateral thoracolumbar radiograph showing numerous calcified disks. The active site of disease is L1-2, where the disk space is narrowed. Calcified disks in situ seldom cause active disease but are likely to herniate later.

away from other dogs or cats. Analgesics or other antiinflammatory drugs should be used at home only when the client agrees to cooperate fully with the instructions for strict cage rest. The most common mistake made by veterinarians is to administer corticosteroids without exercise restriction. Predictably, these animals return in 36 to 48 hours with severe neurologic signs. Generally, dogs should be hospitalized for 1 week. Prednisone, 0.5 mg per kilogram of body weight, is given every 12 hours for 72 hours and then discontinued. Nonsteroidal antiinflammatory drugs (NSAIDs) can then be administered as needed. The animal is sent home with instructions for cage confinement of 3 weeks' duration. If satisfactory progress is made, exercise is restricted to a leash for an

additional 3 weeks. If followed closely, these procedures result in considerable improvement; however, the owner must be aware that further attacks may occur and that the recurrence may be severe. If the animal's signs deteriorate at any time, surgery should be performed immediately. Pain and its control are described in Chapter 14.

Paralyzed animals that have lost deep pain sensation for 48 hours or longer have a grave prognosis (less than a 5% chance for recovery) with or without surgery. The absence of deep pain perception represents a severe, usually irreparable spinal cord injury. Unless the owner definitely wants to try surgery in the face of these odds, the animal should be treated medically. Even with intense therapy, the prognosis is grave. Methylprednisolone sodium succinate (MPSS), 30 mg/kg, is given intravenously (IV) on presentation, followed by a continuous infusion of 5 mg/kg per hour for 24 hours. Other corticosteroids do not have the same effect (see Chapter 12 for a complete discussion of the use of corticosteroids in central nervous system [CNS] trauma). Mannitol, 0.5 g/kg, may also be given. Steroids are not given after 24 hours. They are not likely to be of benefit unless administration is started within a few hours of the onset of the injury to the spinal cord. Physical therapy then is initiated. Euthanasia is indicated for an animal that shows no improvement in clinical signs within 3 weeks. Corticosteroid therapy, if continued longer than 5 to 7 days, can result in gastrointestinal ulceration and can aggravate urinary tract infection in dogs with urine retention from a paralyzed detrusor muscle. Chemonucleolysis with chymopapain and collagenase has been used experimentally and clinically in dogs with disk disease.[4] Controlled studies of the overall effect are lacking, and the procedure is not recommended for most dogs with signs of spinal cord compression.

Surgical Therapy. The various forms of surgical therapy have been reviewed extensively by Hoerlein.[1] General agreement exists that disk fenestration may benefit some animals with recurrent pain and minimal spinal cord compression.

Table 6-7   Treatment of Thoracolumbar Intervertebral Disk Herniation

Therapy	Indications Based on History and Clinical Signs
Medical	Pain only—first episode
	Mild ataxia and paresis—first episode
	Medical condition precludes surgery
	Paralyzed—deep pain response absent ≥48 h
	Progressive myelomalacia
Surgical	Multiple episodes of pain only
Fenestration only	Paresis and ataxia—second episode
Decompression (hemilaminectomy) with fenestration	No improvement or deterioration of signs with medical therapy
	Moderate paresis or paralysis, deep pain response present—first episode
	Paralysis, deep pain response absent <48 h (very guarded prognosis)

Although no decompression occurs, fenestration helps to prevent further protrusion. This surgical procedure may also produce an acute inflammatory process that stimulates phagocytosis (the resorption of necrotic disk material) and the formation of fibrosis, which helps to stabilize the disk. Although these animals may have minimal signs of spinal cord compression, myelographic studies often identify considerable extrusion of disk material. These cases are best treated with surgical decompression, as described in the next section.

Percutaneous laser disk ablation has been successfully used as a replacement for surgical disk fenestration.[5,6] It is indicated for dogs that have multiple episodes of pain and no evidence of spinal cord compression. Using fluoroscopy, hypodermic needles are placed in the nucleus of the disk and a holmium-yttrium-aluminum-garnet laser is guided through the needle into the disk. Bartels and colleagues[6] reported on the outcome and complications associated with prophylactic percutaneous laser disk ablation in dogs. Of 277 dogs treated, only five developed complications in the perioperative period. These researchers contacted 262 owners 1 to 85 months after the procedure; 76% of these owners indicated that their dogs were immediately improved, 22% indicated their dogs were the same, 2% indicated their dogs were worse, and 81% reported their dogs had not had any recurrence of thoracolumbar disk disease.

In dogs with moderate to severe paresis and ataxia, decompressive surgery should be performed immediately. This recommendation is supported by several clinical and experimental studies that compared the speed and duration of spinal cord compression with the rate of recovery. Tarlov and co-workers demonstrated that acute spinal cord compression with a force sufficient to produce complete sensorimotor paralysis results in complete recovery if the compression is less than 2 hours in duration.[7,8] Furthermore, the rate of recovery in Tarlov's study correlated directly with the duration of compression. After 10 minutes of acute compression, 2 to 3 days were required for initial improvement in neurologic function. With 50 to 120 minutes of acute compression, 20 to 30 days were required for initial improvement. Gradual compression of the spinal cord was better tolerated, and irreversible changes developed at a slower rate in these animals. Gradual compression to paralysis in 75 minutes resulted in full recovery if the compressive force was removed within 9 hours; 1 to 3 days were required for initial improvement. Thus, early decompressive surgery may have a positive influence on both the quality of restored function and the rate of recovery. *When indicated, spinal cord decompression should be performed without delay.* Medically treating dogs with moderate to severe paresis or paraplegia for 24 to 48 hours and then performing surgery if no improvement occurs is not recommended. This procedure discounts the experimental data regarding the effects of spinal compression over variable periods and the clinical experience of many veterinary surgeons.[1]

Dogs with acute paralysis and no deep pain responses should undergo decompression within 2 hours for possible functional recovery. Surgery is recommended for dogs with absence of deep pain sensation for up to 48 hours; however, the rate and quality of recovery are much less predictable. After 48 hours, the chance for recovery is probably less than 5%. These dogs are surgically treated only at the owner's insistence.

If a paralyzed dog is to be referred to a surgeon for decompression, the administration of corticosteroids as outlined in the section on medical treatment is indicated.

Supportive Care of the Paraplegic. Supportive care of the "downer dog" is directed at preventing the development of decubital ulcers, urinary tract infection, and muscle atrophy. Physical therapy is described in Chapter 15. Bladder care is described in Chapter 3.

The rate of return to acceptable pelvic limb function and micturition is highly correlated with the duration and rate of the spinal cord compression. Generally, if paraplegia has lasted longer than 48 hours, voluntary motor function, micturition, and normal pain responses return within 2 to 3 weeks. Good voluntary motor activity should return within 4 to 5 weeks, and the unassisted ability to support weight usually is restored within 6 to 8 weeks. Proprioception is the last function to return. *Early decompression hastens the return of neurologic function.* The quality of recovery depends on the severity of secondary injury to the spinal cord. Animals decompressed in the first 24 hours may be walking in the next 24 hours.

Equine Herpesvirus 1 (Rhinopneumonitis) Myeloencephalitis

Equine herpesvirus 1 (EHV-1) myeloencephalitis is an acute progressive neurologic disease that usually affects adult horses and, less commonly, foals.[9] Multifocal neurologic lesions, primarily severe vasculitis and necrosis, occur in the brain and the spinal cord[9]; however, the spinal cord lesions usually produce the majority of clinical signs. Histopathologic examination reveals diffuse to multifocal lymphocytic perivascular cuffing and hemorrhage throughout the spinal cord white matter. The pathogenesis of this disease is not related to direct viral infection of the CNS. An immune-mediated, Arthus-type reaction involving a viral antigen and an antibody may induce the severe neurologic vasculitis characteristic of this disease.

Clinical Signs. Usually EHV-1 myeloencephalitis occurs within 1 to 2 weeks after outbreaks of upper respiratory tract infections or abortions. Pregnant mares may be more susceptible to the development of severe spinal cord lesions and may abort if infected in the last trimester of pregnancy. Neurologic signs develop acutely. The classic clinical signs are those of an ascending myelitis with the pelvic limbs more severely affected than the thoracic limbs. Progression of the signs is variable, depending on the severity of the initial spinal cord lesions. Affected horses may recover in 24 to 48 hours, or they may progress rapidly to severe tetraplegia or paraplegia. Neurologic signs vary according to the area of the spinal cord involved. Usual neurologic signs include dysuria, ataxia of the pelvic limbs, and flaccid anus and tail. Signs may progress to severe pelvic limb paresis or paralysis. A dog-sitting stance is not unusual. Tetraparesis may be severe if cervical spinal cord lesions are extensive. In a few cases, involvement of the cerebral cortex or the brainstem may produce seizures, cranial nerve dysfunction, or vestibular signs. In most cases the clinical signs are those of thoracolumbar cord dysfunction. Both UMN and LMN signs may be noted relative to the site of development of vascular lesions in the spinal cord. In addition, neurologic signs may be symmetric or lateralizing, depending on the site of involvement.

Diagnosis. Whenever neurologic disease appears to follow outbreaks of respiratory tract infection or abortion, EHV-1 myeloencephalitis, a sporadic disease of horses, must be suspected. Analysis of the cerebrospinal fluid (CSF) reveals significant elevations in protein levels (150 mg/dl or greater) with normal or slightly elevated cell counts. The CSF is usually xanthochromic. The definitive diagnosis is made by isolation of the virus from nervous tissue or by serologic methods. Because viral isolation is difficult, comparison of antibody titers at the onset of clinical signs and during convalescence has been recommended for confirming a clinical diagnosis. In experimental studies, a sharp rise in serum antibody neutralization titers occurs within 5 to 7 days after inoculation. Rising serum antibody titers are rarely observed in horses with neurologic disease, however, because the sharp rise in antibody titers occurs during the respiratory phase of the disease some 1 to 2 weeks before the onset of neurologic signs. Antibody titers from CSF higher than those in serum are suggestive of EHV-1 infection. Determination of the albumin quotient and immunoglobulin ratio may help identify intrathecal production of immunoglobulins.

Treatment. No definitive treatment for this disease exists. Because an immune mechanism may be responsible, some have suggested the use of corticosteroids (dexamethasone, 0.1 to 0.25 mg/kg).[9,10] The benefits of this therapy are difficult to document insofar as many animals recover if given supportive nursing care, including catheterization of the urinary bladder. A killed intramuscular (IM) vaccine is available that probably provides immunity to the respiratory disease but not to infection of the placenta or CNS. Therefore, vaccinated animals may still have abortions or neurologic disease.

Equine Protozoal Myeloencephalomyelitis

Equine protozoal myeloencephalomyelitis (EPM) is the most common neurologic disease in horses with multifocal or asymmetric neurologic deficits. The disease is characterized by either *sudden* or *gradual* onset of pelvic limb paresis and ataxia. Because lesions may be multifocal in the spinal cord or brain, neurologic signs may indicate involvement of any part of the CNS. EPM is caused by a sporozoan parasite resembling *Sarcocystis cruzi.*[9,11] This organism has been named *Sarcocystis neurona,*[12] but DNA studies strongly suggest that it is identical to *Sarcocystis falcatula.* The opossum is the definitive host for *S. falcatula* and harbors the sexual stages of the protozoa within its gastrointestinal tract. Infective sporocysts are shed in the feces. Birds can serve as intermediate hosts. After ingestion of the sporocysts, sarcocysts develop in the bird's muscles. The cycle is completed when opossums eat infected birds. Although Koch's postulates have yet to be fulfilled, horses may be aberrant hosts that become infected after accidental ingestion of sporocysts shed in opossum feces or, possibly, of feed contaminated by dead birds. In horses, the organism invades and multiplies in the CNS rather than encysting in muscle. Early reports suggested that the disease was most common in the eastern United States, but it has been reported in many other locations and may occur anywhere in North America.[9,12-16] It has not been reported in Europe or in locations without opossums.

Lesions within the CNS are focal or multifocal and usually are asymmetric. The histopathologic lesion is a nonsuppurative myelitis affecting both gray and white matter. The disease is most common in young to middle-aged horses of the light breeds.

Clinical Signs. No typical presentation or characteristic set of neurologic signs have been established for EPM, and symmetric neurologic disease does not preclude its diagnosis.[16] Clinical signs usually develop suddenly and progress slowly over days to weeks. Rapid progression sometimes also occurs. Asymmetric ataxia and paresis of the pelvic limbs are the usual predominant manifestations.

Because lesions may be multifocal, however, a mixture of UMN and LMN signs may be present in the pelvic and thoracic limbs, and brainstem signs also may be present. If the lesion occurs in the brachial intumescence, the thoracic limb signs may be worse than the pelvic limb signs. These animals move with the thoracic limbs extended forward and the head held low. The clinical signs may resemble those observed in the equine wobbler syndrome and EHV-1 myeloencephalitis; however, the asymmetry that is seen helps in the clinical differentiation of protozoal myelitis-encephalitis from the other two diseases.

Diagnosis. In EPM, unlike EHV-1 encephalomyelitis, few CSF abnormalities occur. Mildly increased concentrations of mononuclear cells and protein occasionally are found. Cervical radiographs are normal, differentiating this disease from equine wobbler syndrome. Electromyography (EMG) can help to identify multifocal LMN damage, which is more common in this disease than in the others that resemble it. Analysis of serum or CSF using Western blot technology for the presence of antibody to EPM is currently the method for confirming the diagnosis, but controversy exits regarding its specificity.[16,17] Its low specificity indicates that false-positive test results are likely[17]; however, its high sensitivity indicates that a negative test result is useful in ruling out EPM. Furthermore, there appears to be no advantage in testing CSF versus serum. Antigen-specific antibody can be detected in the CSF of normal horses in which antigen has not been administered intrathecally.[18] Finally, serum and CSF from normal foals born to seropositive mares will test positive for EPM for up to days after birth.[19] Identification of EPM antigen in CSF via polymerase chain reaction is available, but the sensitivity and specificity await clarification.[12]

Treatment. Therapy may be effective, especially if it is started before profound signs are present. Although no definitive therapy is known, pyrimethamine (not licensed for horses) is given in a loading dose of 0.5 mg/kg orally, followed by 0.1 to 2.5 mg/kg once daily and trimethoprim and sulfadiazine at 15 to 20 mg/kg given orally twice daily. This regimen should be continued for 1 to 3 months.[9,16] The hemogram should be monitored for depression of blood cell production. Vitamin B complex can be given to help counteract folic acid inhibition.

Verminous Migration

Equine. The migration of several parasites through the spinal cord of horses has been described.[9,20,21] The most important of these organisms includes *Halicephalobus deletrix, Strongylus vulgaris, Draschia megastoma,* and *Hypoderma lineatum. S. vulgaris* is the most common organism to cause

verminous myelitis and the one most likely to affect the spinal cord.[20] *H. deletrix* may be the most common cause of verminous meningoencephalitis, but it usually affects the brain and not the spinal cord. Both *Draschia* and *Hypoderma* organisms tend to affect the brain. The clinical signs depend on the location of the parasite and may be asymmetric, focal, or multifocal. Embolization of *S. vulgaris* larvae into spinal or cerebral arteries may produce severe acute progressive or nonprogressive clinical signs.

A confirmed clinical diagnosis is difficult to make. The CSF may contain increased concentrations of eosinophils, neutrophils, macrophages, and red blood cells.[15] It may be mildly to moderately xanthochromic.

No definitive therapy is known. In suspected cases, thiabendazole (440 mg/kg), oxfendazole (10 mg/kg), fenbendazole (50 mg/kg daily for 3 days), diethylcarbamazine (50 mg/kg), or ivermectin (200 µg/kg) have been recommended.[9,20] Glucocorticosteroids and dimethyl sulfoxide can be used to decrease the inflammatory response to the dying worms. Many animals will have permanent disability, but the response can be good if treatment is started early.

Bovine. The larvae of *Hypoderma bovis* migrate through the epidural space of cattle. Infestation usually occurs during the months of July through October. If the larvae die or are killed while in the epidural space, a severe immunologic reaction occurs, resulting in spinal cord injury. The clinical signs usually appear in cattle treated with organophosphate insecticides during the period of epidural larva migration. Clinical signs develop acutely hours to days after treatment and usually are caused by thoracolumbar spinal cord injury. Prominent signs include pelvic limb ataxia and paresis. If the lumbosacral cord is involved, LMN signs may be detected in the pelvic limbs. The signs are usually asymmetric.

The diagnosis is based on the history and the clinical signs. The CSF changes reflect signs of degeneration (moderate increases in protein and cell concentrations). Eosinophils may not be present in the CSF. Affected animals should be treated with corticosteroids or phenylbutazone to reduce the inflammatory reaction. If signs develop several days to weeks after organophosphate application, the possibility of organophosphate intoxication should be considered.

Ovine, Caprine. Sheep and goats may serve as aberrant hosts for the meningeal worm of white-tailed deer, *Parelaphostrongylus tenuis.* Migration of this parasite through the CNS produces a variety of clinical signs that include pelvic limb paresis and ataxia. The clinical course is variable and may include progression, stasis, or improvement in clinical signs. Affected animals have a history of grazing in pastures that have been exposed to white-tailed deer. The CSF of these animals usually contains increased concentrations of protein and cells. A mononuclear and eosinophilic pleocytosis is usually encountered. Treatment with diethylcarbamazine, levamisole, or thiabendazole is recommended. The prognosis is guarded.

Porcine. The kidney worm of swine, *Stephanurus dentatus,* may migrate through the spinal cord, producing pelvic limb paresis and ataxia. This organism must be considered in individual swine that develop acute paraparesis, particularly swine residing on farms in the southeastern United States.

Viral Leukoencephalomyelitis of Goats (Caprine Arthritis-Encephalomyelitis)

This disease affects goats 1 to 4 months of age and probably is caused by a lentivirus. The disease causes perivenous demyelination and nonsuppurative granulomatous leukomyelitis. As in other viral diseases, lesions may develop anywhere in the spinal cord, producing focal or multifocal asymmetric neurologic signs. The clinical signs of this disease include a progressive paraparesis that eventually involves the thoracic limbs. More than one kid is affected in most cases. Weight loss, arthritis, pneumonitis, and hard udder may be present in one or more animals. Neurologic signs may reflect multifocal disease, including involvement of the brain. The CSF usually contains markedly increased concentrations of mononuclear cells and modestly increased concentrations of protein; however, an eosinophilic pleocytosis is not present. EMG may indicate some LMN loss. Serologic tests (enzyme-linked immunosorbent assay [ELISA] and agar gel immunodiffusion) can be helpful if positive. Many affected animals, however, have negative results. No effective treatment is available. The neurologic syndrome is permanent and may be fatal.[9]

Acute Nonprogressive Diseases, T3-L3

Spinal Cord Trauma

Spinal cord trauma, usually the result of automobile accidents, is a common neurologic injury.[22] The incidence is much greater in areas where leash laws are poorly enforced. Spinal cord trauma is more frequent in large animals when they are young but may occur in mature animals as a result of falls, trailer accidents, or overcrowding in chutes. The management of spinal cord trauma has been discussed extensively by others.[23-25] This section provides a concise review. Veterinarians have two primary obligations in these cases. First, they

must diagnose and treat shock, major abdominal or thoracic hemorrhage, visceral rupture, or ventilation abnormalities. Second, they must be able to give owners accurate prognoses for the animal's recovery of neurologic function.

First Aid and Emergency Medical Treatment. An injury of sufficient force to produce spinal cord trauma may result in another life-threatening injury.[22,26] Maintenance of a patent airway is of the utmost importance. The mouth is cleared of fluid or blood, the tongue is pulled forward, and the unconscious animal is intubated. Adequate ventilation is of great importance because hypoxia aggravates CNS edema. Shock, if present, must be treated. IV lactated Ringer's solution is given to restore vascular volume. MPSS is given IV at a dosage of 30 mg/kg over a 10-minute period.[25,28] This drug is beneficial in the prevention and treatment of CNS edema and secondary biochemical reactions in the nervous tissue.[25] To be effective, the initial dose of MPSS must be given within 8 hours post injury. Administration of corticosteroids after the 8-hour window has closed may be detrimental. Fluid therapy must be carefully monitored to prevent overhydration, which can aggravate CNS edema, but the patient must have fluid volume restored and maintained.

After providing first aid and treating shock, the veterinarian must perform a thorough physical examination. Abdominal or thoracic trauma may be difficult to appreciate immediately after an injury; therefore, visceral function must be monitored for several days. Little benefit exists in successfully repairing the spinal fracture only to have the animal die several days later from a diaphragmatic hernia or a ruptured urinary bladder; however, spinal cord trauma must be treated without delay to improve the odds of recovery. Once circulatory problems are corrected, mannitol therapy is instituted (see Chapter 12 for details on the management of edema).

During the period of early evaluation and treatment, the animal must be restrained to prevent further spinal cord injury. Animals should be transported on a rigid stretcher or a board. Movement should be discouraged, especially if vertebral fractures or luxations are suspected.

Neurologic Examination. Most spinal cord injuries are the result of vertebral fracture, vertebral luxation, or traumatic disk extrusion and are likely to produce severe, irreversible neurologic deficits, especially if early treatment has not been provided. Localization of the spinal cord lesion and the prognosis based on the severity of the injury are determined by the neurologic examination. The spinal column should be gently palpated for alterations in vertebral conformation because these changes have good localizing value. The principles

Table 6-8 **Signs of Complete Spinal Cord Transection**

Spinal Cord Segments	Signs Caudal to Lesion		
	Motor	**Sensory**	**Autonomic**
C1–C4	Tetraplegia (UMN)	Anesthesia	Apnea, no micturition
C5–C6	Tetraplegia (UMN), LMN suprascapular nerve	Anesthesia, hyperesthesia—mid cervical	Apnea—phrenic nerve, LMN, no micturition
C7–T2	Tetraplegia or paraplegia (UMN), LMN brachial plexus	Anesthesia, hyperesthesia—brachial plexus	Diaphragmatic breathing only, no micturition
T3–L3	Paraplegia (UMN), Schiff-Sherrington syndrome	Anesthesia, hyperesthesia—segmental	Diaphragmatic, some intercostal and abdominal respiration, depending on level of lesion, no micturition
L4–S1	Paraplegia with LMN lumbosacral plexus	Anesthesia, hyperesthesia—segmental	No micturition; S1 = anal sphincter may be atonic
S1–S3	Knuckling of hind foot, paralysis of tail	Anesthesia, hyperesthesia—segmental	No micturition, sphincters atonic
Cd1–Cd5	Paralysis of tail	Anesthesia, hyperesthesia—segmental	None

C, Cervical; *T*, thoracic; *L*, lumbar; *S*, sacral; *Cd*, caudal; *LMN*, lower motor neuron; *UMN*, upper motor neuron.

of lesion localization were reviewed earlier. Table 6-8 summarizes the signs of complete spinal cord transection at various levels of the cord.

The prognosis of a spinal cord injury depends on the severity and duration of the compressive force and the extent of secondary vascular responses to the injury.[23,25] The most important factor is reversibility. The spinal cord may be anatomically or physiologically transected. In most cases, physiologic transection is the most common cause of irreversibility. Sudden compression of the spinal cord is far worse than gradual compression. Acute experimental compression of the spinal cord with a force sufficient to produce paralysis, and loss of deep pain perception results in irreversible spinal cord injury if the duration of compression exceeds 4 hours. Most experimental studies documenting effective medical therapy of spinal cord trauma indicate that treatment must be given in the first hour. The key to prognosis is the *perceptual response* to noxious stimuli applied caudally to the lesion. In the absence of deep pain perception, the duration of the injury becomes the critical factor related to prognosis. The absence of deep pain perception is a very unfavorable sign, especially if the injury has been present for longer than 4 hours. Other neurologic signs that correlate with severe thoracolumbar spinal cord injury include spinal shock (temporary loss of spinal reflexes), crossed extensor reflexes, and the Schiff-Sherrington phenomenon. The presence of these signs does *not* indicate that the lesion is irreversible because these signs may occur in the presence of deep pain perception. Assuming that the skeletal lesion can be stabilized, injured animals are categorized as shown in Table 6-9.

Special Examinations. Radiographs of the spinal column are necessary if surgical treatment is contemplated. Radiographs define the precise location and type of skeletal lesion (Figure 6-7). These findings dictate the surgical procedure needed to decompress and stabilize the injury. Spinal radiographs are not useful for evaluating the functional status of the spinal cord. The amount of displacement visualized on radiographs is frequently the least displacement that occurred at the time of the injury. The functional status is determined by the neurologic examination. Somatosensory-evoked potentials may be of benefit to define spinal cord integrity more precisely (see Chapter 4).

Table 6-9 **Prognosis of Acute Spinal Cord Injuries**

Group	Signs	Duration of Injury	Prognosis
Group 1	Good pain response	<24 h	Fair to good
Group 2	No pain response	<4 h	Poor
Group 3	No pain response	>4 h	Grave

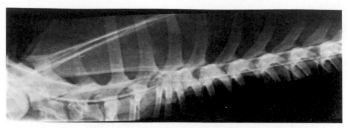

Figure 6-7 Myelogram of a dog with a compression fracture of T3. The compression of the spinal cord was not apparent on survey films.

Medical Therapy. Corticosteroids are given as part of the emergency treatment for shock. MPSS is given in an initial dose of 30 mg/kg, followed by a continuous infusion of 5 mg/kg per hour for 24 hours. None is given after 24 hours.[24-30] To be effective, MPSS should be administered within 8 hours post injury.[25] A hypertonic osmotic diuretic such as 20% mannitol solution should be administered immediately after hypovolemia has been corrected. Mannitol acts quickly to reduce spinal cord edema and is indicated in addition to corticosteroids. Mannitol is given at a dosage of 0.5 g/kg body weight over the course of 30 minutes. Vomiting and severe hemolysis of red blood cells may occur if the rate of administration is too rapid. The mannitol therapy is repeated in 2 to 3 hours and then is discontinued. Dimethyl sulfoxide (DMSO) is often recommended, especially for large animals.[9] Most controlled studies do not indicate efficacy, but the literature is controversial.[31] In large animals it is used at an IV dose of 1.0 g/kg, 10% DMSO in 5% dextrose.

One study of 211 dogs and cats with vertebral fractures found minimal difference between medical and surgical management.[32,33] Although clearly many vertebral fractures can be managed medically, surgery is indicated for unstable fractures.

Surgical Therapy. Two major indications exist for spinal surgery in the animal with a traumatic injury: decompression of the spinal cord and stabilization of the vertebra. The decision for decompression is based on the clinical signs. Animals with paralysis almost always need decompression and usually need stabilization. Animals with mild paresis and ataxia may need stabilization, but decompression may not be required in all cases. Decompression should be performed within 4 to 6 hours for animals with complete paralysis. Animals in groups 1 and 2 described in Table 6-9 should undergo early surgery. Surgery is not recommended for animals in group 3.

The decision as to the method of stabilization is based on the findings of clinical and radiographic examinations and on observations made during the operation. Flexible plates, body plates, segmental spinal instrumentation, and vertebral body pins

with methylmethacrylate are the most commonly used equipment and usually are superior to any form of external support.[34-38] Compression fractures of the vertebral body and fractures of the transverse spinous processes without displacement may be stable. Fractures of the vertebral body with luxation or fractures involving the articular facets require reduction and stabilization. When decompression and stabilization are simultaneously indicated, hemilaminectomy is the favored approach for decompression because any method of fixation can be used with this procedure and because it creates less instability. Dorsal laminectomy must be used in the lumbosacral region (Figure 6-8). The reader is referred to other texts and references for in-depth descriptions of the various surgical techniques.[39]

Supportive Care and Rehabilitation. Few animals become ambulatory during the first week after surgery following severe trauma. Most remain paretic or paralyzed and require attentive nursing care and physical therapy and a rehabilitation period. In general, the procedures for supportive care of the paraplegic with disk disease should also be followed up after spinal surgery. Animals should improve within 2 to 3 weeks, and significant improvement should be seen in a month. Failure to show improvement during this time is strongly correlated with permanent spinal cord damage; however, every clinician encounters a few dogs that regain functional use of the pelvic limbs when the initial outlook has seemed hopeless. Unfortunately, in veterinary medicine, the outcome of the case often depends on the dedication and financial cooperation of the owner. Surprisingly, some dogs regain the ability to walk without regaining deep pain perception.[33]

Chronic Progressive Diseases, T3-L3

Chronic progressive diseases of the T3-L3 region are characterized by insidious onset and slow progression of the neurologic signs. Degenerative, neoplastic, and inflammatory diseases are the most important of the various etiologic categories. Although the diseases listed in the right-hand

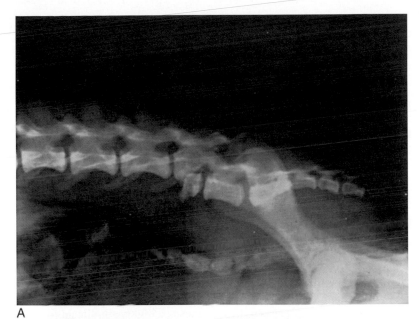

A

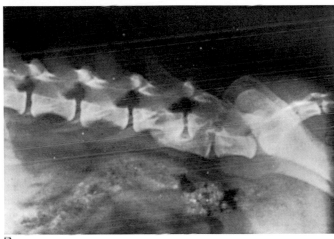

B

Figure 6 8 A, Lumbosacral lateral radiograph demonstrating a fracture of L6. These injuries entrap the spinal nerve roots that form the sciatic, pelvic, pudendal, and caudal nerves. **B,** Follow-up postsurgical radiograph of the same dog. The fracture site was decompressed, and the nerves in the vertebral canal were freed from compression. A callus had bridged the fracture site, although no internal stabilization had been provided.

column of Tables 6-1 through 6-3 may start in the T3-L3 spinal cord segments, progression into other regions may occur. With long-standing disease, cervical spinal cord involvement may cause tetraparesis or hemiparesis. These problems are discussed in Chapter 7.

Degenerative Myelopathy

Degenerative myelopathy is a slowly progressive degenerative disease that involves primarily the long tracts of the canine thoracolumbar spinal cord. The disease was first described by Averill in 1973, and subsequent workers have reported various clinical and pathologic findings.[40-43] The disease appears to be most prevalent in older German shepherd dogs and has been termed German shepherd

myelopathy and progressive myelopathy.[42,44,45] Griffiths and co-workers have termed this disorder *degenerative radiculomyelopathy* because of dorsal root involvement in several of their cases.[43]

A degenerative myelopathy also has been described in horses. Unlike the canine disease, the equine syndrome is seen in young animals, is characterized by an acute progressive course, and involves primarily the cervical cord, although thoracolumbar lesions also occur. The equine disease is discussed in Chapter 7.

Pathologic Findings. In Averill's study, 22 dogs with progressive ataxia and paresis had diffuse degeneration of spinal cord myelin and axons in all spinal cord funiculi.[41] These changes were most extensive in the midthoracic region and were not associated with intervertebral disk extrusion, spondylosis deformans, or dural ossification. Griffiths and Duncan[43] reported their findings with 16 dogs. In addition to confirming many of Averill's observations, these workers reported extensive lesions in the lumbar dorsal columns and involvement of the dorsal nerve roots. They reported that the lesions suggested a "dying-back" process of axons confined to the CNS. In another study, Braund and Vandevelde[35] studied 14 German shepherd dogs affected with this disease. Although this study reconfirmed many of the earlier observations, it did not support the dying back hypothesis. Dogs with degenerative myelopathy have some cell-mediated immunologic abnormalities, and the lesions are similar in some respects to those of multiple sclerosis.[40,44,45] Other hypotheses include a nutritional problem involving vitamins B and E. Dogs with degenerative myelopathy have decreased serum tocopherol levels, but therapy with vitamin B complex and E has not been effective. The immune hypothesis is the most attractive one at present. The predisposition of German shepherd dogs to this syndrome suggests that genetic factors may be involved in the pathogenesis.

Clinical Signs. Clinical signs generally are first recognized in affected dogs at 6 to 9 years of age, although the disease has been documented in a few at 4 years of age. Degenerative myelopathy occurs almost exclusively in large breeds, predominantly German shepherd dogs or shepherd dog cross-breeds. Similar syndromes have been seen in other breeds, however, including a miniature poodle,[46] Siberian huskies,[47] and other large breeds.[48] One cat with a similar syndrome has been reported.[49] Early clinical signs include mild ataxia and paresis of the pelvic limbs. The onset is insidious, and an owner may not seek veterinary assistance for several months, believing that the dog has mild coxofemoral arthritis. The outstanding clinical sign is pelvic limb ataxia. Knuckling of the feet, dragging of the toes, and dysmetria are common signs. The pelvic limbs may cross when the animal walks, and swaying movements of the rear quarters are apparent. If forced to turn quickly, many dogs fall in an outward direction. Clinical signs are bilateral; however, they may not be symmetric. One limb may be affected more severely than another. Urinary or fecal incontinence is uncommon. Most animals appear healthy in other respects. In chronic cases, atrophy of the caudal paraspinal and pelvic limb muscles may occur.

The neurologic examination usually suggests a lesion in spinal cord segments T3-L3. Postural reactions such as proprioceptive positioning, hopping, placing, and the extensor postural thrust are deficient. The degree of proprioceptive dysfunction is usually greater than the degree of motor dysfunction. Flexor (withdrawal) reflexes are normal and, in more advanced cases, may be clonic. Crossed extensor reflexes may be present. In many dogs, the knee jerk reflex is normal or exaggerated. In some dogs, the knee-jerk reflex is depressed or absent even though the (1) leg can be extended readily at the stifle, (2) crossed extensor reflex may be present, and (3) pain is perceived normally from areas innervated by the saphenous branch of the femoral nerve. Involvement of the dorsal roots of the femoral nerve may inhibit sensory impulses from stretch receptors located in the quadriceps muscle. Electrophysiologic and pathologic studies have not detected LMN abnormalities, thus confirming clinical observations that the motor reflex pathways are intact.[43] When present, this clinical finding is highly suggestive of degenerative myelopathy (radiculomyelopathy). Pain perception from the pelvic limbs is normal, and no evidence exists of hyperesthesia, a highly significant finding. Abnormalities of micturition are uncommon. Muscle atrophy develops slowly and is clinically apparent only in long-standing cases. Hyperesthesia is absent. Although mild lesions occur in the cervical spinal cord, the thoracic limbs usually retain normal function.

Diagnosis. The clinical signs and the neurologic findings suggest a slowly progressive compression of the spinal cord. In fact, this disease originally was attributed to spinal cord compression from dural ossification, Hansen type II disk protrusions, or thoracolumbar spondylosis. Degenerative myelopathy must be differentiated radiographically from type II (slow) disk protrusions and spinal neoplasia. Survey radiography and myelography should be performed to rule out the presence of compressive (potentially surgically correctable) diseases. CSF is collected at the time of myelography to help exclude the presence of inflammatory diseases. Mild increases in CSF protein concentrations may be seen, especially if the fluid is collected at the lumbar subarachnoid space. Vertebral spondylosis and dural ossification are common radiographic findings in older large-breed dogs. They seldom cause neurologic dysfunction, and their presence does not correlate with clinical signs or pathologic findings in dogs with degenerative myelopathy.[41] The presence of a type II disk protrusion does not rule out degenerative myelopathy; therefore, the prognosis is guarded, especially for German shepherd dogs. Lumbosacral degenerative stenosis can usually be differentiated by the significant hyperesthesia at the lumbosacral region.

Depressed cell-mediated immune responses to concanavalin A, phytohemagglutinin P, and pokeweed mitogens occur in most affected dogs.[40]

These tests are not routinely available but could be useful, especially in the dog with a positive finding on myelography, to help rule out the presence of concurrent degenerative myelopathy. MRI may also be useful in identifying the lesions and monitoring their progression.[40]

Treatment. Because the cause is unknown, no specific treatment is available. The animal responds poorly, if at all, to corticosteroids, NSAIDs, or B complex vitamins. Clemmons[40] reported some therapeutic benefit from aminocaproic acid (Amicar, Lederle), 500 mg every 8 hours given orally. The proposed mechanism involves an antiprotease action that blocks the final common pathway of tissue inflammation. Progression of the degenerative process was slower in about 50% of treated dogs, and improvement occurred in some. Benefits usually occurred within 8 weeks. Intrathecal interferon therapy has also been proposed. Some veterinarians recommend antioxidant therapy, but no controlled studies have demonstrated a positive effect.

The owner must be warned as to the hopeless prognosis for cure; however, with supportive care, many dogs can be maintained for several months before euthanasia becomes necessary.

Type II Disk Disease

Pathophysiology. Type II disk disease occurs primarily in older (5 to 12 years of age) large-breed, nonchondrodystrophoid dogs. Similar protrusions are sometimes seen in smaller dogs and in cats.[1,50,51] The pathologic change within the intervertebral disk is a fibroid degeneration and a weakening of the dorsal annulus (see Figure 6-3).[52] Recurrent partial disk protrusion produces a dome-shaped mass that eventually becomes large enough to compress the spinal cord or to irritate meninges and nerve roots. The neurologic signs and spinal cord lesions are those of a compressive myelopathy.

Clinical Signs. The clinical signs are similar to those of degenerative myelopathy in that type II disk protrusions result in slowly progressive signs of ataxia and paresis. With type II disk protrusions, pain in the area of the protruded disk may be present, in contrast to the lack of hyperesthesia in degenerative myelopathy. Many of these animals are not in pain, however, presumably because of the slow progression of the syndrome. In addition, voluntary micturition may be affected by the compressive myelopathy, whereas micturition usually remains normal in cases of degenerative myelopathy.

Neurologic abnormalities in the pelvic limbs reflect the level of the disk protrusion and can be similar to the findings in dogs with degenerative myelopathy or spinal neoplasia. Disk protrusions involving cord segments T3-L3 result in UMN signs, whereas protrusions involving segments caudal to L3 can produce a mixture of UMN and LMN signs. The cutaneous reflex may be decreased caudal to the level of the lesion. The presence of these signs has great localizing value and helps to differentiate type II disk disease from degenerative myelopathy. The response to deep pain stimuli is usually normal in both diseases.

Diagnosis. Type II disk disease is differentiated from degenerative myelopathy by radiography of the spine. Survey radiographs rarely reveal the lesion, although suggestive changes may be seen. Increased density in the vertebral canal and narrowing of the disk space are not consistently present in type II disk protrusions. Myelography, CT, or MRI is usually necessary to demonstrate the compressive nature of the disk in question (Figure 6-9). As in cases of degenerative myelopathy, dural ossification and spondylosis are common radiographic findings. These radiographic lesions should not be construed as the cause of the dog's neurologic dysfunction.

Treatment. Patients with early and mild signs may respond temporarily to antiinflammatory drugs such as corticosteroids or NSAIDs; however, the signs soon recur and progressively worsen. Dogs with pain as the only clinical sign can be treated medically, but decompressive surgery with removal of the protruded disk is more satisfactory in most cases. Decompressive surgery is indicated for all dogs with paresis and ataxia. Surgery should be performed early to prevent further neurologic deterioration. The prognosis with surgery is good in that most dogs regain normal neurologic function. All owners should be cautioned that concurrent degenerative myelopathy is always a risk, especially in German shepherd dogs.

Neoplasia

Pathophysiology. Tumors affecting the vertebrae, meninges, nerve roots, or spinal cord may result in neurologic signs. These tumors are classified according to tumor type as primary, metastatic, lymphoreticular, or skeletal and according to location as extradural, intradural-extramedullary, or intramedullary (Table 6-10). Primary CNS tumors are classified in Table 15-6. In general, the most common tumors are extradural and affect structures that house the spinal cord, such as the vertebrae or other tissues, and produce a compressive myelopathy when the mass expands on or around the cord. Most tumors slowly compress the spinal cord, producing signs similar to those of degenerative myelopathy and type II disk disease (Table 6-11). Extradural tumors frequently cause pain, often before significant paresis occurs.[53] Intradural-extramedullary tumors are usually meningiomas or nerve sheath tumors and may be painful. A unique

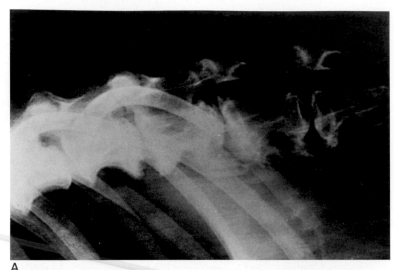

Figure 6-9 A, Survey lateral thoracolumbar radiograph of a dog with slowly progressive paraparesis. Note the extensive spondylosis. This radiographic finding is common in older large breed dogs; however, it is seldom a clinical problem. **B,** Myelogram of the same dog. Note the prominent extramedullary compression at T13-L1 from a type II disk protrusion. (From Kneller SK, Oliver JE, Lewis RE: Differential diagnosis of progressive caudal paresis in an aged German shepherd dog, *J Am Anim Hosp Assoc* 11:414, 1975.)

A

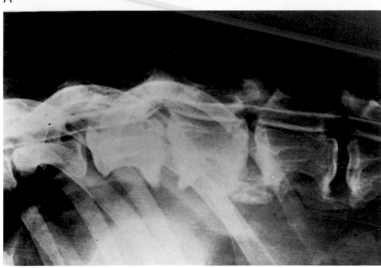

B

intradural-extramedullary blast cell tumor that affects the T10-L2 spinal cord segments has been reported in young dogs 6 months to 3 years of age.[54,55] Intramedullary tumors are either metastatic or primary tumors of nervous tissue. Gliomas and ependymomas are the most common.[46] Sudden onset of signs of a transverse myelopathy may be seen with intramedullary neoplasms affecting the spinal cord, presumably when blood vessels are compromised. Some tumors such as lymphosarcoma may embolize arteries of the spinal cord.

Skeletal (Vertebral) Tumors. Vertebral tumors may be primary or may arise from metastases. Generally, as the tumors grow into the vertebral canal, the spinal cord is compressed slowly, producing signs of a slowly progressive myelopathy. Occasionally, the tumor causes considerable verte-

bral destruction without cord compression. These vertebrae are weakened and may fracture, resulting in acute spinal cord compression. Vertebral tumors are usually painful because of periosteal and, perhaps, meningeal and nerve root irritation. Primary vertebral tumors include osteomas, osteosarcomas (Figure 6-10), fibrosarcomas, hemangiosarcomas, chondromas, chondrosarcomas, and plasma cell myelomas (Figure 6-11). A variety of carcinomas and sarcomas metastatic to vertebrae have been reported. Survey radiographs of the spine are usually diagnostic. Treatment is usually palliative, although total vertebral removal with spinal column fixation has been advocated for certain benign tumors. Malignant tumors may be surgically debulked and then treated with radiation therapy; this approach is also usually palliative.

Table 6-10 **Characteristics of Spinal Cord Tumors**

Characteristic	Tumor Loaction		
	Extradural	**Intradural-Extramedullary**	**Intramedullary**
Frequency	50%	35%	15%
Tumor types	Bone tumors	Neurofibromas	Gliomas
	Metastatic tumors	Meningiomas	Ependymomas
	Lymphosarcoma	Blastomas	
Rate of growth	Rapid	Slow	Usually slow
Clinical signs			
Pain	Early severe	Early, variable	Unusual, late
Paresis	Early, rapidly progressive, usually bilateral	Late, slowly progressive, may be unilateral	Late, rapidly progressive, usually bilateral
Sensation	Usually intact until late	Usually intact until late	Usually intact until late
Course	Acute onset, rapid progression	Very slow progression	Insidious onset, rapid progression
Diagnosis			
CSF	Increased protein, normal cells	Increased protein, normal cells	Increased protein, normal cells, may be xanthochromic
Radiography	Skeletal lesions	Possibly large intervertebral foramen (neurofibroma)	Possible widened vertebral canal
Myelography	Extradural compression	Variable, may be cupping of dye column	Widened spinal cord, attenuated dye column

Modified with permission from Prata RG: Diagnosis of spinal cord tumors in the dog. *Vet Clin North Am* 7:165–185, 1977.

Table 6-11 **Differential Diagnosis of Spinal Cord Tumors**

Characteristic	Spinal Cord Tumor	Degenerative Myelopathy	Inflammation		Type II Disk
			Meningitis and Myelitis	**Diskospondylitis**	
Age	Adult to old	>5 yr	Any	Any	>6 yr
Progression	Usually slow	Slow	Variable	Variable	Slow
Focal signs	Yes, unless metastatic; may be painful	T3–L3, not painful	Sometimes early, later progresses to other areas; frequently painful	Yes, may be multifocal; usually painful	Yes, may be painful
Radiography					
Survey	Sometimes vertebral changes	Normal, frequently have spondylosis because of age and breed	Normal	Characteristic, osteomyelitis	May be normal, frequently have spondylosis because of age and breed
Myelography	Defines extent: extradural, intradural, intramedullary	Normal	Normal	May demonstrate extradural compression	Extradural compression at disk space
CSF	Increased protein, normal cells	Increased protein (variable), normal cells	Increased protein, increased cells	Variable, may be normal	Increased protein (variable), normal cells

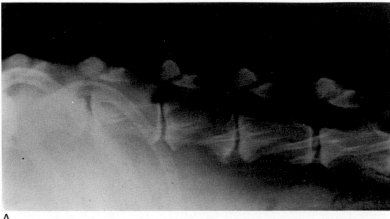

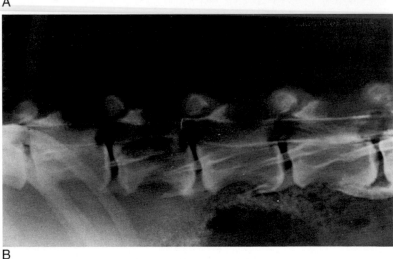

Figure 6-10 A, Osteogenic sarcoma of L2 in a dog with paraplegia and severe back pain. **B,** Myelogram of the thoracolumbar area of the same dog, demonstrating extradural compression at L2.

A

B

Lymphoreticular Tumors. These tumors grow in the vertebral canal and are considered epidural. They do not arise from a vertebra or from the meninges. Lymphosarcoma involving the vertebral canal is frequently encountered in cats and cattle but is uncommon in dogs and horses.

Tumor growth within the vertebral canal produces a compressive myelopathy. Several segments of the spinal cord may be involved, but lesions in the feline and the bovine are most common in thoracolumbar segments. Spinal lymphosarcoma must be considered in any cat or in older cows with a history of progressive neurologic dysfunction of the pelvic limbs. In addition to pelvic limb ataxia and paresis, regional hyperesthesia may be present. Survey radiographs are usually normal. Myelography may reveal extensive compression because the tumor may fill the vertebral canals of several vertebrae. In a study of 21 cases of lymphoma in the vertebral canal of cats, 85% of

Figure 6-11 Lateral thoracolumbar radiograph demonstrating multiple areas of bone lysis in several vertebrae. These changes are characteristic of plasma cell myeloma.

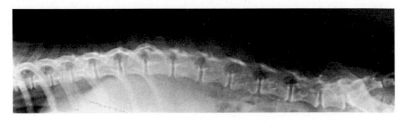

the 13 animals necropsied had lymphoma in other organs. Of 19 cats tested for feline leukemia virus, 16 (84.2%) tested positive.

Analysis of the CSF yields variable results. The CSF is normal when the tumor is outside the meninges. In some animals the CSF may contain malignant lymphocytes and may have increased protein concentrations. Samples taken from the lumbar cistern may be more diagnostic when the thoracolumbar cord is affected.[56] In cats, lymphosarcoma must be differentiated from the neurologic form of feline infectious peritonitis, which may also affect the thoracolumbar spinal cord and results in progressive pelvic limb paresis and ataxia. In feline infectious peritonitis, the CSF usually contains a marked increase in protein, neutrophils, and some mononuclear cells. Fluoroscopically guided percutaneous fine-needle aspiration of epidural masses is an effective method for establishing a definitive diagnosis.[57] Therapy for epidural lymphosarcoma may provide some benefit. Chemotherapy or surgical excision and chemotherapy may result in remission.[58] Treatment for intradural lymphosarcoma is usually ineffective. Corticosteroids may alleviate some of the clinical signs temporarily.

Metastatic Tumors. Malignant tumors may metastasize to the vertebrae and, rarely, to the spinal cord. Neurologic signs result from spinal cord compression secondary to vertebral instability or direct compression by the neoplastic mass. Malignant mammary tumors, prostatic adenocarcinomas, and hemangiosarcomas are the tumors that most frequently metastasize to a vertebra. The rare tumor multiple myeloma also may involve one or more vertebrae, sometimes producing multifocal signs. Spinal radiographs are usually diagnostic (see Figure 6-11). The tumor type is confirmed by histopathology; treatment is palliative.

Primary Tumors. Primary tumors affecting the spinal cord may be intramedullary or intradural-extramedullary.[53] Extramedullary tumors may arise from nerve roots (nerve sheath tumors) or from meninges (meningiomas). Nerve sheath tumors, including schwannomas and neurofibromas, arise from nerve roots or peripheral nerves. They may be extradural or intradural. Early extramedullary neurofibromas result in clinical signs that are restricted to the distribution of the affected nerve root. These early signs may remain undetected if nerve roots T3-L3 are affected. These nerve roots innervate the muscles of the trunk, which are difficult to examine for neurologic dysfunction. If the nerve roots forming the brachial or lumbosacral plexus are involved, neurologic signs of monoparesis develop. As these tumors grow, they follow the nerve proximally to invade or compress the spinal cord, resulting in asymmetric neurologic signs caudal to the lesion. Survey radiographs may show an enlarged intervertebral foramen, whereas myelography may demonstrate spinal cord compression (Figure 6-12). Many of these tumors are inoperable because the tumor either has invaded the spinal cord or involves multiple nerve roots that cannot be sacrificed at surgery. In some cases, the tumor and the affected nerve root can be removed; however, recurrence is frequent because of residual tumor cells. Amputation with complete resection of nerve roots is often the best hope for successful treatment.

Meningiomas usually grow slowly and cause progressive compression of the spinal cord. The site of the lesion may be painful. The clinical course usually resembles that of type II disk disease or degenerative myelopathy. Myelography is necessary for detection of extramedullary spinal cord compression. These lesions should be surgically explored because many meningiomas can be completely removed if detected early.

Medullary tumors of the spinal cord are rare. Initial signs may be unilateral; however, as the tumor grows, bilateral signs develop. Myelography is helpful for differentiating extramedullary compression

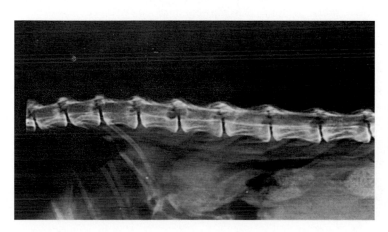

Figure 6-12 Lateral thoracolumbar myelogram of a cat with progressive paraparesis. Note the enlarged intervertebral foramen at L2-3, suggesting a mass in this area. These changes are characteristic of nerve sheath tumors (the eventual diagnosis in this case).

from intramedullary tumors (see Figure 6-10, *B* and Figure 6-13, *A*). The prognosis is poor because these tumors are generally inoperable, although newer microsurgical techniques may allow resection in some cases (see Figure 6-13, *B*).

Spinal Dural Ossification

Dural ossification, also known as *ossifying pachymeningitis,* is a common radiographic or necropsy finding in middle-aged or older dogs (Figure 6-14). Plaques of bone develop on the inner dural surface in response to an unidentified factor. The lesion is most common in large-breed dogs and is often identified in association with vertebral spondylosis. The disease most commonly affects the cervical and lumbar areas. At one time, the clinical signs of degenerative myelopathy and canine wobbler syndrome were attributed to dural ossification. Later studies have demonstrated no relationship between

the bony plaques and the clinical signs. The bony plaques are of little clinical importance except in rare cases in which they entrap a nerve root or cause pain. We have observed one dog with extensive dural ossification that developed clinical signs of pelvic limb paralysis after trauma. No antemortem or necropsy evidence of vertebral fracture or luxation was found. At necropsy, a large subdural hematoma was present, which apparently resulted from a fracture of a large dural bony plaque. Spinal cord compression from this hematoma probably produced the neurologic signs.

Rarely, large dural plaques cause local spinal cord edema, necrosis, or fibrosis. Radiographs are useful for establishing the diagnosis. Myelographic evidence of compression warrants exploratory decompression of the lesion. Medical treatment is nonspecific and is directed at relief of pain. Clinicians should make every attempt to find other

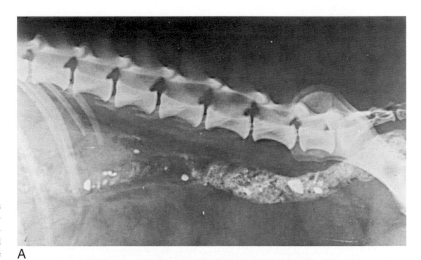

A

Figure 6-13 A, Lateral radiograph of a dog with progressive lower motor neuron paraparesis, constipation, and urinary incontinence. Note the enlarged vertebral canal of L4 and L5. These changes are characteristic of expanding intramedullary tumors. **B,** Spinal cord section from the same dog, which was affected with an intramedullary tumor. The expanding tumor produced the radiographic changes in **A.**

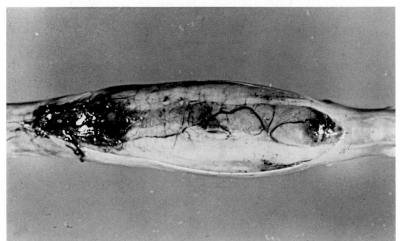

B

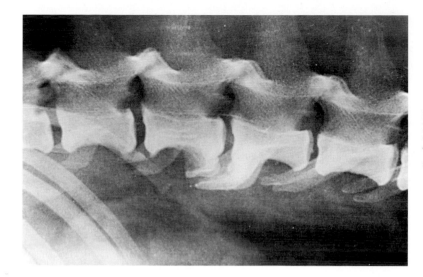

Figure 6-14 Severe spondylosis of the lumbar vertebrae and dural ossification were incidental findings in this dog. These changes seldom cause neurologic signs.

causes for the neurologic signs before assuming that dural ossification is the cause.

Spondylosis Deformans (Hypertrophic Spondylosis)

This noninfectious, nonseptic condition is a common finding during routine radiographic or necropsy examinations. Spondylosis deformans is characterized by the formation of bony spurs and bridges at the intervertebral spaces (see Figure 6-9, *A* and Figure 6-14). The term *spondylitis* originally was used to describe this condition because investigators believed that inflammation produced the bony reaction. Further work suggested that the condition was a noninflammatory process associated with degeneration of the annulus fibrosus of the intervertebral disk.[59] The term *spondylosis* is therefore preferred. Although degeneration of the annulus may be important in the pathogenesis, nuclear degeneration and disk protrusion are not. The presence of spondylosis at a disk space is not proof of disk protrusion. The condition may be present anywhere in the spine but is most common in the caudal thoracic and caudal lumbar vertebrae. Spondylosis occurs in most species but is most frequent in dogs, bulls, and pigs.[6,60,61]

Morgan found that osteophyte formation within the vertebral canal is very rare and seldom, if ever, results in spinal cord compression.[59] In addition, osteophyte formation does not constrict spinal nerves and usually is present without detectable clinical signs. Spondylosis rarely causes neurologic signs; however, occasionally it causes spinal pain, especially after exercise. Spondylosis is frequently present at L7-S1 in dogs and may be associated with stenosis of the vertebral canal or intervertebral foramina that produce pain and LMN signs (see Degenerative Lumbosacral Stenosis). As with dural ossification, clinicians must search for other causes of the neurologic signs before assuming that spondylosis is the cause. Radiographic examinations can differentiate this condition from the true inflammatory spinal disorders (osteomyelitis, diskospondylitis) that produce severe neurologic and musculoskeletal signs. NSAIDs may be required to help alleviate spinal discomfort in animals with severe ankylosing spondylosis.

Multiple Cartilaginous Exostoses

Multiple cartilaginous exostoses, also known as *osteochondromatoses, osteocartilaginous exostoses,* and *multiple osteochondromas,* are conditions that occur in dogs, cats, and horses. The disease is a benign proliferation of cartilage and bone that affects the bones formed by endochondral ossification. In addition to the appendicular skeleton, lesions may develop in the vertebral bodies or the dorsal spinous processes (Figure 6-15, *A*). The ribs are also commonly affected (see Figure 6-15, *B*). A small percentage of cartilaginous exostoses may undergo malignant transformation into chondrosarcomas. Clinical evidence indicates that the condition may be inherited in the dog and horse.[62,63]

Clinical signs appear during the period of active bone growth. Pain or loss of function develops when adjacent structures are compressed or distorted by the bony lesions.[64] Vertebral involvement is frequent in dogs. Spinal cord compression with neurologic deficits caudal to the lesion is common (see Figure 6-15, *C*). In most dogs studied, progressive paraparesis was the most common neurologic finding; however, compressive lesions in the cervical spine may produce progressive tetraparesis. Radiographically, the bony exostoses are

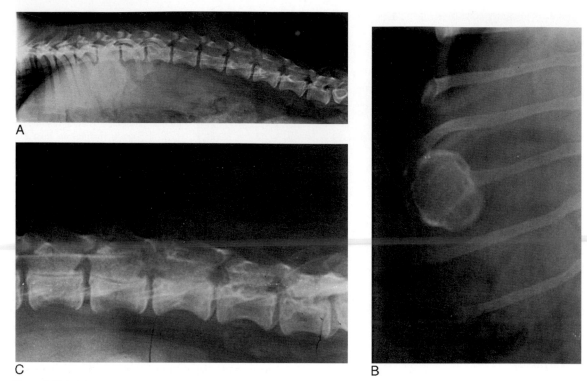

Figure 6-15 A, Multiple cartilaginous exostoses affecting the vertebrae of a young dog. Note the cyst-like structures within the vertebrae. **B,** Radiograph of a cystlike bone lesion in the rib of the same dog. These bony, bullae-like structures are diagnostic of multiple cartilaginous exostoses. **C,** Myelogram demonstrating severe spinal cord compression from L4 to L6. Occasionally, these lesions undergo malignant transformation to chondrosarcoma.

characterized as variably sized radiopaque densities with large radiolucent areas. Vertebral lesions tend to be circular in shape. Radiography provides strong supportive evidence of the diagnosis; however, a definitive diagnosis of multiple cartilaginous exostoses is based on typical biopsy findings. Microscopic examination of a tissue specimen is needed to differentiate the condition from malignant vertebral neoplasia.

The exostoses apparently stop growing after physeal closure. Surgical removal of the lesion should be attempted if skeletal or neurologic dysfunction is present.

Afghan Hound Myelopathy

In 1973, Cockrell and co-workers[65] described a demyelinating malacic spinal cord disease in related, young Afghan hounds. The age at onset varied from 3 to 13 months, and the clinical course was 2 to 6 weeks. Affected dogs developed progressive pelvic limb ataxia and paresis. Spinal reflexes were usually normal or exaggerated. In some dogs, mild thoracic limb deficits were detected. The disorder progressed to tetraplegia and death from respiratory failure in 2 to 6 weeks. Severe destruction of myelin with relative sparing

of axons was found in the ventral, lateral, and sometimes dorsal funiculi. The lesions were prominent in spinal cord segments C5-L3. The most severe changes were found in the cranial thoracic spinal cord.

The pathogenesis is unknown, although a genetic basis may be important. De Lahunta proposes that the lesion is a primary leukodystrophy with a hereditary basis.[66] No effective treatment is known.

Diskospondylitis and Vertebral Abscess

Pathologic Findings. Diskospondylitis is an intervertebral disk infection with concurrent osteomyelitis of contiguous vertebrae (Figure 6-16). Various causes are known, including foreign-body migration and bacterial or fungal infection. In dogs, the most common causes are *Staphylococcus intermedius* and, occasionally, *Streptococcus* spp. Gram-negative rods and *Brucella canis*.[67] Diskospondylitis is associated with urinary tract infection and bacteremia. Infection of the intervertebral disks and the vertebrae usually occurs secondary to infection of one of these primary foci. Infrequently, infection may occur secondary to surgical fenestration of the disks. The infection may

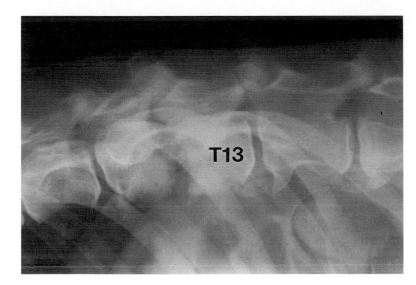

Figure 6-16 Lateral radiograph of the vertebral column of a 5-year-old female German shepherd dog with progressive paraparesis. Lysis of the caudal end-plate of T12 and the cranial end plate of T13 is seen. Osteophytes extend from the ventral aspects of the vertebral bodies at the T13-L1 and L1-L2 interspaces. A diagnosis of diskospondylitis at T12-T13 and spondylosis deformans at T13-L1 and L1-2 was made. (From Kornegay JN: Vertebral diseases of large breed dogs. In Kornegay JN, editor: *Neurologic disorders: Contemporary issues in small animal practice,* vol 5. New York, 1986, Churchill Livingstone.)

involve cervical or thoracolumbar vertebrae; however, it most frequently develops in the lumbosacral, thoracolumbar, cervicothoracic, and midthoracic disk spaces (Figure 6-17). Multifocal lesions may also occur.

Vertebral abscesses are formed primarily in young or debilitated large animals. An association is often present with omphalophlebitis (navel ill) in calves and foals, tail docking in lambs, erysipelas arthritis in swine,[68] pneumonia in cattle,[69] and enteric *Salmonella* infections in horses. The bacteria-producing vertebral abscesses in foals include *Salmonella* spp., *Streptococcus* spp., *Actinobacillus equuli, Eikenella corrodens,* and *Rhodococcus equi.*

In adult horses, *Brucella abortus* and *Mycobacterium tuberculosis* are reported.[9] In food animals, *Corynebacterium pyogenes* is the bacterium most commonly isolated, but *Spherophorus* spp. and *Staphylococcus* spp. in cattle and streptococci and *Erysipelothrix insidiosa* in swine are also common.[9]

Neurologic signs develop from encroachment on the spinal cord or nerve roots by the expanding tissues, causing severe pain and, eventually, paresis. Destruction of the vertebrae may cause spinal instability with secondary compression of the spinal cord. Paresis or paralysis and ataxia caudal to the lesion result from the spinal cord compression.

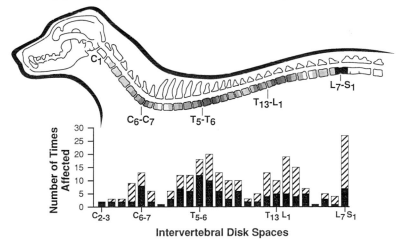

Figure 6-17 Histogram and schematic of frequency of intervertebral disk space involvement in 56 dogs with diskospondylitis evaluated at the University of Georgia College of Veterinary Medicine between 1976 and 1981 (solid bars) and 75 affected dogs evaluated at the North Carolina State University College of Veterinary Medicine between 1983 and 1990 (hatched bars). Some dogs had multiple infected sites. Combined data are expressed in the schematic of the vertebral column, with darker regions identifying areas affected most frequently. (From Kornegay JN: Diskospondylitis. In Slatter DH, editor: *Textbook of small animal surgery,* ed 2. Philadelphia, 1993, WB Saunders.)

Clinical Signs. Diskospondylitis can affect dogs of any age but is more common in adults. In one study, the mean age was 5.1 years.[70] This disease is apparently more frequent in male dogs than in female dogs (2:1 ratio). In all animals, clinical signs may develop acutely and progress rapidly; however, the usual course is chronic and progressive. Most animals have systemic signs including anorexia, depression, and pyrexia. In dogs, signs of urinary tract infection or endocarditis-myocarditis occasionally are detected. Dogs with brucellosis may have signs suggesting this disease (orchitis, epididymitis, abortion, infertility, and so forth). Systemic signs, however, usually are not localizing to any body system.

Frequently encountered clinical signs are directly referable to the musculoskeletal and nervous systems. These signs include hyperesthesia in the area of vertebral involvement, stiff gait, and paresis or paralysis if spinal cord compression occurs. The syndrome is quite similar to intervertebral disk disease except animals with diskospondylitis frequently are systemically ill and have a more chronic disease course. Large-breed dogs with type II disk disease rarely are in as much pain as those with diskospondylitis. Specific neurologic signs are related to the site of involvement. Cervical lesions may cause tetraparesis and severe neck pain. Thoracolumbar lesions cause back pain and pelvic limb paresis and ataxia.

Diskospondylitis and vertebral abscesses always are suspected in animals with fever, depression, anorexia, vertebral pain, and pelvic limb ataxia or paresis.

Diagnosis. A definitive diagnosis is made with conventional radiography of the spine. Occasionally, radiographic abnormalities are not detected in early lesions, even though typical clinical signs are present.[71] Radiographically evident lesions may lag behind the onset of clinical signs for 2 to 3 weeks. Typical radiographic findings include concentric lysis of adjacent vertebral end plates and various degrees of vertebral lysis and bone production (see Figure 6-16). Vertebral bodies may be shortened, and intervertebral disk spaces may be narrowed. Severely destructive lesions may cause vertebral luxation and spinal cord compression. Radionuclide scintigraphy may be useful if diskospondylitis is strongly suspected and no vertebral lesions are seen on survey radiographs. Radiographic changes may not be apparent for about 2 weeks after infection, whereas scintigraphy may demonstrate the lesion within 3 days.[67]

Affected dogs occasionally have leukocytosis and pyuria. Leukocytosis is more common in dogs with associated endocarditis. The CSF is usually normal, although elevations in protein concentration and mononuclear cells are occasionally encountered. Blood cultures are positive in about 45% of cases, and *Staphylococcus intermedius* is the most common bacterium isolated.[71] Urine cultures also may be positive, and *S. intermedius* usually is isolated in these tests as well. The tube agglutination test is usually positive in dogs affected with *Brucella canis*. Aspiration of lesions may be accomplished with fluoroscopic guidance in small animals and directly in large animals. Cultures of this material can establish a definitive diagnosis.[9,72]

Treatment. Antibiotic therapy is based on sensitivity testing of bacteria isolated from urine or blood or from infected tissues (see Chapter 15). Antibiotic therapy alone is suggested unless severe spinal cord compression is present or if after 5 days no response to therapy occurs. Therapy should be continued for at least 4 to 6 weeks. Compressive lesions require decompression, curettage, and stabilization in addition to long-term antibiotic therapy. Brucellosis is difficult to resolve and warrants a guarded prognosis. Owners should be advised of the risk of transmission to humans.

In large animals, antibiotic therapy is based on culture and sensitivity testing. In horses, surgical curettage and drainage of infected vertebrae are beneficial. Dogs that respond favorably in the first week have a good prognosis. The lesions should be monitored radiographically for several months for signs of progression.

Spinal Arachnoid Cysts

Arachnoid cysts involving the spinal cord can cause a progressive compressive myelopathy. Arachnoid cysts occur in the cervical and thoracolumbar spinal cord. Large-breed dogs appear to develop cervical lesions more frequently, and small breed dogs develop them more frequently in the thoracolumbar region.[73] The neurologic signs relate to the region of spinal cord affected. In the thoracolumbar region, clinical signs and course may be protracted over weeks to years. Most dogs develop UMN paraparesis and urinary incontinence. In the cervical region, neurologic signs include ataxia, tetraparesis, and hypermetria of the thoracic limbs. The lesions can be delineated with myelography, CT, and MRI. Various surgical procedures for treating the disorder have been described.[73]

Compressive Myelopathy in Shiloh Shepherd Dogs

An unusual degenerative joint disease that affects the articular processes of the thoracolumbar spinal cord has been described in Shiloh Shepherd dogs.[74] Clinical signs develop from 9 weeks to 16 months of age and include UMN paraparesis and ataxia.

Proliferative lesions involving the articular facets from T11 to L2 were demonstrated radiographically and were responsible for a dorsal compressive myelopathy. Surgery was beneficial in two cases and not beneficial in one case. One dog partially responded to medical treatment consisting of exercise restriction and a reduced protein diet. The disease may be inherited.

Acute Progressive Diseases, L4-S3

The acute progressive diseases that affect the caudal lumbar and sacral spinal cord segments are listed by etiologic category in Tables 6-4 through 6-6. Most of these diseases have been discussed in the previous sections that considered T3-L3 disorders. Remember that some of these diseases initially occur as pelvic limb paresis but may progress to involve the cervical spinal cord. Tetraparesis (tetraplegia) may develop as the disease progresses (see Chapter 7).

Acute Nonprogressive Diseases, L4-S3

In this section two diseases are described: fibrocartilaginous embolism and lumbosacral trauma. Although fibrocartilaginous embolism can affect any spinal cord segment, it occurs most frequently in the caudal lumbar area and less frequently in the midcervical to caudal cervical spinal cord. For this reason, we have elected to discuss it with the other L4-S3 disorders. Fibrocartilaginous embolism has a brief progressive course (a few hours) and then becomes nonprogressive. We have therefore classified it as a nonprogressive disease.

Fibrocartilaginous Emboli and Spinal Cord Infarction

Pathophysiology. Although emboli to the nervous system can develop from a variety of sources such as endocarditis, sepsis, and fat, the most common form causing spinal cord infarction is a fibrocartilaginous material that stains in a manner similar to nucleus pulposus. The cause of this disease is unknown. Fibrocartilaginous emboli occur in dogs, horses, cats, pigs, sheep, and humans.[75,76] Fibrocartilaginous material found in spinal cord arterioles and veins results in an ischemic necrotizing myelopathy (Figure 6-18). Exactly how this material is distributed into the spinal cord circulation is not known, but several theories have been proposed. Most of these are based on the belief that fibrocartilaginous emboli originate from the intervertebral disks. The most probable mechanism is herniation of disk material into the body of the vertebra, followed by entrance into a venous plexus and then into an arteriovenous anastomosis. The

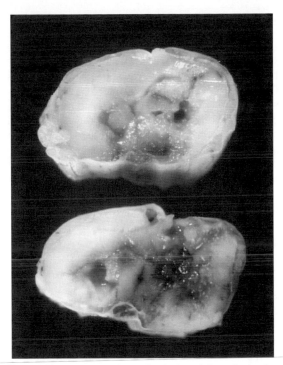

Figure 6-18 Adjacent sections of spinal cord from the lumbar intumescence from a great Dane with acute asymmetric paraplegia resulting from histologically confirmed fibrocartilaginous embolism. Note the right side of the spinal cord is markedly necrotic and contains hemorrhage.

material could then enter the spinal cord in arteries, veins, or both.[75,77]

Clinical Signs. The clinical signs develop acutely and progress rapidly within 1 to 2 hours from initial pain to unilateral or bilateral paralysis. Unilateral or asymmetric signs are common, which is explained by the frequency of unilateral branches of the central branch of the ventral spinal artery. Vigorous exercise may precede the development of signs; however, known trauma is absent. The clinical syndrome is characteristic of acute spinal cord compression from herniated intervertebral disks or vertebral fractures except that hyperesthesia is absent. Lateralization of signs is very suggestive of fibrocartilaginous embolism because spinal cord compression generally causes bilateral signs. Bilateral signs also occur in fibrocartilaginous embolism. The degree and character of the neurologic deficit correspond to the site and the extent of the spinal cord infarction. Infarction of gray matter may cause LMN signs in affected limbs. Larger-breed dogs have been studied most intensely, but spinal cord infarction occurs in smaller dogs as well. Chondrodystrophoid breeds with a predisposition for type I disk disease are affected infrequently.

Diagnosis. The key clinical features of fibrocartilaginous embolism are acute onset, nonprogressive course (except for the first few hours), and nonpainful, asymmetric paresis. A few animals seem to be in pain for 1 or more days. Asymmetry is not found in every case but is a valuable sign when present. Trauma is not in the history, but dogs are frequently reported to be exercising at the time of onset. No definitive diagnostic procedure exists for spinal cord infarction. The diagnosis is supported by evidence that rules out the presence of spinal cord compression. Survey radiography and myelography findings are usually negative. The myelogram may show a slight swelling of the spinal cord for the first few days. The hemogram and the biochemistry values are normal. The CSF may contain a slight increase in protein. Dogs should be evaluated for hypertension and hypothyroidism, conditions that might predispose an animal to CNS vascular occlusion and infarction.

Treatment. Therapy for fibrocartilaginous embolism and spinal cord infarction is aimed largely at reducing spinal cord edema and inflammation with corticosteroids. If therapy can be administered in the first few hours after onset, the protocol described in the section on spinal cord trauma is recommended. If therapy is delayed, it is probably of no benefit. The benefit of anticoagulants is unknown, but because this is not a clotting problem, no reason exists to expect they might be useful. Affected dogs should rest for 1 to 2 weeks. Improvement should be noted within a few days, but functional recovery may require several weeks. The clinical signs of complete paralysis, loss of deep sensation, or LMN involvement are associated with a poor prognosis. If motor neurons are destroyed in an infarcted area of the spinal cord that innervates the limbs or bladder, the deficit is likely to be permanent. Because recovery from white matter damage is more likely to occur, animals with UMN deficits have better prognoses. Many dogs, especially smaller dogs, make satisfactory recoveries, so early euthanasia is discouraged.

Trauma

Pelvic fractures, caudal lumbar fractures, and lumbosacral subluxations are very common skeletal injuries in animals. Traumatic lesions in this area may involve the termination of the spinal cord or the cauda equina. These injuries may compress or entrap the roots of the sciatic, pelvic, and pudendal nerves, resulting in severe neurologic dysfunction of the pelvic limbs, the urinary bladder, and the anal sphincter (Figure 6-19). The assessment of pelvic fractures or lumbosacral subluxations must include a neurologic evaluation of the pelvic limbs, the external anal sphincter, and the urinary bladder. The prognosis for recovery is much better in animals with normal neurologic function. The diagnosis and management of sciatic nerve injury are discussed in Chapter 5.

Sacral and caudal fractures are common, especially in cats, but they also occur in dogs, horses, and cattle. The syndrome in cats is usually caused by a fracture or luxation at the sacrocaudal junction. Traction injury to the cauda equina results in loss of innervation to the tail, perineum, anal sphincter, and urinary bladder. Functional assessment of the anal sphincter affords a good indirect assessment of bladder function; however, some animals have normal anal sphincter function with no bladder function. The mechanism is not clear but may indicate intrapelvic injury to the pelvic nerves. Animals with complete denervation to the perineum, anal sphincter, and bladder have a grave prognosis. We generally recommend medical management for 4 to 6 weeks in case the injury is only temporary (see Chapter 3 for management of neurogenic bladder).

Chronic Progressive Diseases, L4-S3

Degenerative Lumbosacral Stenosis (Cauda Equina Syndrome)

Compression of the cauda equina at the lumbosacral articulation is relatively common and has been reported in dogs of various ages and breeds.

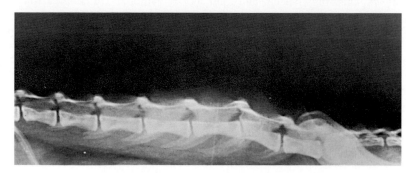

Figure 6-19 Compressive fracture of L6 produced severe paraplegia and loss of deep pain sensation caudal to the lesion. Although little displacement is appreciated radiographically, the fracture had functionally severed the spinal cord.

In several studies, older large-breed dogs such as German shepherd dogs, Labrador retrievers, or crossbreds were affected more frequently.[78,79] Sometimes this disorder is not recognized because of the occurrence of musculoskeletal problems in these breeds.[80-82]

Pathogenesis. Although the cause is unknown, the common initiating factor for the degenerative changes is probably abnormal motion at the lumbosacral articulations. The biomechanical abnormality causes cumulative microtrauma, resulting in proliferation of fibrous connective tissue and osteophytes. Stresses on the annulus fibrosus lead to proliferative changes and bulging of the disk. In essence this is a Hansen type II disk degeneration with additional changes in the articulations and vertebral end plates. Narrowing of the disk causes the intervertebral foramen to be smaller. When osteophytes are around the foramen, the L7 spinal nerve is entrapped (Figure 6-20). In some cases ventral displacement of the sacrum occurs relative to L7, further narrowing the vertebral canal. Proliferation of the soft tissues of the joints, annulus fibrosus, and interarcuate ligament contributes to the compression. Extension of the joint causes additional folding of these tissues, thereby increasing pressure on the nerves (Figure 6-21). A few animals appear to have a narrow canal with shortened pedicles, suggesting a developmental stenosis similar to the cervical spondylopathy in great Danes.

This syndrome appears to have several similarities to canine wobbler syndrome (cervical

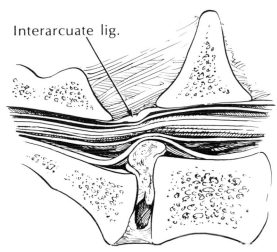

Figure 6-21 Lumbosacral degenerative stenosis. Compression of the cauda equina in a sagittal plane by the combined effects of disk herniation and ventral folding of the interarcuate ligament. Note how extension would increase the compression. (From Chambers JN: Degenerative lumbosacral stenosis in dogs, *Vet Med Rep* 1:166-180, 1989.)

spondylopathy; see Chapter 7). Both syndromes are characterized by a narrowing of the vertebral canal that results from subluxation or stenosis of the vertebral foramen. Altered soft tissue structures and type II disk herniations may narrow the vertebral canal further. Cervical spondylopathy results in spinal cord compression, whereas lumbosacral spondylopathy produces compression or entrapment of the cauda equina or the L7 nerve root. The high incidence in German shepherd dogs suggests a developmental predisposition, even though the clinical signs occur in older dogs.

Clinical Signs. Early clinical signs are related to lumbosacral pain. Dogs may experience difficulty rising, and at this stage the clinical signs are easily confused with hip dysplasia. Recurring lameness of one or both pelvic limbs is common. The owner frequently reports that the dog does not jump or has difficulty going up steps. Exercise often exacerbates the signs. At this stage, various orthopedic problems, including hip dysplasia and stifle injury, are often suspected. Because most of the affected dogs also commonly have hip dysplasia, the primary problem is frequently missed. Rear-limb paresis is not usual unless the condition is advanced. Then the problem is usually weakness in the muscles innervated by the sciatic nerve, causing decreased extension of the hock. Only rarely are significant proprioceptive positioning deficits present. A few animals appear to have paresthesia in the tail or perineal region and may lick or chew the affected area. Frequently the owner may notice a less erect tail carriage.

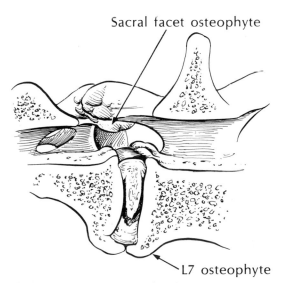

Figure 6-20 Lumbosacral degenerative stenosis. Compromise of intervertebral foramen by articular osteophytes that have formed on facet and vertebral body. (From Chambers JN: Degenerative lumbosacral stenosis in dogs, *Vet Med Rep* 1:166-180, 1989.)

Urinary and fecal incontinence are common associated clinical signs in advanced cases and result from compression of the sacral nerves. The anal sphincter may be atonic, and the perineal reflex may be weak or absent. The urinary incontinence is of the LMN type, resulting in a poor detrusor reflex and a weak urethral sphincter. The bladder usually is easily expressed.

In early cases the examination indicates lameness without paresis, normal to marginally slow postural reactions, and normal spinal reflexes. Some animals appear to have brisk knee jerk reflexes because of loss of resistance from the flexors innervated by the sciatic nerve. The flexion reflex is usually not weak until the condition is severe. The key to clinical diagnosis is localization of hyperesthesia in the lumbosacral region. More than 90% of affected dogs are in pain. The examiner must elicit pain from the lumbosacral region without causing pain from the hips. The examiner first applies pressure on the vertebral column. In contradistinction to the evaluation of most conditions, we prefer to start in the cervical region and work caudally. This establishes the dog's tolerance to deep palpation so that hyperesthesia can be recognized. The typical reaction is increasing anxiety as palpation progresses caudally, with a significant reaction when the lumbosacral area is pressed. Placing the thumbs on the midline, with the fingers on each ilium, allows the examiner direct pressure at the correct location without stressing the dog's hips. If this fails to elicit a reaction, the tail is elevated with continued pressure on the lumbosacral region. Each pelvic limb can also be extended caudally to stress the lumbosacral articulation even further. Remember, extension of the lumbosacral articulation causes maximal compression and pain. Extension of the hips also may cause pain if hip dysplasia is present; however, abduction and rotation of the hips should also cause pain in hip dysplasia but not stress the lumbosacral junction. By comparing the dog's response to lumbosacral extension with the response to hip manipulation, the examiner can distinguish lumbosacral stenosis from hip dysplasia.

Diagnosis. Lumbosacral spondylopathy must be differentiated from disease syndromes with similar clinical signs. These disorders include various causes of compression such as trauma and neoplasia; inflammatory diseases such as diskospondylitis and abscesses; orthopedic diseases such as arthritis, hip dysplasia, and cranial cruciate rupture; and spinal cord diseases such as degenerative myelopathy. Localization is critical to rule out most of these diseases. Those that affect the cauda equina require additional diagnostic tests. EMG can be a valuable tool for mapping the distribution of denervation and localizing the lesion to specific nerve roots. Radiography is useful for establishing whether the skeletal lesions are compatible with stenosis, subluxation, or spondylosis. Myelography, vertebral sinus venography, epidurography, and CT are the primary diagnostic tools recommended by most authorities. Our preference is epidurography and CT. Myelography is useful to help rule out concurrent disease in the spinal cord, but it is not as effective as epidurography in defining lumbosacral compression. Both flexed and extended lateral views must be taken during epidurography to accentuate the compression in animals with minimal change (Figure 6-22). See Chapter 4 and the references for additional discussion and techniques.[80,82-85]

Treatment. The management of lumbosacral spondylopathy is based on an evaluation of the severity and duration of the clinical signs. Rest for 4 to 6 weeks and analgesics are recommended for dogs with an initial episode of pain only. Progression of clinical signs is a strong indication for surgery.

Dorsal laminectomy is recommended if signs continue despite confinement, recur as soon as exercise is allowed (the usual outcome) or become progressively worse, or if significant motor deficits or urinary and fecal incontinence develop. The annulus of the disk is excised and the nucleus is removed. Evidence of L7 nerve root entrapment, most readily recognized on EMG, warrants foraminotomy in addition to laminectomy. Postoperative care includes scrupulous attention to the maintenance of bladder functions if this is a problem (see Chapter 3). Exercise should be restricted for at least 6 weeks. Dogs that become active too early often have episodes of pain. Nonsteroidal analgesics may be given to reduce pain in the postoperative period. Prognosis depends on the severity and duration of signs. Dogs with pain as the only sign have an excellent prognosis for complete recovery, although they may experience episodes of discomfort after vigorous exercise. We have treated dogs that have returned to hunting after surgery. Chambers reported that 13 of 18 dogs with pain only were completely normal after surgery. Three of the remaining four dogs were substantially improved.[80] In another study, 17 of 18 dogs responded well to surgery.[70] Recovery is far less certain when LMN signs, especially with incontinence, are present before surgery.[79, 80-86]

Vertebral Column Malformations

Vertebral Anomalies. Vertebral anomalies are common in dogs with a screw tail, such as the English and French bulldogs and the Boston terrier.[87] They are reported in other species, especially the horse.[88] Incomplete separation of the vertebral

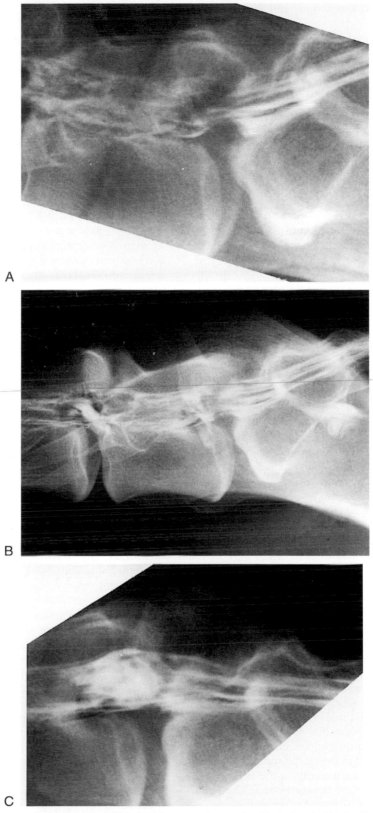

Figure 6-22 Degenerative lumbosacral stenosis. A lateral epidurogram view made with the legs in (**A**) dorsiflexion (extension), (**B**) neutral position, and (**C**) flexion. The lesion is most apparent in the dorsiflexion view. Slight (less than 50%) elevation of the epidural space is seen on the neutral view, and no compression is seen on the flexed view. (From Selcer BA: Radiographic imaging in canine lumbosacral disease, *Vet Med Rep* 1:282-290, 1989.)

bodies, arches, or entire vertebra is called *block vertebrae. Hemivertebra* is potentially of clinical importance. Failure of ossification of one half of the vertebral body may cause unilateral, dorsal, or ventral hemivertebra. Unilateral hemivertebra causes scoliosis, dorsal hemivertebra causes kyphosis, and ventral hemivertebra causes lordosis. *Butterfly vertebra* has a sagittal cleft of the vertebral body. These anomalies are most common in the thoracic area and rarely cause clinical signs. Dorsal displacement of a ventral hemivertebra may induce chronic progressive spinal cord compression. Vertebrae that have properties of two major divisions of the vertebral column are called *transitional vertebrae.* Cervicothoracic transitional vertebrae have transverse processes that resemble ribs. We have seen one dog that had a cervical rib that seemed to cause pain from stretching of the spinal nerve. Thoracolumbar transitional vertebrae may also have spinous processes resembling ribs, absence of a rib on one side, or fusion of the last rib like a transverse process. The major significance is in the location of the correct interspace in spinal surgery, where the T13-L1 interspace is identified as a landmark. Lumbosacral transitional vertebrae may have some association with degenerative lumbosacral stenosis. The last lumbar vertebra may fuse with the first sacral vertebra bilaterally or unilaterally. Unilateral sacralization may cause deviation of the pelvis and possibly nerve root entrapment. The appearance of transverse processes on the first sacral vertebra is called *lumbarization* and may lead to instability.

Spinal Dysraphism. The dysraphic conditions are congenital defects that result from failure of normal closure of the neural tube. They may affect the brain or spinal cord, often with accompanying abnormalities in the surrounding bone and other tissues. Those affecting the vertebral column or the spinal cord in animals include spinal dysraphism, syringomyelia, spina bifida with or without myelomeningocele, and caudal vertebral hypoplasia.

Spinal dysraphism occurs in several breeds of dogs and pigs but has been documented most frequently in the weimaraner.[89] Changes within the spinal cord include absence, distention, or duplication of the central canal. Other changes include hydromyelia, syringomyelia, and anomalies of the ventral median fissure. Fluid-filled cavitations are commonly observed in dysraphic spinal cords, and spinal dysraphism, particularly in the weimaraner breed, has been called *syringomyelia.* The fluid-filled cysts in the dysraphic spinal cords of weimaraners probably result from abnormal vascularization that produces ischemia, degeneration, and cavitation. The thoracic spinal cord is most commonly affected. Because dysraphic lesions are

the cause of the clinical signs, the term *spinal dysraphism* is preferred to the term *syringomyelia.*

Clinical signs are usually apparent at 6 to 8 weeks of age, although in mild cases the dog may not be presented for examination until it is several months old. The classic clinical signs include a symmetric hopping gait with the pelvic limbs (bunny hopping), a crouching posture, and a wide-based stance. Proprioceptive positioning in the pelvic limbs is depressed, and the animal may occasionally knuckle over. The postural reactions are depressed. The spinal reflexes are usually normal, and exaggerated scratch reflexes may be present. Pain perception is usually intact. The neurologic signs are nonprogressive but become more obvious as the animal matures. Less common clinical signs include abnormal hair streams or hair whorls in the dorsal cervical area, kinking of the undocked tail, scoliosis, and depression of the sternum.

Diagnosis is based on typical clinical signs and the breed involved. The clinical signs are nearly pathognomonic in the weimaraner. Spinal radiographs and CSF analysis help eliminate the diagnosis of a treatable disease. No effective treatment is available. Because the syndrome is probably inherited in the weimaraner, owners are advised to cease breeding animals that have produced affected puppies.

Spina Bifida. Spina bifida is the incomplete closure or fusion of the dorsal vertebral arches. In many cases it occurs in association with protrusion of the meninges (meningocele) or the spinal cord and the meninges (myelomeningocele) through the vertebral defect (Figure 6-23). Often these meningeal or spinal cord protrusions adhere to the skin where the neural ectoderm failed to separate from the other ectodermal structures (see Figure 6-23). These adhesions may produce a small depression or dimple in the skin at the site of attachment. In some cases this defect is open and spinal fluid leaks onto the skin, producing epidermal ulceration. Because the meninges are exposed in this situation, meningitis may develop. In most cases that have been investigated, the caudal and some of the sacral nerves are either severely attenuated or incomplete. Associated anomalies may include myeloschisis, tethering of the distal spinal cord, and hydrocephalus.[90,91] Spina bifida may affect any vertebra but is most common in the caudal lumbar and sacral areas. This defect has been observed in the thoracic and lumbar vertebrae in a litter of kittens. Spina bifida is most common in the Manx cat and the bulldog but can occur in all species.[90-92]

Clinical signs may be minimal or extensive, depending on the severity of the involvement of the spinal cord or the cauda equina. Some animals have signs similar to those of spinal dysraphism.

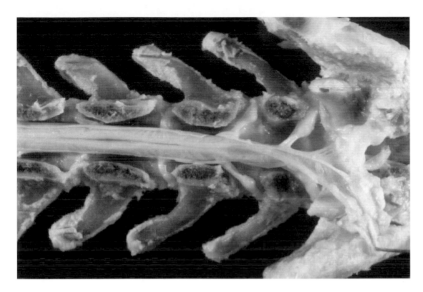

Figure 6-23 Caudal region of the vertebral column, spinal cord, and cauda equina from a 2-year-old female English bulldog with urinary-fecal incontinence since birth. Portions of the cauda equina extend dorsally into a meningeal sac *(arrow),* and a dorsal longitudinal spinal cleft is present. A diagnosis of meningomyelocele with associated myeloschisis was made. (From Kornegay JN: Lesions of the lumbosacral intumescence and cauda equina. In Slatter DH, editor: *Textbook of small animal surgery,* Philadelphia, 1985, WB Saunders.)

In the bulldog, clinical signs often are related to dysfunction in the areas innervated by the cauda equina. Mild to moderate pelvic limb ataxia and paresis may be present. Many animals have decreased innervation of the muscles supplied by the sciatic nerve. The limb may be fixed in extension owing to the unopposed contraction of the quadriceps muscle. Affected dogs consistently have fecal and urinary incontinence, and pelvic limb ataxia is usually present. Pain perception may be decreased in the perineal area and from the distal regions of the pelvic limbs. Spina bifida without myelomeningocele is not associated with any neurologic deficits.

Spina bifida is confirmed radiographically. The presence of meningocele and myelomeningocele can be determined myelographically (Figure 6-24). No specific treatments are available for spina bifida. Surgical correction of the tethered spinal cord has been attempted, but no improvement occurred in the single case reported.[90] The extensive loss of normal nerve supply to bladder and anus makes recovery unlikely in most of these animals. Meningoceles can be closed surgically to prevent the leakage of CSF and to prevent meningeal infection.

Sacrocaudal Hypoplasia in Manx Cats. The Manx cat has been bred selectively to have a bobtail; however, numerous spinal and neural anomalies are encountered in the breed. The Manx factor, or taillessness, is apparently inherited as an autosomal dominant trait.[92] The anomalies are caused by

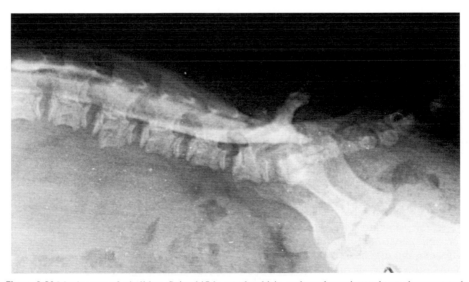

Figure 6-24 Myelogram of a bulldog. Spina bifida, myeloschisis, and myelomeningocele are demonstrated.

incomplete penetrance of the dominant genes for taillessness. In addition to caudal dysgenesis, sacral hypoplasia may occur. Spina bifida is also commonly encountered in this breed. Spinal cord anomalies include dysraphism, syringomyelia, meningocele, and myelomeningocele.[93]

The neurologic signs are related to abnormal development of the nerves in the cauda equina. These signs include LMN deficits to the anus, the urinary bladder, and the pelvic limbs. Urinary and fecal incontinence and fecal retention are major problems. A bunny-hopping gait is characteristic of the breed and is not considered abnormal by Manx breeders. Undoubtedly a certain degree of spinal dysraphism is present in these so-called normal cats. Severely affected cats have pelvic limb paresis or paralysis and ataxia. Primary uterine inertia has also been observed. The clinical signs are present from birth and are nonprogressive. The diagnosis is based on the breed, the clinical signs, and radiographic evidence of sacrocaudal abnormalities (Figure 6-25). Therapy is directed at relieving urinary and fecal retention.

Neuritis of the Cauda Equina (Polyneuritis Equi)

This is a severe, slowly progressive granulomatous LMN disease that primarily affects adult horses. Neuritis of the cauda equina is usually restricted to the caudal spinal cord nerves and nerve roots. The lesion is a demyelination with a granulomatous neuritis and meningitis involving the caudal nerve roots. Cranial nerve involvement may also occur in some cases, hence the term *polyneuritis equi*.[9, 94,95] The lesion resembles allergic neuritis, and the evidence suggests that this is an autoimmune polyneuritis.[96] As in coon hound paralysis and Landry-Guillain-Barré syndromes, a factor such as a virus probably initiates the immune reaction. A history of vaccination or respiratory illness is reported in some cases. Equine adenovirus 1 was isolated from two affected horses.[97] The cause is unknown.

Clinical Signs. Early signs include rubbing the perineal area, urine scalding, and constipation. LMN paresis or paralysis of the tail, the bladder, and the anal sphincter is found on examination. Decreased sensation in the perineal area also occurs and becomes more severe as the disease progresses. In male horses, pudendal paralysis results in a dropped penis or the inability to retract the penis. Hypalgesia to the penis also may occur. Cranial nerves V, VII, and VIII are frequently affected. Signs such as head tilt, nystagmus, and facial paralysis may occur in some horses.

Diagnosis. If both the cauda equina and cranial nerves are affected, the diagnosis is likely. If only the cauda equina is involved, sacral fractures should be ruled out by rectal palpation and radiography.

EMG and evoked potentials may be useful adjuncts if involvement of the cauda equina is in doubt. Collection of spinal fluid at the lumbar cistern is often diagnostic of cauda equina neuritis. Lumbosacral taps reveal moderately increased concentrations of protein (100-300 mg/dl) and cells (>100 cells/mm^3). The cytologic composition is mainly macrophages, neutrophils, and lymphocytes. Antibody to P_2 protein can be demonstrated by ELISA.[98]

Treatment. No specific treatment is known. Evacuation of the bladder and bowel may allow the animal to live for prolonged periods; however, denervation of the genital tract precludes breeding stallions.

Sorghum Cystitis and Ataxia

Degeneration of the spinal cord and spinal nerve fibers occurs in horses, cattle, and sheep that ingest sorghum, Johnson, or Sudan grass. Lesions develop primarily in the lumbar, sacral, and caudal spinal cord segments. Histopathologically these lesions are characterized by focal axonal degeneration and demyelination with associated lipid-laden macrophages. The lesions may result from chronic sublethal doses of hydrocyanic acid found in plants of the genus *Sorghum*. Production of a lathyrogenic principle (nitrile-related amino acid) has also been postulated.[99]

History. Enzootics of this disease occur in horses of all ages that graze in sorghum or Sudan grass pastures. The disease usually occurs when the plants are young and rapidly growing, but mature and second-growth plants also have been incriminated. Apparently the toxins do not persist in cured hay or silage.

Clinical Signs. Although the signs of urinary incontinence are most noticeable in many horses, neurologic signs usually develop first. They include flaccidity of the anus and tail and pelvic limb ataxia. Occasionally, severe LMN paralysis of the pelvic limbs develops within 24 hours after the onset of neurologic signs. In female horses, clinical signs include continual opening and closing of the vulva, perineal paresis, and dribbling of urine. Urine scalds and thick urine deposits occur on the buttocks, the thighs, and the hocks. Male horses drip urine from a relaxed and extended penis. Urinary incontinence is intensified when the animal is forced to move suddenly. Hyporeflexia and proprioceptive deficits are detectable in the pelvic limbs. Clinical signs rarely extend to the thoracic limbs, even though brainstem and cerebral cortical lesions have been reported.

Pregnant mares may abort, and these foals may have severe ankylosis (arthrogryposis). Arthrogryposis also may occur in full-term foals when the dam has grazed hybrid Sudan plants.

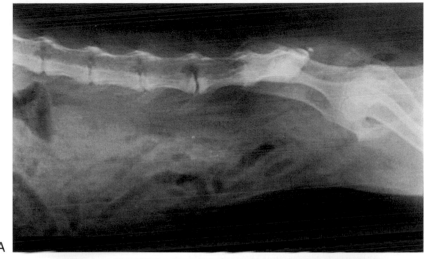

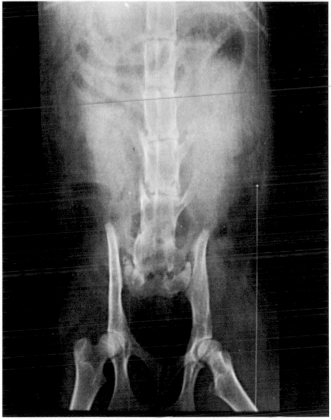

Figure 6-25 Lateral lumbosacral (**A**) and ventrodorsal (**B**) radiographs of a Manx cat with sacrocaudal abnormalities. Note the short, malformed sacrum and the absence of caudal vertebrae.

Diagnosis. The diagnosis is suspected from the history and the clinical signs. Affected horses have a severe fibrinopurulent cystitis secondary to neurogenic urine retention. Several different bacteria have been isolated from the urine of affected horses. Some animals develop severe ascending pyelonephritis from the chronic cystitis. The sensory loss in the perineum is less than that from cauda equina neuritis or sacral fracture.[9] Ancillary diagnostic tests are of little benefit. Mild changes in the CSF are found. Protein elevations are slight (60 to 80 mg/dl), and cell counts range from 5 to 10 mononuclear cells/mm^3. Urine or serum can be tested for high levels of thiocyanate, the major detoxification product of cyanide.

Treatment. No definitive treatment is known. Horses should not be allowed to graze in sorghum pastures while the plants are rapidly growing or are stunted by drought. Plants are generally safe if they are yellow, are more than 2 feet tall, or have formed fruiting heads. Pastures can be checked periodically to determine the amount of cyanide present when toxic forage is suspected.

Aortic Thrombosis (Ischemic Neuromyopathy)

Thromboembolism of the aorta or iliac arteries occurs with moderate frequency in cats and occasionally in dogs and horses. In cats it is associated with cardiomyopathy.[100] Saddle thrombi extend from the aorta into the iliac arteries. Vasoactive substances are believed to be involved in the pathogenesis of the ischemic changes.

Clinically the syndrome is characterized by an acute onset with little progression. Pelvic limb pain and paralysis are common. The femoral pulse is weak or absent. The distal limbs are cool, and pain sensation is absent. Distal limb muscles are affected more than proximal muscles. Although functional recovery may be possible, recurrences are also possible, and cardiomyopathy must be considered. Surgical removal of the thrombus may improve recovery, but its efficacy is controversial.

A similar syndrome is seen in performance horses. Associations with *Strongylus vulgaris* arteritis, thrombotic diseases, and cardiomyopathy have not been conclusively demonstrated.[9]

Case Histories

CASE HISTORY 6A

Signalment

Canine, Saint Bernard, female, 6 years old.

History

Six days ago, the dog suddenly cried out in pain and developed paresis in the pelvic limbs. Within 2 hours she became totally paralyzed in the pelvic limbs. No possibility of trauma was evident. The dog developed signs while under the owner's observation in the backyard.

Physical Examination

No abnormalities were found other than the neurologic problem described in the next section.

Neurologic Examination*

A. Observation
  1. Mental status: Alert

---

*0, Absent; +1, decreased; +2, normal; +3, exaggerated; +4, very exaggerated or clonus; PL, pelvic limb; TL, thoracic limb.

2. Posture: Normal, except gait
  3. Gait: No voluntary movement of either pelvic limb
B. Palpation: Hypertonus in right pelvic limb, hypotonus in left pelvic limb
C. Postural reactions

Left	Reactions	Right
	Proprioceptive positioning	
0	PL	0
+2	TL	+2
+2	Wheelbarrowing	+2
	Hopping	
0	PL	0
+2	TL	+2
0	Extensor postural thrust	0
0	Hemistand-hemiwalk	0
	Placing, tactile	
0	PL	0
+2	TL	+2
	Placing, visual	
2	TL	+2

D. Spinal reflexes

Left	Reflex, Spinal Segment	Right
+1	Quadriceps, L4-L6	+2
+2	Extensor carpi radialis, C7-T1	+2
+2	Triceps, C7-T1	+2
+1	Flexion—PL, L-S1	+3
+2	Flexion—TL, C6-T1	+2
Absent	Crossed extensor	Present
+2	Perineal, S1-S2	+2

E. Cranial nerves: All normal
F. Sensation: Location
  Hyperesthesia: 0
  Superficial pain: +2
  Deep pain: +2
Complete sections G and H before reviewing case summary.
G. Assessment (anatomic diagnosis and estimation of prognosis)
H. Plan (diagnostic)

  Rule-outs   *Procedure*
  1.
  2.
  3.
  4.

CASE HISTORY 6B

Signalment
Canine, Dachshund, female, 7 years old.

History
Two days ago the dog had a sudden onset of difficulty walking in the pelvic limbs and within 6 hours became paralyzed in both pelvic limbs. When the dog was examined initially, the pelvic limb reflexes were present, but pain perception was absent in both pelvic limbs. The thoracic limbs were normal.

Physical Examination
Urinary incontinence, hematuria, and shallow abdominal respirations are present. The dog cries periodically as if it were in pain.

Neurologic Examination*
A. Observation
   1. Mental status: Apprehensive
   2. Posture: Cannot maintain sternal recumbency
   3. Gait: No voluntary movements of pelvic limbs; short, choppy steps with thoracic limbs
B. Palpation: Hypotonus in both pelvic limbs; abdominal muscles are flaccid
C. Postural reactions

Left	Reactions	Right
	Proprioceptive positioning	
0	PL	0
+2	TL	+2
+1 to +2	Wheelbarrowing	+1 to +2
	Hopping	
0	PL	0
+2	TL	+2
0	Extensor postural thrust	0
0	Hemistand-hemiwalk	0
	Placing, tactile	
0	PL	0
+2	TL	+2
	Placing, visual	
+2	TL	+2

D. Spinal reflexes

Left	Reflex, Spinal Segment	Right
0	Quadriceps, L4-L6	0
+2	Extensor carpi radialis, C7-T1	+2
+2	Triceps, C7-T1	+2
0	Flexion—PL, L5-S1	0
+2	Flexion—TL, C6-T1	+2
0	Crossed extensor	0
0	Perineal, S1-S2	0

E. Cranial nerves: All normal
F. Sensation: Location
   Hyperesthesia: Present at T2-T3
   Superficial pain: Absent caudal to scapula
   Deep pain: Absent caudal to scapula.
Complete sections G and H before reviewing case summary.
G. Assessment (anatomic diagnosis and estimation of prognosis)
H. Plan (diagnostic)

   Rule-outs   Procedure
   1.
   2.
   3.
   4.

CASE HISTORY 6C

Signalment
Canine, German Shepherd dog, female, 1.5 years old.

History
Six weeks ago, the dog became lame in the right pelvic limb. Since then, paresis and ataxia have gradually developed in both pelvic limbs, more so on the right side than on the left. Three days ago the dog became completely paralyzed in both pelvic limbs.

Physical Examination
Findings were normal except for the neurologic problem.

Neurologic Examination*
A. Observation
   1. Mental status: Alert
   2. Posture: See Gait
   3. Gait: No voluntary movements in pelvic limbs; thoracic limbs normal
B. Palpation: Muscle atrophy from TL region caudally along spine; increased extensor tone in both pelvic limbs
C. Postural reactions

Left	Reactions	Right
	Proprioceptive positioning	
0	PL	0
+2	TL	+2
+2	Wheelbarrowing	+2

---

*0, Absent; +1, decreased; +2, normal; +3, exaggerated; +4, very exaggerated or clonus; *PL*, pelvic limb; *TL*, thoracic limb.

	Hopping	
0	PL	0
+2	TL	+2
0	Extensor postural thrust	0
0	Hemistand-hemiwalk	0
	Placing, tactile	
0	PL	0
+2	TL	+2
	Placing, visual	
+2	TL	+2

D. Spinal reflexes

Left	Reflex, Spinal Segment	Right
+3	Quadriceps, L4-L6	+3
+2	Extensor carpi radialis, C7-T1	+2
+2	Triceps, C7-T1	+2
+2	Flexion—PL, L5-S1	+2
+2	Flexion—TL, C6-T1	+2
0	Crossed extensor	0
+2	Perineal, S1-S2	+2

E. Cranial nerves: All normal
F. Sensation: Location
   Hyperesthesia: L2-L3
   Superficial pain: Absent caudal to L2
   Deep pain: Blunted caudal to L2-L3
Complete sections G and H before reviewing case summary.
G. Assessment (anatomic diagnosis and estimation of prognosis)
H. Plan (diagnostic)

Rule-outs	Procedure
1.	
2.	
3.	
4.	

CASE HISTORY 6D

Signalment
Canine, bulldog, male, 7 weeks old.

History
Since he became ambulatory the puppy has had a spastic, ataxic gait in the pelvic limbs. Urinary and fecal incontinence have been present for at least 2 weeks.

Physical Examination
Findings are normal except for the neurologic problem. Urinary incontinence is present.

Neurologic Examination*
A. Observation
   1. Mental status: Alert, responsive
   2. Posture: See Gait
   3. Gait: Paretic and ataxic in pelvic limbs; wide-based stance, feet tend to slip from under the dog
B. Palpation: No tone in anal sphincter; small depression in lumbar area just cranial to sacrum
C. Postural reactions

Left	Reactions	Right
	Proprioceptive positioning	
0	PL	0
+2	TL	+2
+2	Wheelbarrowing	+2
	Hopping	
+1	PL	+1
+2	TL	+2
+1	Extensor postural thrust	+1
+1	Hemistand-hemiwalk	+1
+2	Tonic neck	+2
	Placing, tactile	
0	PL	0
+2	TL	+2
	Placing, visual	
+2	TL	+2

D. Spinal reflexes

Left	Reflex, Spinal Segment	Right
+2	Quadriceps, L4-L6	+2
+2	Extensor carpi radialis, C7-T1	+2
+2	Triceps, C7-T1	+2
0 to +1	Flexion—PL, L5-S1	0 to +1
+2	Flexion—TL, C6-T1	+2
0	Crossed extensor	0
+0	Perineal, S1-S2	0

E. Cranial nerves: All normal
F. Sensation: Location
   Hyperesthesia: None
   Superficial pain: Absent in perineal area
   Deep pain: Present but decreased in perineum and tail
Complete sections G and H before reviewing case summary.

---

*0, Absent; +1, decreased; +2, normal; +3, exaggerated; +4, very exaggerated or clonus; PL, pelvic limb; TL, thoracic limb.

G. Assessment (anatomic diagnosis and estimation of prognosis)

H. Plan (diagnostic)

Rule-outs	Procedure
1.	
2.	
3.	
4.	

ASSESSMENT 6A

Anatomic Diagnosis

This dog has paraplegia characterized by UMN signs in the right limb and LMN signs in the left limb, with no hyperesthesia. An asymmetric lesion in the midlumbar spinal cord is probably present (spinal cord segments L2-7). The lesion has spared spinal cord sensory pathways. Acute nonprogressive diseases should be considered.

Diagnostic Plan

(Rule-outs—see Tables 6-1 and 6-4)

1. Spinal cord infarction (fibrocartilaginous embolism): No evidence of spinal cord compression, no hyperesthesia
2. Intervertebral disk disease: Spinal radiography and myelography were both negative.

Therapeutic Plan

1. At 6 days after injury, corticosteroids are very unlikely to be beneficial
2. Supportive care of a paraplegic

Client Education

The prognosis is poor because the lesion is severe and LMN involvement is present. The presence of pain sensation implies that some spinal cord integrity is present, however. Maintain the dog for 2 weeks. If no improvement occurs, consider euthanasia.

Case Summary

1. Diagnosis: Spinal cord infarction
2. Result: No improvement; euthanasia was performed

Spinal cord hemorrhage with infarction from L2-4.

ASSESSMENT 6B

Anatomic Diagnosis

Motor examination reveals severe bilateral LMN disease in both pelvic limbs and the pudendal nerve. The symmetry of the signs suggests severe disease in segments L4-S2. The sensory examination reveals complete analgesia caudal to the shoulders. This finding suggests a severe lesion extending forward to T3. In addition, the LMN neurons to the abdominal and intercostal muscles are involved. Therefore, diffuse symmetric disease of the spinal cord caudal to T3 should be suspected. The history suggests lesion progression insofar as spinal reflexes in the pelvic limbs were present 2 days ago. The lesion involves both gray and white matter throughout the spinal cord caudal to T3.

Diagnostic Plan

(Rule-out—see Tables 6-1 and 6-4)

Ascending/descending myelomalacia secondary to spinal cord compression.

Therapeutic Plan

None.

Client Education

1. The prognosis is hopeless
2. Recommend euthanasia

Case Summary

The diagnosis is severe ascending/descending myelomalacia secondary to a herniated disk at T13-L1.

ASSESSMENT 6C

Anatomic Diagnosis

The neurologic examination reveals bilateral UMN disease to both pelvic limbs, suggesting a lesion in segment T2-L3. The clinical course suggests a progressive disease. The hyperesthesia suggests a lesion at segment L2-L3.

Diagnostic Plan

(Rule-outs—see Table 6-1)

1. Type II disk disease: Spinal radiography and myelography were negative for extradural compression.
2. Neoplasia: Myelography disclosed intramedullary compression of the contrast column at L1-2.
3. Chronic meningomyelitis: CSF contained 1 white blood cell/mm^3, 33.5 mg/dl protein.
4. Diskospondylitis: Survey radiographs were normal.

Therapeutic Plan

1. Chemotherapy, corticosteroids
2. Exploratory laminectomy

Client Education

The prognosis is very poor. The myelogram suggests an intramedullary spinal cord tumor. These tumors are usually inoperable.

Case Summary

1. Diagnosis: Inoperable blast cell tumor at L1-2
2. Euthanasia was performed

ASSESSMENT 6D

Anatomic Diagnosis

LMN signs with blunted pain perception suggest a bilateral lesion in the segment L4-S2 or in the lumbosacral plexus. The urine and fecal incontinence is explained by a lesion in this region. The age and the breed suggest a developmental abnormality.

Diagnostic Plan

(Rule-outs—see Table 6-4)

1. Spina bifida: Radiography of the lumbosacral area
2. Spinal dysraphism: Myelography, EMG of the perineal muscles; a meningomyelocele was demonstrated (see Figure 6-24)

Therapeutic Plan

None.

Client Education

1. The prognosis is poor.
2. This congenital abnormality is a problem in certain lines of bulldogs.

Case Summary

1. The diagnosis was spina bifida with concurrent meningomyelocele (see Figure 6-23).
2. Euthanasia was performed.

References

1. Hoerlein BF: Intervertebral disk disease. In Oliver JE, Hoerlein BF, Mayhew IG, editors: *Veterinary neurology.* Philadelphia, 1987, WB Saunders.
2. Jensen VF, Arnbjerg J: Development of intervertebral disk calcification in the dachshund: A prospective study longitudinal study, *J Am Anim Hosp* 37:274-282, 2001.
3. Griffiths I: The extensive myelopathy of intervertebral disc protrusions in dogs ("the ascending syndrome"), *J Small Anim Pract* 13:425-437, 1972.
4. Fry TR, Johnson AL: Chemonucleolysis of treatment of intervertebral disk disease, *J Am Vet Med Assoc* 199:622-627, 1991.
5. Dickey DT, et al: Use of the holmium yttrium aluminum garnet laser for percutaneous thoracolumbar intervertebral disk ablation in dogs, *J Am Vet Med Assoc* 208:1263-1267, 1996.
6. Bartels KE, et al: Outcome of and complications associated with prophylactic laser disk ablation in dogs with thoracolumbar disk disease: 277 cases (1992-2001), *J Am Vet Med Assoc* 222:1733-1739, 2003.
7. Tarlov I, Klinger H: Spinal cord compression studies, II: Time limits for recovery after acute compression in dogs, *Arch Neurol Psychiatry* 71:271-290, 1954.
8. Tarlov I, Klinger H, Vitale S: Spinal cord compression studies, I: Experimental techniques to produce acute and gradual compression, *Arch Neurol Psych*iatry 70:813-819, 1953.
9. Mayhew IG: *Large animal neurology: A handbook for veterinary clinicians.* Philadelphia, 1989, Lea & Febiger.
10. Ingram JT, Colter SB: How do I treat? Neurologic rhinopneumonitis in the horse, *Prog Vet Neurol* 1:483, 1990.
11. Beech J, Dodd DC: Toxoplasma-like encephalomyelitis in the horse, *Vet Pathol* 11:87-96, 1974.
12. Fenger CK: PCR-based detection of *Sarcocystis neurona:* Implications for diagnosis and research. *Proceedings of the 12th American College of Veterinary Internal Medicine Forum,* 1994, pp 550-552.
13. Dorr TE, Higgins RJ, Dangler CA, et al: Protozoal myeloencephalitis in horses in California, *J Am Vet Med Assoc* 185:801-802, 1984.
14. Clark EG, Townsend HGG, McKenzie NT: Equine protozoal myeloencephalitis: A report of two cases from Western Canada, *Can Vet J* 22:140-144, 1981.
15. Fayer R, Mayhew IG, Baird JD, et al: Epidemiology of equine protozoal myeloencephalitis in North America based on histologically confirmed cases, *J Vet Intern Med* 4:54-57, 1990.
16. Fenger CK: Update on the diagnosis and treatment of equine protozoal myeloencephalitis (EPM). *Proceedings of the 13th American College of Veterinary Internal Medicine Forum,* 1995, pp 597-599.
17. Daft BM, et al: Sensitivity and specificity of western blot testing of cerebrospinal fluid and serum for diagnosis of equine protozoal myeloencephalitis in horses with and without neurologic abnormalities, *J Am Vet Med Assoc* 221:1007-1013, 2002.
18. Furr M: Antigen-specific antibodies in cerebrospinal fluid after intramuscular injection of ovalbumin in horses, *J Vet Intern Med* 16:588-592, 2002.
19. Cook AG, et al: Detection of antibodies against *Sarcocystis neurona* in cerebrospinal fluid from clinically normal neonatal foals, *J Am Vet Med Assoc* 220:208-211, 2002.
20. Lester G: Parasitic encephalomyelitis in horses, *Compend Cont Educ Pract Vet* 14:1624-1631, 1992.
21. Darien BJ, Belknap J, Nietfeld J: Cerebrospinal fluid changes in two horses with central nervous system nematodiasis (*Micronema deletrix*), *J Vet Intern Med* 2:201-205, 1988.
22. Turner WD: Fractures and fracture-luxations of the lumbar spine: A retrospective study in the dog, *J Am Anim Hosp Assoc* 23:459-464, 1987.
23. Rucker NC: Management of spinal cord trauma, *Prog Vet Neurol* 1:397-412, 1990.
24. LeCouteur RA: Central nervous system trauma. In Kornegay JN, editor: *Neurologic disorders.* New York, 1986, Churchill Livingstone.
25. Olby N: Current concepts in the management of acute spinal cord injury, *J Vet Intern Med* 13:399-407, 1999.
26. Oliver JE: Neurologic emergencies in small animals, *Vet Clin North Am* 2:341-357, 1972.
27. Braund KG, Shores A, Brawner WR: The etiology, pathology, and pathophysiology of acute spinal cord trauma, *Vet Med* 85:684-691, 1990.
28. Bracken MB, et al: A randomized, controlled trial of methylprednisolone or naloxone in the treatment of acute spinal-cord injury, *N Engl J Med* 322:1405-1411, 1990.
29. Faden AI: Pharmacotherapy in spinal cord injury: A critical review of recent developments, *Clin Neuropharmacol* 10:193-204, 1987.
30. Hoerlein BF, et al: Evaluation of naloxone, crocetin, thyrotropin-releasing hormone, methylprednisolone, partial myelotomy, and hemilaminectomy in the treatment of acute spinal cord trauma, *J Am Anim Hosp Assoc* 21:67-77, 1985.
31. Hoerlein B, et al: Evaluation of dexamethasone, DMSO, mannitol, and solcoseryl in acute spinal cord trauma, *J Am Anim Hosp Assoc* 19:216-226, 1983.
32. Selcer RR, Bubb WJ, Walker TL: Management of vertebral column fractures in dogs and cats: 211 cases (1977-1985), *J Am Vet Med Assoc* 198:1965-1968, 1991.
33. Olby N, et al: Long-term functional outcome of dogs with severe injuries of the thoracolumbar spinal cord: 87: cases (1996-2001), *J Am Vet Med Assoc* 222:762-769, 2003.
34. Hoerlein B: Methods of spinal fusion and vertebral immobilization in the dog, *Am J Vet Res* 17:685-709, 1956.
35. Yturraspe D, Lumb W: The use of plastic spinal plates for internal fixation of the canine spine, *J Am Vet Med Assoc* 161:1651-1657, 1972.
36. Blass C, Seim H: Spinal fixation in dogs using Steinmann pins and methylmethacrylate, *Vet Surg* 13:203-210, 1984.
37. Walter M, Smith G, Newton C: Canine lumbar spinal internal fixation techniques: A comparative biomechanical study, *Vet Surg* 15:191-198, 1986.
38. McAnulty J, Lenehan T, Maletz L: Modified segmental spinal instrumentation in repair of spinal fractures and luxations in dogs, *Vet Surg* 15:143-149, 1986.
39. Oliver JE, Hoerlein BF, Mayhew IG: *Veterinary neurology.* Philadelphia, WB Saunders, 1987.
40. Clemmons RM: Degenerative myelopathy. In Kirk RW, editor: Current veterinary therapy X: Small animal practice. Philadelphia, 1989, WB Saunders.
41. Averill DR: Degenerative myelopathy in the aging German shepherd dog, *J Am Vet Med Assoc* 162:1045-1051, 1973.
42. Braund KG, Vandevelde M: German shepherd dog myelopathy: A morphologic and morphometric study, *Am J Vet Res* 39:1309-1315, 1978.
43. Griffiths IR, Duncan ID: Chronic degenerative radiculomyelopathy in the dog, *J Small Anim Pract* 16:461-471, 1975.
44. Waxman FJ, Clemmons RM, Hinrichs DJ: Progressive myelopathy in older German shepherd dogs, II: Presence of circulating suppressor cells, *J Immunol* 124:1216-1222, 1980.
45. Waxman FJ, et al: Progressive myelopathy in older German shepherd dogs, I: Depressed response to thymus-dependent mitogens, *J Immunol* 124:1209-1215, 1980.

46. Matthews NS, DeLahunta A: Degenerative myelopathy in an adult miniature poodle, *J Am Vet Med Assoc* 186:1213-1214, 1985.

47. Bichsel P, Vandevelde M: Degenerative myelopathy in a family of Siberian Husky dogs, *J Am Vet Med Assoc* 183:998-1000, 1983.

48. Kornegay JN: Congenital and degenerative diseases of the central nervous system. In Kornegay JN, editor: *Neurologic disorders.* New York, 1986, Churchill Livingstone.

49. Mesfin GM, Kusewitt D, Parker A: Degenerative myelopathy in a cat, *J Am Vet Med Assoc* 176:62-64, 1980.

50. Littlewood J, Herrtage M, Palmer A: Intervertebral disc protrusion in a cat, *J Small Anim Pract* 25:119-127, 1984.

51. Heavner J: Intervertebral disc syndrome in the cat, *J Am Vet Med Assoc* 159:425-428, 1971.

52. Hansen HJ: A pathologic-anatomical study on disk degeneration in the dog, *Acta Orthop Scand* 1952.

53. Kornegay JN: Central nervous system neoplasia. In Kornegay JN, editor: *Neurologic disorders.* New York, 1986, Churchill Livingstone.

54. Ribas JL: Thoracolumbar spinal cord blastoma: A unique tumor of young dogs, *J Vet Intern Med* 4:127, 1990.

55. Summers BA, et al: A novel intradural extramedullary spinal cord tumor in your dogs, *Acta Neuropathol (Berl)* 75:402-410, 1988.

56. Thomson CE, Kornegay JN, Stevens JB: Analysis of cerebrospinal fluid from the cerebellomedullary and lumbar cisterns of dogs with focal neurologic disease: 145 cases (1985-1987), *J Am Vet Med Assoc* 11:1841-1844, 1990.

57. Irving G, McMillan MC: Fluoroscopically guided percutaneous fine-needle aspiration biopsy of thoracolumbar spinal lesions in cats, *Prog Vet Neurol* 1:473-475, 1990.

58. Spodnick GJ, et al: Spinal lymphoma in cats: 21 cases (1976-1989), *J Am Vet Med Assoc* 200:373-376, 1992.

59. Morgan J: Spondylosis deformans in the dog, *Acta Orthop Scand Suppl* 96:1-88, 1967.

60. Romatowski J: Spondylosis deformans in the dog, *Compend Cont Educ Pract Vet* 8:531-534, 1986.

61. Weisbrode S, et al: Osteochondrosis, degenerative joint disease, and vertebral osteophytosis in middle-aged bulls, *J Am Vet Med Assoc* 181:700-705, 1982.

62. Doige C: Multiple cartilaginous exostoses in dogs, *Vet Pathol* 24:276-278, 1987.

63. Shupe JL, et al: Hereditary multiple exostoses, *Am J Pathol* 104:285-288, 1981.

64. Acton CE: Spinal cord compression in young dogs due to cartilaginous exostosis, *Calif Vet* 41:7-26, 1987.

65. Cockrell BY, et al: Myelomalacia in Afghan hounds, *J Am Vet Med Assoc* 162:362-365, 1973.

66. de Lahunta A: *Veterinary neuroanatomy and clinical neurology,* 2nd ed. Philadelphia, 1983, WB Saunders.

67. Kornegay JN: Diskospondylitis revisited. In *Proceedings of the Ninth Annual Veterinary Medical Forum,* New Orleans, 1991, pp 291-293.

68. Doige C: Discospondylitis in swine, *Can J Comp Med* 44:121-128, 1980.

69. Sherman D, Ames T: Vertebral body abscesses in cattle: A review of five cases, *J Am Vet Med Assoc* 188:608-611, 1986.

70. Kornegay J, Barber D: Diskospondylitis in dogs, *J Am Vet Med Assoc* 177:337-341, 1980.

71. Kornegay J: Diskospondylitis. In Kirk RW, editor: *Current veterinary therapy IX: small animal practice.* Philadelphia, 1986, WB Saunders.

72. Kornegay JN: Vertebral diseases of large breed dogs. In Kornegay JN, editor: *Neurologic disorders.* New York, 1986, Churchill Livingstone.

73. Skeen TM, et al: Spinal arachnoid cysts in 17 dogs, *J Am Anim Hosp* 39:271-282, 2003.

74. McDonnell JJ, Knowles KE, deLahunta A, et al.: Thoracolumbar spinal cord compression due to vertebral process degenerative joint disease in a family of Shiloh shepherd dogs, *J Vet Intern Med* 17:530-537, 2003.

75. Penwick RC: Fibrocartilaginous embolism and ischemic myelopathy, *Compend Cont Educ Pract Vet* 11:287-299, 1989.

76. Johnson RC, Anderson WI, King JM: Acute pelvic limb paralysis induced by a lumbar fibrocartilaginous embolism in a sow, *Cornell Vet* 78:231-234, 1988.

77. Gilmore DR, de Lahunta A: Necrotizing myelopathy secondary to presumed or confirmed fibrocartilaginous embolism in 24 dogs, *J Am Anim Hosp Assoc* 23:373-376, 1987.

78. Oliver J, Selcer R, Simpson S: Cauda equina compression from lumbosacral malarticulation and malformation in the dog, *J Am Vet Med Assoc* 173:207-214, 1978.

79. Watt PR: Degenerative lumbosacral stenosis in 18 dogs, *J Small Anim Pract* 32:125-134, 1991.

80. Chambers JN: Degenerative lumbosacral stenosis in dogs, *Vet Med Rep* 1:166-180, 1989.

81. Palmer RH, Chambers JN: Canine lumbosacral diseases, I: Anatomy, pathophysiology, and clinical presentation, *Compend Cont Educ Pract Vet* 13:61-69, 1991.

82. Palmer RH, Chambers JN: Canine lumbosacral diseases, II: Definitive diagnosis, treatment, and prognosis, *Compend Cont Educ Pract Vet* 13:213-222, 1991.

83. Hathcock JT, et al: Comparison of three radiographic contrast procedures in the evaluation of the canine lumbosacral spinal canal, *J Vet Radiol* 29:4-15, 1988.

84. Selcer BA: Radiographic imaging in canine lumbosacral disease, *Vet Med Rep* 1:282-290, 1989.

85. Lang J: Flexion-extension myelography of the canine cauda equina, *Vet Radiol* 29:242-257, 1988.

86. Chambers JN, Selcer BA, Oliver JE: Results of treatment of degenerative lumbosacral stenosis in dogs by exploration and excision, *Vet Comp Orthop Trauma* 3:130-133, 1988.

87. Bailey CS: An embryological approach to the clinical significance of congenital vertebral and spinal cord abnormalities, *J Am Anim Hosp Assoc* 11:426-434, 1975.

88. Braund KG: Degenerative and developmental diseases. In Oliver JE, Hoerlein BF, Mayhew IG, editors: *Veterinary neurology.* Philadelphia, WB Saunders, 1987.

89. McGrath JT: Spinal dysraphism in the dog, *Pathol Vet Suppl* 2:1-36, 1965.

90. Fingeroth JM, et al: Neuroradiographic diagnosis and surgical repair of tethered cord syndrome in an English Bulldog with spina bifida and myeloschisis, *J Am Vet Med Assoc* 194:1300-1302, 1989.

91. Wilson JW, et al: Spina bifida in the dog, *Vet Pathol* 16:165-179, 1979.

92. Kitchen H, Murray RE, Cockrell BY: Animal model for human disease, spina bifida, sacral dysgenesis and myelocele, *Am J Pathol* 68:203-206, 1972.

93. Leipold HW, et al: Congenital defects of the caudal vertebral column and spinal cord in Manx cats, *J Am Vet Med Assoc* 164:520-523, 1974.

94. Rousseaux C, Futcher K, Clark E, et al: Cauda equina neuritis: A chronic idiopathic polyneuritis in two horses, *Can Vet J* 25:214-218, 1984.

95. Wright JA, Fordyce P, Edington N: Neuritis of the cauda equina in the horse, *J Comp Pathol* 97:667-675, 1987.

96. Cummings J, de Lahunta A, Timoney J: Neuritis in the cauda equina, a chronic idiopathic polyradiculoneuritis in the horse, *Acta Neuropathol* 46:17-24, 1979.
97. Edington N, Wright J, Patel J, et al: Equine adenovirus 1 isolated from cauda equina neuritis, *Res Vet Sci* 37:252-254, 1984.
98. Fordyce P, Edington N, Bridges G, et al: Use of an ELISA in the differential diagnosis of cauda equina neuritis and other equine neuropathies, *Equine Vet J* 19:55-59, 1987.
99. Osweiler GD, et al: *Clinical and diagnostic veterinary toxicology,* 3rd ed. Dubuque, IA, 1985, Kendall/Hunt Publishing.
100. Braund KG: Diseases of peripheral nerves, cranial nerves, and muscle. In Oliver JE, Hoerlein BF, Mayhew IG, editors: *Veterinary neurology.* Philadelphia, 1987, WB Saunders.

Chapter 7

Tetraparesis, Hemiparesis, and Ataxia

Tetraparesis (-plegia) (quadriparesis, quadriplegia) refers to partial (-paresis) or complete (-plegia) loss of voluntary motor function in all four limbs. The paresis may be manifested as a gait abnormality or as postural reaction deficits. The term *hemiparesis* refers to motor dysfunction of two limbs on the same side. Ataxia is a frequently associated problem. Lesion localization is discussed in Chapter 2, summarized in Figure 7-1, and reviewed briefly in this chapter.

LESION LOCALIZATION

Animals with tetraparesis usually have neurologic disease. Diffuse muscle or skeletal diseases may result in tetraparesis, which at times is difficult to differentiate from a true neurologic lesion. In addition, tetraparesis of neurologic origin must be differentiated from generalized muscle weakness or depression associated with severe metabolic disease (e.g., adrenal insufficiency, hypoglycemia). When initially presented with a tetraparetic animal, the clinician must decide which systems are involved (i.e., nervous, musculoskeletal, or general metabolic). Results of the history, physical examination, and laboratory tests usually provide sufficient evidence for the practitioner to make this differentiation. In this chapter, primary consideration is given to lesions involving the nervous and musculoskeletal systems.

Neurologic lesions that produce tetraparesis may involve the cerebral cortex or thalamus (forebrain), the brainstem, the cervical spinal cord, or the lower motor neurons (LMNs). Lesion localization is based on the decisions outlined in Figure 7-1. Although the motor cortex is important for the performance of learned reactions and to help initiate gait (see Chapters 1 and 2), it does not maintain locomotion in domestic animals. Diffuse brainstem centers coordinate these functions with reinforcement from the cerebral cortex. Animals with diffuse, bilateral forebrain disease, therefore, often

have little or no gait abnormality once the gait is initiated. Postural reactions are generally abnormal contralateral to the lesion. Other signs of forebrain dysfunction, such as altered mental status, seizures, or blindness, may be present and may help in lesion localization.

Lesions involving the brainstem and the cervical spinal cord result in an abnormal gait because motor signals from brainstem centers to the LMNs of the spinal cord are disrupted. Tetraparesis develops if the lesion is bilateral, and hemiparesis (usually ipsilateral) develops if the lesion is unilateral. Altered sensory function (ataxia, hypesthesia) frequently is associated with the motor dysfunction because lesions usually disrupt sensory pathways from the limbs and body.

Lesions in the brainstem and C1-5 spinal cord segments result in upper motor neuron (UMN) signs in the limbs. As explained in Chapter 2, disruption of UMN signals that inhibit the segmental spinal reflexes results in "release," or hyperactivity, of the LMNs. Brainstem and cranial cervical cord lesions are differentiated by examination of the head because lesions in either region can result in identical abnormalities in the limbs. The brainstem can be described as a cervical spinal cord that is modified by the presence of nuclei. Evidence of dysfunction in these nuclei indicates brainstem disease. Paresis associated with vestibular signs, altered mental status, or abnormal cranial nerve function strongly suggests a lesion in the brainstem.

Lesions involving the C6-T2 spinal segments result in tetraparesis. LMN signs may be present in the thoracic limbs if the motor neurons forming the brachial plexus are injured. In addition, Horner's syndrome may develop if the LMNs in segments T1-3 that form the sympathetic nerve are injured. UMN signs develop in the pelvic limbs because spinal pathways are disrupted as they pass through the caudal cervical spinal cord. Sensory function is invariably altered with significant lesions at C6-T2.

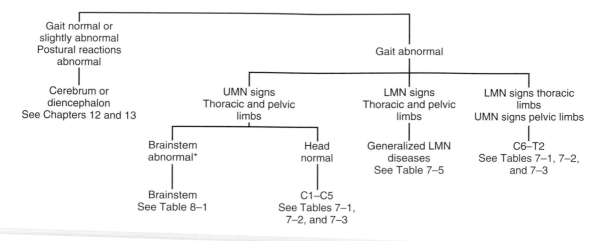

*Brainstem involvement: one or more signs involving the head are present, e.g., head tilt, nystagmus, cranial nerve signs, seizures, and so forth.

Figure 7-1 Algorithm for the diagnosis of tetraparesis, hemiparesis, and ataxia.

Animals with tetraparesis associated with diffuse LMN signs involving both the thoracic and pelvic limbs can have lesions involving the motor neurons located in the spinal cord, the axonal processes (ventral spinal root, spinal nerve, peripheral nerve), or the neuromuscular end plates (motor end plates). Peripheral neuropathies and motor end plate disorders are commonly encountered in animals, whereas neuronopathies are rare. Lesions involving motor neurons, ventral nerve roots, or neuromuscular end plates do not produce sensory dysfunction. Peripheral neuropathies may cause sensory dysfunction because most peripheral nerves contain both motor and sensory fibers. Animals with tetraparesis, LMN signs in the limbs, and normal sensation usually have a disease that involves the ventral nerve roots or the neuromuscular junctions. Those with neurologic signs that are episodic (e.g., exacerbated by exercise) usually have motor end plate disease. Animals with diffuse muscle disease occasionally develop clinical signs consistent with diffuse LMN disease, and these signs may be episodic. Careful muscle palpation, laboratory tests, and biopsy are usually necessary to differentiate primary muscle disease from primary neurologic disease.

DISEASES

The diseases discussed in this chapter include those that commonly affect the cervical spinal cord and those that diffusely affect the LMN system. Diseases that affect the cerebral cortex and the brainstem are discussed in Chapters 8 through 15. This section is organized according to the anatomic

location of the lesion and the course of the disease (acute versus chronic, progressive versus nonprogressive). The disorders that affect spinal cord segments C1-T2 in small animals are presented in Table 7-1. Cervical cord diseases of Equidae are presented in Table 7-2, and the cervical cord lesions of food animals are listed in Table 7-3. Diffuse LMN diseases are listed in Table 7-4. Each table indicates the chapter in which the disease is discussed.

Acute Progressive Diseases

Cervical Disk Disease

The pathophysiology of intervertebral disk disease is discussed in Chapter 6. Hansen type I disk protrusions in the cervical area occur most frequently in the chondrodystrophoid breeds (small poodle, dachshund, beagle, cocker spaniel) but also occur in certain large-breed dogs, such as the Doberman pinscher. Disk protrusions rarely cause clinical signs in other species, primarily cats and horses.[1-4] The incidence of cervical disk disease is lower than that of thoracolumbar disk disease. About 14% of all disk lesions in the dog occur in the cervical area.[1] Intervertebral spaces C2-3 and C3-4 are most frequently involved.

Unlike thoracolumbar disk disease, cervical disk herniations less commonly result in compressive myelopathy sufficient to cause paresis or paralysis. Although many factors may account for this finding, the larger diameter of the vertebral canal in the cervical area is probably the most important explanation. Because of the greater

Table 7-1 **Small Animal C1-T2 Spinal Cord Diseases: Differential Diagnosis Based on Clinical Course and Etiologic Categories***

Etiologic Category	Acute Nonprogressive	Acute Progressive	Chronic Progressive
Degenerative	None	Type I disk disease (6,7) Hemorrhagic myelomalacia (6)	Type II disk disease (6, 7) Cervical vertebral spondylopathy (7) Spondylosis deformans (6) Afghan hound myelopathy (6) Demyelinating diseases (7) Axonopathies and neuronopathies (7) Storage diseases (15) Extradural synovial cysts (7)
Anomalous	None	None	Spinal dysraphism (6) Vertebral anomalies (6) Atlantoaxial luxation (7)
Neoplastic (6)	None	Metastatic Primary Skeletal Lymphoreticular	Primary Lymphoreticular Skeletal Metastatic
Nutritional	None	None	Hypervitaminosis A (cats) (15)
Inflammatory	None	Distemper myelitis (15) Bacterial myelitis (15) Diskospondylitis (6) Protozoal myelitis (15) Mycotic myelitis (15)	Feline infectious peritonitis (15) Granulomatous meningoencephalomyelitis (15) Immune-mediated meningoencephalomyelitis (15)
Traumatic	Fractures (6) Luxations (6) Contusions (6) Intervertebral disk rupture (6)	Hemorrhagic myelomalacia (6) Intervertebral disk rupture (6)	None
Vascular	Fibrocartilaginous embolism (6) Vascular malformations (7)	None	None

*Numbers in parentheses refer to chapters in which the entities are discussed.

Table 7-2 **Equine C1-T2 Spinal Cord Diseases: Differential Diagnosis Based on Clinical Course and Etiologic Categories***

Etiologic Category	Acute Nonprogressive	Acute Progressive	Chronic Progressive
Degenerative	None	Degenerative myeloencephalopathy (7)	Cervical spondylopathy (7) Neuronopathies (7) Demyelinating diseases (7) Axonopathies (7)
Anomalous	None	None	Vertebral anomalies (6) Occipitoatlantoaxial malformation (7) Atlantoaxial luxation (7)
Neoplastic (6)	None	Metastatic Primary Skeletal Lymphoreticular	Primary Skeletal Lymphoreticular
Nutritional	None	Degenerative myeloencephalopathy (7)	
Inflammatory	None	Herpesvirus (6) Protozoal myelitis (6) Verminous migrations (6) Vertebral osteomyelitis (6) Mycotic myelitis (6)	See acute progressive
Traumatic	Fractures (6) Luxations (6)	None	None
Vascular	Embolic myelopathy (6) Fibrocartilaginous emboli (6) Postanesthetic myelopathy	None	None

*Numbers in parentheses refer to chapters in which the entities are discussed.

space surrounding the cervical cord, disk herniations in this area are less likely to result in focal compressive myelopathy. Likewise, the syndrome of ascending-descending myelomalacia rarely results from cervical disk herniation.

Clinical Signs. The most prominent sign in cervical disk protrusions is pain that arises from meningeal or nerve-root irritation, even though most dogs with only neck pain have some myelographic evidence of spinal cord compression.[5] The head is usually held low, and the neck may be extended rigidly. Dogs may resist any attempt to move their head or neck. Occasionally, affected dogs with lateral extrusions develop lameness of one thoracic limb as a result of nerve-root compression ("nerve root signature"; see Chapter 5).[6] Forced movement of the limb may cause considerable pain. Dogs that are in pain have a stiff, short-strided gait and may cry or whine if forced to change direction suddenly. Most dogs are reluctant, or refuse, to descend stairs or jump. The clinical signs resulting from pain are similar to those associated with meningitis (see Chapters 14 and 15).

Occasionally, cervical disk extrusions sufficiently compress the cervical cord to cause paresis and ataxia of the thoracic and pelvic limbs.[7] Rarely, a massive or acute disk herniation produces tetraplegia or hemiplegia with associated hemorrhagic necrosis in the spinal cord.[8,9] Tetraplegia with loss of deep pain sensation is not seen because respiration would be impaired with such a lesion. Cranial cervical disk extrusions, however, can cause dysphonia or respiratory dysfunction if edema extends to the caudal brainstem.[10] Disk protrusions affecting the cervical spinal cord may produce Horner's syndrome as a result of the involvement of descending UMNs that control sympathetic LMNs. Caudal cervical disk herniation may produce LMN signs in one or both thoracic limbs. The presence of neurologic signs other than pain strongly suggests spinal cord compression. Evidence of severe pain or spinal cord compression is an indication for decompressive surgery.

Diagnosis. The clinical diagnosis of cervical disk disease is confirmed by radiographic examination of the cervical area (Figures 7-2 and 7-3). Radiographs are taken for all surgical candidates. Anesthesia is required for proper positioning. If conventional radiographs do not reveal a lesion, cerebrospinal fluid (CSF) should be obtained to

Table 7-3 **Food Animal C1-T2 Spinal Cord Diseases: Differential Diagnosis Based on Clinical Course and Etiologic Categories***

Etiologic Category	Acute Nonprogressive	Acute Progressive	Chronic Progressive
Degenerative	None	None	Progressive ataxia of Charolais cattle—B (7)
			Degenerative myeloencephalopathy—B (7)
			Spondylosis deformans—all (6)
			Arthrogryposis—all (7)
			Demyelinating diseases—B (7)
			Neuronopathies—O (7)
			Occipitoatlantoaxial malformations—B, O (6)
Anomalous	None	Occipitoatlantoaxial malformations—B, O (6)	Vertebral anomalies—all (6)
Neoplastic (6)	None	Metastatic	Primary
		Primary	Lymphoreticular
		Skeletal	Skeletal
		Lymphoreticular	Metastatic
Nutritional	None	None	Enzootic ataxia, copper deficiency—C, O (15)
Inflammatory	None	Caprine arthritis-encephalomyelitis—C (6)	Visna-Maedi—O (15)
		Bacterial myelitis—all (15)	Verminous migration—all (6)
		Vertebral osteomyelitis—all (6)	
		Protozoal myelitis (15)	
		Mycotic myelitis (15)	
Toxic	None	Selenium—P (15)	
Traumatic	Fractures (6)	None	None
	Luxations (6)		
	Contusions (6)		
Vascular	Fibrocartilaginous embolism—P (6)	None	None

*Numbers in parentheses refer to chapters in which the entities are discussed.
B, Bovine; *C*, caprine; *O*, ovine; *P*, porcine.

179

Table 7-4 **Diffuse Lower Motor Neuron Diseases**

Acute Progressive Disorders
Polyradiculoneuritis
Tick paralysis
Botulism
Aminoglycoside paralysis

Chronic Progressive Disorders
Motor neuronopathies
   Spinal muscle atrophy of Brittany spaniels
   Swedish Lapland dog paralysis
   Stockard's paralysis
   Spinal muscle atrophy of pointers
   Spinal muscle atrophy of German shepherd dogs
   Spinal muscle atrophy of rottweilers
   Multisystem neuronal degenerations
   Equine motor neuron disease
Polyneuropathy (see Table 7-6)
Polymyopathy (see Table 7-7)

Episodic Progressive Disorders
Myasthenia gravis
Metabolic (polysystemic) disorders (see Chapter 15)
   Hypoglycemia
   Hyperkalemia
   Hypercalcemia
   Hypocalcemia
   Hypomagnesemia
Chronic relapsing polymyositis

rule out meningomyelitis. If the CSF is normal, myelography should be done to demonstrate potential spinal cord compression (Figure 7-4). Many surgeons prefer to perform a myelogram and or computed tomography (CT) for all cervical disk protrusions to define the lateralization and extent of the disk material. Oblique projections may be useful to identify lateral extrusions on both survey radiographs and myelography.[6] Dogs with an initial episode of pain may be treated medically, and in such cases conventional radiographs are not necessary. Because the signs of cervical disk protrusion are virtually identical to those of meningitis, animals that do not respond promptly to medical therapy should be anesthetized and evaluated with conventional radiography, CSF analysis, and myelography (if the CSF is normal).

Treatment. Many dogs with cervical disk disease respond at least temporarily to medical therapy (see next section). Because the risk of severe, permanent neurologic dysfunction is not great, cervical disk disease is usually not a neurosurgical emergency. Fenestration of the disks at an early stage in the disease prevents recurrences in type I disk disease. Because severe herniations require decompression and recurrences are frequent, early fenestration is recommended. Decisions regarding medical or surgical therapy are based on the clinical signs and the chronicity of the problem.

Medical Therapy. Medical therapy for cervical disk disease, as with thoracolumbar disk herniations, should be restricted to dogs with an initial episode of neck pain. Therapy must support normal healing processes, keep the animal reasonably comfortable, and not cause serious complications. The most important part of the treatment is strict confinement to keep movement to a minimum. The more the dog moves the neck, the more disk material is extruded. Confining the dog to an airline crate is preferred. Exercise for bladder and bowel evacuation is done on a leash with a harness. Collars are avoided. If the animal is confined but still has considerable pain, analgesics, glucocorticoids (prednisolone, 0.25 mg/lb every 12 hours for 72 hours), or nonsteroidal antiinflammatory drugs

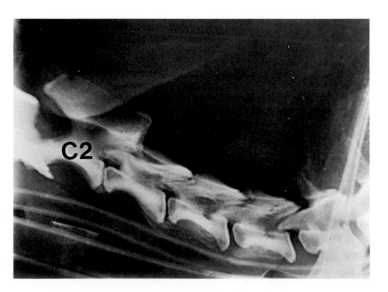

Figure 7-2 Lateral cervical radiograph of a dog with cervical disk disease. Note the narrow spaces at C2-3 and C3-4. The condition responded to ventral fenestration.

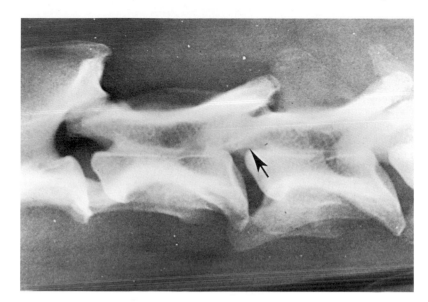

Figure 7-3 Lateral cervical radiograph showing massive disk herniation *(arrow)* at C3-4. Decompressive surgery is indicated in this case.

may be used (see Chapter 14). Pain relief must be accompanied by strict confinement because otherwise the animal may become too active. The owner is instructed to maintain confinement for at least 2 weeks, regardless of how much the dog improves. If signs worsen, the dog should be reevaluated for surgery. Most dogs that are treated medically improve but relapse later. Owners must be cautioned that clinical signs often recur after medical therapy.

Surgical Therapy. The various forms of surgical therapy have been reviewed extensively by Hoerlein.[1] General agreement exists that fenestration reduces the likelihood of recurrence.[11] The procedure is easy to perform and causes little postoperative reaction. Because disk material in the vertebral canal is not removed, however, clinical signs may persist or worsen.[12] One study concluded that decompression is superior to fenestration

except in the rates of intraoperative and postoperative complications.[13] We generally recommend cervical radiographs, CSF evaluation, and myelography for dogs that acutely lose the ability to walk and in those with cervical hyperesthesia that does not respond to 2 weeks of medical management.

Decompressive surgery, usually cervical slot, is recommended for dogs with spinal cord compression. Fenestration is done concomitantly to lessen the likelihood of recurrence. Dorsal laminectomy or hemilaminectomy may be done in dogs with asymmetric lesions or in small dogs in which a slot provides only limited exposure.[6,14] The prognosis for functional recovery after decompression of most type I cervical disk protrusions is excellent. In large-breed dogs with type II disk protrusions, recovery may be slow and may entail considerable physical therapy (see Cervical Spondylopathy: Therapy).

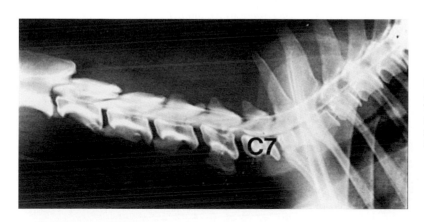

Figure 7-4 Cervical myelogram of a dog with a disk protrusion at C6-7. The lesion was not visualized on survey radiographs. The condition responded to ventral decompressive surgery.

Cervical Meningomyelitis

Inflammation of the meninges caused by bacterial, viral, rickettesial, or fungal agents or subsequent to idiopathic diseases, such as granulomatous meningoencephalomyelitis (GME), may produce clinical signs that are similar to those of cervical disk disease. Cervical pain is common with meningitis. Involvement of the white or gray matter of the spinal cord results in paresis, paralysis, and sensory ataxia. These diseases are sometimes characterized by polysystemic signs and multifocal neurologic lesions. In many cases, the course becomes chronic and progressive after the acute development of neurologic signs. Diagnosis is primarily based on CSF abnormalities. These disorders are discussed in Chapters 14 and 15.

Equine Degenerative Myeloencephalopathy

Equine degenerative myeloencephalopathy, or a similar condition, occurs in light breeds of horses, captive Przewalski horses, zebras, and a few ruminant species. The disease is characterized by acute, progressive, symmetric ataxia and paresis in young animals up to 24 months of age. Chronic progressive forms of the disease have been described. Histopathologically, the disease is characterized by diffuse myeloencephalopathy of variable severity.[15,16] Consistent degeneration of white matter occurs in all spinal cord funiculi, especially in the sensory (proprioceptive) relay nuclei in the medulla oblongata and spinal cord. A similar, potentially familial, form of neuroaxonal dystrophy is seen in Morgan horses.[17] The cause of degenerative myeloencephalopathy is unknown. Some studies showed evidence of vitamin E deficiency,[16,18] but this finding was not substantiated.[19] The disease must be differentiated clinically from cervical spondylopathy and protozoal myeloencephalitis.

Clinical Signs. Signs develop in horses that are younger than 2 years of age and include symmetric UMN and proprioceptive deficits in all four limbs. Deficits tend to be more severe in the pelvic limbs.[15] Cutaneous and cervical reflexes, such as with the slap test, may be decreased. Although the disease is progressive, tetraplegia is rare. The early onset of signs, at a mean age of 0.4 years, and the marked disparity in gait deficit between the thoracic and pelvic limbs help to differentiate degenerative myeloencephalopathy from focal cervical myelopathies.

Diagnosis. Antemortem diagnosis is difficult. Radiology of the cervical spine is useful for distinguishing equine degenerative myeloencephalopathy from cervical spondylopathy if rigid criteria are followed (see Cervical Spondylopathy: Diagnosis). Serum vitamin E concentrations should be greater than 1.5 mg/ml in normal horses.[15] Levels in affected horses may be half that or less. The fact that CSF of horses with degenerative myeloencephalopathy is relatively normal helps to differentiate this disease from protozoal encephalomyelitis.

Treatment. Vitamin E supplementation is recommended at a level of 1000 to 2000 U daily. Providing fresh green forage with an adequate vitamin E content may be better.[15] The prognosis is poor for complete resolution of signs, although they may stabilize. A familial predisposition may occur.

Acute Nonprogressive Diseases, C1-T2

Fibrocartilaginous Embolism

This syndrome is described in Chapter 6. The disease can occur in the cervical spinal cord and seems to occur more commonly in small-breed dogs. The clinical signs develop acutely and progress rapidly in 1 to 2 hours from initial pain to tetraparesis or hemiparesis if only one side of the cord is involved. Signs are compatible with acute cervical spinal cord compression, except affected dogs often have dramatic asymmetry and experience much less pain. Lesions at C6-T2 frequently result in LMN signs in the thoracic limbs and UMN signs in the pelvic limbs. Diagnosis and management are discussed in Chapter 6.

Cervical Spinal Cord Trauma

Traumatic compression of the cervical spinal cord, in contrast to that in the thoracolumbar area, is more likely to cause pain with little motor dysfunction; however, extensive compression results in severe motor and sensory dysfunction. Injuries cranial to C5 may cause sudden death through disruption of the respiratory pathways to the phrenic and intercostal motor neurons. Tetraplegia with loss of deep pain sensation caudal to the lesion, therefore, is rare, because affected animals die of respiratory failure. The pathophysiology, diagnosis, and management of spinal cord trauma are discussed in Chapter 6.

Chronic Progressive Diseases, C1-5

Atlantoaxial Subluxation

Slowly progressive subluxation of the atlantoaxial articulation was originally described in 10 small-breed dogs.[20] The condition is seen rarely in other species.[21] A variety of lesions involving the atlas and the axis have been reported.[22,23] Most cause dorsal displacement of the axis into the vertebral canal, resulting in compression of the cervical spinal cord.[22] These lesions include luxations with either an intact or a congenitally malformed dens and fractures of the axis or atlas. Some congenital malformations that involve the atlas, axis, and occipital bone are discussed in the next section.

Pathophysiology. Disorders of the atlantoaxial articulation usually result from a congenital malformation, traumatic fracture of the dens, or traumatic tearing or stretching of the transverse atlantal ligament. The normal atlantoaxial articulation allows rotational movement. The dens projects from the body of the axis and is bound to the ventral arch of the atlas by a strong transverse ligament (Figure 7-5). This attachment prevents flexion between the atlas and the axis (Figure 7-6, *A*). Disorders of this attachment allow the axis to rotate dorsally. The spinal cord is then compressed between the axis and the dorsal arch of the atlas (see Figure 7-6, *B*). Cervical flexion accentuates the degree of spinal cord compression.

Atlantoaxial luxation with an intact dens results from traumatic rupture or malformation of the transverse atlantal ligament.[24] The spinal cord is severely compressed between the intact dens and the dorsal atlantal arch (see Figure 7-6, *B*). Luxations caused by a fracture or congenital malformation of the dens usually produce less severe neurologic signs because less compression of the spinal cord occurs. Fractures of the body of the axis produce neurologic signs similar to those of acute traumatic luxation. Neurologic signs result from

acute or chronic progressive compressive myelopathy. The congenital disorders are usually more chronic with gradual progression of neurologic signs. They occur most frequently in the toy or miniature breeds.

Clinical Signs. Traumatic luxations or fractures of C1-2 result in cervical pain, tetraparesis, and ataxia. Neurologic signs may be asymmetric. Dogs with congenital lesions usually show signs during the first year of life; however, older dogs also may develop signs. Some dogs may not show clinical signs because adequate vertebral support by other fibrous and muscular structures prevents C1-2 luxation. With age these structures may weaken, allowing the axis to rotate dorsally and to compress the spinal cord. In the congenital form of the disorder, the initial clinical sign is usually cervical pain. The signs progress from pain to minor motor dysfunction to severe paresis or paralysis.[20,24]

The displaced axis may be palpated as a firm swelling just caudal to the occiput.[22] Because flexing the neck causes severe pain and accentuates motor dysfunction, it must be done cautiously. Respiratory failure occurs when these pathologic events compromise respiratory pathways. *When atlantoaxial luxation or fractures are suspected, extension of the neck must be maintained, especially during anesthesia.*[22]

Diagnosis. Atlantoaxial lesions must be suspected in all toy or miniature dogs with cranial cervical pain, neck rigidity, and paresis or paralysis. Spinal radiography is useful for revealing the C1-2 malalignment (Figure 7-7, *A* and *B*). Survey spinal radiographs should be taken while the animal is awake. The fact that anesthetized dogs do not maintain cervical muscle tension increases the possibility of neck flexion and severe spinal cord compression. Lateral and ventrodorsal views should be taken. If the survey films reveal minor displacement, a definitive diagnosis can be made with radiographs taken with the dog anesthetized just before surgical fixation.[22] Careful neck flexion may be needed to demonstrate the luxation.

Treatment. Atlantoaxial luxations and most fractures require immediate surgical immobilization. Medical management with external stabilization has been reported, but we prefer surgical stabilization. Therapy to resolve spinal cord edema may be necessary for animals with traumatic lesions or during surgery (see Chapters 6 and 12).

Surgery has included simple decompression and various forms of stabilization and fusion.[22,25-33] Most surgeons now stabilize C1-2 using a ventral approach.[25,26] Screws or pins are placed across the C1-2 joint (see Figure 7-7, *C* and *D*). The ventral approach allows fusion of the articulation with a bone graft potentially to provide permanent

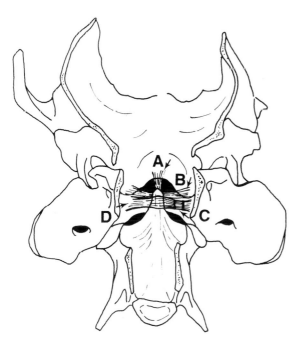

Figure 7-5 The ligamentous attachments of the dens. **A,** Apical. **B,** Alar. **C,** Lateral. **D,** Transverse atlantal. (From Oliver JE Jr, Lewis RE: Lesions of the atlas and axis in dogs, *J Am Anim Hosp* Assoc 9:307, 1973.)

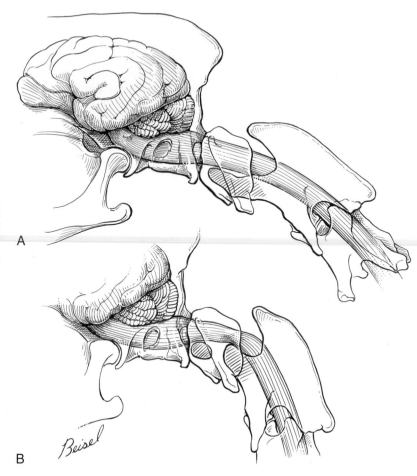

Figure 7-6 A, Drawing of the normal atlantoaxial articulation. **B,** Drawing of atlantoaxial luxation resulting from separation of the dens from the body of the axis. Note the dorsal displacement of the axis, compressing the spinal cord at this level.

fixation. Luxations can also be stabilized by securing the arch of the atlas to the dorsal process of the axis with wire,[22,27] suture,[28] or the nuchal ligament.[29] A metallic clip positioned around the cranial aspect of the lamina of the atlas and anchored to the axis has also been used to stabilize luxations.[30] Dorsal stabilization techniques may not eliminate rotation and shear forces acting across the joint and are more prone to failure.[33]

The risk factors that can affect the outcome of surgery for atlantoaxial subluxation have been studied in dogs. Dogs younger than 24 months of age and those with signs of less than 10 months duration generally had better outcomes.[34] Severity of neurologic signs before surgery was only marginally predictive of a successful outcome. Residual neurologic signs were detected in a greater percentage of dogs following dorsal procedures, but the success rates of both procedures were nearly identical.[34]

Occipitoatlantoaxial Malformations

These congenital malformations are reported in horses, cattle, cats, and dogs.[15,35] Congenital asymmetric occipitoatlantoaxial malformations and asymmetric atlantooccipital fusion are presumed to be inherited in Arabian horses.[15] Ataxia, tetraparesis, and a stiff neck may be found in neonates or in weanling foals. The abnormal cervical articulations usually can be palpated. A wide variety of anomalies have been reported. Dorsal angulation of the dens is seen in dogs.[36] Fusion of the atlas to the occipital bone as part of the malformation is seen in horses, cattle, and cats.

Occipitoatlantal Luxations

Traumatic luxations of the occipitoatlantal joint are rare. They have been reported in dogs, a cat, and a goat.[37-41] In two dogs and one cat, the luxations were managed by manual reduction and application of a cast with the neck in flexion. Two dogs and a goat were treated surgically. This rare injury would be expected to cause death in most cases, but these animals had relatively minimal neurologic deficits.

Cervical Vertebral Anomalies

Malformations, with or without secondary spinal cord compression, affect the cervical vertebrae as

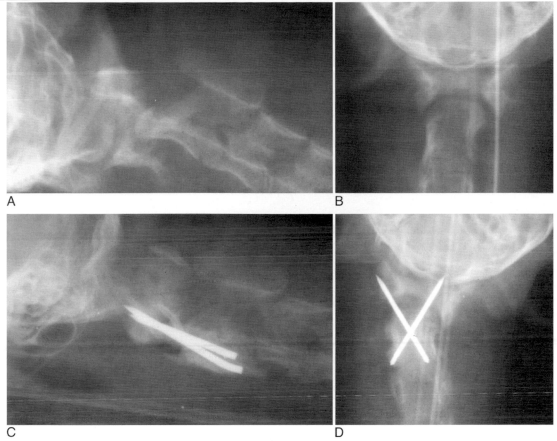

A B C D

Figure 7-7 Radiographs of the cervical region of a miniature pinscher with cervical hyperesthesia and atlantoaxial subluxation taken before (**A** and **B**) and after (**C** and **D**) stabilization with pins placed across the joint ventrally. Note the marked dorsal luxation of the axis relative to the atlas preoperatively, with subsequent reduction. The odontoid process is absent. (From Kornegay JN: The nervous system. In Hoskins JD, editor: *Veterinary pediatrics,* 2nd ed. Philadelphia, 1995, WB Saunders.)

elsewhere in the spine (see Chapter 6 for a description of these anomalies). Malformations may be a component of the "wobbler" syndrome, which we term *cervical spondylopathy.*

Cervical Spondylopathy

The growing popularity of giant-breed dogs and performance horses during the past 20 years is probably responsible for the increased interest in this neurologic syndrome. The disorder appears with greater frequency in great Danes, Doberman pinschers, and thoroughbred horses, but it has been recognized in several other breeds of dogs and horses. Controversy still exists regarding proper terminology for this syndrome. Currently, *cervical spondylopathy, cervical spondylomyelopathy, cervical vertebral malformation-malarticulation,* and *cervical vertebral stenotic myelopathy* appear to be the most useful names encompassing the forms of the disease in all affected animals. Some investigators prefer to group all breeds together, whereas others prefer to characterize each breed separately. Our objective is to describe similarities and differences in the pathologic lesions and management of cervical spondylopathy in each affected breed.

Pathophysiology. The pathologic lesions responsible for the clinical signs in young great Danes, Doberman pinschers, and thoroughbreds form the basic model with which the disease in other animals is compared. In affected animals, neurologic signs develop because of progressive spinal cord compression from surrounding vertebral bony and soft tissue structures. Abnormalities of the midcervical to the caudal cervical vertebrae or their articulations, or both, are usually revealed radiographically (Figure 7-8) or at necropsy (Figure 7-9). Because the exact cause is unknown, the term *cervical spondylopathy* is used broadly to encompass the various vertebral abnormalities.

Early studies suggested that excessive mobility of the caudal cervical vertebrae was primarily responsible for cord compression. Subsequent

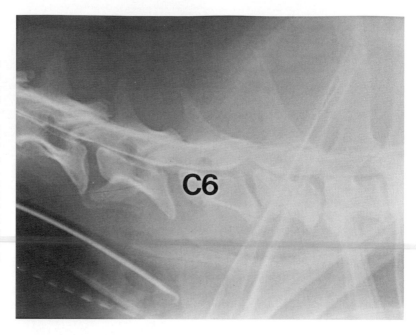

Figure 7-8 Lateral cervical myelogram from an 8-year-old female Doberman pinscher with progressive tetraparesis. The intervertebral disk space at C6-7 is narrow and the cranial aspect of the vertebral body of C7 is displaced dorsally. Marked dorsal deviation of the ventral contrast column overlying the C6-7 interspace occurs with attenuation of the dorsal contrast column at this same site. Changes are typical of those seen with cervical spondylopathy in middle-aged Doberman pinschers. (From Kornegay JN: Vertebral diseases of large breed dogs. In Kornegay JN, editor: *Neurologic disorders.* [*Contemporary issues in small animal practice,* vol 5.] Philadelphia, 1986, WB Saunders.)

studies demonstrated that malformation of the cervical vertebrae resulted in stenosis of the vertebral canal.[42-46] These changes are more consistently present in young great Danes and include narrowing and dorsoventral flattening of the cranial vertebral foramina of C5, C6, and C7. The sixth cervical vertebra is usually most severely affected. In young thoroughbred horses and basset hounds, these findings are more common at C3 and C4.

Abnormalities in the size, shape, or position of the articular processes may be present. In some cases, hyperostosis of the articular facets may cause direct spinal cord compression. The vertebral malformation tends to lead to malarticulation and vertebral instability. Instability without severe

malformation is seen in young Doberman pinschers. Apparently, in an attempt to correct the instability, soft tissues that support and strengthen the cervical articulations proliferate. In dogs and in some horses, hypertrophy of the interarcuate ligament, dorsal longitudinal ligament, or dorsal annulus may compress the spinal cord at the vertebral articulations. In older Doberman pinschers, type II degeneration and protrusion of the caudal cervical intervertebral disks contribute to the clinical signs and radiographic, surgical, and necropsy findings (see Figures 7-8 and 7-9).[44,47,48] This finding suggests that the syndrome affecting older Doberman pinschers differs from that affecting young great Danes.

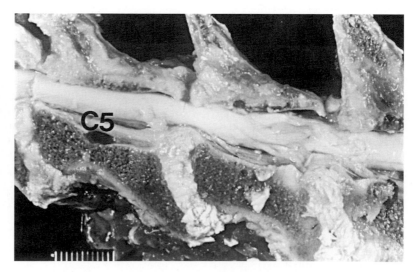

Figure 7-9 Lateral view, at necropsy, of the caudal cervical vertebral column from a 6-year-old male Doberman pinscher with progressive tetraparesis and cervical hyperesthesia. The spinal cord is compressed ventrally at both C5-6 and C6-7 by soft tissue proliferation of either the dorsal annulus fibrosus or the dorsal longitudinal ligament, or both. Scale is in millimeters. (From Kornegay JN: Vertebral diseases of large breed dogs. In Kornegay JN, editor: *Neurologic disorders.* [*Contemporary issues in small animal practice,* vol 5.] Philadelphia, 1986, WB Saunders.)

Although many, perhaps genetically controlled, factors may contribute to cervical spondylopathy, the exact cause is unknown. Many of the large and giant breeds have been selected for their size and rapid growth. The disease occurs primarily in horses that are large for their age and breed. The very large head of certain breeds of dogs may exert an unusual force on the midcervical to caudal cervical vertebrae. Great Danes in particular have been selected for a prancing, high-stepping gait that some consider to be a mild form of hypermetria. Breeding for this gait actually may select for this neurologic-musculoskeletal disorder. One study of great Danes established a relationship between excessive nutrition and several skeletal changes that also involved the cervical vertebrae.[49] The exact cause of the disorder awaits further classification. Vertebral pathologic lesions are quite similar in young great Danes and thoroughbred horses.

Clinical Signs. In most affected great Danes and horses, and in some Doberman pinschers, clinical signs develop at 3 to 18 months of age. Clinical signs develop later in life at 3 to 8 years of age in most Doberman pinschers. The disease usually occurs in horses less than 3 years old.[15] There is no sex predilection. Dogs typically develop mild pelvic limb ataxia that progresses to severe bilateral ataxia and hypermetria. Compression of ascending proprioceptive pathways is responsible for these neurologic signs. With increasing compression, involvement of descending motor pathways causes UMN paresis or paralysis.

Although the cervical spinal cord is compressed, clinical signs usually remain more severe in the pelvic limbs in both dogs and horses. Ataxia and paresis in the thoracic limbs may be pronounced in some cases but are sometimes detected only by careful neurologic examination. Forcing the dog to wheelbarrow with its head extended so that it cannot see the floor accentuates proprioceptive deficits in the thoracic limbs. Some tetraparetic dogs and horses may have LMN signs in the thoracic limbs because of cervical gray matter involvement. Neck pain is usually absent unless the disorder is associated with cervical disk protrusion. Extension of the neck may cause pain. Signs worsen progressively, and urinary incontinence may occur as a late manifestation in dogs. In some animals, trauma may precede the development of acute signs. Deep pain responses are usually preserved. Unlike most dogs, most horses have acute ataxia, paresis, and spasticity of all four limbs. After an initial period of progression, the equine disease usually stabilizes. The abnormalities of the pelvic limbs are usually one grade worse than those of the thoracic limbs.[15]

Diagnosis. The diagnosis of cervical spondylopathy is confirmed radiographically (Figures 7-8 and 7-10). Changes observed on survey radiographs include the following:

1. Changes in shape or density, or both, of the intervertebral disk or disk space, or both; this change is more common in the older Doberman pinscher
2. Changes in shape or density, or both, of the articular facets to sclerosis and exostosis
3. Vertebral displacement (subluxation); however, diagnosis of subluxation based on survey radiographs is not definitive because of considerable variability in normal dogs
4. Stenosis of the vertebral canal
5. Malformed or misshapen vertebral bodies
6. Misshapen dorsal spinous processes[43,49,50]

Stressed (flexion, extension) survey radiographs are not useful without myelography. The range of normal variability is large, and danger exists of further damaging the spinal cord. Myelography is necessary to identify minor changes in vertebral canal architecture, soft tissue compression, and disk protrusions and to define multiple lesions and the exact site or cause of spinal cord compression (see Figures 7-8 and 7-10). Myelograms made with the neck extended dorsally often reveal dynamic soft tissue or bony compression that may be missed if the neck is imaged in normal positions (Figure 7-11). This dynamic compression often is alleviated by ventral cervical flexion or traction. Based on the myelographic

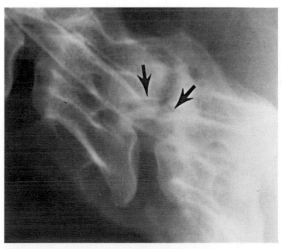

Figure 7-10 Myelogram of the cervical spine in dorsal extension. Note the dorsal compression of the spinal cord from ligamentous proliferation in this area *(arrows)*. Myelograms are needed to demonstrate compression by soft tissues in certain cases of cervical spondylopathy.

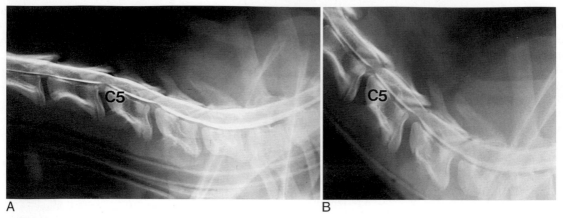

Figure 7-11 Lateral cervical myelogram from a 6-month-old male Doberman pinscher with progressive tetraparesis. Radiographs were taken without traction or extension (A) and with dorsal extension (B). Attenuation of both the dorsal and ventral contrast columns at C4-5 and C5-6 is seen in each radiograph; however, the degree of compression is more pronounced with extension. (From Kornegay JN: Vertebral diseases of large breed dogs. In Kornegay JN, editor: *Neurologic Disorders*. [*Contemporary issues in small animal practice,* vol 5.] Philadelphia, 1986, WB Saunders.)

results, rational surgical therapy can be instituted. Myelography is mandatory in older Doberman pinschers to exclude disk disease as the primary cause of the neurologic signs (see Figure 7-8). Myelography combined with CT provides additional information, particularly on the degree of spinal cord atrophy.[51]

In horses, cervical spondylopathy must be differentiated from degenerative myeloencephalopathy and protozoal myeloencephalitis. Vertebral changes may be demonstrated on survey cervical radiographs. In one study, determination of the ratio of the minimum sagittal diameter of the vertebral canal to the sagittal width of the vertebral body had a sensitivity and specificity of ≥89% for diagnosis of cervical spondylopathy.[52] This finding suggests that vertebral canal stenosis plays a critical role in affected horses. Myelography is necessary for accurate assessment.

Therapy. Some dogs improve with cage rest, physiatry, and analgesics.[53] Neurologic status usually deteriorates with resumption of normal activity. Corticosteroids are contraindicated in young, growing animals. The best long-term benefits are provided by surgical stabilization or decompression, or both.[48,54-61] Ventral[54,55] or dorsal[56,57] decompression may be indicated, depending on the sites of compression. Distraction techniques are used by many surgeons when the compression is dynamic and relieved by traction.[58-61] Surgical treatment of dogs with multiple lesions is particularly problematic. Dorsal laminectomy extending over the entire area of involvement has been advocated.[56,57] Distraction techniques can also be applied at adjacent disks. Regardless of the procedure, surgical results largely depend on the degree of preexisting spinal cord damage.

Medical therapy for equine cervical spondylopathy is similar to that for dogs. Early in the course of the disease, young horses may improve when fed a balanced, minimal-growth diet.[15] Ventral cervical fusion is indicated for horses with cord compression caused by cervical vertebral instability. Dorsal decompression is used to treat stenotic lesions that cause cord compression, irrespective of neck position.[15,62,63] Results of surgery depend, to some degree, on the severity, distribution, and duration of cervical cord compression.

Prognosis. In general, the prognosis for full recovery is poor in tetraplegic dogs and guarded in others. Factors that contribute to poor recovery include (1) irreparable spinal cord damage, (2) failure to provide adequate decompression or stabilization, (3) development of compression at sites adjacent to the initial lesions, and (4) postsurgical complications caused by difficulty in rehabilitating large, recumbent dogs. Published results suggest that about 75% of dogs improve subsequent to most surgical techniques. The prognosis is better in dogs in which the clinical signs result primarily from cervical disk protrusion or herniation. Most affected animals respond to ventral decompression or distraction with stabilization. Some dogs that initially improve subsequently develop compression at adjacent sites.[54,64] Certain stabilization procedures actually may increase stress forces at adjacent intervertebral sites. Owners should be warned that the surgery is difficult to perform and that the results may not be satisfactory.

In horses, the prognosis is poor without surgery. The results of ventral cervical fusion appear to be better than those with subtotal dorsal decompression.[62,63]

Extradural Synovial Cysts

Extradural synovial cysts have been reported in dogs and horses and may cause compressive myelopathy. Compressive cervical myelopathy has been reported in young great Danes and mastiffs.[65] Affected dogs were males 15 to 18 months of age that had progressive tetraparesis and ataxia from 1 week to 3 months before examination. The neurologic signs were suggestive of cervical spondylopathy, and all dogs exhibited cervical pain. Survey cervical radiographs revealed degenerative joint disease of the articular facets from C2-3 to C6-7. Myelographic studies revealed lateral compression of the cervical spinal cord medial to the articular facets. CSF analysis revealed increased protein concentrations. All dogs responded well to dorsal laminectomy and cyst removal.

Diseases With Diffuse Lower Motor Neuron Signs

Diseases that affect one or more components of the LMNs (Figure 7-12) result in hyporeflexic or areflexic paresis or paralysis. Sensory function may be normal or decreased. Hyperesthesia occasionally is present. The various diseases listed in Table 7-4 can be classified as acute progressive, chronic progressive, or episodic. All are characterized by diffuse symmetric or asymmetric involvement of LMNs. The neurologic examination must be done carefully and thoroughly in these patients. In the early stages of more chronic diseases, LMN signs are subtle. Decreased strength of the flexion reflex may be the most prominent sign.

Acute Progressive Diseases

Acute Idiopathic Polyradiculoneuritis (Coonhound Paralysis). This acute neurologic syndrome has been recognized largely in hunting dogs that have been exposed to raccoons, but it also has been observed in dogs with no exposure to raccoons.[66-68] The disease is remarkably similar to acute polyneuritis in humans (Landry-Guillain-Barré syndrome). *Pathophysiology.* Immune-mediated segmental demyelination and degeneration of axons are found in dogs exposed to raccoons. Apparently, a transmissible substance in raccoon saliva produces the disease.[69] Other inflammatory neuropathies occasionally are reported in dogs and some other animals, including a cat[70] and a goat[71] (see discussion of chronic polyradiculoneuritis in cats). Polyneuritis equi (cauda equina neuritis) is relatively common and is discussed in Chapter 6. Chronic polyneuropathies are discussed separately. The Landry-Guillain-Barré syndrome in humans has been induced by several diseases, including respiratory infections and influenza vaccinations. Postvaccinal polyradiculoneuritis has also been seen in a dog.[72]

The disease attacks primarily the ventral roots and spinal nerves. Characteristic microscopic lesions include segmental demyelination, degeneration of both myelin and axons, leukocyte infiltration, secondary degeneration of the ventral horn cells, and neurogenic muscle atrophy.[68,73] Neurologic signs develop because motor signal transmission from the spinal cord to the muscle fibers is blocked. *Clinical Signs.* Neurologic signs develop in some dogs 7 to 14 days after raccoon exposure. Early clinical signs include pelvic limb paresis and hyporeflexia. Ascending weakness or paralysis develops quickly. Affected dogs become tetraparetic 24 to 48 hours after the neurologic signs first develop. Spinal reflexes are severely depressed or absent. Passive flexion and extension of the limbs reveal severe hypotonus of affected muscles. Cerebral responses to painful stimuli are normal or exaggerated. Diffuse hyperesthesia is occasionally

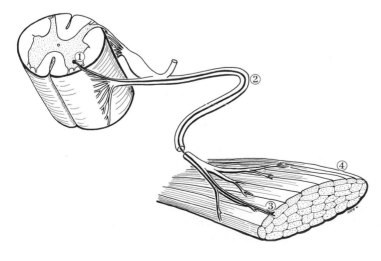

Figure 7-12 Schematic of anatomic sites of neuromuscular disease. *(1)* Neuronal cell bodies (neuronopathy), *(2)* peripheral nerves (neuropathy), *(3)* neuromuscular junction (junctionopathy), and *(4)* muscles (myopathy). (From Kornegay JN: *Feline neurology.* [*Problems in veterinary medicine series.*] Philadelphia, 1991, JB Lippincott.)

seen. Dogs with rapidly progressive disease may develop respiratory paralysis. Cranial nerve involvement is uncommon, although the dog's bark may be weak. Swallowing, gag reflex, and esophagus are normal. The patient remains alert, responsive, and afebrile. Defecation, urination, and tail mobility usually are normal because the sacral and caudal nerve roots are relatively spared. Muscle atrophy can be detected by direct palpation 10 to 14 days after the onset of paresis. Occasionally, the initial clinical signs are detected in the thoracic limbs and progress to the pelvic limbs. The thoracic limbs may remain preferentially involved in some acute forms of polyradiculoneuritis.[74,75] The clinical course is usually 3 to 6 weeks but is sometimes 2 to 4 months or longer.[76] Improvement begins by the third week, and complete recovery may take 6 to 8 weeks. In patients that develop severe muscle atrophy, recovery may not be complete.

Diagnosis. The differential diagnosis should include tick paralysis and botulism because these diseases produce clinical signs that are essentially identical to those of the early stages of polyradiculoneuritis. Polyradiculoneuritis is suspected when no ticks are found on physical examination and exposure to botulism toxin is not possible. Laboratory and radiographic studies are normal. CSF collected from the lumbar subarachnoid space shows an increase in protein concentration with a normal cell count. A diagnosis of polyradiculoneuritis is supported by electromyographic (EMG) evidence of diffuse denervation of affected muscles. These changes occur 5 to 7 days after injury of the motor axon. The EMG abnormalities include increased insertion activity, fibrillation potentials, and positive sharp waves. Evoked potentials are slightly reduced in amplitude and may be polyphasic, but are not as severely affected as with botulism or tick paralysis.[77] Nerve conduction velocities are reduced later in the course of the disease. F-waves are delayed and dispersed after paralysis has developed fully.[78] An enzyme-linked immunosorbent assay using raccoon saliva as the antigen shows some promise as a diagnostic test.[78] Table 7-5 compares the diagnostic features of polyradiculoneuritis, tick paralysis, and botulism.

Treatment. No specific treatment for polyradiculoneuritis exists. Controlled trials of treatment with corticosteroids have not been reported. One study in humans with chronic inflammatory demyelinating polyradiculoneuropathy demonstrated mild but significant improvement with prednisone.[79] Another study did not show benefit of high-dose intravenous methylprednisolone early in Landry-Guillain-Barré syndrome.[80] We do not routinely give corticosteroids. Chronic glucocorticoid

therapy may cause urinary tract infection, muscle wasting, and delayed healing of decubital ulcers. Plasmapheresis has been effective in human patients with Landry-Guillain-Barré syndrome,[81] has been used in other immune-mediated diseases of dogs,[82] and could be beneficial in dogs with polyradiculoneuritis.

Supportive care consists of attentive nursing that (1) prevents decubital ulcers, (2) minimizes muscle atrophy and contractures, (3) prevents urinary tract infection, (4) prevents pneumonia, and (5) supports respiratory function. Animals should be bedded on deep straw or hay, air mattresses, sealed foam, or waterbeds; turned frequently; and kept clean. Voluntary micturition usually is preserved; however, many dogs cannot produce a normal abdominal press and may fail to empty their bladders. Gentle manual expression of the bladder is helpful. Physical therapy consisting of muscle massage and passive manipulation of the limbs is important. Hydrotherapy is helpful for preventing muscle atrophy and contractures and for keeping the dog clean.

The prognosis for recovery is usually good. Recurrences have been observed. Some dogs appear to be particularly susceptible to recurrences. The course of the illness is 3 to 6 weeks. Neurologic signs usually abate in the reverse order of development.

Botulism. For many years, this disease was suspected in dogs but was never documented. Carrion eaters and some carnivores, including dogs, were thought to be resistant to botulism toxin. In 1978 Barsanti and co-workers[83] documented an outbreak of type C botulism in foxhounds in Georgia. Botulism also has been reported in dogs in Great Britain, the European continent, and Australia.[84-87] Before a detailed description of polyradiculoneuritis was published, many hunting dogs with acute progressive LMN disease were thought to have botulism. After the Cummings and Haas report[68] on coonhound paralysis, most dogs were believed to have this disorder. Both conditions are now known to exist in dogs, but it can be difficult to make a differential diagnosis.

In large animals, botulism results from ingestion of toxin or from the contamination of an ulcerated gastrointestinal tract with proliferating *Clostridium botulinum* spores. Outbreaks in cattle occur as a result of the ingestion of hay, silage, or water that has been contaminated by dead rodents.[88] The shaker foal syndrome occurs most frequently in foals 2 to 5 weeks of age. Foals that are given highly nutritious feed develop gastrointestinal ulcers. These ulcers are colonized by *C. botulinum*, which then produces the offending toxin.[89-91] Botulism can also occur from wound infection.[92]

Table 7-5 **Diagnostic Comparison of Acute Progressive Lower Motor Neuron Disorders**

	Polyradiculoneuritis	Tick Paralysis	Botulism
History	Single case; previous exposure to raccoon in some cases	Single case–engorged tick	Multiple cases are very suggestive; access to carrion or spoiled food
Pathophysiology	Nonsuppurative nerve root inflammation and demyelination	Interference with action potential release of acetylcholine and action potential production	Block of neuromuscular transmission
Autonomic signs	Rare	Rare	Common
Cranial nerve involvement	Rare	Rare	Usual
Electromyography	Fibrillation potentials and positive sharp waves	No denervation	Usually no denervation
Conduction velocity	Normal to decreased	Normal to slightly decreased	Normal
Evoked potentials	Reduced	Reduced	Reduced; reduction in amplitude on repetitive stimulation
Special tests	None	None	Toxin in feces and serum
Treatment	Supportive	Tick removal	Supportive
Recovery time	3-6 wk	24-48 hr	2-3 wk

Pathophysiology. Clinical signs develop when the preformed *C. botulinum* toxin is ingested. Several different strains of exotoxin-producing organisms have been identified. Types A, B, and E are most commonly associated with human disease. Types C and D, found in carrion, cause most cases of botulism in birds and mammals other than humans. All cases reported in dogs were caused by type C. Most of those in large animals were caused by type B. Botulinal toxin produces generalized neuromuscular blockade by inhibiting the release of acetylcholine from the terminals of cholinergic nerve fibers.[93] The exact mechanism is unknown.

Clinical Signs. The incubation period is less than 6 days. Clinical signs are those of a progressive, symmetric, generalized LMN disorder. Severity varies with the amount of toxin ingested and ranges from mild generalized weakness to tetraplegia with respiratory failure. Both cranial and spinal nerves are affected.[83,84] Facial paralysis, megaesophagus, intestinal ileus, anisocoria, detrusor atony, and changes in the bark are more common than with polyradiculoneuritis. In dogs, the usual clinical course is less than 14 days.

Diagnosis. Botulism must be suspected in animals with acute progressive LMN disease. *Botulism is especially likely when multiple animals are affected.* Tick paralysis and polyradiculoneuritis are sporadic diseases that involve individual animals. EMG studies may help to differentiate botulism from polyradiculoneuritis, but some similarity exists, depending on the stage of disease. Electrodiagnostic findings in affected humans include normal motor nerve-conduction velocity, decreased M-wave amplitude, decrement/increment of the M wave with slow/rapid repetitive nerve stimulation, and increased "jitter" with single fiber EMG.[94] Electrophysiologic evidence of peripheral nerve involvement has been collected from dogs.[95]

Identification of toxin in the food, carrion, serum, feces, or vomitus of an affected animal confirms the diagnosis. The organism can be isolated from the viscera and feces of clinically normal animals.

Treatment. Treatment of botulism is largely supportive. To be effective, the specific antitoxin must be administered before the botulinal toxin binds to receptors at the myoneural junction. This approach is rarely possible because signs usually are present before the animal is treated. Polyvalent products that contain type C antitoxin generally are not available. The efficacy of antibiotic therapy has not been proven. The prognosis for recovery is generally good unless the dog develops severe, rapidly progressive signs. Artificial respiration may be necessary in some dogs. Mildly affected animals recover without therapy.[83]

Tick Paralysis. This disease has been recognized worldwide, but most in-depth reports have come from the United States and Australia. The clinical signs are similar to those of polyradiculoneuritis and botulism.

Pathophysiology. A neurotoxin secreted by engorged feeding female ticks either inhibits depolarization in the terminal portions of motor nerves or blocks the release of acetylcholine at the neuromuscular junction. The toxin may affect both motor and sensory nerve fibers by altering ionic fluxes that mediate action potential production.[96] In the United States, *Dermacentor andersoni* and *D. variabilis* are the primary ticks involved. In Australia, the disease is produced by *Ixodes holocyclus*, although *I. cornuatus* and *I. hirsti* are also incriminated.[97]

Clinical Signs. Clinical signs develop 7 to 9 days after attachment of the tick. The earliest clinical sign is marked ataxia with rapid progression to paresis, paralysis, areflexia, and hypotonus. In the United States, cranial nerve involvement is rare. Nystagmus is occasionally observed. Death can occur from respiratory failure if the ticks are not removed. Painful stimuli normally are perceived. In Australia, affected dogs or cats develop more severe signs. Respiratory failure and autonomic signs occur with greater frequency in these animals than in those from the United States. In the Australian syndrome, clinical signs may progressively worsen, even though the ticks have been removed.[98,99] In the U.S. syndrome, dramatic improvement follows tick removal.

Diagnosis. Tick paralysis is diagnosed by rapid improvement after tick removal. In unusual cases, EMG can be used to differentiate this disease from acute polyradiculoneuritis.[77] In tick paralysis, no EMG evidence of denervation exists and the amplitude of evoked motor potentials is markedly reduced. Repetitive stimulation does not cause further decrement in the amplitude. Nerve-conduction velocities may be slightly slower than normal, and terminal conduction times may be prolonged.[96]

Treatment. In the U.S. syndrome, removal of the tick results in marked improvement within 24 hours and complete recovery within 72 hours. Animals must be examined thoroughly for ticks. The areas evaluated should include the ear canals and interdigital spaces. Ticks are removed carefully so that the head is not left embedded in the animal's skin. The toxin probably comes from the salivary glands of the tick. Failure to remove the head may cause worsening of the clinical signs. When tick paralysis is suspected and ticks cannot be found, insecticide solutions should be sponged over the entire dog. The prognosis for complete recovery is good. In Australian tick paralysis, tick removal does not prevent further progression of the disease. Hyperimmune dog serum has been advocated to prevent death from respiratory failure.[97]

Aminoglycoside Toxicity. The aminoglycoside antibiotics, when given parenterally, can cause neuromuscular blockade.[100] Their effects are similar to those of curare. We observed one animal that developed severe muscle weakness and hyporeflexia after 5 days of gentamicin therapy for deep pyoderma. The clinical signs resolved within 48 hours after the drug was discontinued.

Chronic Progressive Diseases

Motor Neuronopathies. These diseases (see Table 7-4) are characterized by progressive degeneration of motor neurons in the gray matter of the spinal cord and nuclei of the brainstem. Progressive denervation of muscle fibers results in paresis, paralysis, and severe muscle atrophy. The diseases in dogs resemble the inherited spinal muscular atrophies of humans.

Brittany Spaniel Spinal Muscular Atrophy. This inherited disease was first reported in 1979 in a family of Brittany spaniels in the southeastern United States.[101] The signs typically develop by 4 months of age. Characteristic signs include severe atrophy of the paraspinal and proximal pelvic girdle muscles. Affected animals walk with a crouched, waddling gait in the pelvic limbs. The thoracic limbs are less severely affected. Cranial nerves V, VII, and XII are involved in some dogs. The distal appendicular muscles tend to be spared. The disease is inherited as an autosomal dominant trait and has three phenotypic forms: accelerated, intermediate, and chronic. Homozygous dogs have the accelerated form. Signs are seen by 6 to 8 weeks of age, with severe paralysis developing by 3 to 4 months. Dogs with the chronic form may live for several years. Pathologic studies have established that degeneration of motor neurons produces the clinical signs. Some dogs, however, have relatively normal numbers of neurons, although the neurons are smaller than normal. These neurons may be dysfunctional.[102,103] The condition is nearly identical to juvenile spinal muscular atrophy of children. No effective treatment is available.

Hereditary Neuronal Abiotrophy of the Swedish Lapland Dog. Dogs with this disorder develop weakness at 5 to 7 weeks of age and are unable to stand within 2 weeks.[104] Either the pelvic or thoracic limbs may be preferentially affected at the onset of disease, but then involvement becomes uniform. Weakness and atrophy are most conspicuous in the distal muscles. The disease shows little tendency to progress after the initial 2 weeks. The trait may be inherited in an autosomal recessive manner. No effective treatment exists.

Rottweiler Spinal Muscular Atrophy. This disease is similar to the condition of Brittany spaniels. Two affected pups studied had megaesophagus and were tetraplegic by 8 weeks of age, when they were euthanized. Accumulation of neurofilaments was not seen. The mode of inheritance is not known.[105,106]

Pointer Spinal Muscular Atrophy. Another disease similar to Brittany spaniel spinal muscular atrophy occurs in pointers and is inherited as an autosomal recessive trait. Inclusions found in motor neurons suggest that this may be a storage disease.[107,108]

German Shepherd Spinal Muscular Atrophy. Two German shepherd dog pups had focal degeneration of motor neurons in the brachial intumescence. Denervation of thoracic limb muscles caused weakness and atrophy. The lesions resembled other spinal muscular atrophies but were localized.[109]

Equine Motor Neuron Disease. A spontaneous motor neuron disease has been characterized in horses, primarily in the northeastern United States.[110,111] Various breeds and ages are affected. Characteristic initial signs include weight loss, excessive recumbency, and trembling. Constant shifting of weight in the pelvic limbs, abnormally low head carriage, and muscle fasciculations are also seen. Serum muscle-derived enzyme levels are increased. Spontaneous activity is consistently seen on EMG, particularly in the proximal thoracic limbs.[112] Environmental risk factors include absence of grazing for more than 1 year and provision of poor quality hay.[107] The cause is not known. Vitamin E levels were significantly lower in affected horses. Together with other findings, this suggests that oxidative insults may be responsible.[111] Some horses have improved after being allowed on pasture and given supplemental vitamin E. Lesions are similar to those of the other spinal muscular atrophies.[110] A tentative antemortem diagnosis can be established by demonstrating degeneration of myelinated axons in biopsy samples of the ventral branch of the spinal accessory nerve.[113]

Stockard's Paralysis. This syndrome causes paraplegia in the offspring of great Dane–bloodhound or great Dane–Saint Bernard matings.[114] The pelvic limbs are selectively involved. Signs of pelvic limb paresis develop when the dog is 11 to 14 weeks of age and progressively worsen for a few days. Thereafter, the signs remain rather constant. Preferential distal pelvic limb muscle involvement occurs.

Bovine Spinal Muscular Atrophy. Brown Swiss cattle have an inherited disease in which ventral horn cells of the spinal cord and UMNs degenerate.[115] Calves develop progressive weakness and neurogenic muscle atrophy within the first few weeks of life. Brown Swiss cattle also develop progressive degenerative myeloencephalopathy ("weaver" syndrome)[116] and congenital axonopathy.[117]

Multisystem Neuronal Degenerations. Progressive neuronopathy has been characterized in 4- to 7-month-old cairn terriers.[118-120] Pelvic limb paresis progresses to tetraplegia in weeks to months. Signs of cerebellar dysfunction and cataplexy also may be seen. Spinal and brainstem neurons are chromatolytic. Wallerian degeneration was noted in peripheral nerves. One dog had symmetrical thoracolumbar myelomalacia in the dorsal horns and adjoining white matter.[120] A hereditary basis is assumed but not proven. Four cocker spaniels had neuronal degeneration of multiple areas of the brain, causing a syndrome of behavioral changes, ataxia, dysmetria, and normal spinal reflexes.[121] Pedigree analysis suggested a hereditary cause.

Polyneuropathy. These diseases (Table 7-6) are recognized more frequently in dogs now than a few years ago, but they are relatively uncommon in other species. The chronic neuropathies have an insidious onset and progress slowly over several months. Attacks of the disease may be interrupted by periods of spontaneous improvement. Definition of the cause of chronic polyneuropathy is often elusive. Better diagnostic techniques, especially electrophysiologic tests and histopathologic assessment of muscle and nerve biopsy samples, have contributed to a greater understanding of this problem.[122-126]

Chronic Idiopathic Polyneuritis. This syndrome affects primarily mature dogs.[127,128] Cats may also be involved.[129,130] Signs of lameness, muscle atrophy, paresis, and eventually paralysis develop slowly over several months. The neurologic findings vary with the stage of the illness. Postural reactions, spinal reflexes, and muscle strength are decreased. Cranial nerves V and VII may be involved. Hypalgesia may occur later when sensory nerves become involved. The clinical course varies from several months to years. Signs of this disease can resemble those of primary muscle disorders.

The diagnosis is made by muscle and nerve biopsy. EMG and nerve-conduction velocity studies are useful but do not provide evidence of inflammation. Pathologic studies suggest that nonsuppurative inflammation, perhaps with an immune basis, is responsible for the disease.[127,128] The dorsal root ganglia and cranial nerves are affected in some cases, causing sensory deficits; this condition has been called *ganglioradiculitis* (see discussion of sensory neuropathies).[131] Some animals appear to benefit from corticosteroid therapy but then relapse and continue to worsen. Because of the disease's waxing-waning character, the benefit of corticosteroids is not proved (see discussion of acute polyradiculoneuritis).

Degenerative Hereditary Neuropathies. The hereditary neuropathies are rare diseases with chronic progressive courses.

Table 7-6 **Causes of Polyneuropathy***

Congenital or Hereditary (see Appendices for Complete List by Species and Breed)
 Peripheral neuropathies (motor or sensory)
  Progressive axonopathy in boxers
  Giant axonal neuropathy in German shepherd
   dogs
  Neurofibrillary accumulations
  Hypertrophic neuropathy in Tibetan mastiffs
  Sensory neuropathy in longhaired dachshunds,
   pointers, golden retrievers, Doberman pinschers,
   Siberian huskies, whippets, Scottish terriers
  Storage diseases (e.g., sphingomyelinosis in the cat,
   globoid leukodystrophy in cairn and West
   Highland white terriers; see Chapter 15)
  Demyelinating diseases
  Laryngeal paralysis in horses, Siberian huskies,
   Bouvier des Flandres (see Chapter 9)
  Polyneuropathy of Alaskan malamutes
  Distal axonopathy of Birman cats
  Familial neuropathy of Gelbvieh calves
 	
 Metabolic
 Endocrine
  Beta-cell tumor
  Diabetes mellitus
  Hypothyroidism
 Metabolic defects
  Hyperchylomicronemia in cats
  Hyperoxaluria in cats
 Kangaroo gait in ewes
 	
 Neoplastic
 Paraneoplastic neuropathies
 	
 Nutritional
 Copper deficiency in lambs and kids
	Idiopathic
	 Distal denervating disease in dogs
	 Neurofibrillary accumulations
	 Dysautonomia in cats and dogs (see Chapter 9)
	 Distal symmetric polyneuropathy in dogs
	 Stringhalt in horses (see Chapter 10)
	
	 Inflammatory and Immune Mediated
	 Acute polyradiculoneuritis
	 Coonhound paralysis
	 Idiopathic
	 Chronic polyneuritis
	 Ganglioradiculoneuritis
	 Brachial plexus neuritis (see Chapter 5)
	 Neuritis of the cauda equina in horses (see Chapter 6)
	 Protozoal polyradiculoneuritis
	
	 Toxic (Including Drugs)
	 Aminoglycosides
	 Vincristine
	 Heavy metals
	  Lead
	  Mercury
	  Thallium
	  Copper, antimony, zinc
	 Organophosphate compounds
	 Industrial
	  Trichlorethylene
	  N-Hexane
	  Acrylamide
	
	 Vascular
	 Ischemic neuromyopathy (see Chapter 6)
	 Aortoiliac thrombosis (see Chapter 6)

*All have a chronic progressive course except acute idiopathic polyneuritis, vascular neuropathies, and aminoglycoside toxicity.

Progressive Axonopathy of Boxer Dogs. This disease is usually apparent by 2 to 3 months of age.[132,133] Pelvic limb ataxia is noted first, followed by involvement of the thoracic limbs. Postural reactions are abnormal, muscle tone and spinal reflexes are decreased, and ocular tremor or head bobbing may be present. Clinical signs tend to stabilize after 1 to 2 years, and dogs can lead a reasonably normal life. Axonal swellings are seen in the nerve roots, with distal atrophy of the axons. Demyelination and remyelination are present, probably secondary to the axon changes.[122] Progressive axonopathy is inherited as an autosomal recessive trait. It has been reported only in the United Kingdom.

Giant Axonal Neuropathy of German Shepherd Dogs. Axons of both the central and peripheral nervous systems are affected in a disease reported in one family of German shepherd dogs in the United Kingdom.[122,134,135] It is believed to be inherited as

an autosomal recessive trait. Swollen axons are noted in the distal portions of long tracts and peripheral nerves. Pelvic limb nerves are more severely affected than those of the thoracic limbs. Multiple swellings containing disoriented neurofilaments occur along the course of a single fiber. Both sensory and motor fibers are affected. Signs begin at 14 to 16 months of age and progress over several months' time. Proprioceptive deficits are noted first. Regurgitation, because of megaesophagus, occurs at about 18 months. Pain sensation may be reduced before 2 years of age.

Neurofibrillary Accumulations. Neurofilaments accumulate in neurons and axons in a number of degenerative central nervous system (CNS) diseases, including some that affect LMNs. Additional cases in which LMNs are involved have been described in pigs,[136] calves,[137] a cat,[138] a collie pup,[139] and a zebra.[140] Neurofilaments may accumulate because of disordered axon transport.[141]

Hypertrophic Neuropathy of Tibetan Mastiff Dogs. Tibetan mastiff pups developed generalized weakness and decreased reflexes at 7 to 12 weeks of age and were tetraplegic within 3 weeks of onset.[142] Nerve-conduction velocities were decreased. The primary lesion was demyelination of peripheral nerves, with little axonal degeneration. Autosomal recessive inheritance was suggested. A similar syndrome was seen in one mongrel dog.[143]

Polyneuropathy of Alaskan Malamutes. This syndrome has been seen in Norway and is thought to be inherited as an autosomal recessive trait.[144] Paraparesis that progresses to tetraparesis, coughing, dyspnea, and regurgitation is noted as early as 7 months of age but usually between 12 and 18 months of age. Shoulder and thigh muscles are atrophied. The patellar, cranial, tibial, and panniculus reflexes are depressed to absent. Megaesophagus may be seen. Spontaneous activity is present on EMG evaluation, and motor-nerve-conduction velocity is reduced. Neurogenic muscle atrophy and axonal degeneration are seen. Dogs may stabilize and then deteriorate.

Distal Axonopathy of Birman Cats. Cats with this disease have progressive paraparesis with a plantigrade posture and gait in the pelvic limbs.[145] Reduced numbers of myelinated axons were seen in distal axons of both the peripheral and central nervous systems.

Peripheral Neuropathy and Glomerulopathy of Gelbvieh Calves. Calves affected with this disease initially have paraparesis and ataxia that progresses to tetraparesis and recumbency within days to several weeks.[146] At the time of examination, calves ranged in age from 5 weeks to 13 months. Degenerative lesions were severe in peripheral nerves and nerve roots and less severe in dorsal fasciculi of the spinal cord. Glomerular lesions included mild mesangial hypercellularity to glomerulosclerosis. This disease is likely inherited.

Distal Symmetric Polyneuropathy. This disease of dogs is characterized by degeneration of the distal axons of peripheral nerves. Only intramuscular branches may be affected. This condition is common in the United Kingdom but not elsewhere.[122,147] Signs develop over a period of 1 to 4 weeks. Tetraparesis varies in severity. The neck muscles may be weak, but cranial nerves and pain sensation are not affected. Muscle biopsy and examination of intramuscular nerve fibers often reveal distal nerve degeneration. More proximal portions of the nerve may be normal. Most dogs recover. No breed or age predisposition exists.

A distal neuropathy has also been reported in Doberman pinschers and is termed *dancing Doberman disease.*[148] Pelvic limb weakness is noted initially. The dogs are 6 months to 7 years old at onset, and the disease progresses slowly for at least 5 years. Typically, affected dogs flex one pelvic limb while standing. Eventually both pelvic limbs are affected so that the dog alternately flexes each limb as if it is dancing. Signs are similar to those seen in horses with stringhalt (see discussion that follows). Pelvic limb tendon reflexes often are hyperactive. Histopathologic changes of both axonopathy and myopathy have been reported. The gastrocnemius muscles are preferentially involved.

Polyneuropathy has been recognized in rottweilers between 1.5 and 4 years of age.[149] Affected dogs develop paraparesis that progresses to tetraparesis, spinal hyporeflexia, hypotonia, and neurogenic appendicular muscle atrophy. Signs may resolve and then recur. Myelinated axons are lost in both sensory and motor nerves.

Distal axonopathy, with associated neurogenic muscle atrophy, has been identified in horses with Australian stringhalt.[150] Affected horses flex one or both pelvic limbs excessively during attempted movement. In contrast to classic stringhalt, this disease has a seasonal incidence, and affected horses may recover spontaneously.

Sensory Neuropathies. Hereditary sensory neuropathies occur in long-haired dachshunds[151] and pointers.[152] A single case was described in a border collie pup.[153] Ganglioneuritis, with involvement of sensory ganglia, has been described in a number of dogs.[131,154] Siberian huskies may be predisposed.[155] In the Dachshund, abnormalities of proprioception, pain sensation, and urinary function begin as early as 8 weeks of age. Paresis and muscular atrophy are not seen. Affected dogs are severely incontinent by 1.5 years of age. EMG and motor-nerve-conduction velocities are normal, but severe depletion of both large myelinated and unmyelinated fibers occurs. No treatment is known, and an inherited basis is presumed.

The syndrome in pointers is characterized by self-mutilation beginning at about 4 months of age. Dogs lick and chew their paws to the point of digital amputation. Pain sensation is reduced distally. Primary sensory neurons in the dorsal root ganglia are depleted. Substance P is reduced in the ganglia.[156] The condition is inherited. No treatment exists.

Initial signs in dogs with the inflammatory sensory neuropathies include pelvic limb ataxia, difficulty in eating, regurgitation, dysphagia, and mutilation/hyperesthesia.[155] Patellar reflexes often are reduced or absent.

Based on electrophysiologic abnormalities, one investigator suggested that dogs with acral lick dermatitis may have a mild sensory axonal polyneuropathy.[157]

Hypothyroid Neuropathy. Hypothyroidism causes polyneuropathy in dogs. Dogs may have signs of LMN dysfunction, peripheral vestibular dysfunction, megaesophagus, or laryngeal paralysis.[158,159] In most animals, both cranial and spinal peripheral nerves are affected. The early stages are often missed because the signs are mild. Diffuse evidence of neuropathy is seen with EMG examination. Many affected animals do not have obvious signs of hypothyroidism. Presenting complaints include weakness, intermittent lameness, and signs of cranial nerve VII, VIII, IX, and X dysfunction (see Chapters 8 and 9). The diagnosis of hypothyroidism in affected dogs is based on serum levels of free thyroxine (T_4) and thyroid-stimulating hormone (TSH). Degenerative changes may be seen in nerve biopsy specimens. Hypothyroidism also may cause histologic changes of myopathy[160] and has been associated with acquired myasthenia gravis in dogs.[161] The rate and degree of recovery subsequent to levothyroxine treatment depend on the severity of the denervation. Actual improvement of motor function usually takes several months. Animals with severe, generalized denervation have not done well. Some dogs that fail to respond have mononuclear cellular infiltration of their peripheral nerves, perhaps reflecting a systemic immune-mediated disease directed against both the thyroid gland and nerves.

Diabetic Neuropathy. Peripheral neuropathy has been documented in association with diabetes mellitus in both cats and dogs.[162-165] Axons are affected primarily, with secondary demyelination. Distal axons are particularly susceptible. The pelvic limbs may be preferentially involved. Affected cats characteristically have a plantigrade stance and decreased patellar reflexes. Signs of neuropathy may occur in advance of those more typically associated with diabetes mellitus. Subclinical electrophysiologic abnormalities may be present in diabetic animals.[166] Sensory nerves may be preferentially involved. Clinical signs may resolve within 6 to 12 months of serum glucose stabilization with insulin therapy.

Paraneoplastic Neuropathies. Neoplasia can affect peripheral nerves because of either direct involvement or paraneoplastic ("remote") effects.[167] Effects on peripheral nerves may be difficult to distinguish from those caused by chemotherapy or irradiation.[168] Paraneoplastic effects are thought to be immune mediated.[167] Subclinical pathologic evidence of peripheral neuropathy has been identified in dogs with distant neoplasia.[169] Clinical involvement occurs rarely.[170] Beta-cell tumors cause profound hypoglycemia that affects the metabolism of the CNS, causing seizures, behavioral abnormalities, and other signs of forebrain

disease (see Chapters 12 and 13). In addition, polyneuropathy is a rare complication.[171-173] Paraparesis that progresses to tetraparesis, with muscle atrophy and reduced spinal reflexes and muscle tone, has been reported. Whereas hypoglycemia may play a role in the development of lesions, an immune-mediated pathogenesis may be involved, and dogs might benefit from corticosteroid therapy independent of their hyperglycemic properties.[173]

Hyperchylomicronemia in Cats. Cats with inherited lipoprotein lipase deficiency develop hyperlipemia, lipemia retinalis, and peripheral neuropathies.[174,175] Plasma triglyceride and cholesterol levels are increased. Peripheral nerves are compressed by lipid granulomas that probably develop subsequent to trauma.[174]

Hyperoxaluria in Cats. Hereditary renal failure due to deposition of oxalate crystals in the kidney causes paresis with reduced reflexes.[176] Axons in the spinal cord, ventral roots, and intramuscular nerves are distended with neurofilaments. Human patients with a similar condition (primary hyperoxaluria type 2) and affected cats have decreased levels of the enzyme D-glycerate dehydrogenase. The cause of the axonal swellings is not known.

Kangaroo Gait in Ewes. Polyneuropathy that primarily affects the radial nerve has been reported in lactating ewes in the United Kingdom and New Zealand.[177] The thoracic limbs are primarily affected. Minimal involvement is seen outside the brachial plexus. Most ewes recover. The cause is unknown.

Protozoal Polyradiculoneuritis. *Neospora caninum* and *Toxoplasma gondii* can cause inflammation of the peripheral nerves, muscles, or CNS.[178-181] *Neospora* is the likely causative agent in many cases originally thought to be toxoplasmosis. In the peripheral nervous system, the spinal nerve roots are more severely affected. The syndrome is usually seen in young dogs. Pelvic limb extensor rigidity (genu recurvatum) is a classic feature of protozoal muscle and nerve infection. *N. caninum* and *T. gondii* infections can be distinguished using serologic, immunohistochemical, and morphologic criteria,[178] although the clinical significance of this distinction is not clear. Because infections may be subclinical, evidence of seroconversion 2 or more weeks after the initial immunoglobulin G (IgG) antibody titer is required for a diagnosis (see Chapter 15). All dogs with clinical neosporosis have had serum titers greater than 1:200, but titers greater than 1:800 have been seen in clinically normal dogs.[181] Treatment should include trimethoprim-sulfadiazine (15 mg/kg, orally, every 12 hours for 4 weeks) and pyrimethamine (1 mg/kg, orally, every 24 hours for 4 weeks) or clindamycin (10 mg/kg, orally, every 8 hours for 2 to 6 weeks).[181] Early treatment may be beneficial, but if muscle contracture is present, recovery is unlikely.

Toxic Neuropathies. Table 7-6 lists some toxins that may cause neuropathy. None of these is common. The potential for toxicity varies among species. Decreased metabolism or excretion of the toxin, as with hepatic disease in dogs receiving vincristine, may increase the likelihood of toxicity.[168]

Diffuse Muscle Disorders. Diseased muscles are usually weak. Muscle pain (myalgia), failure of muscles to relax (myotonia), and sudden muscle contraction (cramp) also suggest muscle disease. Myopathies include disorders characterized by weakness that does not have a neurogenic basis. A myopathy may be a result of inflammation (myositis) or degeneration. Inflammatory muscle diseases may be infectious or immune mediated. Degenerative diseases are either acquired or congenital. Nutritional, endocrine, metabolic, and vascular diseases cause acquired forms of muscle diseases. Most of the congenital diseases are inherited. Muscular dystrophies are progressive, inherited degenerative myopathies. The signs of diffuse muscle disease are very similar to those of diffuse polyneuropathies. Because of ambiguities in the diagnosis, increasing attention has been given to evaluation of serum enzyme levels, EMG and nerve-conduction velocity studies, and muscle biopsy.[182-184] Animal myopathies are classified in Table 7-7 and are discussed briefly in subsequent sections of this chapter.

Polymyositis. Polymyositis is classified as diffuse muscle inflammation of infectious or immune-mediated origin (see Table 7-7).[183] Infectious polymyositis is rare but may be seen with toxoplasmosis, neosporosis, or leptospirosis. Clostridial infections are relatively common in large animals but usually affect only one limb. Polymyositis may occur in association with systemic lupus erythematosus, as a paraneoplastic syndrome, or with some drugs, notably trimethoprim-sulfadiazine in Doberman pinschers and D-penicillamine in humans.[182,183,185,186] Dogs are most commonly affected[187,188]; cats may also develop polymyositis.[189] Adults are usually involved, although one report described two 7-month-old German wire-haired pointer littermates as being affected.[190] The most common clinical signs include muscle pain, weakness, stilted gait, and fever. Muscle atrophy, depression, anorexia, weight loss, and bark change occur less frequently.[187,188] Regurgitation may develop in dogs with megaesophagus.[187] Clinical signs may occur acutely, followed by periods of spontaneous remission, or they may occur chronically. Signs resemble those of chronic polyneuritis

or myasthenia gravis. Acute, painful episodes must be differentiated from those of meningitis and skeletal diseases.

Criteria to diagnose polymyositis in animals have been extrapolated from those in humans.[187] A definitive diagnosis is based on (1) evidence of muscle pain or weakness; (2) elevations in the concentrations of serum muscle enzymes (creatine kinase [CK], lactic dehydrogenase, aspartate aminotransferase [AST]); (3) EMG abnormalities;

Table 7-7 **Causes of Polymyopathy in Animals**

Inflammatory
Infectious
  Toxoplasma gondii
  Neospora caninum
  Leptospira icterohaemorrhagiae
  Clostridium spp.
  Hepatozoan canis
  Microfilariasis
Noninfectious
  Idiopathic polymyositis
  Masticatory myositis
  Systemic lupus erythematosus—polymyositis
  Eosinophilic myositis
  Dermatomyositis in collies and border collies
  Extraocular myositis
Paraneoplastic thymoma—associated
Drug-induced
  Trimethoprim-sulfadiazine
  D-Penicillamine

Degenerative
Inherited
  Muscular dystrophy in multiple species and breeds
  Myotonic myopathy in chow chows, Staffordshire terriers, great Danes, Rhodesian ridgebacks, Cavalier King Charles spaniels, goats, Shropshire lambs (various horses, inheritance not proven) (see Chapter 10)
  Myopathy of Pietrain pigs (creeper)
  Periodic paralysis
  Exertional rhabdomyolysis
Nutritional (white muscle disease)
  Vitamin E deficiency
  Selenium deficiency
Endocrine
  Hyperadrenocorticism (steroid myopathy)
  Hypothyroidism
  Hypokalemia
  Hyperkalemia
Metabolic
  Exertional rhabdomyolysis
  Malignant hyperthermia
  Postanesthetic myopathy (large animals)
  Mitochondrial myopathies
  Periodic paralysis
Vascular
  Ischemic neuromyopathy (see Chapter 6)

and (4) histopathologic evidence of muscle necrosis and inflammation. A probable diagnosis can be made when three of these four findings are present. Little correlation exists between muscle-enzyme concentrations and either the severity of clinical signs or the degree of muscle necrosis or inflammation seen on examination of biopsy specimens.[187] EMG changes include fibrillation potentials, positive sharp waves, polyphasic motor-unit potentials, motor-unit potentials of decreased duration, complex repetitive discharges, and increased insertional activity. Fading of evoked motor-unit potentials, reversed with neostigmine, has been reported.[187] Pathologic changes may include muscle fiber necrosis, as evidenced by hyaline fibers and myophagocytosis, variable fiber size, and regeneration. Inflammatory cells include lymphocytes and some neutrophils. Eosinophilic inflammation has been reported.[188] Serologic tests for toxoplasmosis and neosporosis should be done.

Idiopathic polymyositis should be treated with prednisone (2.0 mg/kg per day) until remission is achieved. Alternate-day therapy then is instituted to maintain remission. A lesser dosage may be adequate; treatment can be discontinued in some dogs without recurrence of signs. Dogs with megaesophagus may develop aspiration pneumonia. Management of these cases is difficult, and the prognosis for regaining normal esophageal function is guarded.

Masticatory Muscle Myositis. Inflammation affecting primarily the muscles of mastication is seen more commonly in dogs than is polymyositis.[191-193] Eosinophilic and atrophic myositis may represent acute and chronic forms of this disease. In the acute stages of masticatory myositis, the temporal and masseter muscles are firm, swollen,

and painful. Chronic trismus and marked masticatory muscle atrophy are seen. Selective involvement of the masticatory muscles is due to differences in histochemical and biochemical properties of the masticatory muscles. Antibodies are produced against a specific myosin isoform in type-2M fibers of the masticatory muscles.[191] The autoimmune reaction may be initiated by a bacterial antigen.[183] The diagnosis and treatment are the same as that for polymyositis; 13 of 14 dogs treated with corticosteroids in one study either had a complete or partial response.[193] Dogs treated for 2 weeks or longer responded better.

Bilateral myositis restricted to the extraocular muscles was reported in two unrelated golden retrievers.[194] Exophthalmos was seen clinically. One of the dogs responded to glucocorticoids treatment. Five other dogs, including two golden retrievers, had similar signs that also responded to glucocorticoids.

Dermatomyositis. Collies and shetland sheepdogs have an inherited inflammatory skin and muscle disease.[195,196] The dermatitis is most severe on the ears, face, tail, and distal extremities. Myositis is often subclinical, but atrophy, weakness, and EMG changes may be seen. The muscles of mastication may be preferentially involved. An autosomal-dominant inherited, immune-mediated pathogenesis is suspected.[196] A similar syndrome was described in a Pembroke Welsh corgi.[197]

Muscular Dystrophies. The muscular dystrophies are inherited primary myopathies characterized by progressive degeneration of skeletal muscle.

X-linked Muscular Dystrophy. This form of muscular dystrophy is similar to Duchenne muscular dystrophy in humans and has been reported in golden retrievers (Figure 7-13), Irish terriers,

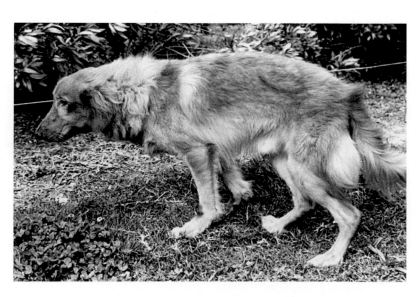

Figure 7-13 Dog with golden retriever muscular dystrophy at approximately 18 months of age with characteristic kyphosis, plantigrade stance, and temporalis muscle atrophy. (From Sharp NJH, Kornegay JN, Lane SB: The muscular dystrophies. *Semin Vet Med Surg (Small Anim)* 4:133-140, 1989.)

Samoyeds, rottweilers, Belgian tervurens, a miniature schnauzer, and domestic cats.[184,198-200] A similar syndrome was described in a foal, but testing to confirm the diagnosis was not done.[201] A membrane-associated muscle protein, *dystrophin*, is decreased or absent in affected animals (Figure 7-14) and humans. Molecular testing confirms the nature of the underlying genetic lesion[202,203] and may be used to identify carriers.[204] Affected pups are weak at birth and may die before a diagnosis is made. Stilted gait, trismus, muscle atrophy, stunted growth, and drooling may be seen as early as 6 weeks of age. Debilitating muscle contractures develop subsequently. Signs often stabilize to some extent after 6 months of age in golden retrievers but ultimately progress. Cats develop marked muscle hypertrophy.[200] Serum muscle enzymes are dramatically elevated in affected animals; creatine kinase values greater than 20,000 U/L are seen at 1 day of age. Complex repetitive discharges are noted on EMG. Histopathologic changes include myofiber necrosis and phagocytosis, variation in myofiber size, and myofiber mineralization. Colonies of affected golden retrievers and cats have been established.

Labrador Retriever Myopathy. The Labrador retriever has an autosomal-recessive form of muscular dystrophy.[205-207] Signs develop between 6 weeks and 7 months of age and are generally much less severe than those in the X-linked dystrophies. Affected dogs may have a stilted gait and advance their pelvic limbs simultaneously. The temporalis muscles are often atrophied. Affected dogs have cervical ventroflexion. Tendon reflexes, particularly the patellar, are depressed or absent. Signs generally stabilize by 6 to 8 months of age. Some dogs develop megaesophagus. Pathologic changes include variation in fiber size, myofiber group atrophy, and angular fibers. These changes are compatible with neural involvement, but underlying lesions have not been identified. Type-2 myofibers may be preferentially involved in some muscles.

Bouvier des Flandres Myopathy. Degeneration of the pharyngeal and esophageal muscles, with normal nerves, has been identified in Bouviers with dysphagia.[208,209] Regurgitation occurs beginning around 2 years of age.

Merino Sheep. The muscular dystrophy of Merino sheep is inherited as an autosomal-recessive trait. Signs develop at 3 to 4 weeks of age and are similar to the canine diseases.[210,211]

Hereditary Myopathy of Devon Rex Cats. Affected cats develop cervical ventroflexion, dorsal protrusion of the scapulae, megaesophagus, and tetraparesis at 3 to 23 weeks of age.[212] Serum muscle-enzyme levels are normal. Muscle lesions include variation in fiber size and increased numbers of internal nuclei. Four of six affected cats died because of laryngospasm after obstruction of the pharynx with food.

Distal Myopathy of Rottweilers. Affected dogs have plantigrade and palmigrade stance, hock hyperflexion, and splayed forepaw digits.[214] Histopathologic changes include myofiber atrophy and mild necrosis; endomysial fibrosis and fatty deposition occur. Plasma and muscle carnitine levels are decreased.

Metabolic Myopathies. The metabolic myopathies include diseases in which either a primary biochemical defect involving skeletal muscle or a generalized metabolic or endocrine disorder causes muscle dysfunction. Major endocrine myopathies are discussed later in this chapter.

The glycogen-storage diseases result from deficiencies of specific enzymes involved in glycogenolysis. Glycogen accumulates intracellularly; skeletal

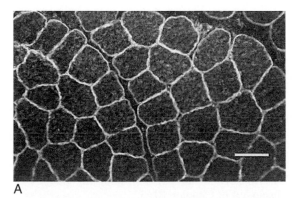

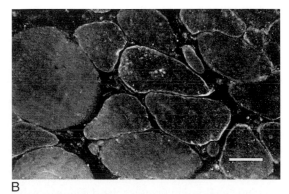

A   B

Figure 7-14 Characteristic subsarcolemmal staining pattern of dystrophin in a normal dog (**A**) and relative absence of staining in a littermate affected with golden retriever muscular dystrophy (**B**). Several myofibers show focal peripheral staining in **B**. Marked variation in myofiber size is also noted in the affected dog. Bar = 75 μm in **A** and 38 μm in **B**. Immunofluorescence: C-terminal domain antibody. (From Kornegay JN: The X-linked muscular dystrophies. In Kirk RW, Bonagura JD, editors: *Current veterinary therapy XI.* Philadelphia, 1992, WB Saunders.)

muscle often is affected. Glycogen storage disease type II (Pompe's disease) with associated myopathy has been reported in Lapland dogs.[215] Acid α-glucosidase activity was reduced in peripheral blood leukocytes in one dog. Affected dogs had progressive weakness, vomiting, regurgitation, and dysphonia. Prolonged insertional activity and complex repetitive discharges were noted on EMG. Electrocardiographic changes also occurred. All dogs were euthanized before 18 months of age because of the severity of clinical involvement. Shorthorn calves also have been affected.[216] Episodic weakness was noted as early as 4 months of age in German shepherds with suspected glycogen-storage disease type III (Cori's disease).[217] Norwegian forest cats with glycogen storage disease type IV (Andersen's disease) developed clinical disease after 4 months of age.[218,219] Branching enzyme activity was reduced. The trait was inherited in an autosomal-recessive manner. Glycogen-storage disease type V (McArdle's disease), resulting from deficiency of phosphorylase, was reported in Charolais calves that became weak and recumbent after minimal exercise.[220] Serum creatine kinase (CK) and aspartate aminotransferase (AST) levels were markedly elevated. Numerous myofibers in one calf were necrotic, depleted of glycogen, and contained degenerate mitochondria, indicating recent rhabdomyolysis. Pedigree analysis suggested autosomal-recessive inheritance.

Phosphofructokinase deficiency (glycogen-storage disease type VII; Tarui's disease) is inherited as an autosomal-recessive trait in English springer spaniels and causes sporadic intravascular hemolysis with hemoglobinuria. Affected dogs have disordered energy metabolism in skeletal muscles[221] but typically have neither clinical nor morphologic evidence of a myopathy. Episodic weakness and mild muscle atrophy occurred in one 11-year-old dog late in life.[222]

Some horses with exertional rhabdomyolysis (see following discussion) have a form of glycogen-storage disease (polysaccharide storage myopathy, PSSM).[223] Affected horses have characteristic stiffness, painful muscular cramping, and myoglobinuria after mild to strenuous exercise. Serum muscle enzymes are elevated. Autosomal-recessive inheritance is suspected.[224,225] Rhabdomyolysis may occur as early as 6 months of age, but definitive diagnosis of PSSM by histopathology of muscle biopsies may take up to 3 years.[225]

Another subgroup of metabolic myopathies, the mitochondrial myopathies, has been reasonably well characterized in humans[226] and, to a lesser degree, in animals. Disordered energy metabolism in affected individuals typically causes weakness and cramping with minimal exercise. Inherited enzymatic defects within the mitochondrial electron-transport (respiratory) chain generally are responsible. Typical histopathologic changes include bizarre mitochondria on ultrastructural evaluation and histochemical evidence of "ragged red" fibers. Intermediary metabolites, most often glycogen or lipid, typically also accumulate within some myofibers. Episodic weakness with associated exertional lactic acidosis was noted in two male Old English sheepdog littermates.[227] Exercise intolerance occurred within the first year of life. Serum CK level was markedly elevated. Complex repetitive discharges occurred on EMG. Myofiber necrosis and scattered "ragged red" fibers were noted histologically. Occasional fibers contained material that was periodic acid–Schiff positive. Mitochondria and glycogen were increased on electron microscopic evaluation. Some mitochondria were vacuolated. Reduced cytochrome oxidase deficiency was identified in fibroblast cultures.[228] Somewhat similar syndromes have been described in Clumber, Sussex, and Cavalier King Charles spaniels in the United Kingdom.[229] Dyserythropoiesis, cardiomegaly, and polymyopathy characterized by gross muscle atrophy and histologic evidence of myofiber size variation and poorly defined inclusions have been reported in English Springer spaniels.[230]

Nemaline Myopathy. An apparently inherited myopathy potentially analogous to the adult onset form of nemaline myopathy of humans has been described in five related cats.[231] The cats became weak between 6 and 18 months of age and later developed a characteristic rapid, choppy, hypermetric gait. The skin twitched vigorously when two of the cats were examined. Patellar reflexes were depressed. Flexor reflexes and pain sensation were normal. The scapular and gluteal muscle groups were atrophied. General deterioration necessitated euthanasia in each cat. Type-1 and 2A fibers were atrophied. Type-1 fibers were reduced in some muscles. Characteristic nemaline rods were common.

Myopathy of Pietrain Pigs (Creeper). This autosomal-recessive inherited trait occurs in Pietrain pigs. Muscular weakness is noted at 3 weeks and progresses to recumbency by 12 weeks. Atrophy of type-1 myofibers is prominent in proximal muscles. No treatment exists.[15,232]

Myotonic Myopathies. Contraction of muscle that persists after the cessation of voluntary effort or stimulation is called *myotonia* (if generalized) or *cramp* (if localized). Myotonic myopathies are discussed in Chapter 10.

Nutritional Myopathies (White Muscle Disease). White muscle disease, a degenerative myopathy of many species caused by dietary deficiency of α-tocopherol or selenium,[15] occurs most frequently in calves and lambs, less frequently in pigs, and rarely in other large animals, cats, and dogs. Acute and chronic forms of the disease occur. The acute form is characterized by sudden death that occurs during exertion and is due to cardiac muscle degeneration. The chronic form is marked by a gradual onset of tetraparesis in calves 2 weeks of age or older. Lambs develop a stiff gait and tetraparesis at 10 days to 2 months of age. Muscles may be swollen and painful. Foals may have pain around the base of the tail, beneath the mane, and in the tongue and submandibular tissues. Other diseases linked to selenium deficiency include mulberry heart disease in baby pigs, white muscle disease in foals, equine tying-up syndrome (see following discussion), and retained placenta in cattle.

The diagnosis is based on clinical signs, histologic examination of biopsy samples from affected muscles, quantitation of glutathione peroxidase levels, and response to therapy.[233] In the skeletal muscle form, degeneration is characterized by symmetric grayish or white streaks. Selenium and vitamin E are beneficial if the signs are severe. Diets should be corrected if selenium deficiencies are found. Selenium can be highly toxic if used at high concentrations.

Steroid-induced Myopathy. Dogs with spontaneous and iatrogenic Cushing's disease resulting from glucocorticoid excess[234,235] develop muscle atrophy and weakness. The muscle changes may be subclinical, but some develop an associated myotonia-like syndrome.[236,237] High-frequency discharges that do not wax and wane are typical on EMG. The exact biochemical cause of steroid-induced myopathy is not known. Disturbances of calcium metabolism have been suggested. Myopathic changes include fiber atrophy, necrosis, regeneration, and increased muscle fat and connective tissue. Withdrawal of exogenous steroids or suppression of endogenous steroids may be beneficial. Dogs with severe disease may not improve even after plasma steroid levels are decreased. Dogs that improve with appropriate therapy may have persistent high-frequency discharges on EMG.[234]

Splayleg, a muscular weakness in newborn pigs, may be due to glucocorticoid excess resulting from stress and hormonal imbalance in the sow.[238]

Hypothyroid Myopathy. Weakness and muscle degeneration have been seen in hypothyroid dogs.[159,160] These changes are less pronounced than those of the neuropathy previously described. Varied neonatal musculoskeletal abnormalities, including ruptured tendons, angular limb deformities, forelimb contractures, and mandibular prognathisms, have been found in foals with hypothyroidism.[239]

Exertional Rhabdomyolysis. This disorder of racing greyhounds and horses, also known as Monday morning disease, tying-up, and paralytic myoglobinuria, develops from local muscle ischemia.[15,124,240] A similar syndrome in exotic animals is called *capture syndrome*. Altered glycogen storage (see Metabolic Myopathies), electrolyte abnormalities including hypokalemia,[241] and other factors seem to be the initiating cause. The final events appear to be muscle swelling and necrosis. The cause in some horses is PSSM.[223,225]

Horses may become stiff and in pain after exercising or may suddenly stop while exercising. Myoglobinuria is often seen. The muscles are painful and swollen on palpation. Serum muscle-enzyme levels are commonly increased. Muscle atrophy may persist after recovery. Gannon[240] has categorized the clinical signs in dogs as hyperacute, acute, and subacute. Factors that lead to the syndrome include (1) lack of physical fitness, (2) excitement before racing, (3) hot and humid conditions, and (4) excessive frequency of running. In the more acute forms of the disease, clinical signs are observed during the race. The most severe signs include generalized muscle pain, hyperpnea, and heavy myoglobinuria. Death may occur within 48 hours. Recumbent horses usually die.[15] In the milder (subacute) form of the disease, muscle pain is confined to the longissimus thoracis muscle and may not be apparent for 24 to 72 hours after the race. Myoglobinuria is rarely observed in subacute exertional rhabdomyolysis.

The hyperacute and acute forms of the disease are treated similarly. Intravenous fluids are given to treat or prevent hypovolemic shock and to aid in renal excretion of myoglobin. Sodium bicarbonate is added to the fluid to combat muscle acidosis and to help prevent precipitation of myoglobin in renal tubules. The patient is cooled to remove excess heat. Other potential treatments include anabolic steroids, oral sodium bicarbonate, B vitamins, and analgesics.

Prophylactic therapy may include (1) installation of air conditioning in kennels, (2) reduction of body temperature with cool-water baths before racing, (3) administration of oral bicarbonate-glucose solutions before kenneling for racing, (4) alkalinization of the urine with sodium bicarbonate or potassium citrate, (5) administration of an oral potassium supplement, and (6) reduction in the frequency of racing.[240] Recommendations are similar for horses. Sodium bicarbonate added to the diet may be beneficial. Deficiencies of vitamin E or selenium have not been demonstrated.[15] In quarter-horse foals, increasing the amount of daily turnout for free exercise seems to decrease muscle stiffness and the extent of rhabdomyolysis compared with foals given strict stall rest.[225]

Malignant Hyperthermia. This disease is seen in pigs (porcine stress syndrome) and more rarely in dogs, cats, or horses.[15,124] The trait is apparently inherited in Pietrain, Poland China, and Landrace pigs. After stressors such as anesthesia, hot weather, exercise, or restraint, pigs exhibit stiffness, reluctance to move, and difficult respiration. Sudden death may occur. A hypersensitive calcium-release mechanism that causes high levels of myoplasmic calcium apparently initiates the increased muscle activity and hyperthermia. Muscles are pale, soft, and exudative on necropsy. Halothane may be used diagnostically to detect susceptible pigs. Dantrolene sodium may be helpful, but death usually occurs. Reducing stress and selective breeding are recommended for prevention.[15]

Postanesthetic Myopathy. Heavy, large animals have pain and swelling of groups of muscles after prolonged anesthesia.[15] Nerves also may be affected. The condition is caused, at least in part, by a compartment syndrome of affected muscles. Prolonged recumbency causes increased pressure in the muscle, with subsequent ischemia and necrosis. Treatment includes supporting the animal in a sling, administering intravenous fluids and electrolytes, and providing analgesics for relief of pain. Massage and passive manipulation of the limbs help to increase blood flow and reduce the risk of decubital ulcers. The prognosis is good if the horse is standing. Recumbent animals may have severe muscle atrophy. Preventive measures include careful padding, elevation of the uppermost limb, and avoidance of hypotension during anesthesia.[15]

Hypokalemic Myopathy. Potassium depletion can occur in any species, causing muscle weakness (see also Chapter 15). A generalized polymyopathy of cats has been characterized.[189, 242-246] Affected cats have signs of muscular weakness, including cervical ventroflexion, exercise intolerance, a stiff gait, and in some cases muscle pain on palpation. Tiring and lethargy may be observed before obvious weakness is noticed. Mechanisms to account for the weakness are not fully understood. In severe hypokalemia, the myofiber membrane is hypopolarized and severe muscle weakness and rhabdomyolysis may occur. The condition is apparently caused by chronic renal dysfunction with excessive potassium loss. Hypokalemia induces further renal dysfunction, establishing a vicious cycle of renal dysfunction and hypokalemia. Some diets were also low in potassium, but they have subsequently been corrected. Acidification of the urine, as is often done for management of urinary calculi, also accelerates potassium excretion. The diagnosis is based on clinical signs, serum potassium levels less than 3.0 mEq/L, increased serum CK levels, and assessment of renal function.

Nonspecific EMG and muscle pathologic changes are seen. Cats with muscle weakness are treated with oral potassium gluconate. The initial dosage is 2.0 to 6.0 mEq per day in divided doses. Rapid correction of dehydration with fluids that are not supplemented with potassium may lead to exacerbation of hypokalemia. Severely affected cats should be given potassium chloride (diluted in lactated Ringer's solution) at a rate of 0.5 to 1.0 mEq/kg per hour.

Ventral neck flexion and episodic weakness affecting primarily the pelvic limbs were associated with hypokalemia in Burmese cats at 2 to 6 months of age.[247] A similar syndrome was reported earlier in Burmese cats, but serum potassium levels were not measured.[248]

Episodic Progressive Diseases

Diseases in which episodes of weakness are interspersed with periods of normalcy are perplexing because many different body systems may be involved. Episodic weakness usually results from cardiovascular, metabolic, or neuromuscular diseases (Table 7-8). The primary neuromuscular disorder, myasthenia gravis, is discussed in this section. Several myopathies that may cause episodic weakness have been discussed previously. Other endocrine-metabolic causes are discussed in Chapter 15.

Myasthenia Gravis

Pathophysiology. Myasthenia gravis (MG) involves the motor end plate and results in progressive loss of muscle strength with exercise. Acetylcholine receptors (AChR) at neuromuscular junctions are decreased. This disorder is most commonly due to an autoimmune attack but may also be inherited.[183,249,250] Human myasthenic muscles have a 70% to 90% reduction in the number of AChR per motor end plate. The decreased number of available receptors reduces the probability that acetylcholine molecules will react with muscle receptor sites. The safety margin of neuromuscular transmission is greatly reduced in MG. With repeated nerve stimulations of the motor end plate, severe muscle weakness results. In humans and animals, MG has been associated with several thymic disorders and other autoimmune diseases.[250-253] Decreased muscle AChR and antibodies fixed to AChR have been documented in dogs. MG occurs in dogs and cats, but it has not been documented in large animals.[15]

Congenital MG, a rare disease involving no antibodies to AChR, has been documented in springer spaniels, Jack Russell terriers, smooth fox terriers, Samoyeds, and cats.[250,254,255] The congenital form is caused by reduced AChR. Myasthenic syndrome, in which a presynaptic defect interferes

Table 7-8 **Episodic Progressive Diseases**

Diseases	Diagnostic Tests
Metabolic Disorders (see Chapter 15)	
Hyperkalemia	Serum potassium levels, electrocardiogram (ECG)
Adrenal insufficiency	Plasma cortisol levels
Severe acidosis	Blood gases and pH
Severe renal failure	Blood urea nitrogen levels, urinalysis
Periodic paralysis (equine)	Genetic
Hypokalemia	Serum potassium levels
Chronic renal failure	Serum potassium levels, blood urea nitrogen levels, urinalysis
Hypocalcemia	Serum calcium and phosphorus levels
Hypoparathyroidism	Serum parathyroid hormone (PTH) assays
Hypercalcemia	Serum calcium levels
Primary hyperparathyroidism	Serum PTH assay, parathyroid mass
Pseudohyperparathyroidism	Evidence of lymphosarcoma or myeloma
Hypoglycemia	Fasting blood glucose levels
Functional beta-cell tumor	Amended glucose-insulin ratio
Glycogen-storage disease	Glucagon response test
Adrenal insufficiency	Plasma cortisol levels
Cardiovascular Disorders (see Chapter 13)	
Arrhythmias	ECG
Conduction disturbances	ECG
Congestive heart failure	ECG, thoracic radiographs, auscultation
Dirofilariasis	Thoracic radiographs, Knott test
Respiratory Disorders	Auscultation, thoracic radiographs
Neuromuscular Disorders	
Myasthenia gravis	Repetitive nerve stimulation, anticholinesterase test, antibodies against acetylcholine receptors
Polymyositis	Serum muscle enzyme levels, muscle biopsy, EMG
Inherited myopathies	See Table 7-7
Narcolepsy	See Chapter 13

with release of acetylcholine, has been described in the Gammel Dansk Honschund dog.[256] Conditions are inherited as autosomal recessive traits in the two terrier breeds and the Gammel Dansk Honsehund.[255,256]

Clinical Signs. Except in acute fulminating MG,[257] the neurologic examination is normal when the animal is rested. With exercise, muscle weakness becomes progressively worse. This phenomenon is most apparent in the appendicular muscles. Animals become fatigued, develop a shortened stride, and then lie down to rest. Strength returns with rest. Ptosis of the upper eyelids and drooping of the lips occur in some dogs with weak facial muscles. Sialosis, regurgitation of food, and dysphagia develop in a high percentage of cases. Megaesophagus is one of the most common initial clinical signs of MG.[258] Aspiration pneumonia occurs in many dogs with megaesophagus. Some dogs with idiopathic megaesophagus or laryngeal paralysis without generalized muscle weakness have MG.[258,259] Thymoma is found in a small portion of cases but appears to be associated more commonly with megaesophagus.[253] Other immune-mediated diseases such as polymyositis may occur concomitantly, particularly in dogs with thymoma.[253] Third-degree atrioventricular block was seen in four dogs with acquired MG, although a cause-and-effect relationship was not proved.[260]

Diagnosis. Diagnosis is aided by the exclusion of cardiovascular and metabolic diseases with appropriate laboratory or electrophysiologic tests. Exercise-induced weakness, a decremental response to repetitive nerve stimulation, and a positive response to anticholinesterase drugs support the diagnosis. Definitive diagnosis is made by detection of AChR antibodies or immune complexes at the neuromuscular junction.[249,258]

The EMG findings are usually normal in myasthenia gravis, although variability in amplitude of motor units and occasional fibrillations may be seen. Repetitive nerve stimulation at 3 Hz does not cause any decrement in the amplitude or area of the evoked muscle action potential in normal animals.[261] In MG the response decreases by at least 10% in the first ten responses. Definitive studies on large numbers of myasthenic dogs, however, have not been reported. Based on studies in humans, the decrement is maximal in the first two responses. Any decrement is suspect. Variation in results makes a definitive diagnosis difficult. At least two muscles should show a decrement.[262] The muscle should be kept warm during the test. If a decrement is demonstrated, administration of the short-acting anticholinesterase edrophonium chloride (Tensilon) intravenously should cause a normal response for a few minutes. Although the decremental response is abnormal in most myasthenic animals, both false-positive and false-negative results may occur. Single-fiber EMG analysis of jitter is reported to be the most definitive electrodiagnostic test for establishing a diagnosis of MG.[263]

In field testing, the diagnosis of MG has been supported by the administration of edrophonium chloride intravenously after weakness has been induced by exercise.[264] Weakness should resolve for about 15 minutes in animals with MG. Care must be exercised in both the performance and interpretation of the test results. Edrophonium is not effective in some dogs with MG[265]; in contrast, dogs with other neuromuscular diseases such as polymyositis may improve. A definitive diagnosis must be based on serologic techniques. Anticholinesterase drugs also may cause excessive muscle depolarization (cholinergic crisis), vomiting, salivation, and defecation. Accordingly, atropine should be given before edrophonium to block muscarinic receptors.

Serum autoantibodies to AChR provide the strongest evidence for a diagnosis. About 90% of dogs with acquired MG have AChR antibodies.[266,267] Seronegative dogs often have immune complexes at the neuromuscular junction.[249]

Treatment. Once the diagnosis has been confirmed, initial therapy should include anticholinesterase agents (pyridostigmine bromide, 0.5 to 3.0 mg/kg, two to three times daily, orally).[249,264] If the animal does not respond, glucocorticoids (prednisone, 0.5 to 1.0 mg/kg daily; increase to 1.0 to 2.0 mg/kg daily after a few days) should be added. Once remission is achieved, alternate-day steroid therapy is continued at a dosage of 2.0 mg/kg. The dosage of anticholinesterase drugs and glucocorticoids is gradually decreased and, if possible, eliminated. Drastic changes in the therapy should not occur. Thymectomy should be considered for dogs with thymoma or those that respond poorly to medical therapy.[253] AChR antibody levels may persist despite clinical improvement after thymectomy.

Other forms of immunosuppressive therapy, such as cyclosporine alone or with plasmapheresis, may be beneficial.[268,269] Some dogs with apparent MG improve spontaneously, or the condition resolves after several weeks. Megaesophagus may resolve in some dogs subsequent to treatment.[270]

In human patients, in contrast, the disease tends to worsen.

Hyperkalemic Periodic Paralysis. This disease causes episodic weakness and muscle trembling in quarter horses and is caused by an autosomal-dominant sodium channel defect.[15,271-273] Episodes last minutes to hours and may be precipitated by exercise. Horses are normal between episodes. The signs range from mild muscle tremors to complete recumbency. Pharyngeal and laryngeal dysfunction may occur alone, particularly in foals.[274,275] Blood samples taken during an episode show hemoconcentration and hyperkalemia (5.0-11.7 mEq/L).[271] Some affected horses have normal potassium levels. Other parameters are not remarkable. Evidence of complex repetitive discharges on EMG is suggestive of the disease. A diagnosis also is suggested by inducing signs through administration of potassium chloride (0.1 g/kg, orally, initially; increase in 0.025 g/kg increments every 48 hours to a total of 0.2 g/kg), but this can cause death.[272] Genetic testing is available and is preferred.[273] Acute episodes should be treated by intravenous administration of sodium bicarbonate, dextrose, or calcium solutions. Diuretic therapy (acetazolamide; 2.2 mg/kg orally, two to three times daily) may lessen the frequency and severity of attacks.[271] A similar syndrome has been reported in one dog.[276]

Exercise Intolerance and Collapse in Labrador Retrievers. This syndrome has been seen with increasing frequency in young Labrador retrievers, especially excitable, hard-driving dogs bred for field trials.[277] Clinical signs develop between 7 months and 2 years of age. There is no sex or coat color predilection. After 5 to 15 minutes of strenuous exercise, dogs hyperventilate, become weak, uncoordinated, and then collapse. Body temperatures are usually severely elevated during episodes but are normal at rest. Inability to regulate body temperature does not initiate the episodes. The diagnosis of exercise intolerance and collapse is made by ruling out other muscle disorders and cardiovascular diseases. There is no specific treatment, but most dogs respond well to avoiding strenuous exercise and excitement.

Case Histories

CASE HISTORY 7A

Signalment

Canine, mixed breed, male, 6 months old.

History

An acute onset of tetraparesis progressed rapidly to total paralysis. The dog has been paralyzed for 24 hours.

Physical Examination
Nothing significant was found except for the neurologic problems.

Neurologic Examination*
A. Observation
1. Mental status: Alert
2. Posture: Recumbent
3. Gait: The dog cannot support weight or maintain sternal recumbency; tetraplegia. The dog can wag his tail
B. Palpation: The limbs have decreased muscle tone and strength
C. Postural reactions

Left	Reactions	Right
	Proprioceptive positioning	
0	PL	0
0	TL	0
0	Wheelbarrowing	0
	Hopping	
0	PL	0
0	TL	0
0	Extensor postural thrust	0
0	Hemistand-hemiwalk	0
	Placing, tactile	
0	PL	0
0	TL	0
	Placing, visual	
0	TL	0

D. Spinal reflexes

Left	Reflex (Spinal Segment)	Right
	Quadriceps (L4-6)	
0		0
	Extensor carpi radialis (C7-T1)	
+1		+1
	Flexion, PL (L5-S1)	
0 to +1		0 to +1
	Flexion, TL (C6-T1)	
0 to +1		0 to +1
0	Crossed extensor	0
	Perineal (S1-2)	
+2		+2

E. Cranial nerves

Left	Nerve—Function (Response/Test)	Right
+2	CN II—vision (menace)	+2
Normal	CN II, III—pupil size	Normal
+2	(Stimulus left eye)	+2
+2	(Stimulus right eye)	+2
Normal	CN II—fundus	Normal
	CN III, IV, VI	
0	(Strabismus)	0
0	(Nystagmus)	0
+2	CN V—sensation	+2
Normal	CN V—mastication	Normal
Normal	CN VII—facial muscles	Normal
+2	(Palpebral)	+2
+2	CN IX, X—swallowing	+2
Normal	CN XII—tongue	Normal

F. Sensation: Location
   Hyperesthesia: None
   Superficial pain: +2
   Deep pain: +2
Complete sections G and H before reviewing the case summary.
G. Assessment (anatomic diagnosis and estimation of prognosis)
H. Plan (diagnostic)

   Rule-outs   *Procedure*
   1.
   2.
   3.
   4.

CASE HISTORY 7B

Signalment
Canine, miniature schnauzer, male, 6 years old.

History
The dog had a sudden onset of falling to the right with paresis of both pelvic limbs and paralysis of the right thoracic limb. No previous trauma. The signs began 7 days ago and were not progressive from the onset.

Physical Examination
Negative except for the neurologic problem.

Neurologic Examination*
A. Observation
1. Mental status: Alert
2. Posture: Lateral recumbency

---

*0, Absent; +1, decreased; +2, normal; +3, exaggerated; +4, very exaggerated or clonus; *PL*, pelvic limb; *TL*, thoracic limb.

*0, Absent; +1, decreased; +2, normal; +3, exaggerated; +4, very exaggerated or clonus; *PL*, pelvic limb; *TL*, thoracic limb.

3. Gait: The dog can stand if assisted for a short time; he knuckles severely on the right limbs.
B. Palpation: Atrophy of the right supraspinatus, deltoid, and triceps muscles
C. Postural reactions

Left	Reactions	Right
	Proprioceptive positioning	
+2	PL	0
+2	TL	+1
+2	Wheelbarrowing	+1
	Hopping	
+2	PL	0
+2	TL	+1
+2	Extensor postural thrust	0
+2	Hemistand-hemiwalk	0
	Placing, tactile	
+2	PL	0
+2	TL	+1
	Placing, visual	
+2	TL	+1

D. Spinal reflexes

Left	Reflex (Spinal Segment)	Right
+2	Quadriceps (L4-6)	+3
+2	Extensor carpi radialis (C7-T1)	+1
+2	Flexion, PL (L5-S1)	+2
+2	Flexion, TL (C6-T1)	+1
0	Crossed extensor	Present
+2	Perineal (S1-2)	+2

E. Cranial nerves

Left	Nerve—Function (Response/Test)	Right
+2	CN II—vision (menace)	+2
Normal	CN II, III—pupil size	Normal
+2	(Stimulus left eye)	+2
+2	(Stimulus right eye)	+2
Normal	CN II—fundus	Normal
0	CN III, IV, VI (Strabismus)	0
0	(Nystagmus)	0
Normal	CN V—sensation	Normal
+2	CN V—mastication	+2
Normal	CN VII—facial muscles	Normal
+2	(Palpebral)	+2
Normal	CN IX, X—swallowing	Normal
+2	CN XII—tongue	+2

F. Sensation: Location
Hyperesthesia: None
Superficial pain: +2
Deep pain: +2
Complete sections G and H before reviewing the case summary.
G. Assessment (anatomic diagnosis and estimation of prognosis)
H. Plan (diagnostic)

Rule-outs	Procedures
1.	
2.	
3.	
4.	

CASE HISTORY 7C

Signalment
Canine, miniature poodle, male, 11 years old.

History
One month ago lameness developed in the left thoracic limb, progressing to both thoracic limbs within 7 days. Two weeks later the dog developed ataxia of both pelvic limbs; 1 week ago he developed severe paresis of both pelvic limbs. The dog does not wag his tail.

Physical Examination
Grade IV/VI holosystolic mitral murmur. Fluid lung sounds. Severe periodontal disease.

Neurologic Examination[*]
A. Observation
1. Mental status: alert
2. Posture: Recumbent (sternal)
3. Gait: Tetraparesis
B. Palpation: Extensor rigidity of thoracic limbs; hypertonus of pelvic limbs
C. Postural reactions

Left	Reactions	Right
	Proprioceptive positioning	
0	PL	0
0	TL	0
0	Wheelbarrowing	0

---

[*]*0*, Absent; *+1*, decreased; *+2*, normal; *+3*, exaggerated; *+4*, very exaggerated or clonus; *PL*, pelvic limb; *TL*, thoracic limb.

	Hopping	
0	PL	0 to +1
0	TL	0 to +1
0	Extensor postural thrust	0
0	Hemistand-hemiwalk	0
	Placing, tactile	
0	PL	0
0	TL	0
0	Placing, visual TL	0

D. Spinal reflexes

Left	Reflex (Spinal Segment)	Right
+2	Quadriceps (L4-6)	+3
+2	Extensor carpi radialis (C7-T1)	+3
+2	Flexion, PL (L5-S1)	+2
+2	Flexion, TL (C6-T1)	+2
0	Crossed extensor	0
+2	Perineal (S1 2)	+2

E. Cranial nerves

Left	Nerve—Function (Response/Text)	Right
+2	CN II—vision (menace)	+2
Normal	CN II, III—pupil size	Normal
+2	(Stimulus left eye)	+2
+2	(Stimulus right eye)	+2
Normal	CN II—fundus	Normal
0	CN III, IV, VI (Strabismus)	0
0	(Nystagmus)	0
Normal	CN V—mastication	Normal
Normal	CN VII—facial muscles	Normal
+2	(Palpebral)	+2
Normal	CN IX, X—swallowing	Normal
Normal	CN XII—tongue	Normal

F. Sensation: Location
   Hyperesthesia: Moderate on palpation of cervical area
   Superficial pain: +2
   Deep pain: +2

Complete sections G and H before reviewing the case summary.
G. Assessment (anatomic diagnosis and estimation of prognosis)
H. Plan (diagnostic)

   Rule-outs   *Procedure*
   1.
   2.
   3.
   4.

CASE HISTORY 7D

Signalment
Canine, toy poodle, male, 1 year old.

History
Five weeks ago the dog experienced severe pain and could not walk up or down the stairs. The head was slightly flexed, and the neck was stiff. One week ago the dog bumped his head, cried out in pain, fell down, and became stiff. He cries out when the head is moved.

Physical Examination
Negative except for 5% dehydration and the neurologic problem.

Neurologic Examination*
A. Observation
   1. Mental status: Alert; cries out if manipulated
   2. Posture: Lateral recumbency; neck is slightly extended and rigid
   3. Gait: Severe tetraparesis
B. Palpation: The thoracic limbs are in extensor rigidity; persistent fontanelle
C. Postural reactions

Left	Reactions	Right
	Proprioceptive positioning	
+1	PL	+1
+1 to +2	TL	+1 to +2
+1	Wheelbarrowing	+1
	Hopping	
+1	PL	+1
+1	TL	+1
+1	Extensor postural thrust	+1
+1	Hemistand-hemiwalk	+1
	Placing, tactile	
0	PL	0
+1	TL	+1
	Placing, visual	
+1	TL	+1

*0, Absent; +1, decreased; +2, normal; +3, exaggerated; +4, very exaggerated or clonus; *PL*, pelvic limb; *TL*, thoracic limb.

D. Spinal reflexes

Left	Reflex (Spinal Segment)	Right
+3	Quadriceps (L4-6)	+3
+3	Extensor carpi radialis (C7-T1)	+3
+2	Flexion, PL (L5-S1)	+2
+2	Flexion, TL (C6-T1)	+2
0	Crossed extensor	0
+2	Perineal (S1-2)	+2

E. Cranial nerves

Left	Nerve-Function (Response/Test)	Right
+2	CN II—vision (menace)	+2
Normal	CN II, III—pupil size	Normal
+2	(Stimulus left eye)	+2
+2	(Stimulus right eye)	+2
Normal	CN II—fundus	Normal
	CN III, IV, VI	
0	(Strabismus)	0
0	(Nystagmus)	0
Normal	CN V—sensation	Normal
Normal	CN V—mastication	Normal
Normal	CN VII—facial muscles	Normal
+2	(Palpebral)	+2
Normal	CN IX, X—swallowing	Normal
Normal	CN XII—tongue	Normal

F. Sensation: Location
Hyperesthesia: Cervical; resists movement, painful on palpation of cranial cervical area
Superficial pain: +2
Deep pain: +2
Complete sections G and H before reviewing the case summary.
G. Assessment (anatomic diagnosis and estimation of prognosis)
H. Plan (diagnostic)

Rule-outs	Procedure
1.	
2.	
3.	
4.	

CASE HISTORY 7E

Signalment
Canine, Doberman pinscher, male, 8 years old.

History
For several months the dog has had knuckling, ataxia, and paresis in the pelvic limbs. He occasionally knuckles on the thoracic limbs. He has been treated with intramuscular injections of corticosteroids that gave temporary improvement. He recently developed paralysis of the right pelvic limb.

Physical Examination
Negative except for the neurologic signs described below.

Neurologic Examination*
A. Observation
   1. Mental status: Alert
   2. Posture: Ambulatory
   3. Gait: Paraparesis and ataxia; occasionally knuckles on the thoracic limbs
B. Palpation: Stiff neck; muscle atrophy is severe in the right pelvic limb distal to the stifle; abrasions are present on the dorsal surface of the right pelvic foot
C. Postural reactions

Left	Reactions	Right
	Proprioceptive positioning	
0	PL	0
+2	TL	+2
Knuckles	Wheelbarrowing	Knuckles
	Hopping	
+1	PL	0
+2	TL	+2
+1	Extensor postural thrust	+1
+1	Hemistand-hemiwalk	+1
	Placing, tactile	
+1	PL	0
+2	TL	+2
	Placing, visual	
+2	TL	+2

D. Spinal reflexes

Left	Reflex (Spinal Segment)	Right
+3	Quadriceps (L4-6)	+3
+3	Extensor carpi radialis (C7-T1)	+3
+2	Flexion, PL (L5-S1)	0; flexes at hip

*0, Absent; +1, decreased; +2, normal; +3, exaggerated; +4, very exaggerated or clonus; *PL*, pelvic limb; *TL*, thoracic limb.

	Flexion, TL (C6-T1)	
+2		+2
0	Crossed extensor	0
+2	Perineal (S1-2)	+2

E. Cranial nerves

Left	Nerve—Function (Response/Test)	Right
+2	CN II—vision (menace)	+2
Normal	CN II, III—pupil size	Normal
+2	(Stimulus left eye)	+2
+2	(Stimulus right eye)	+2
Normal	CN II—fundus	Normal
	CN III, IV, VI	
0	(Strabismus)	0
0	(Nystagmus)	0
Normal	CN V—sensation	Normal
Normal	CN V—mastication	Normal
Normal	CN VII—facial muscles	Normal
+2	(Palpebral)	+2
Normal	CN IX, X—swallowing	Normal
Normal	CN XII—tongue	Normal

F. Sensation: Location
   Hyperesthesia: Mild in midcervical area
   Superficial pain: +2, except absent in right pelvic foot
   Deep pain: +2, except absent in right pelvic foot
Complete sections G and H before reviewing the case summary.
G. Assessment (anatomic diagnosis and estimation of prognosis)
H. Plan (diagnostic)

   Rule-outs   *Procedure*
   1.
   2.
   3.
   4.

CASE 7F

Signalment
Rottweiler, male, 10 years old.

History
Generalized weakness of 3 weeks' duration. Slowly progressive tetraparesis for several days, and now signs are static. There is no history of recent trauma, and the dog has had excellent veterinary care. Two other dogs at home are normal. Referring veterinarian has diagnosed degenerative joint disease in right stifle, left hip, and right elbow. Hips certified as good several years ago. No systemic signs are reported by the owner.

Physical Examination
Nothing abnormal noted except for generalized weakness.

Neurologic Examination*
A. Observation
   1. Mental status: Dog is bright, alert and responsive. There is no history of seizure activity.
   2. Posture: No head tilt or circling noted.
   3. Gait: Dog is profoundly weak in pelvic limbs and moderately weak in thoracic limbs. No ataxia is noted.
B. Palpation: mild muscle atrophy is noted in distal muscles of the pelvic limbs.
C. Postural reactions:

Left	Reactions	Right
	Proprioceptive positioning	
+1 - +2	PL	+1 - +2
+2	TL	+2
+1-+2	Wheelbarrowing	+1- +2
	Hopping	
+1	PL	+1
+1	TL	+1 - +2
NE	Extensor postural thrust	NE
+1	Hemistand-hemiwalk	+1
	Placing-tactile	
NE	PL	NE
	TL	
	Placing-visual	
NE	TL	NE

D. Spinal reflexes:

Left	Reflexes (Spinal Segment)	Right
+1 - +2	Quadriceps (L4-6)	+1 - +2
+2	Extensor carpi radialis (C7-T1)	+2
+2	Triceps (C7-T1)	+2
+1	Flexion-PL (L5-S1)	+1
+1	Flexion-TL (C6-T1)	+1
absent	Crossed extensor	absent
+2	Perineal	+2

*0, Absent; +1, decreased; +2, normal; +3, exaggerated; +4, very exaggerated or clonus; *PL*, pelvic limb; *TL*, thoracic limb.

E. Cranial nerves

Left	Nerve-function (Response, test)	Right
+2	CN II—vision (menace)	+2
+2 +2	CN II, III—pupil size (Stimulate left eye) (Stimulate right eye)	+2 +2
Normal	CN II—fundus	Normal
None None	CN III, IV, VI (Strabismus) (Nystagmus)	None None
+2	CN V—sensation	+2
+2	CN V—mastication	+2
Normal +2	CN VII—facial muscles (Palpebral)	Normal +2
NE	CN IX, X—swallowing	NE
+2	CN XII—tongue	+2

F. Sensation: Location
Hyperesthesia: Mild cervical resistance is noted
Superficial pain: Normal
Deep pain: Normal
Complete sections G and H before reviewing the case summary.
G. Assessment (anatomic diagnosis and estimation of prognosis)
H. Plan (diagnostic)

Rule-outs	Procedure
1.	
2.	
3.	
4.	

ASSESSMENT 7A

Anatomic Diagnosis
Generalized LMN signs are present, and pain perception is preserved. Generalized neuropathy or motor end plate disease should be suspected.

Diagnostic Plan (Rule-outs)
1. Tick paralysis: Examine for ticks (present)
2. Botulism: History, EMG, toxin analysis
3. Polyradiculoneuritis: EMG
4. Other polyneuropathies

Therapeutic Plan
1. Remove ticks.
2. Support the dog with attentive nursing care.

Client Education
The prognosis is good.

Case Summary
Tick paralysis was diagnosed. The ticks were removed; the dog improved within 24 hours and was normal in 36 hours. This is a typical recovery for tick paralysis.

ASSESSMENT 7B

Anatomic Diagnosis
This dog has a right hemiparesis with a normal left thoracic limb and a nearly normal left pelvic limb. The right hemiparesis is characterized by LMN signs in the thoracic limb and UMN signs in the pelvic limb. The lesion is most likely at C6-T2.

Diagnostic Plan (Rule-outs)
1. Trauma: History, cervical radiography (negative)
2. Cervical disk disease: Myelography (negative)
3. Myelitis: Cerebrospinal fluid examination (negative)
4. Cervical spinal cord infarction: Supported by negative diagnostic tests

Therapeutic Plan
1. Prescribe cage rest, prevent decubital sores, and perform hydrotherapy.
2. Corticosteroid therapy is of questionable value at this stage of the spinal cord infarct.

Client Education
The prognosis for recovery in the right thoracic limb is poor because of LMN involvement. The tracts frequently recover, but neurons do not. The prognosis for recovery of pelvic limb function is more favorable but still guarded.

Case Summary
A severe hemorrhagic vascular lesion on the right (C7-T1 cord segments) was diagnosed. The dog did not improve, and euthanasia was performed. Necropsy confirmed the presence of the lesion. The cause of the infarction was not found.

ASSESSMENT 7C

Anatomic Diagnosis
The dog has UMN tetraparesis with no evidence of brainstem disease. This finding localizes the lesion to spinal cord segments C1-5.

Diagnostic Plan (Rule-outs)
The disease is acutely progressive in course, and hyperesthesia is present in the cervical area.
1. Cervical disk disease: Radiology (disk herniation at C2-3; myelography revealed significant compression of the spinal cord)
2. Cervical neoplasia: Myelography (negative)
3. Cervical myelitis: Cerebrospinal fluid analysis (protein 35 mg/dl, two white blood cells; not indicative of inflammatory disease)

Therapeutic Plan
Although this dog had other medical problems, surgery was done because of the severity of the signs and the compression of the spinal cord on myelography.

Client Education
The prognosis is fair to poor. If the dog were in excellent health, the prognosis would be good.

Case Summary
Cervical disk disease was diagnosed. The dog did well in surgery and went home significantly improved.

ASSESSMENT 7D

Anatomic Diagnosis
Severe tetraparesis is present with UMN signs in all four limbs. Cervical pain and the absence of brainstem signs localize the lesion to spinal cord segments C1-5.

Diagnostic Plan (Rule-outs)
The dog has hyperesthesia in the cranial cervical region and is a toy breed but is very young for disk disease. Inflammatory disease is a possibility, but atlantoaxial luxation should be ruled out before any manipulation of the neck is done.
1. Atlantoaxial subluxation: Cervical radiography (atlantoaxial subluxation is present)
2. Cervical disk: Myelography (not performed)
3. Meningomyelitis: Cerebrospinal fluid examination (not performed)

Therapeutic Plan
Surgical stabilization.

Client Education
The prognosis is fair to good.

Case Summary
Atlantoaxial subluxation was diagnosed. After surgery, the patient recovered.

ASSESSMENT 7E

Anatomic Diagnosis
Two lesions must be present to explain the clinical findings in this case. LMN disease and hypalgesia are present in the right pelvic limb, suggesting a selective sciatic nerve injury (probably a needle injury from intramuscular injection). The other neurologic signs suggest a cervical lesion.

Diagnostic Plan (Rule-outs)
1. Cervical spondylopathy: Cervical radiography and myelography (negative)
2. Cervical disk: Type II compression of the spinal cord at C5-6
3. Cervical myelitis: Cerebrospinal fluid analysis (normal)
4. Injection neuritis: EMG (denervation potentials in the flexors of the stifle and all muscles distal to the stifle)

Therapeutic Plan
1. Ventral cervical decompression or distraction and stabilization of C5-6
2. Physical therapy and a boot for the right pelvic limb

Client Education
The prognosis is very guarded.

Case Summary
Cervical disk compression and sciatic injury were diagnosed. The UMN deficits improved so that the gait was nearly normal. The right pelvic limb improved more than 50% in the first 4 months after surgery.

ASSESSMENT CASE 7F

Anatomic Diagnosis
The dog has generalized weakness with no signs of sensory dysfunction. In addition, spinal reflexes are decreased, especially withdrawal reflexes. Distal muscle atrophy is present in the pelvic limbs. A generalized LMN disorder or myopathy should be suspected. The signs cannot be explained by degenerative joint disease.

Dignostic Plan (Rule-outs)
1. Degenerative polyneuropathy: EMGs, nerve-conduction velocities, nerve-muscle biopsy (not performed)
2. Chronic polyneuritis: EMGs, nerve-muscle biopsy (not performed)
3. Degenerative myopathy: muscle enzymes, muscle biopsy (not performed)

In the course of diagnostic evaluation, a blood glucose concentration of 50 mg/dl was found on biochemical profile. Further diagnostic testing revealed hypoglycemia secondary to functional beta-cell tumor (insulin levels elevated relative to blood glucose concentration and mass detected in pancreas by ultrasonography). CK was normal.

Diagnosis
Functional beta cell tumor (insulinoma) with paraneoplastic polyneuroopathy.

Treatment
1. Surgical resection of pancreatic mass (histopatholgy confirmed diagnosis)
2. Chemotherapy

Client Education
The prognosis for long-term survival is guarded because beta-cell carcinomas are malignant and frequently metastasize to the liver and regional lymph nodes.

Case Summary
One week following surgery, the dog's weakness and neurological function improved dramatically and the dog continued to improve over the next 3 weeks. Although likely, a paraneoplastic polyneuropathy was not proven in this case.

References

1. Hoerlein BF: Intervertebral disk disease. In Oliver JE, Hoerlein BF, Mayhew IG, editors: *Veterinary neurology*. Philadelphia, 1987, WB Saunders.
2. Stadler P, Van den Berg SS, Tustin RC: Servikale intervertebrale diskus prolaps in 'n perd, *J South Afr Vet Assoc* 59:31-32, 1987.
3. Foss R, et al: Cervical intervertebral disc protrusion in two horses, *Can Vet J* 24:188-191, 1983.
4. Nixon A, et al: Cervical intervertebral disk protrusion in a horse, *Vet Surg* 13:154-158, 1984.
5. Morgan PW, Parent JM, Holmberg DL: Cervical pain secondary to intervertebral disk disease in dogs: radiographic findings and surgical implications, *Prog Vet Neurol* 4:76-80, 1993.
6. Felts J, Prata R: Cervical disk disease in the dog: Intraforaminal and lateral extrusions, *J Am Anim Hosp Assoc* 19:755-760, 1983.
7. Waters DJ: Nonambulatory tetraparesis secondary to cervical disk disease in the dog, *J Am Anim Hosp Assoc* 25:647-653, 1989.
8. Olsson SE: The dynamic factor in spinal cord compression: A study on dogs with special reference to cervical disc protrusions, *J Neurosurg* 15:308-321, 1958.
9. Griffiths IR: A syndrome produced by dorsolateral "explosions" of the cervical intervertebral discs, *Vet Rec* 87:737-741, 1970.

10. Bagley RS, et al: Dysphonia in two dogs with cranial cervical intervertebral disk extrusion, *J Am Anim Hosp Assoc* 29:557-559, 1993.

11. Russell SW, Griffiths RC: Recurrence of cervical disc syndrome in surgically and conservatively treated dogs, *J Am Vet Med Assoc* 153:1412-1417, 1968.

12. Tomlinson J: Tetraparesis following cervical disk fenestration in two dogs, *J Am Vet Med Assoc* 187:76-77, 1985.

13. Fry TR, et al: Surgical treatment of cervical disc herniations in ambulatory dogs: Ventral decompression vs. fenestration, 111 cases (1980-1988), *Prog Vet Neurol* 2:165-173, 1991.

14. Gill PJ, Lippincott CL, Anderson SM: Dorsal laminectomy in the treatment of cervical intervertebral disk disease in small dogs: Retrospective study of 30 cases, *J Am Anim Hosp Assoc* 32:77-80, 1996.

15. Mayhew IG: *Large animal neurology: A handbook for veterinary clinicians*. Philadelphia, 1989, Lea & Febiger.

16. Mayhew I, et al: Equine degenerative myeloencephalopathy: A vitamin E deficiency that may be familial, *J Vet Intern Med* 1:45-50, 1987.

17. Beech J, Haskind M: Genetic studies of neuraxonal dystrophy in the Morgan, *Am J Vet Res* 48:109-113, 1987.

18. Blythe LL, et al: Serially determined plasma α-tocopherol concentrations and results of the oral vitamin E absorption test in clinically normal horses and in horses with degenerative myeloencephalopathy, *Am J Vet Res* 52:908-911, 1991.

19. Dill SG, et al: Serum vitamin E and blood glutathione peroxidase values of horse with degenerative myeloencephalopathy, *Am J Vet Res* 50:166-168, 1989.

20. Geary JC, Oliver JE, Hoerlein BF: Atlanto-axial subluxation in the canine, *J Small Anim Pract* 8:577-582, 1967.

21. Shelton SB, et al: Hypoplasia of the odontoid process and secondary atlantoaxial luxation in a Siamese cat, *Prog Vet Neurol* 2:209-211, 1991.

22. Oliver JE, Lewis RE: Lesions of the atlas and axis in dogs, *J Am Anim Hosp Assoc* 9:304-313, 1973.

23. Bailey CS: An embryological approach to the clinical significance of congenital vertebral and spinal cord abnormalities, *J Am Anim Hosp Assoc* 11:42-434, 1975.

24. Watson AG, de Lahunta A: Atlantoaxial subluxation and absence of transverse ligament of the atlas in a dog, *J Am Vet Med Assoc* 195:235-237, 1989.

25. Sorjonen DC, Shires PK: Atlantoaxial instability: A ventral surgical technique for decompression, fixation and fusion, *Vet Surg* 10:22-29, 1981.

26. Denny HR, Gibbs C, Waterman A: Atlantoaxial subluxation in the dog: A review of thirty cases and an evaluation of treatment by lag screw fixation, *J Small Anim Pract* 29:37-47, 1988.

27. Cook JR, Oliver JE: Atlantoaxial luxation in the dog, *Compendium Continuing Educ Pract Vet* 3:242-252, 1981.

28. Chambers JN, Betts CW, Oliver JE: The use of nonmetallic suture material for stabilization of atlantoaxial subluxation, *J Am Anim Hosp Assoc* 13:602-604, 1977.

29. LeCouteur RA, et al: Stabilization of atlantoaxial subluxation in the dog, using the nuchal ligament, *J Am Vet Med Assoc* 177:1011-1017, 1980.

30. Kishigami M: Application of an atlantoaxial retractor for atlantoaxial subluxation in the cat and dog, *J Am Anim Hosp Assoc* 20:413-419, 1984.

31. Owen RAR, Maxie LLS: Repair of fractured dens of the axis in a foal, *J Am Vet Med Assoc* 173:854-856, 1978.

32. Nixon AJ, Stashak TS: Laminectomy for relief of atlantoaxial subluxation in four horses, *J Am Vet Med Assoc* 193:677-682, 1988.

33. van Ee RT, Pechman R, Van Ee RM: Failure of the atlantoaxial tension band in two dogs, *J Am Anim Hosp Assoc* 25:707-712, 1989.

34. Beaver DP, et al: Risk factors affecting the outcome of surgery for atlantoaxial subluxation in dogs: 46 cases (1978-1998), *J Am Vet Med Assoc* 216:1104-1109, 2000.

35. Jaggy A, et al: Occipitoatlantoaxial malformation with atlantoaxial subluxation in a cat, *J Small Anim Pract* 32:366-372, 1991.

36. Parker AJ, Park RD, Cusick PK: Abnormal odontoid process angulation in a dog, *Vet Rec* 93:559-561, 1973.

37. DeCamp CE, Schirmer RG, Stickle RL: Traumatic atlanto-occipital subluxation in a dog, *J Am Anim Hosp Assoc* 27:415-418, 1991.

38. Lappin MR, Dow S: Traumatic atlanto-occipital luxation in a cat, *Vet Surg* 12:30-32, 1983.

39. Greenwood KM, Oliver JE: Traumatic atlanto-occipital dislocation in two dogs, *J Am Vet Med Assoc* 173:1324-1327, 1978.

40. Crane SW: Surgical management of traumatic atlanto-occipital instability in a dog, *Vet Surg* 7:39-42, 1978.

41. Sorjonen DC, et al: Ventral surgical fixation and fusion for atlanto-occipital subluxation in a goat, *Vet Surg* 12:127-129, 1983.

42. Powers B, et al: Pathology of the vertebral column of horses with cervical static stenosis, *Vet Pathol* 23:392-399, 1986.

43. Trotter E: Canine wobbler syndrome. In Kirk RW, editor: *Current veterinary therapy IX*. Philadelphia, 1986, WB Saunders.

44. Chambers J, Betts C: Caudal cervical spondylopathy in the dog: A review of 20 clinical cases and the literature, *J Am Anim Hosp Assoc* 13:571-576, 1977.

45. Selcer R, Oliver J: Cervical spondylopathy: Wobbler syndrome in dogs. *J Am Anim Hosp Assoc* 11:175-179, 1975.

46. Fraser H, Palmer A: Equine incoordination and wobbler disease of young horses, *Vet Rec* 80:338-355, 1967.

47. Lewis DG: Cervical spondylomyelopathy ("wobbler" syndrome) in the dog: A study based on 224 cases, *J Small Anim Pract* 30:657-665, 1989.

48. Seim HB: Wobbler syndrome in the Doberman pinscher. In Kirk RW, editor: *Current veterinary therapy X*. Philadelphia, 1989, WB Saunders.

49. Hedhammer A, et al: Overnutrition and skeletal disease: An experimental study in growing Great Dane dogs, *Cornell Vet* 64:1-160, 1974.

50. VanGundy T: Canine wobbler syndrome, Part I: Pathophysiology and diagnosis. *Compendium Continuing Educ Pract Vet* 11:144-158, 1989.

51. Sharp NJH, et al: Computed tomography in the evaluation of caudal cervical spondylopathy of the Doberman pinscher, *Vet Radiol Ultrasound* 36:100-108, 1995.

52. Moore BR, et al: Assessment of vertebral canal diameter and bony malformations of the cervical part of the spine in horses with cervical stenotic myelopathy, *Am J Vet Res* 55:5-13, 1994.

53. Speciale J, Fingeroth JM: Use of physiatry as the sole treatment for three paretic or paralyzed dogs with chronic compressive conditions of the caudal portion of the cervical spinal cord, *J Am Vet Med Assoc* 217:43-47, 2000.

54. Bruecker KA, Seim HB III, Withrow SJ: Clinical evaluation of three surgical methods for treatment of caudal cervical spondylomyelopathy of dogs, *Vet Surg* 18:197-203, 1989.

55. Goring RL, Beale BS, Faulkner RF: The inverted cone decompression technique: A surgical treatment for cervical vertebral instability "wobbler syndrome" in Doberman pinschers, Part 1, *J Am Anim Hosp Assoc* 27:40-409, 1991.

56. Lyman RL, Seim HB: Viewpoint: Wobbler syndrome. *Prog Vet Neurol* 2:143-150, 1991.

57. Lyman R: Continuous dorsal laminectomy for the treatment of caudal cervical vertebral instability and malformation. In *Proceedings of the 13th Annual Kal-Kan Symposium,* Columbus, OH, 1989, pp 13-16.

58. McKee WM, et al: Vertebral distraction-fusion for cervical spondylopathy using a screw and double washer technique, *J Small Anim Pract* 31:22-27, 1990.

59. Bruecker KA, Seim HB, Blass CE: Caudal cervical spondylomyelopathy: Decompression by linear traction and stabilization with Steinmann pins and polymethyl methacrylate, *J Am Anim Hosp Assoc* 25:677-683, 1989.

60. Ellison GW, Seim HB, Clemmons RM: Distracted spinal fusion for management of caudal cervical spondylomyelopathy in large-breed dogs, *J Am Vet Med Assoc* 193:447-453, 1988.

61. Dixon BC, Tomlinson JL, Kraus KH: Modified distraction-stabilization technique using an interbody polymethyl methacrylate plug in dogs with caudal cervical spondylopathy, *J Am Vet Med Assoc* 208:61-68, 1996.

62. Wagner P, et al: Evaluation of cervical spinal fusion as a treatment in the equine wobbler syndrome, *Vet Surg* 8:84-88, 1979.

63. Nixon AJ: Surgical management of equine cervical vertebral malformation, *Prog Vet Neurol* 2:183-195, 1991.

64. Wilson ER, Aron DN, Roberts RE: Observation of a secondary compressive lesion after treatment of caudal cervical spondylomyelopathy in a dog, *J Am Vet Med Assoc* 205:1297-1299, 1994.

65. Levitski RE, Chauvet AE, Lipsitz D: Cervical myelopathy associated with extradural synovial cysts in 4 dogs, *J Vet Intern Med* 13:181-186, 1999.

66. Northington J, Brown M: Acute canine idiopathic polyneuropathy: A Guillain-Barré-like syndrome in dogs, *J Neurol Sci* 56:259-272, 1982.

67. Northington J, et al: Acute idiopathic polyneuropathy in the dog, *J Am Vet Med Assoc* 179:375-379, 1981.

68. Cummings JF, Haas DC: Coonhound paralysis: An acute idiopathic polyradiculoneuritis in dogs resembling Landry Guillain Barré syndrome, *J Neurol Sci* 4:51-81, 1967.

69. Holmes D, et al: Experimental coonhound paralysis: Animal model of Guillain-Barré syndrome. *Neurology* 29:1186-1187, 1979.

70. Lane JR, de Lahunta A: Polyneuritis in a cat, *J Am Anim Hosp Assoc* 20:1006-1008, 1984.

71. MacLachlan N, Gribble D, East N: Polyradiculoneuritis in a goat, *J Am Vet Med Assoc* 180:166-167, 1982.

72. Schrauwen E, Van Ham L: Postvaccinal acute polyradiculoneuritis in a young dog, *Prog Vet Neurol* 6:68-70, 1995.

73. Cummings J, et al: Coonhound paralysis: Further clinical studies and electron microscopic observations, *Acta Neuropathol* 57:167-178, 1982.

74. Alexander JW, de Lahunta A, Scott DW: A case of brachial plexus neuropathy in a dog, *J Am Anim Hosp Assoc* 10:515-517, 1974.

75. Bright RM, Crabtree BJ, Knecht CD: Brachial plexus neuropathy in the cat: A case report, *J Am Anim Hosp Assoc* 14:612-615, 1978.

76. Duncan I: Polyradiculoneuritis: Coonhound paralysis revisited. In *Proceedings of an American College of Veterinary Internal Medicine Forum,* San Diego, 1987, pp 334-337.

77. Chrisman C: Differentiation of tick paralysis and acute idiopathic polyradiculoneuritis in the dog using electromyography, *J Am Anim Hosp Assoc* 11:455-458, 1975.

78. Cuddon PA: Electrophysiological and immunological evaluation in coonhound paralysis. In *Proceedings of the Eighth Annual Veterinary Medical Forum,* Washington, DC, 1990, pp 1009-1012.

79. Dyck P, et al: Prednisone improves chronic inflammatory demyelinating polyradiculoneuropathy more than no treatment, *Ann Neurol* 11:136-141, 1982.

80. Guillain Barré Syndrome Steroid Trial Group: Double-blind trial of intravenous methylprednisolone in Guillain-Barré syndrome, *Lancet* 341:586-590, 1993.

81. The Guillain-Barré Syndrome Study Group: Plasmapheresis and acute Guillain-Barré syndrome, *Neurology* 35:109-1104, 1985.

82. Matus RE, et al: Plasmapheresis in five dogs with systemic immune-mediated disease, *J Am Vet Med Assoc* 187:595-599, 1985.

83. Barsanti J, et al: Type C botulism in American foxhounds, *J Am Vet Med Assoc* 172:809-814, 1978.

84. Cornelissen J, Haagsma J, van Nes J: Type C botulism in five dogs, *J Am Anim Hosp Assoc* 21:401-404, 1985.

85. Farrow B, et al: Type C botulism in young dogs, *Aust Vet J* 60:374-377, 1983.

86. Darke P, et al: Suspected botulism in foxhounds, *Vet Rec* 99:98-99, 1976.

87. Marlow G, Smart JL: Botulism in foxhounds, *Vet Rec* 111:242, 1982.

88. Ricketts SW, et al: Thirteen cases of botulism in horses fed big bale silage, *Equine Vet J* 16:515-518, 1984.

89. Swerczek T: Toxicoinfectious botulism in foals and adult horses, *J Am Vet Med Assoc* 176:217-220, 1980.

90. Swerczek T: Experimentally induced toxicoinfectious botulism in horses and foals, *Am J Vet Res* 41:348-350, 1980.

91. Kelly AP, et al: Outbreak of botulism in horses, *Equine Vet J* 16:519-521, 1984.

92. Bernard W, et al: Botulism as a sequel to open castration in a horse, *J Am Vet Med Assoc* 191:73-74, 1987.

93. Kao I, Drachman D, Price D: Botulinum toxin: Mechanism of presynaptic blockade, *Science* 193:1256-1258, 1976.

94. Pickett JB: AAEE Case report #16: Botulism, *Muscle Nerve* 11:1201-1205, 1988.

95. van Nes J, van der Most van Spijk D: Electrophysiology evidence of peripheral nerve dysfunction in six dogs with botulism type C, *Res Vet Sci* 40:372-376, 1986.

96. Swift TR, Ignacio OJ: Tick paralysis: Electrophysiologic studies, *Neurology* 25:1130-1133, 1975.

97. Ilkiw JE: Tick paralysis in Australia. In Kirk RW, editor: *Current veterinary therapy VIII.* Philadelphia, 1983, WB Saunders.

98. Farrow BRH: Tick paralysis and botulism. In *Proceedings of the Sixth Annual Veterinary Medical Forum,* Washington, DC, 1988, pp 61-63.

99. Ilkiw J, Turner D: Infestation in the dog by the paralysis tick *Ixodes holocyclus,* 2: Blood gas and pH, haematological and biochemical findings, *Aust Vet J* 64:139-142, 1987.

100. Osweiler GD, et al: *Clinical and diagnostic veterinary toxicology,* 3rd ed. Dubuque, IA, 1985, Kendall/Hunt Publishing.

101. Lorenz MD, et al: Hereditary muscular atrophy in Brittany spaniels: Clinical manifestations, *J Am Vet Med Assoc* 175:833-839, 1979.

102. Cork LC, et al: Pathology of motor neurons in accelerated hereditary canine spinal muscular atrophy, *Lab Invest* 46:89-99, 1982.

103. Cork LC, et al: Neurofilamentous abnormalities in motor neurons in spontaneously occurring animal disorders, *J Neuropathol Exp Neurol* 47:420-431, 1988.

104. Sandefeldt E, et al: Hereditary neuronal abiotrophy in the Swedish Lapland dog, *Cornell Vet* 63:1-71, 1973.

105. Shell L, Jortner B, Leib M: Spinal muscular atrophy in two Rottweiler littermates, *J Am Vet Med Assoc* 190:878-880, 1987.

106. Shell L, Jortner B, Leib M: Familial motor neuron disease in Rottweiler dogs: Neuropathologic studies, *Vet Pathol* 24:135-139, 1987.

107. Inada S, et al: Canine storage disease characterized by hereditary progressive neurogenic muscular atrophy: Breeding experiments and clinical manifestation, *Am J Vet Res* 47:2294-2299, 1986.

108. Inada S, et al: A clinical study on hereditary progressive neurogenic muscular atrophy in pointer dogs, *Jpn J Vet Sci* 40:539-547, 1978.

109. Cummings JF, et al: Focal spinal muscular atrophy in two German shepherd pups, *Acta Neuropathol* 79:113-116, 1989.

110. Cummings JF, et al: Equine motor neuron disease: A preliminary report, *Cornell Vet* 80:357-379, 1990.

111. Divers TJ, et al: Equine motor neuron disease: Findings in 28 horses and proposal of a pathophysiological mechanism for the disease, *Equine Vet J* 26:409-415, 1994.

112. Podell M, et al: Electromyography in acquired equine motor neuron disease, *Prog Vet Neurol* 6:128-134, 1995.

113. Jackson CA, et al: Spinal accessory nerve biopsy as an antemortem diagnostic test for equine motor neuron disease, *Equine Vet J* 28:215-219, 1996.

114. Stockard C: An hereditary lethal factor for localized motor and preganglionic neurons, *Am J Anat* 59:1-53, 1936.

115. Troyer D, et al: Upper motor neurone and descending tract pathology in bovine spinal muscular atrophy, *J Comp Pathol* 107:305-317, 1992.

116. Leipold HW, El Hamidi M, Troyer D: Pathogenic studies of bovine progressive degenerative myelencephalopathy (Weaver) of Brown Swiss cattle, *Bovine Practitioner* 24:145-146, 1989.

117. Kwiechien JM, et al: Congenital axonopathy in a Brown Swiss calf, *Vet Pathol* 32:72-75, 1995.

118. Palmer AC, Blakemore WF: A progressive neuronopathy in the young cairn terrier, *J Small Anim Pract* 30:101-106, 1989.

119. Cummings JF, de Lahunta A, Moore JJ: Multisystemic chromatolytic neuronal degeneration in a cairn terrier pup, *Cornell Vet* 78:301-314, 1988.

120. Cummings JF, de Lahunta A, Gasteiger EL: Multisystemic chromatolytic neuronal degeneration in Cairn terriers. A case with generalized cataplectic episodes, *J Vet Intern Med* 5:91-94, 1991.

121. Jaggy A, Vandevelde M: Multisystem neuronal degeneration in cocker spaniels, *J Vet Intern Med* 2:117-120, 1988.

122. Duncan ID: Peripheral neuropathy in the dog and cat, *Prog Vet Neurol* 2:111-128, 1991.

123. Duncan I: Etiology and classification of peripheral neuropathies. In *Proceedings of an American College of Veterinary Internal Medicine Forum,* San Diego, 1987, pp 325-329.

124. Braund KG: Diseases of the peripheral nerves, cranial nerves, and muscle. In Oliver JE, Hoerlein BF, Mayhew IG, editors: *Veterinary neurology.* Philadelphia, 1987, WB Saunders.

125. Braund KG: Nerve and muscle biopsy techniques, *Prog Vet Neurol* 2:35-56, 1991.

126. Shelton GD: Diagnosis and treatment of disorders of peripheral nerve, muscle, and neuromuscular junction. In *Proceedings of the 13th Annual Kal-Kan Symposium,* Columbus, OH, 1989, pp 7-11.

127. Cummings J, de Lahunta A: Chronic relapsing polyradiculoneuritis in a dog: A clinical, light and electron microscopic study, *Acta Neuropathol* 28:191-204, 1974.

128. Bichsel P, et al: Chronic polyneuritis in a Rottweiler, *J Am Vet Med Assoc* 191:991-994, 1987.

129. Flecknell PA, Lucke VM: Chronic polyradiculoneuritis in a cat, *Acta Neuropathol (Berl)* 41:81-84, 1978.

130. Shores A, Braund KG, McDonald RK: Chronic relapsing polyneuropathy in a cat, *J Am Anim Hosp Assoc* 23:569-573, 1987.

131. Cummings J, de Lahunta A, Mitchell W: Ganglioradiculitis in the dog: A clinical, light- and electron-microscopic study, *Acta Neuropathol (Berl)* 60:29-39, 1983.

132. Griffiths IR: Progressive axonopathy: An inherited neuropathy of boxer dogs, 1: Further studies of the clinical and electrophysiological features, *J Small Anim Pract* 26:381-392, 1985.

133. Griffiths IR, Duncan ID, Barker J: A progressive axonopathy of boxer dogs affecting the central and peripheral nervous system, *J Small Anim Pract* 21:29-43, 1980.

134. Duncan ID, Griffiths IR: Canine giant axonal neuropathy: Some aspects of its clinical, pathological and comparative features, *J Small Anim Pract* 22:491-501, 1981.

135. Griffiths IR, et al: Further studies of the central nervous system in canine giant axonal neuropathy, *Neuropathol Appl Neurobiol* 6:421-432, 1980.

136. Higgins RJ, et al: Spontaneous lower motor neuron disease with neurofibrillary accumulation in young pigs, *Acta Neuropathol (Berl)* 59:288-294, 1983.

137. Rousseaux CG, Klavano GG, Johnson ES: "Shaker" calf syndrome: A newly recognized inherited neurodegenerative disorder of horned Hereford calves, *Vet Pathol* 22:104-111, 1985.

138. Vandevelde M, Greene C, Hoff E: Lower motor neuron disease with accumulation of neurofilaments in a cat, *Vet Pathol* 13:428-435, 1976.

139. de Lahunta A, Shively GN: Neurofibrillary accumulation in a puppy, *Cornell Vet* 65:240-247, 1975.

140. Higgins RJ, et al: Neurofibrillary accumulation in the Zebra (*Equus burchelli*), *Acta Neuropathol (Berl)* 37:1-5, 1977.

141. Gajdusek DC: Hypothesis: Interference with axonal transport of neurofilament as a common pathogenetic mechanism in certain diseases of the central nervous system, *N Engl J Med* 312:714-719, 1985.

142. Cooper BJ, et al: Canine inherited hypertrophic neuropathy: Clinical and electrodiagnostic studies, *Am J Vet Res* 45:1172-1177, 1984.

143. Cummings J, de Lahunta A: Hypertrophic neuropathy in a dog, *Acta Neuropathol (Berl)* 20:325-336, 1974.

144. Moe L: Hereditary polyneuropathy of Alaskan Malamutes. In Kirk RW, Bonagura JD, editors: *Current veterinary therapy XI: small animal practice.* Philadelphia, 1992, WB Saunders.

145. Moreau PM, et al: Peripheral and central distal axonopathy of suspected inherited origin in Birman cats, *Acta Neuropathol (Berl)* 82:143-146, 1991.

146. Panciera RJ, et al: A familial peripheral neuropathy and glomerulopathy in Gelvieh calves, *Vet Pathol* 40:63-70, 2003.

147. Griffiths I, Duncan I: Distal denervating disease: A degenerative neuropathy of the distal motor axon in dogs, *J Small Anim Pract* 20:579-592, 1979.

148. Chrisman CL: Dancing Doberman disease: Clinical findings and prognosis, *Prog Vet Neurol* 1:83-90, 1990.

149. Braund KG, et al: Distal sensorimotor polyneuropathy in mature Rottweiler dogs, *Vet Pathol* 31:316-326, 1994.

150. Slocombe RF, et al: Pathological aspects of Australian stringhalt, *Equine Vet J* 24:174-183, 1992.

151. Duncan ID, Griffiths IR, Munz M: The pathology of a sensory neuropathy affecting longhaired dachshund dogs, *Acta Neuropathol* 58:141-151, 1982.

152. Cummings JF, et al: Animal model of human disease: Hereditary sensory neuropathy. Nociceptive loss and acral mutilation in pointer dogs: Canine hereditary sensory neuropathy, *Am J Pathol* 112:136-138, 1983.

153. Wheeler SJ: Sensory neuropathy in a border collie puppy, *J Small Anim Pract* 28:281-289, 1987.

154. Wouda W, et al: Sensory neuronopathy in dogs: A study of four cases, *J Comp Pathol* 93:437-450, 1983.

155. Duncan ID, Cuddon PA: Sensory neuropathy. In Kirk RW, editor: *Current veterinary therapy X: small animal practice*. Philadelphia, 1992, WB Saunders.

156. Cummings JF, et al: Reduced substance P-like immunoreactivity in hereditary sensory neuropathy of pointer dogs, *Acta Neuropathol (Berl)* 63:33-40, 1984.

157. Nes J: Electrophysiological evidence of sensory nerve dysfunction in 10 dogs with acral lick dermatitis, *J Am Anim Hosp Assoc* 22:157-160, 1986.

158. Jaggy A, et al: Neurologic manifestations of hypothyroidism: A retrospective study of 29 dogs, *J Vet Intern Med* 8:328-336, 1994.

159. Indrieri R, et al: Neuromuscular abnormalities associated with hypothyroidism and lymphocytic thyroiditis in three dogs, *J Am Vet Med Assoc* 190:544-548, 1987.

160. Braund KG, et al: Hypothyroid myopathy in two dogs, *Vet Pathol* 18:589-598, 1981.

161. Dewey CW, et al: Neuromuscular dysfunction in five dogs with acquired myasthenia gravis and presumptive hypothyroidism, *Prog Vet Neurol* 16:117-123, 1995.

162. Wolff A: Neuropathy associated with transient diabetes mellitus in 2 cats, *Modern Vet Pract* 65:726-728, 1984.

163. Kramek B, et al: Neuropathy associated with diabetes mellitus in the cat, *J Am Vet Med Assoc* 184:42-45, 1984.

164. Johnson C, Kittleson M, Indrieri R: Peripheral neuropathy and hypotension in a diabetic dog, *J Am Vet Med Assoc* 183:1007-1009, 1983.

165. Katherman A, Braund K: Polyneuropathy associated with diabetes mellitus in a dog, *J Am Vet Med Assoc* 182:522-524, 1983.

166. Steiss J, Orsher A, Bowen J: Electrodiagnostic analysis of peripheral neuropathy in dogs with diabetes mellitus, *Am J Vet Res* 42:2061-2064, 1981.

167. Posner JB, Furneaux HM: Paraneoplastic syndromes. In Waksman BH, editor: *Immunologic mechanisms in neurologic and psychiatric disease*. New York, 1990, Raven Press.

168. Hamilton TA, et al: Vincristine-induced neuropathy in a dog, *J Am Vet Med Assoc* 198:635-638, 1991.

169. Braund K, et al: Peripheral neuropathy associated with malignant neoplasms in dogs, *Vet Pathol* 24:16-21, 1987.

170. Presthus J, Teige J: Peripheral neuropathy associated with lymphosarcoma in a dog, *J Small Anim Pract* 27:463-469, 1986.

171. Braund KG, et al: Insulinoma and subclinical peripheral neuropathy in two dogs, *J Vet Intern Med* 1:86-90, 1987.

172. Schrauwen E, et al: Peripheral polyneuropathy associated with insulinoma in the dog: Clinical, pathological, and electrodiagnostic features, *Prog Vet Neurol* 7:16-19, 1996.

173. Van Ham L, et al: Treatment of a dog with an insulinoma-related peripheral polyneuropathy with corticosteroids, *Vet Rec* 141:98-100, 1997.

174. Jones B, et al: Peripheral neuropathy in cats with inherited primary hyperchylomicronaemia, *Vet Rec* 119:268-272, 1986.

175. Peritz LN, et al: Characterization of a lipoprotein lipase class III type defect in hypertriglyceridemic cats, *Clin Invest Med* 13:259-263, 1990.

176. McKerrell RE, et al: Primary hyperoxaluria (L glyceric aciduria) in the cat: A newly recognized inherited disease, *Vet Rec* 125:31-34, 1989.

177. O'Toole D, et al: Radial and tibial nerve pathology of two lactating ewes with kangaroo gait, *J Comp Pathol* 100:245-258, 1989.

178. Dubey JP, et al: Newly recognized fatal protozoan disease of dogs, *J Am Vet Med Assoc* 192:1269-1285, 1988.

179. Cuddon P, et al: *Neospora caninum* infection in English springer spaniel littermates: Diagnostic evaluation and organism isolation, *J Vet Intern Med* 6:325-332, 1992.

180. Knowler C, Wheeler SJ: *Neospora caninum* infection in three dogs, *J Small Anim Pract* 36:172-177, 1995.

181. Ruehlmann D, et al: Canine neosporosis: A case report and literature review, *J Am Anim Hosp Assoc* 31:174-183, 1995.

182. Shelton GD: Differential diagnosis of muscle diseases in companion animals, *Prog Vet Neurol* 2:27-33, 1991.

183. Shelton G, Cardinet H: Pathophysiologic basis of canine muscle disorders, *J Vet Intern Med* 1:36-44, 1987.

184. Kornegay JN: Disorders of the skeletal muscles. In Ettinger SJ, Feldman EC, editors: *Textbook of veterinary internal medicine*, 4th ed. Philadelphia, 1995, WB Saunders.

185. Krum SH, et al: Polymyositis and polyarthritis associated with systemic lupus erythematosus in a dog, *J Am Vet Med Assoc* 170:61-64, 1977.

186. Giger U, et al: Sulfadiazine-induced allergy in six Doberman pinschers, *J Am Vet Med Assoc* 186:47-484, 1985.

187. Kornegay JN, et al: Polymyositis in dogs, *J Am Vet Med Assoc* 176:431-438, 1980.

188. Smith MO: Idiopathic myositides in dogs, *Semin Vet Med Surg* 4:156-160, 1989.

189. Schunk KL: Polymyopathy. In *Proceedings of an American College of Veterinary Internal Medicine Forum*, 1984, Washington, DC, pp 197-200.

190. Presthus J, Lindboe CF: Polymyositis in two German wirehaired pointer littermates, *J Small Anim Pract* 29:239-248, 1988.

191. Shelton GD, Bandman E, Cardinet GH: Electrophoretic comparison of myosins from masticatory muscles and selected limb muscles in the dog, *Am J Vet Res* 46:493-498, 1985.

192. Shelton GD, Cardinet GH III, Bandman E: Canine masticatory muscle disorders: A study of 29 cases, *Muscle Nerve* 10:753-766, 1987.

193. Gilmour MA, Morgan RV, Moore FM: Masticatory myopathy in the dog: A retrospective study of 18 cases, *J Am Anim Hosp Assoc* 28:300-305, 1992.

194. Carpenter JL, et al: Canine bilateral extraocular polymyositis, *Vet Pathol* 26:510-512, 1989.

195. Hargis AM, et al: A skin disorder in three shetland sheepdogs: Comparison with familial canine dermatomyositis of collies, *Compendium Continuing Educ Pract Vet* 7:306-315, 1985.

196. Haupt KH, Prieur DJ, Moore MP, et al: Familial canine dermatomyositis: Clinical, electrodiagnostic, and genetic studies, *Am J Vet Res* 46:1861-1869, 1985.

197. White SD, et al: Dermatomyositis in an adult pembroke Welsh corgi, *J Am Anim Hosp Assoc* 28:398-401, 1992.

198. Kornegay JN: The X-linked muscular dystrophies. In Kirk RW, Bonagura JD, editor: *Current veterinary therapy XI*. Philadelphia, 1992, WB Saunders.

199. Van Ham LML, Roels SLMF, Hoorens JK: Congenital dystrophy-like myopathy in a Brittany spaniel puppy, *Prog Vet Neurol* 6:135-138, 1995.

200. Gaschen FP, et al: Dystrophin deficiency causes lethal muscle hypertrophy in cats, *J Neurol Sci* 110:149-159, 1992.

201. Sarli G, Salda LD, Marcata PS: Dystrophy-like myopathy in a foal, *Vet Rec* 135:156-160, 1994.

202. Sharp NJH, et al: An error in dystrophin mRNA processing causes golden retriever muscular dystrophy, an animal homologue of Duchenne muscular dystrophy, *Genomics* 13:115-121, 1992.

203. Winand NJ, et al: Deletion of the dystrophin muscle promoter in feline muscular dystrophy, *Neuromuscul Disord* 4:433-445, 1994.

204. Bartlett RJ, et al: Mutation segregation and rapid carrier detection of X-linked muscular dystrophy in dogs, *Am J Vet Res* 57:650-654, 1996.

205. Kramer JW, Hegreberg GA, Hamilton MJ: Inheritance of a neuromuscular disorder of Labrador retriever dogs, *J Am Vet Med Assoc* 179:380-381, 1981.

206. McKerrell R, Braund K: Hereditary myopathy in Labrador retrievers: Clinical variations, *J Small Anim Pract* 28:479-489, 1987.

207. McKerrell RE, Braund KG: Hereditary myopathy of Labrador retrievers. In Kirk RW, editor: *Current veterinary therapy X: small animal practice*. Philadelphia, 1989, WB Saunders.

208. Braund KG, et al: Investigating a degenerative polymyopathy in four related Bouvier des Flandres dogs, *Vet Med* 85:558-570, 1990.

209. Peeters ME, et al: Dysphagia in Bouviers associated with muscular dystrophy: Evaluation of 24 cases, *Vet Q* 13:65-73, 1991.

210. Richards RB, et al: Ovine congenital progressive muscular dystrophy: Mode of inheritance, *Aust Vet J* 65:93-94, 1988.

211. Richards R, et al: Ovine congenital progressive muscular dystrophy: Clinical syndrome and distribution of lesions, *Aust Vet J* 63:396-401, 1986.

212. Malik R, et al: Hereditary myopathy of Devon rex cats, *J Small Anim Pract* 34:539-546, 1993.

213. Reference deleted in pages.

214. Hanson SM, et al: Juvenile-onset distal myopathy of Rottweiler dogs. In *Proceedings of the 14th American College of Veterinary Internal Medicine Forum,* San Antonio, TX, 1996, p 755.

215. Walvoort HC, et al: Canine glycogen storage disease type II: A clinical study of four affected Lapland dogs, *J Am Anim Hosp Assoc* 20:279-286, 1984.

216. Jolly RD, et al: Generalized glycogenosis in beef shorthorn cattle—heterozygote detection, *Aust J Exp Biol Med Sci* 55:14-50, 1977.

217. Ceh L, et al: Glycogenosis type III in the dog, *Acta Vet Scand* 17:210-222, 1976.

218. Fyfe JC, et al: Glycogen storage disease type IV: Inherited deficiency of branching enzyme activity in cats, *Pediatr Res* 32:719-725, 1992.

219. Coates JR, et al: A case presentation and discussion of type IV glycogen storage disease in a Norwegian forest cat, *Prog Vet Neurol* 7:5-11, 1996.

220. Angelos S, et al: Myophosphorylase deficiency associated with rhabdomyolysis and exercise intolerance in 6 related Charolais cattle, *Muscle Nerve* 18:736-740, 1995.

221. Giger U, et al: Metabolic myopathy in canine muscle-type phosphofructokinase deficiency, *Muscle Nerve* 11:1260-1265, 1988.

222. Harvey JW, et al: Polysaccharide storage myopathy in canine phosphofructokinase deficiency (type VII glycogen storage disease), *Vet Pathol* 27:1-8, 1990.

223. Valberg SJ, et al: Polysaccharide storage myopathy associated with exertional rhabdomyolysis in the horse, *Neuromuscul Disord* 2:351-359, 1992.

224. Valberg SJ, et al: Familial basis of exertional rhabdomyolysis in quarter horse-related breeds, *Am J Vet Res* 57:286-290, 1996.

225. De La Corte F, et al: Developmental onset of polysaccharide storage myopathy in 4 quarter horse foals, *J Vet Inten Med* 216:581-587, 2002.

226. Harding AE, Holt IJ: Mitochondrial myopathies, *Br Med Bull* 45:760-771, 1989.

227. Breitschwerdt EB, et al: Episodic weakness associated with exertional lactic acidosis and myopathy in Old English Sheepdog littermates, *J Am Vet Med Assoc* 201:731-736, 1992.

228. Vijayasarathy C, et al: Canine mitochondrial myopathy associated with reduced mitochondrial mRNA and altered cytochrome c oxidase activities in fibroblasts and skeletal muscle, *Comp Biochem Physiol* 109:887-894, 1994.

229. Wright JA, et al: A myopathy associated with muscle hypertonicity in the Cavalier King Charles spaniel, *J Comp Pathol* 97:559-565, 1987.

230. Holland CT, et al: Dyserythropoiesis, polymyopathy, and cardiac disease in three related English springer spaniels, *J Vet Intern Med* 5:151-159, 1991.

231. Cooper BJ, et al: Nemaline myopathy of cats, *Muscle Nerve* 9:618-625, 1986.

232. Wells GAH, Pinsent PJN, Todd JN: A progressive, familial myopathy of the Pietrain pig: The clinical syndrome, *Vet Rec* 106:556-558, 1980.

233. Roneus B: Glutathione peroxidase and selenium in the blood of healthy horses and foals affected by muscular dystrophy, *Nord Vet Med* 34:350-353, 1982.

234. Greene CE, et al: Myopathy associated with hyperadrenocorticism in the dog, *J Am Vet Med Assoc* 174:1310-1315, 1979.

235. Braund KG, Dillon AR, Mikeal RL: Experimental investigation of glucocorticoid-induced myopathy in the dog, *Exp Neurol* 68:50-71, 1980.

236. Braund KG, et al: Subclinical myopathy associated with hyperadrenocorticism in the dog, *Vet Pathol* 17:134-148, 1980.

237. Duncan ID, Griffiths IR, Nash AS: Myotonia in canine Cushing's disease, *Vet Rec* 100:30-31, 1977.

238. Jirmanova I: The splayleg disease: A form of congenital glucocorticoid myopathy? *Vet Res Commun* 6:91-101, 1983.

239. McLaughlin B, Doige C, McLaughlin P: Thyroid hormone levels in foals with congenital musculoskeletal lesions, *Can Vet J* 27:264-267, 1986.

240. Gannon JR: Exertional rhabdomyolysis (myoglobinuria) in the racing greyhound. In Kirk RW, editor: *Current veterinary therapy VII*. Philadelphia, 1980, WB Saunders.

241. Bain FT, Merritt AM: Decreased erythrocyte potassium concentration associated with exercise-related myopathy in horses, *J Am Vet Med Assoc* 196:1259-1261, 1990.

242. Dow SW, et al: Potassium depletion in cats: Hypokalemic polymyopathy, *J Am Vet Med Assoc* 191:1563-1568, 1987.

243. Dow SW, et al: Potassium depletion in cats: Renal and dietary influences, *J Am Vet Med Assoc* 191:1569-1575, 1987.

244. Dow SW, et al: Hypokalemia in cats: 186 cases (1984-1987), *J Am Vet Med Assoc* 194:1604-1608, 1989.

245. LeCouteur RA, Dow SW, Sisson AF: Metabolic and endocrine myopathies of dogs and cats, *Semin Vet Med Surg* 4:146-155, 1989.

246. Dow SW: Potassium depletion in cats. In *Proceedings of the Sixth Annual Veterinary Medical Forum,* Washington, DC, 1988, pp 33-35.

247. Gruffydd TJ, et al: Hypokalemic episodic weakness in Burmese cats. In *Proceedings of the Fourteenth Annual Veterinary Medical Forum,* San Antonio, TX, 1996, p 757.

248. Mason K: A hereditary disease in Burmese cats manifested as an episodic weakness with head nodding and neck ventroflexion, *J Am Anim Hosp Assoc* 24:147-151, 1988.

249. Shelton GD: Disorders of neuromuscular transmission, *Semin Vet Med Surg* 4:126-132, 1989.

250. Wheeler SJ: Disorders of the neuromuscular junction, *Prog Vet Neurol* 2:129-135, 1991.

251. O'Dair HA, et al: Acquired immune-mediated myasthenia gravis in a cat associated with a cystic thymus, *J Small Anim Pract* 32:198-202, 1991.

252. Scott Moncrieff JC, Cook JR Jr, Lantz GC: Acquired myasthenia gravis in a cat with thymoma, *J Am Vet Med Assoc* 196:1291-1293, 1990.

253. Klebanow ER: Thymoma and acquired myasthenia gravis in the dog: A case report and review of 13 additional cases, *J Am Anim Hosp Assoc* 28:63-69, 1992.

254. Joseph RJ, Carrillo JM, Lennon VA. Myasthenia gravis in the cat, *J Vet Intern Med* 2:75-79, 1988.

255. Wallace ME, Plamer AC: Recessive mode of inheritance in myasthenia gravis in the Jack Russell terrier, *Vet Rec* 114:350, 1984.

256. Flagstad A, Trojaborg W, Gammeltoft S: Congenital myasthenic syndrome in the dog breed Gammel Dansk Honsehund: Clinical, electrophysiological, pharmacological and immunological comparison with acquired myasthenia gravis, *Acta Vet Scand* 30:89-102, 1989.

257. King LG, Vite CH: Acute fulminating myasthenia gravis in five dogs, *J Am Vet Med Assoc* 212:830-834, 1998.

258. Shelton GD, Schule A, Kass PH: Risk factors for acquired myasthenia gravis in dogs: 1,154 cases (1991-1995), *J Am Vet Assoc* 211:1428-1431, 1997.

259. Shelton GD, et al: Acquired myasthenia gravis: Selective involvement of esophageal, pharyngeal, and facial muscles, *J Vet Intern Med* 4:281-284, 1990.

260. Hackett TB, et al: Third degree atrioventricular block and acquired myasthenia gravis in four dogs, *J Am Vet Med Assoc* 206:1173-1176, 1995.

261. Sims MH, McLean RA: Use of repetitive nerve stimulation to assess neuromuscular function in dogs: A test protocol for suspected myasthenia gravis, *Prog Vet Neurol* 1:311-319, 1990.

262. Kimura J: *Electrodiagnosis in diseases of nerve and muscle: Principles and practice,* 2nd ed. Philadelphia, 1989, FA Davis.

263. Hopkins AL, et al: Stimulated single fibre electromyography in normal dogs, *J Small Anim Pract* 34:271-276, 1993.

264. Shelton GD: How do I treat? Acquired myasthenia gravis in the dog and cat, *Prog Vet Neurol* 1:343-344, 1990.

265. Shelton GD: Myasthenia gravis—1000 cases later. In *Proceedings of the 14th American College of Veterinary Internal Medicine Forum,* San Antonio, TX, 1996, p 658.

266. Lennon VA, et al: Acquired and congenital myasthenia gravis in dogs—a study of 29 cases. In Satoyoshi E, editor: *Myasthenia gravis: pathogenesis and treatment.* Tokyo, 1981, Tokyo University Press.

267. Lennon VA, et al: Myasthenia gravis in dogs: Acetylcholine receptor deficiency with and without anti-receptor antibodies. In Rose NR, Bigazzi PE, Warner RL, editor: *Genetic control of autoimmune disease.* New York, 1978, Elsevier North Holland.

268. Tindall RS, et al. Preliminary results of a double-blind, randomized, placebo controlled trial of cyclosporine in myasthenia gravis, *N Engl J Med* 316:719-724, 1987.

269. Bartges JW, et al: Clinical remission following plasmapheresis and corticosteroid treatment in a dog with acquired myasthenia gravis, *J Am Vet Med Assoc* 196:1276-1278, 1990.

270. Shelton GD: Pathogenesis of canine megaesophagus: Neuromuscular disorders. In *Proceedings of the 14th American College of Veterinary Internal Medicine Forum,* San Antonio, TX, 1996, pp 581-582.

271. Spier SJ, et al: Hyperkalemic periodic paralysis in horses, *J Am Vet Med Assoc* 197:1009-1017, 1990.

272. Naylor JM, Jones V, Berry S-L: Clinical syndrome and diagnosis of hyperkalaemic periodic paralysis in quarter horses, *Equine Vet J* 25:227-232, 1993.

273. Rudolph JA, et al: Periodic paralysis in Quarter Horses: A sodium channel mutation disseminated by selective breeding, *Nature Genet* 2:144-147, 1992.

274. Traub-Dargatz JL, et al: Respiratory stridor associated with polymyopathy suspected to be hyperkalemic periodic paralysis in four Quarter Horse foals, *J Am Vet Med Assoc* 201:85-89, 1992.

275. Guglick MA, MacAllister CG, Breazile JE: Laryngospasm, dysphagia, and emaciation associated with hyperkalemic periodic paralysis in a horse, *J Am Vet Med Assoc* 209:115-117, 1996.

276. Jezyk PF: Hyperkalemic periodic paralysis in a dog, *J Am Anim Hosp Assoc* 18:977-980, 1982.

277. Taylor SM, et al: The syndrome of exercise-induced collapse in Labrador retrievers. In *Proceedings of the Twentieth Annual Veterinary Medical Forum,* Dallas, TX, 2002.

Chapter 8

Ataxia of the Head and the Limbs

Ataxia is a lack of coordination that may be present without spasticity, paresis, or involuntary movements. Paresis, when present, is especially useful in localizing lesions. Ataxia is characterized by a broad-based stance and uncoordinated movements of the head, trunk, or limbs. Lesion localization of ataxic animals is described in Chapter 2 and is summarized in Figure 8-1. A brief review is presented in this chapter.

LESION LOCALIZATION

Ataxia is a sign of specific sensory dysfunction. For clinical purposes, it can be classified into three major categories: sensory, vestibular, and cerebellar. Clinical signs result when a disease interferes with the recognition or coordination of position changes involving the head, trunk, or limbs. Key neurologic signs that are useful for localizing the lesion may be observed. Figure 8-2 is an algorithm for the formulation of a differential diagnosis of ataxia. This algorithm is based largely on a few key differential signs. For example, abnormal movements of the head or the eyes indicate that the lesion is not in the spinal cord but rather in the vestibular system, brainstem, or cerebellum.

Sensory Ataxia

Loss of proprioceptive signals from the limbs and, in some cases, the trunk produces sensory ataxia. For the purpose of localization, abnormalities of proprioception in the limbs are interpreted in exactly the same way as motor dysfunction (see Chapters 2, 6, and 7). For example, loss of proprioception in the pelvic limbs with normal proprioception in the thoracic limbs indicates a lesion caudal to T2 involving the sensory long tracts, spinal nerves, or peripheral nerves. Further localization is achieved by examining the spinal reflexes and segmental pain responses. Sensory ataxia is frequently associated with paresis because the pathways for each are closely related throughout the nervous system. The primary spinal cord

pathways for transmission of proprioception are the spinocerebellar tracts and the dorsal columns.

Vestibular Ataxia

The vestibular system detects linear acceleration and rotational movement of the head. This system does not initiate motor activity; however, its sensory input is used to modify and coordinate movement. The vestibular system primarily controls the muscles involved in maintaining equilibrium, positioning the head, and regulating eye movement. Sensory receptors are located in the inner ear in the vestibular labyrinth. Two kinds of receptors are present: maculae in the utriculi and sacculi and cristae in the semicircular canals. The maculae are arranged approximately at right angles to each other. They function to detect head position with respect to gravity and linear acceleration and help to maintain equilibrium. The cristae in the semicircular canals detect the onset of angular or rotational acceleration. These receptors predict loss of balance and maintain equilibrium. Input to the brain is by way of the vestibular division of cranial nerve (CN) VIII. The cell bodies of the vestibular nerve are in a ganglion in the petrosal bone. The nerve terminates in one of four vestibular nuclei or in the cerebellum via the cerebellar peduncles. Pathways from the vestibular nuclei project to other brainstem centers and the cerebellum, cerebral cortex, and spinal cord.

Vestibular projections to the nuclei of nerves controlling eye movements travel by way of the medial longitudinal fasciculus (MLF) in the brainstem. This system controls normal physiologic nystagmus, and it can be demonstrated in the normal animal by moving its head from side to side or up and down. When this control mechanism is disrupted, nystagmus occurs independently of head movement *(pathologic nystagmus)*. Projections to the emetic center in the brainstem are important in the development of motion sickness *(visual-vestibular sensory dissociation)*. The vestibular apparatus works in close association with the

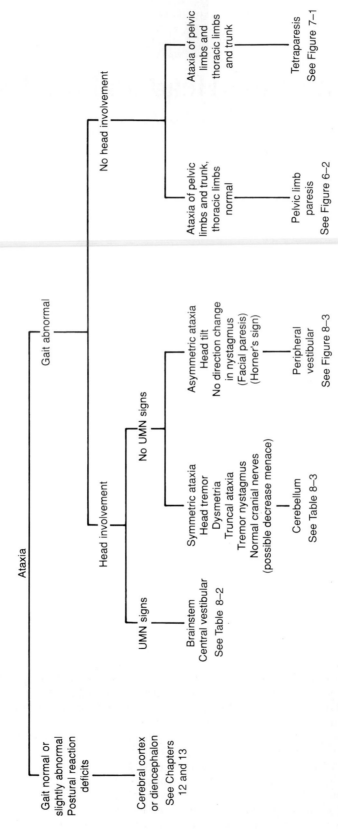

Figure 8-1 Algorithm for the diagnosis of ataxia based on gait, head involvement, and motor function of the limbs.

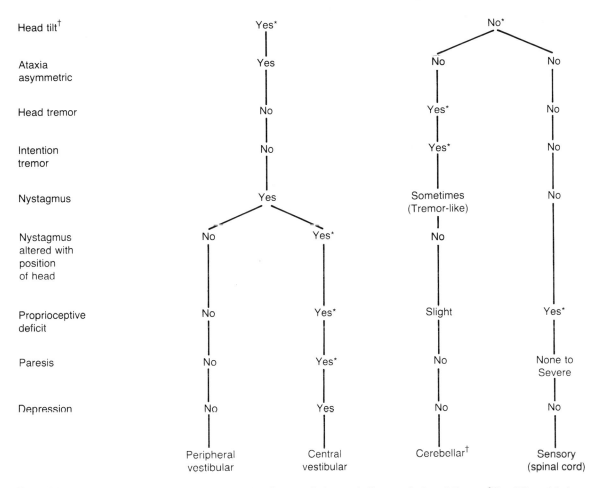

Head tilt†	Yes*		No*	
Ataxia asymmetric	Yes		No	No
Head tremor	No		Yes*	No
Intention tremor	No		Yes*	No
Nystagmus	Yes		Sometimes (Tremor-like)	No
Nystagmus altered with position of head	No	Yes*	No	
Proprioceptive deficit	No	Yes*	Slight	Yes*
Paresis	No	Yes*	No	None to Severe
Depression	No	Yes	No	No
	Peripheral vestibular	Central vestibular	Cerebellar†	Sensory (spinal cord)

Figure 8-2 Algorithm for the diagnosis of ataxia resulting from vestibular, cerebellar, or spinal cord disease. *Key differential signs. Lesion in the brainstem can cause central vestibular, cerebellar, and sensory signs. Lesions involving the cerebellar flocculonodular lobe may cause head tilt. When the caudal cerebellar peduncle is involved, head tilt may be opposite the side of the lesion.

cerebellum to maintain balance and coordination. Pathways project from the vestibular nuclei through the cerebellar peduncles to several cerebellar centers. Vestibular impulses reach the cerebral cortex and inform the animal of its position during movement.

Vestibular information is transmitted to the somatic muscles via the vestibulospinal tracts. These pathways are important for the regulation of antigravity muscles of the limbs and trunk. Most importantly, the vestibulospinal tracts stimulate the ipsilateral extensor muscles. Unilateral vestibular lesions cause a loss of ipsilateral extensor tone, and animals fall in this direction because extensor tone on the contralateral side is not antagonized by extensor muscle tone on the ipsilateral side.

A head tilt indicates vestibular system disease. In most cases the head tilts toward the side of the lesion. The ataxia is generally asymmetric unless bilateral lesions are present. The animal usually falls or drifts toward the side of the lesion. Turning in tight circles is usually a vestibular sign, although exceptions have been observed. The movement is usually toward the side of the lesion, but movement in the opposite direction has been observed with central vestibular lesions (*paradoxical vestibular disease;* see the following discussion). On the basis of a neurologic examination, vestibular ataxia can be localized to peripheral (labyrinth) or central (brainstem) vestibular disease. Signs of paresis or proprioceptive deficits of the limbs associated with a head tilt indicate central vestibular (brainstem) disease. Paresis in central vestibular disease is caused by injury of the motor tracts that project through the brainstem. Thus, a major way to differentiate central and peripheral vestibular disease is to evaluate the animal critically for evidence of motor dysfunction or sensory ataxia. Careful assessment of postural reactions, especially the hopping response, is the key factor in localizing vestibular lesions.

Nystagmus may be present in central or peripheral vestibular disease. In peripheral vestibular disease, the nystagmus may be horizontal or rotatory, with the quick phase directed away from the side of the lesion. With a central vestibular lesion, the nystagmus may be similar to that described for peripheral lesions; however, nystagmus that changes direction with alterations in head position or that is vertical in direction strongly suggests a central vestibular lesion, although exceptions may occur. Facial and sympathetic nerve function may be impaired with either peripheral or central vestibular disease. The facial nerve exits the brainstem in close association with the vestibular nerve and separates from it in the petrosal bone. The facial nerve does not cross through the middle ear.[1] The sympathetic nerve courses through the middle ear in dogs and cats and often is affected in otitis media with associated Horner's syndrome. Brainstem lesions affecting the sympathetic pathways typically affect other structures, and additional signs are seen. Dysfunction of other cranial nerves associated with head tilt suggests a central vestibular lesion that involves other areas of the brainstem. Some syndromes that cause peripheral vestibular dysfunction, however, also affect other cranial nerves. Thus, evidence of multiple cranial nerve involvement does not necessarily indicate central vestibular disease. Physiologic nystagmus may be depressed or absent with vestibular lesions. Caloric tests and assessment of postrotatory nystagmus are difficult to perform and interpret and are usually not needed in the evaluation of vestibular disease. Animals with central lesions may be depressed because of involvement of the reticular activating system in the brainstem. Severely affected animals may be stuporous or comatose. Ventral strabismus is seen ipsilateral to the lesion when the head is elevated in either peripheral or central vestibular disease.

Paradoxical vestibular disease is evidenced by one or more vestibular signs (e.g., head tilt, nystagmus) that are in the direction opposite the other localizing signs. These signs generally are caused by lesions that involve the flocculonodular lobes or the caudal cerebellar peduncles.[2] Postural reaction deficits usually occur ipsilateral to the lesion, whereas the head tilt is contralateral. Bilateral vestibular disease does not cause a head tilt. The animal often walks slowly and in a crouched position, tends to avoid sudden movements, and exhibits a characteristic side-to-side swaying of the head. Vestibular eye movements are absent.

Cerebellar Ataxia

The cerebellum functions as a major coordinator of motor activity. It compares the intent of motor activity with the performance required to complete the activity. The cerebellum receives sensory input through three paired peduncles. The caudal cerebellar peduncles carry sensory fibers from the vestibular system, basal nuclei, and spinal cord. The middle cerebellar peduncles transmit information from the cerebral cortex by way of brainstem centers. Cerebellar output to the cerebral cortex, brainstem, and spinal cord travels through the rostral and caudal cerebellar peduncles. A disease of the cerebellum or its peduncles results in characteristic clinical signs. The cerebellum performs below the level of consciousness to control muscle movements accurately, assist in maintaining equilibrium, and control posture.

Most diseases that affect the cerebellum are relatively slow in onset, but vascular lesions such as infarction of cerebellar blood vessels may cause acute, nonprogressive clinical signs. Clinical signs described subsequently are related to these diseases. Because the cerebellum does not initiate motor activity, paresis is not a sign of cerebellar dysfunction unless the brainstem is also affected. Symmetric ataxia characterized by a hypermetric, base-wide gait, truncal ataxia, and intention tremor that is most pronounced in the head is very suggestive of cerebellar disease. The head tremor is most obvious when the animal attempts a purposeful movement such as eating or drinking. Unlike vestibular disorders, cerebellar dysfunction rarely produces head tilt or circling. Lesions of the flocculonodular lobe of the cerebellum, however, can cause vestibular dysfunction (see previous discussion).[2] Nystagmus, when present, is tremor like (rapid eye flutter). Menace response may be impaired in animals with diffuse cerebellar disease, even though vision and facial nerve function are normal. Behavior and level of consciousness are not affected by cerebellar lesions.

Acute cerebellar dysfunction from trauma or vascular disease has a different clinical picture. The animal develops decerebellate posture: opisthotonus, tonic extension of the thoracic limbs, and clonic movements of the pelvic limbs. The pelvic limbs may also be extended if the ventral aspect of the rostral lobe is affected. Spinal reflexes may be exaggerated in the early stages.[2] Rigidity decreases after a few days, and the other signs of chronic lesions, including tremor and ataxia, develop over a period of several weeks to months.

The flocculonodular lobes of the cerebellum are important in vestibular reactions. Lesions of these lobes cause vestibular signs, often paradoxical, as described in the discussion of vestibular disease.

DISEASES

This chapter discusses diseases that commonly affect the brainstem, cerebellum, and peripheral vestibular system. The disorders that produce sensory ataxia because of spinal cord disease are described in Chapters 6 and 7. Diseases with involuntary movement as the primary sign (e.g., tremor, spasticity) are discussed in Chapter 10. As in previous chapters, this section is organized according to the anatomic location of the lesion and the course of the disease (acute versus chronic, progressive versus nonprogressive).

Peripheral Vestibular Diseases

A diagnostic approach to peripheral vestibular disorders is outlined in Figure 8-3. Using otoscopic, radiographic, and advanced imaging examinations of the ear canal and the osseous bulla, the clinician must decide whether abnormalities exist. If no lesions are detected, a search is made for evidence of ototoxic drugs. If these agents have not been administered, the patient's history is used to place the condition in one of two categories: chronic progressive or acute nonprogressive. If the initial otoscopic or radiographic examination is positive,

the disorder is classified as inflammatory or noninflammatory based on the results of myringotomy, cytology, and culture and sensitivity testing. Certain inflammatory and neoplastic diseases can fall into either broad category, depending on the propensity of the disease to produce grossly visible or radiographically detectable lesions.

Otitis Media Interna

The most common cause of peripheral vestibular disease in dogs and cats is an inner ear infection that has progressed from the middle ear. Of 83 cases of peripheral vestibular disease in the dog, 49% were attributed to infection.[3] Otitis media interna is also common in food animals but not in horses.[4] Otitis externa caused by bacteria is the most common cause of otitis media in small animals. Otitis media interna may develop in animals with no history or physical evidence of otitis externa, especially large animals. In these cases, retrograde infection through the auditory tube from the pharynx or hematogenous infection is suspected. Extension of guttural pouch mycosis in horses is a rare cause of vestibular signs. Most commonly, otitis media in animals is caused by bacteria, although yeast and fungal organisms are encountered occasionally. The causative bacteria in small animals include staphylococci, *Proteus* spp., *Pseudomonas* spp., *Pasteurella* spp., and *Escherichia coli*. In horses, *Streptococcus* spp.,

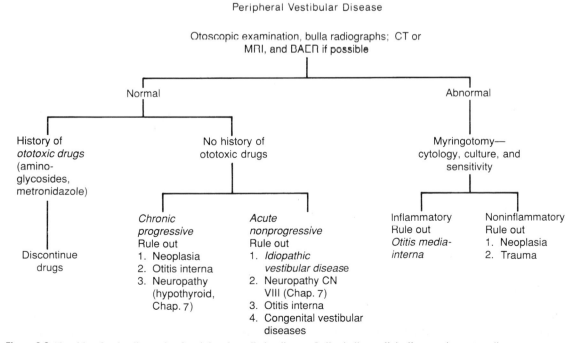

Peripheral Vestibular Disease

Figure 8-3 Algorithm for the diagnosis of peripheral vestibular disease. Italics indicate clinically most important diseases.

Actinobacillus spp., and *Staphylococcus* spp. are most frequent. Lambs and cattle more often have *Pasteurella* spp., *Streptococcus* spp., or *Corynebacterium* spp.[5] *Streptococcus* organisms are most likely to be found in swine.[6] Breeds of dogs that are predisposed to chronic otitis externa (cocker spaniels, poodles, and German shepherd dogs) or animals with chronic *Otodectes* infection are at increased risk of otitis media interna. Occasionally, otic foreign bodies such as grass awns, foxtail awns, or spear grass predispose dogs to otitis externa with progression to otitis media interna. Recurrent episodes are common.

Clinical Signs. Otitis media interna may cause the clinical signs of vestibular ataxia as discussed earlier. Head shaking, aural pain, and inflammatory discharge also are often present in cases of primary otitis externa. Torticollis, circling, ataxia, positional ventral strabismus, and nystagmus are specific neurologic signs that are suggestive of otitis interna *if the patient has no demonstrable paresis.* Unilateral facial nerve paralysis is common because the inflammatory process often extends to the facial nerve as it passes through the petrosal bone. Otitis media, with no involvement of the inner ear, does not cause vestibular dysfunction or facial paralysis. Complete or partial Horner's syndrome can be seen on the affected side if the sympathetic nerve in the middle ear is involved. Because the sympathetic nerves do not enter the middle ear in large animals, Horner's syndrome is not seen with otitis media interna in these species.

Diagnosis. The diagnosis of otitis media interna is confirmed by otoscopic examination and skull imaging. If purulent otitis externa is present, the external ear is cultured for bacteria and the ear then is cleaned gently but thoroughly. Deep sedation or anesthesia aids in critical otoscopic examination. The tympanic membrane is examined carefully for hyperemia, edema, hemorrhage, and erosion. Fluid in the middle ear makes the tympanic membrane appear opaque and produces bulging of the membrane into the external auditory canal. If the tympanic membrane is ruptured or eroded, fluid is aspirated gently from the middle ear for cytologic and bacteriologic examination. If the tympanic membrane is intact but abnormal, myringotomy is performed with a 3-inch, 18- to 20-gauge spinal needle or with a sterile myringotomy knife. If aspiration of the middle ear fails to yield a small quantity of fluid for evaluation, 0.25 to 0.5 ml of sterile saline is injected and then aspirated. The fluid is examined for cells and bacteria and cultured.

Radiographic examination of the skull is a valuable aid in the diagnosis and prognosis of chronic otitis media interna. Radiographic projections include lateral, dorsoventral, open-mouth, and oblique views of each tympanic bulla. Positive findings include fluid density in the bulla and exostosis, sclerosis, or erosion in the bulla (Figure 8-4). Lysis of the bulla or surrounding structures is more often associated with neoplasia. Stress fractures of the petrosal bone and periosteal proliferative changes around the bulla and hyoid bones may be seen in horses.[7-9] Unfortunately, normal radiographs do not rule out middle ear disease.[10] Despite positive findings on otoscopic examination, radiographs may be normal. Computed tomography (CT) or magnetic resonance imaging (MRI) should be performed in these situations.

Treatment. The medical treatment of otitis media interna consists of long-term systemic antibiotics chosen on the basis of positive culture and sensitivity results. Penicillinase-resistant penicillins, cephalosporins, and chloramphenicol are appropriate. Long-term chloramphenicol therapy is used with caution in cats because of its propensity to cause anorexia, depression, weight loss, and occasional blood dyscrasia. We prefer long-term bactericidal antibiotic therapy. In chronic cases, therapy for 6 to 8 weeks is recommended. Therapy with systemic aminoglycosides must be performed with caution because ototoxic signs are masked by the existing disease. Antibiotics and corticosteroids instilled in the external ear canal rarely reach the middle ear and therefore are seldom useful for resolving the inner ear infection. Because ototoxic agents can penetrate into the inner ear from the middle ear, they should be avoided. Unfortunately, this excludes most of the common topical medications (see subsequent discussion of Ototoxicity).[11]

In chronic disease involving the middle ear and the bulla, surgical debridement and drainage often are needed to resolve the infection. Various techniques have been described; however, we prefer the ventral bulla osteotomy because it affords the best visibility and exposure for biopsy, debridement, and drainage. After surgery drains are left in place for 10 days, and medical therapy is followed as described previously. Total ear canal ablation combined with bulla osteotomy may be required in dogs with chronic otitis externa and media.[12,13] Nasopharyngeal polyps of the middle ear may result in recurrent infections and must be removed (see subsequent discussion).

Therapy for otitis media interna must resolve the infection and prevent extension to the brainstem. The prognosis for recovery depends on several factors: (1) the resistance of the organism, (2) the chronicity of disease, (3) the extent of bone involvement, and (4) the reversibility of the neurologic damage. In chronic otitis interna, neurologic deficits may be irreversible; however, most animals soon compensate for their vestibular deficits. Facial

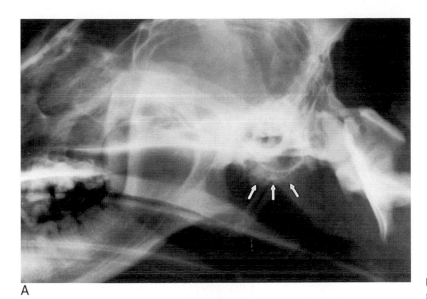

A

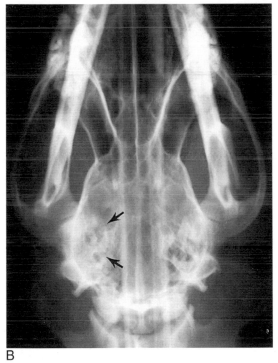

B

Figure 8-4 A, Lateral skull radiograph of a dog with severe otitis media interna. Note the proliferative bony reaction of the osseous bulla *(arrows).* **B,** Ventrodorsal skull radiograph of the same dog. Note the opacity of the right tympanic bulla *(arrows).* A bulla osteotomy was performed to curette the diseased bone and to establish drainage from the middle ear.

paralysis is usually irreversible. Resulting keratoconjunctivitis sicca requires long-term therapy with artificial tears.

Idiopathic Vestibular Diseases

Feline Vestibular Syndrome. An acute, idiopathic, nonprogressive vestibular disturbance has been recognized in cats. The condition occurs sporadically and is not associated with other infectious diseases. The incidence seems to be highest in July and August in the northeastern United States; these observations have not been substantiated in the southern United States,[14] leading some to speculate that the syndrome may be caused by cuterebra fly larvae. In a review of 75 cases, including two necropsies, one cat had hemorrhage in the labyrinth on the affected side, and the other cat had mild nonsuppurative leptomeningitis but no lesions directly involving the vestibular system.[14]

An analogous syndrome has been termed *lizard poisoning* in some areas and is believed to be related to the ingestion of blue-tailed lizards;

however, these lizards are not present in the Northeast, where the incidence seems high.

Clinical Signs. Clinical signs develop acutely and are usually unilateral, although bilateral involvement has been observed. Signs of otitis externa are lacking, and affected cats are usually healthy in all other respects. No sex, breed, or age predilection is apparent. Cats with unilateral disease develop severe head tilt, disorientation, falling, rolling, and nystagmus. In bilateral disease, affected cats have little head tilt but have difficulty moving because of severe disorientation. The head may swing in wide excursions from side to side. The cat usually remains in a crouched posture with the limbs widely abducted and may cry out as if extremely frightened. Nystagmus may not be present; however, vestibular eye movements are depressed bilaterally. Some affected cats vomit and are anorectic.

Diagnosis. The diagnosis is based on the clinical signs and the absence of evidence supporting a diagnosis of bacterial otitis externa, media, or interna of other causes.

Treatment. No specific therapy is available. Affected cats spontaneously improve within 72 hours and are usually normal in 2 to 3 weeks. Antiemetics are indicated in cats that vomit but do not ease the vestibular signs. Sedation may be necessary during the acute phase of the disease to suppress crying or thrashing. Although bacteria are not incriminated in the pathogenesis of this disease, antibiotics should be considered in cases in which differentiation from acute bacterial otitis media interna is difficult. The prognosis for recovery is excellent. Residual vestibular dysfunction is uncommon.

Canine Vestibular Syndrome. Acute, idiopathic vestibular syndromes are recognized in older dogs. In a review of 83 cases of peripheral vestibular disease, 39% were considered idiopathic.[3] The disease is not associated with any known infectious agent.

Clinical Signs. Signs develop acutely and on occasion may be preceded by vomiting and nausea. The signs are similar to those described in the section on the feline syndrome.

Diagnosis. The diagnosis is based on the clinical signs and the absence of evidence supporting a diagnosis of bacterial otitis media interna or other disease. We have seen dogs with peripheral vestibular disease that are hypothyroid and recover with thyroid supplementation. Because the idiopathic disease is usually self-limiting, cause and effect are difficult to prove. See the discussion of hypothyroidism in Chapter 7.

Treatment. No specific therapy is available. Dogs spontaneously improve in 72 hours and are usually normal in 7 to 10 days. Head tilt may persist in some cases but usually does not interfere with function.

Congenital Vestibular Syndromes

Congenital vestibular syndromes occur sporadically in litters of purebred dogs and cats. They have been reported in beagles, German shepherd dogs, Doberman pinschers, cocker spaniels, smooth fox terriers, Akitas, and several other breeds. Affected Siamese, Burmese, and Tonkinese cats also have been identified.[15-19] Vestibular signs develop from the time of birth until the animal is several weeks of age. Deafness may accompany the vestibular disease and may be unilateral or bilateral. The pathogenesis of the lesion is unknown. Although most of the conditions are assumed to be inherited, a definite pattern has not been identified. Lymphocytic labyrinthitis was identified histologically in two litters of affected Doberman pinschers.[19] Some animals gradually improve, whereas others have persistent head tilt and deafness. No effective therapy is known.

The pendular nystagmus of Siamese cats is caused by an abnormality of the visual pathways rather than vestibular disease (see Chapter 11). Pendular nystagmus of Holstein and Jersey cattle with no other clinical signs could be a similar syndrome.[4]

Neoplastic Diseases

Primary tumors initially can cause peripheral vestibular dysfunction if the tumor originates from or compresses the vestibular nerve. Neurofibromas rarely develop in this nerve; when present, a slowly progressive course of vestibular disease evolves over several months. Eventually this tumor grows into the brainstem, and central vestibular signs become apparent. Other tumors, particularly meningioma and choroid plexus papilloma, occur at the cerebellopontine angle and cause vestibular dysfunction as well as deficits referable to involvement of CN V and VII and evidence of brainstem disease (see Chapter 15). Tumors of the osseous bullae or the labyrinth (fibrosarcomas, chondrosarcomas, osteosarcomas) may destroy structures in the inner ear. Squamous cell carcinoma may arise from the epithelial lining of either the middle or inner ear.[20] Bony lysis may be seen on skull radiographs. CT or MRI provides greater anatomic detail (Figure 8-5). Brainstem auditory-evoked potentials can also be used to assess the degree of brainstem involvement.[21]

Polyps have been identified within the nasopharynx, the external ear canal, or a combination of these sites in numerous cats.[22,23] Most of these polyps appear to originate within the auditory tube. Affected cats are generally less than 2 years

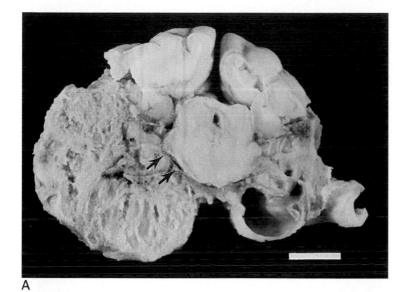

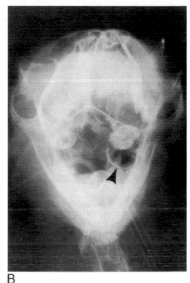

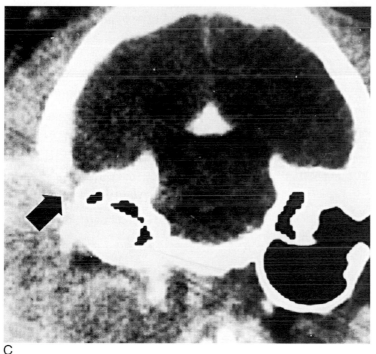

Figure 8-5 Transverse pathologic section of brain and skull (**A**), survey skull radiograph (**B**), and computed tomography image (**C**) from a 5-year-old female domestic cat with initial signs of otitis externa and peripheral vestibular disease and subsequent clinical evidence of brainstem involvement. A mass was palpated at the base of the left ear. A mass has obliterated the left tympanic bulla and invaded the calvaria *(arrows in A and C)*. The left tympanic bulla in B is obscured compared with the right tympanic bulla, which can be clearly seen *(arrowhead)*. However, the nature of the underlying lesion is poorly defined in the survey radiograph. The cat was euthanized and squamous cell carcinoma was diagnosed on microscopic examination of the lesion. Bar in A = 1 cm. (From Kornegay JN: *Feline neurology.* [Problems in Veterinary Medicine Series.] Philadelphia, 1991, JB Lippincott.)

of age. Polyps that originate in the auditory tube apparently block drainage of middle ear secretions and otorrhea, and signs of otitis externa result. Middle ear involvement and subsequent otitis interna lead to peripheral vestibular dysfunction. Other cats may have signs of upper respiratory involvement. Polyps typically can be seen in the external ear canal or oropharynx. Most polyps are attached by only a narrow stalk to the auditory tube and can be removed by traction. Lateral ear resection and bulla osteotomy may be necessary to remove others.

Ototoxicity

A large variety of drugs can cause ototoxicity, affecting vestibular function, hearing, or both. Most of these agents initially cause damage to the receptors and eventually cause degeneration of the nerve. Toxicity can occur from either systemic or topical therapy. Topical application is probably safe if the tympanic membrane is intact. Ototoxic agents are listed in Table 8-1.

The aminoglycoside antibiotics are most frequently incriminated in ototoxicity. The signs may

Table 8-1 Ototoxic Drugs and Chemicals

Antibiotics
  Aminoglycosides
    Streptomycin
    Dihydrostreptomycin
    Gentamicin
    Neomycin
    Kanamycin
    Amikacin
    Tobramycin
  Other
    Polymixin B
    Minocycline
    Erythromycin
    Vancomycin
    Chloramphenicol

Antiseptics
  Ethanol
  Iodine and iodophors
  Benzalkonium chloride
  Chlorhexidine
  Centrimide

  Benzethonium
    chloride

Antineoplastics
  Cisplatin
  Nitrogen mustard

Diuretics
  Bumetanide
  Ethacrynic acid
  Furosemide

Heavy Metals
  Arsenic
  Lead
  Mercury

Miscellaneous
  Ceruminolytic agents
  Detergents
  Quinine
  Propylene glycol
  Salicylates

Data from Mansfield PD: Ototoxicity in dogs and cats, *Compendium Continuing Educ Pract Vet* 12:332-337, 1990.

be unilateral or bilateral. High doses of these drugs, therapy for longer than 14 days, or their use in treating patients with impaired renal function are factors that contribute to ototoxicity. Patients receiving these drugs should be monitored closely for signs of renal toxicity and ototoxicity. In patients with decreased renal function, dosages are reduced or the drugs are replaced by other nontoxic antibiotics. Vestibular signs usually improve once the offending antibiotics are discontinued; however, deafness may be permanent.

Central Vestibular Diseases

A diagnostic approach to central vestibular (brainstem) disorders is outlined in Table 8-2. Of the various categories listed, neoplastic, chronic degenerative, and inflammatory conditions are most common. These disorders are discussed in Chapter 15. Localization of lesions to the caudal brainstem has been discussed previously.

Cerebellar Diseases

Table 8-3 outlines the diagnostic approach to cerebellar disorders. Of the categories listed, the

Table 8-2 Etiology of Central Vestibular (Brainstem) Disease*

Etiologic Category	Acute Nonprogressive	Acute Progressive	Chronic Progressive
Degenerative			Storage diseases (15) Neuronopathies (15) Demyelinating diseases (15)
Metabolic		Hypoglycemia (15)	
Neoplastic (15)		Metastatic	Primary Meningioma Medulloblastoma Glioma Choroid plexus papilloma Epidermoid cyst
Inflammatory (15)		Viral Distemper Equine encephalomyelitis Feline infectious peritonitis Bacterial Listeriosis Various bacteria Rickettsial Protozoal Granulomatous meningoencephalitis	Viral Distemper Feline infectious peritonitis Bacterial Protozoal Mycotic Granulomatous meningoencephalitis
Toxic (15)		Lead Hexachlorophene	Lead Hexachlorophene
Traumatic (12)	Head injury		
Vascular (12)	Hemorrhage Infarction		

*Numbers in parentheses refer to chapters in which entities are discussed.

Table 8-3 **Etiology of Cerebellar Disease***

Etiologic Category	Acute Nonprogressive	Acute Progressive	Chronic Progressive
Degenerative			Abiotrophies Neuroaxonal dystrophies Demyelinating disease (15) Storage diseases (15) Spongiform encephalopathies (10)
Anomalous	Cerebellar hypoplasia Dysmyelinogenesis (10)		

Neoplastic (15)		Metastatic	Primary
			   Medulloblastoma
			   Choroid plexus papilloma
			   Epidermoid cyst
			   Glioma
			   Meningioma

Nutritional (15)		Thiamine deficiency	
Inflammatory (15)	Steroid responsive tremor syndrome (10)	Distemper FIP Scrapie Louping ill Protozoal Rickettsial GME	Distemper FIP Protozoal Mycotic GME
Toxic (15)		Ivermectin	Lead Hexachlorophene Organophosphates Plants
Traumatic (12)	Head injury		
Vascular (12)	Infarction Septic emboli Hemorrhage		

*Numbers in parentheses refer to chapters in which entities are discussed.

chronic degenerative conditions, malformations, and inflammatory conditions are most common. Those diseases likely to produce multifocal neurologic lesions are discussed in Chapter 15. Steroid-responsive tremor syndrome (idiopathic cerebellitis) is discussed in Chapter 10. Disorders confined largely to the cerebellum are discussed in the following sections. These conditions are largely congenital; the abnormality occurs during gestation or before normal ambulation. In a review of congenital cerebellar diseases, de Lahunta[24] grouped these disorders into three categories: (1) in utero or neonatal viral infections; (2) malformations of genetic or unknown cause; and (3) degenerative diseases, referred to as *abiotrophies*. Tables 8-4 and 8-5 list the congenital disorders occurring in animals. The appendix also has these diseases listed by breed and species.

Neonatal Syndromes

Clinical signs are present at birth or in the early postnatal period before normal ambulation. These syndromes are characterized by symmetric signs and nonprogressive courses.

Viral-induced Cerebellar Hypoplasia

Feline Parvovirus. The parvovirus responsible for feline infectious enteritis (panleukopenia) can produce a variety of cerebellar malformations, including cerebellar hypoplasia. In utero or perinatal infection of the brain adversely affects development of the cerebellum. Destruction of the external germinal cell layer causes hypoplasia of the granular cell layer. Growing Purkinje neurons also may be destroyed. The destruction may be so severe that the size of the cerebellar cortex is grossly reduced (hence the term *cerebellar hypoplasia*) (Figure 8-6). Granule and Purkinje cells are reduced microscopically (Figure 8-7). The resulting lesions are irreversible.[25-27] Some affected kittens have concomitant hydrocephalus or hydranencephaly.[28]

In some litters all kittens are affected, whereas in other litters only one kitten or a portion of the litter are affected. Symmetric, nonprogressive cerebellar signs are present in affected kittens at the time of ambulation. Some kittens appear to improve, apparently because of accommodation through other senses, such as vision and conscious

Table 8-4 **Congenital Cerebellar Diseases in Dogs and Cats**

Diseases and Species	Diseases and Breeds	Inherited	References
Neonatal Syndromes			
Viral infections			
Dogs	Canine herpes virus	No	23,29
Cats	Feline panleukopenia	No	24-27, 31
Malformations			
Dogs	Cerebellar hypoplasia (dysplasia) with lissencephaly		
	Wire-haired Fox terriers	Possible	24, 31
	Irish Setters	Possible	24, 31
	Cerebellar hypoplasia		
	Chow chows	AR	32
	Miniature poodles	Unknown	64,65
	Various breeds	Single case	34-36
Cats	Vermian hypoplasia	Single case	66
Abiotrophies			
Dogs	Australian kelpies	Unknown	67
	Beagles	Possible	24
	Bull mastiff (with hydrocephalus)	AR	68
	English pointer	X-linked	69
	Irish setter	AR	37,70
	Labrador retriever	Unknown	71
	Miniature poodles	Unknown	72
	Samoyeds	Unknown	24
Cats	Olivopontocerebellar atrophy	Unknown	16,24
	Cerebellar degeneration	AR	73
Postnatal Syndromes			
Dogs	Akitas	Unknown	38
	Airedale terriers	Unknown	74
	Beagles	Unknown	75
	Bern running dogs	Possible	24
	Bernese mountain dogs	Unknown	38
	Border collies	Unknown	76
	Brittany spaniels	Unknown	77,78
	Cairn terriers	Unknown	79
	Clumber spaniel	Unknown	38
	Cocker spaniels	Unknown	80
	Finnish terriers	Unknown	81
	Fox terriers	Unknown	38
	Golden retrievers	Unknown	24
	Gordon setters	Possible	42-44,82
	Great Dane	Unknown	24
	Kerry Blue terrier	AR	39-41
	Labrador retriever	Unknown	24
	Miniature poodle	Unknown	31
	Miniature schnauzer-beagle crosses	Unknown	83
	Mixed breeds	Unknown	38
	Rhodesian ridgeback	Unknown	84
	Rough-coated collie	AR	45
	Old English sheepdog	AR	50
	Rottweiler	Unknown	48,49
	Strattfordshire terriers	Unknown	
Cats	GM$_1$-Gangliosidosis (type II)		
	Domestic	Unknown	51
	Siamese		

AR, Autosomal recessive; *Unknown,* single or multiple litters; *Possible,* substantial evidence present.

Table 8-5 **Congenital Cerebellar Diseases in Large Animals**

Diseases and Species	Diseases and Breeds	Inherited	References
Neonatal Syndromes			
Viral infections			
Cattle	Bovine virus diarrhea		24,30,85
	Akabane virus		24
	Bluetongue virus		24
Sheep	Akabane virus		24
	Bluetongue virus		24
Swine	Hog cholera virus		24,86
Malformations			
Cattle	Cerebellar hypoplasia		
	Hereford	AR	4,24
	Short horn	AR	4,24
	Ayrshire, Angus, other breeds	Suspected	4,87
	Vermian hypoplasia		88
Sheep	Various malformations		24
Horses	Vermian hypoplasia	Unknown	89
Abiotrophies			
Cattle	Hereford	Probable	24
Sheep	Welsh mountain	AR	24
	Corriedale	AR	24
Swine	Saddleback-large white crosses	Probable	90
Postnatal syndromes			
Abiotrophies			
Horses	Arabian	R (?)	24,91
	Gotland pony	AR	24,92
	Oldenburg	Unknown	4
	Thoroughbred	Unknown	93
Cattle	Holstein-Friesian	R (?)	24,46
	Polled Hereford	Probable	94
	Angus	Probable	38
Sheep	Merino	Unknown	95
Swine	Yorkshire	R (?)	24

A, Autosomal; *AR,* autosomal recessive; *Probable,* good evidence present; *R,* recessive.

proprioception. No systemic signs of panleukopenia are present. Kittens that are infected with the virus after 2 weeks of age rarely develop neurologic signs, even though systemic signs may be severe. In addition to the virulent virus, a modified live vaccine virus also may produce this syndrome. Pregnant queens and kittens less than 3 weeks of age should be given killed virus vaccines. The presence of nonprogressive signs of strict cerebellar disease in young kittens strongly suggests a diagnosis of cerebellar hypoplasia. No effective therapy for this disease exists. Some kittens can function as pets; however, others have incapacitating disease and should be euthanized.

Canine Herpesvirus. This virus affects puppies less than 2 weeks of age. The disease is characterized by generalized systemic signs, including sudden death. Rarely, puppies survive the systemic effects of the virus and develop residual cerebellar ataxia. This form of cerebellar disease should be suspected in puppies that survive

systemic herpes infection. The cerebellar signs are nonprogressive.[24,29]

Bovine Virus Diarrhea. Fetal calves infected with this virus between 100 and 200 days of gestation develop severe cerebellar degeneration and hypoplasia. Ocular lesions include retinal atrophy, optic neuritis, cataracts, and microphthalmia with retinal dysplasia. At birth, affected calves have symmetric, nonprogressive cerebellar signs. Some calves improve as they compensate for the cerebellar disease. No treatment is known. The disease can be prevented by vaccinating appropriately.[4,30]

Akabane Virus. This virus produces severe destruction of germinal cells in the brains of fetal lambs and calves. Hydranencephaly also may be seen. The disease has been observed in Australia, Japan, and Israel. Clinical signs are related to the cerebral and cerebellar lesions.[4,24]

Bluetongue Virus. This virus produces severe destruction of germinal cells in the brains of fetal lambs and calves. Hydranencephaly and cerebellar

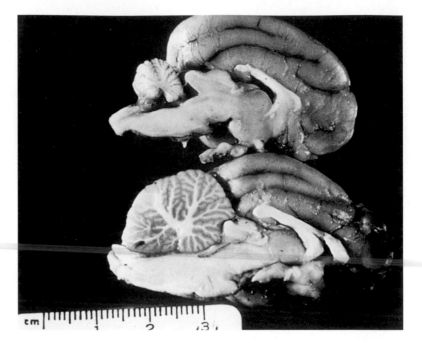

Figure 8-6 Cerebellar hypoplasia in a kitten affected in utero with panleukopenia virus *(top).* Note the small cerebellum, compared with that of a normal cat *(bottom).*

atrophy are the usual lesions. Lambs develop the most severe lesions when infected at 50 to 58 days of gestation.[4,24]

Hog Cholera Virus. Hog cholera vaccine virus, when administered to susceptible pregnant sows, produces numerous lesions in fetal pigs, including lesions in the cerebellum. The clinical signs are those of a diffuse whole-body tremor (see Chapter 10).

Cerebellar Malformation. Numerous breed-specific syndromes and individual cases of cerebellar dysplasia or hypoplasia have been described in dogs and other animals. In some affected animals, the cerebellum is malformed at birth, and further clinical or pathologic deterioration is not apparent. Progressive degeneration of differentiated cells in the cerebellum, with associated clinical deterioration, occurs in other animals. This latter progressive group of diseases is discussed in the section on abiotrophies.

Dysplasia of the cerebrum and the cerebellum has been reported in wire fox terriers and Irish setters.[24,31] The clinical signs do not progress. Generalized seizures developed in one dog after 1 year of age and were associated with lissencephaly.

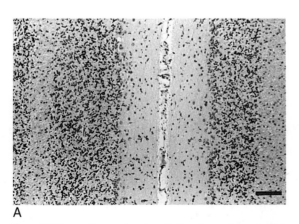

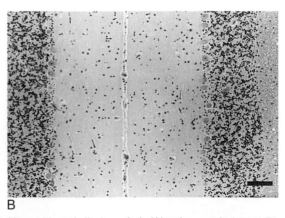

A **B**

Figure 8-7 Photomicrographs of cerebellum from a 6-week-old female kitten with cerebellar hypoplasia **(A)** and a normal adult cat **(B).** The cerebellar folia of the affected kitten are hypoplastic. Note particularly the relative thickness of the molecular cell layers at the center of each figure. Granule cell and Purkinje cell numbers are reduced in the affected kitten. Hematoxylin and eosin. Bar = 30 μm in each. (From Kornegay JN: Cerebellar hypoplasia. In August JR, editor: *Consultations in feline internal medicine.* Philadelphia, 1991, WB Saunders.)

The cerebellum is symmetrically small as a result of abnormal development of the cerebellar cortex. The cause is unknown, but a genetic mode is suspected.

Microscopic cerebellar hypoplasia has been reported in chow chow pups.[32] Cerebellar ataxia was present at birth and persisted as the pups developed. Purkinje neurons and granular cells were depleted. An autosomal recessive mode of inheritance was suspected. This syndrome should not be confused with a similar syndrome in chow chow pups that results from dysmyelinogenesis. Dogs with dysmyelinogenesis tend to improve over time (see Chapter 10).

Individual cases of cerebellar hypoplasia have occurred in most species.[4,29,33 36] Animals often have selective loss of the caudal vermis, similar to the Dandy Walker syndrome in humans (Figure 8-8).[35,36] Mechanisms responsible for preferential caudal cerebellar vermis involvement have not been defined. The primitive caudal medullary velum may be abnormally impermeable to cerebrospinal fluid (CSF), thus leading to distention of the embryonic fourth ventricle so that the caudal vermis fails to differentiate properly from the metencephalic alar plates. Some of these animals also have hydrocephalus.

Neonatal syndromes characterized principally by Purkinje cell degeneration and clinical signs at the time of ambulation have been characterized in several breeds, including beagles,[24] Samoyeds,[24] and Irish setters.[37] Severe ataxia, tremor, and dysmetria are the predominant signs. Microscopic lesions include swollen axons and diffuse absence of Purkinje neurons. Irish setters are blind and nonambulatory. Delayed neuronal degeneration and clinical onset are compatible with the abiotrophies (see subsequent discussion).

Degenerative Postnatal Syndromes

Several degenerative diseases that affect the cerebellum have been described in dogs. Cerebellar abiotrophy has been the most frequently reported.

The term *abiotrophy* denotes premature death of neurons caused by disruption of the metabolic processes necessary for cell vitality and function.[38] After a variable period of normal neurologic function, cerebellar signs develop and may progress slowly or rapidly. Purkinje neuron degeneration is most pronounced histologically. Occasionally, granular cells, cerebellar medullary nuclei, and brainstem nuclei are affected.[24] These diseases have been studied most extensively in Kerry blue terriers and Gordon setters in the United States and in rough-coated collies in Australia. Other affected breeds are listed in Table 8-4.

Kerry Blue Terrier Abiotrophy. This syndrome was reported in 1968 in nine dogs from New York and California.[39] Since then additional dogs have been evaluated.[40,41] Pups develop progressive cerebellar dysfunction at 9 to 16 weeks of age. The earliest signs include pelvic limb stiffness and mild head tremor. Hypermetria develops later. Most animals are unable to stand by 10 to 12 months of age. Progressive cerebellar cortical degeneration, with loss of Purkinje cells, has been demonstrated. Degenerative lesions also have been observed in the olivary nuclei, substantia nigra, and caudate nuclei. Autosomal recessive inheritance has been proposed.

Gordon Setter Abiotrophy. This syndrome has been studied in dogs from several states.[42-44] Slowly progressive cerebellar ataxia develops at 6 to 24 months of age. The ataxia worsens but does not prevent the dog from standing. Early signs include mild thoracic limb stiffness, hypermetria, and stumbling. Signs progress slowly and at times even appear static. Diffuse degeneration of cerebellar cortical neurons is seen histologically. Autosomal recessive inheritance is suspected.

Rough-coated Collie Abiotrophy. This syndrome has been noted in dogs in Australia.[45] Signs develop when the dog is 4 to 12 weeks of age and progress fairly rapidly for 1 to 4 weeks. In addition to cerebellar cortical degeneration, lesions also occur in cerebellar and brainstem nuclei. Autosomal recessive inheritance is suspected.

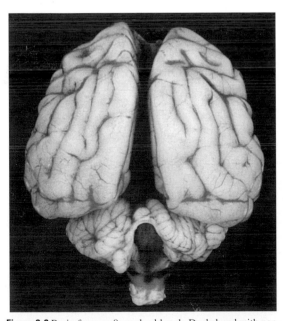

Figure 8-8 Brain from an 8-week-old male Dachshund with nonprogressive ataxia and intention tremor. The caudal vermis is hypoplastic. (From Kornegay JN: Congenital cerebellar diseases. In Kirk RW, editor: *Current veterinary therapy X.* Philadelphia, 1989, WB Saunders.)

Arabian Horse Abiotrophy. Signs of cerebellar ataxia may occur from 1 to 6 months of age.[4,24] The signs may progress rapidly and then stabilize or progress slowly. Most affected foals can walk but have symmetric spasticity of all four limbs and head tremor. The menace reaction may be absent. Nystagmus and opisthotonos are absent. A hereditary basis is suspected. A similar syndrome has been described in Gotland ponies and Oldenberg foals.

Holstein-Friesian Cattle Abiotrophy. Acute cerebellar ataxia has been noted in Holstein cattle, beginning when calves are 3 to 8 months of age.[46] The signs are first rapidly progressive and then become static or slowly progressive. The neck is extended with the ears retracted. Head tremor is common. Dorsomedial strabismus and nystagmus may be present. The menace reaction is often absent. Recessive inheritance is suspected.

Yorkshire Swine Abiotrophy. Acute pelvic limb stiffness and cerebellar ataxia have been observed in Yorkshire pigs at 1 to 5 weeks of age.[24] The clinical signs progress over a few days. Recessive inheritance is suspected.

Neuroaxonal Dystrophy. This abiotrophy affects the neurons of multiple systems, including the cerebellum and associated pathways. Signs may be primarily cerebellar in origin in some dogs (rottweilers, collies, Chihuahuas) and in domestic cats. Similar lesions, predominantly in the spinal cord, are seen in German shepherd dogs, boxers, Suffolk sheep, and Morgan horses (see Chapter 15). Neurons degenerate with prominent axonal swellings called *spheroids*. The age of onset is 5 weeks in cats, 7 weeks in Chihuahuas, 2 to 4 months in collies, and 1 to 2 years in rottweilers. All affected animals have signs of cerebellar ataxia with tremor. Autosomal recessive inheritance is suspected.[38,47]

Neuronal Vacuolation and Degeneration in Rottweilers. This progressive disease affects rottweiler puppies, with neurologic signs developing at 6 to 8 weeks of age.[48,49] It has been reported in rottweilers from the United States and Europe. The onset of clinical signs is characterized by an ataxic and hypermetric gait with severe paraparesis. In some puppies, head ataxia was present, but no cranial nerve deficits were detected. The disease was rapidly progressive, and by 16 to 18 weeks of age, puppies developed quadriparesis, severe placing deficits, and inspiratory dyspnea. At necropsy, no gross lesions were detected. The most prominent histopathologic lesion was widespread central nervous system (CNS) neuronal vacuolation. The lesions were most prominent in the cerebellum, brainstem, and

spinocerebellar tracts. Diagnostic tests did not support a scrapie agent–associated spongiform encephalopathy.[47]

Cerebellar Degeneration in Old English Sheepdogs. This progressive disease affects adult Old English sheep dogs. Clinical signs develop at 6 to 40 months of age and are slowly progressive.[50] Predominant clinical signs include hypermetria of the thoracic limbs, a base wide stance, and an absence of menace response. Later dogs develop truncal ataxia, and some have a fine head tremor. Degenerative changes in the cerebellar cortex consists of localized loss of Purkinje cells, gliosis, and thinning of the molecular layer. Pedigree analysis suggests that the disease is inherited as a simple autosomal recessive defect. Some animals survive for long periods before neurologic deterioration requires euthanasia.

GM_1-Gangliosidosis (Type 2) in Cats. Inherited lysosomal storage diseases can cause progressive cerebellar degeneration.[51] GM_1-gangliosidosis (type 2) occurs in domestic and Siamese cats. Neurologic signs are typically present at 4 to 5 months of age and are characterized by truncal and limb ataxia and intention and muscular tremors. Ocular examination may reveal corneal leukoma. Vacuolation of blood lymphocytes may be detected. Cytoplasmic vacuoles occur throughout the nervous system, eye, and viscera. There is no known treatment.

Adult-onset Cerebellar Abiotrophy of Strattfordshire Terriers. This disease was recently recognized in the United States. It is a slowly progressive degenerative disease with clinical signs developing at 4 to 6 years of age. Early clinical signs are subtle and may include only mild limb ataxia. More typical cerebellar signs develop in weeks to months.

Occipital Dysplasia

Enlargement of the foramen magnum and congenital shortening of C1, most often seen in toy-breed dogs, has been called *occipital dysplasia*.[52,53] Concomitant hydrocephalus has been observed. In severe cases the cerebellum and brainstem are exposed, making these structures vulnerable to compression. The clinical signs reported included cranial neck pain, personality change, and cerebellar ataxia. Many dogs remain asymptomatic. Often the clinical signs are more related to hydrocephalus. The diagnosis was confirmed by radiographs of the skull and cervical vertebrae. Other causes of the signs should be pursued because many normal animals have an enlarged foramen magnum.[54] Marked variation in the shape of the foramen magnum was found in a study of 48 beagle skulls. No impairment of function could be attributed to the change. No brain or spinal cord anomalies were found. An apparent correlation of the larger opening and brachycephalic skulls was noted.[55]

Neoplasia

Primary and secondary tumors can affect the cerebellum. Medulloblastomas selectively arise in the cerebellum in all species and are most likely to occur in younger animals.[29] Choroid plexus papillomas can occur in any part of the ventricular system but are most common in the fourth ventricle. Gliomas and meningiomas may occur in the caudal fossa affecting the cerebellum, but they are more frequent in the rostral fossa. Lymphosarcoma affecting only the cerebellum has been reported in dogs.[56] Neurologic signs were typical of cerebellar disease. Necropsy and histopathologic examination revealed no evidence of lymphosarcoma in other organs.

Signs of cerebellar neoplasia usually progress slowly, but acute exacerbation may follow hemorrhage or obstruction of CSF flow with secondary increased intracranial pressure.

The diagnosis should be made with CT or MRI. Spinal puncture for CSF analysis is contraindicated because of the risk of herniation. Surgical resection of these tumors is difficult because of limited exposure, but debulking and radiation therapy or chemotherapy can provide an alternative to euthanasia.

Vascular Infarction

Occlusion of the rostral cerebellar artery causes infarction of the cerebellum and brainstem, producing a paradoxical vestibular syndrome.[57] The disorder is most commonly observed in older dogs. The clinical signs are preacute, severe, lateralizing, and nonprogressive after the first few hours. Neurologic signs include acute ataxia, head tilt, menace deficit, ventrolateral vestibular strabismus, mild lateralizing proprioceptive deficits, and nystagmus. Diagnosis is based on MRI examination of the brain. Diagnostic findings include hyperintense wedge-shaped lesions in the rostral cerebellum that may extend into the dorsal medulla. CSF may be normal or mild increases in mononuclear cells and protein may be present. The lesions correspond to the distribution of the rostral cerebellar artery. We have observed similar cases in our hospital. Affected dogs usually improve within 5 to 7 days and may totally recover. There is no definitive treatment, and the use of corticosteroids is controversial. Affected dogs should be carefully evaluated for hypertension and hypothyroidism, conditions that predispose to vascular disease and thrombosis.

Miscellaneous Ataxias

Plant-induced Ataxias

Table 15-14 lists common plants that may cause ataxia, tremors, tetany, and other signs related, at least in part, to cerebellar involvement. For a complete discussion, other references should be consulted.[58,59]

Ergotism (Dallis Grass Staggers). This acute disorder occurs in cattle, sheep, and, rarely, horses that ingest Dallis grass or rye infected with the fungus *Claviceps paspali*.[60] The sclerotium of the fungus develops in the seed head of Dallis grass and is present in highest concentrations during wet summers. Toxic fungal alkaloids, found primarily in the mature sclerotia, cause the neurologic signs. A similar syndrome has been described in cattle grazing on Bermuda grass pastures in Louisiana.

Affected animals have an uncoordinated gait when stimulated. Tremors, twitching, and dysmetria are apparent. Affected animals are bright and alert and gradually recover when removed from toxic pastures. Severely affected animals may develop extensor rigidity, opisthotonos, and clonic convulsions. Cattle should be removed from affected pastures. Control of the disorder is achieved by grazing cattle before the seed heads develop or by mowing affected pastures to remove the seed heads. Similar syndromes are seen after grazing on ryegrass and Bermuda grass.[59]

Case Histories

CASE HISTORY 8A

Signalment
Canine, spitz, female, 3 years old.

History
The owner reports a severe lack of coordination and loss of balance since the dog was 6 weeks old. The signs have been nonprogressive.

Physical Examination
Negative except for the neurologic problem.

Neurologic Examination*
A. Observation
  1. Mental status: Alert
  2. Posture: Severe symmetric truncal ataxia; head tremors; no head tilt or circling
  3. Gait: Severe hypermetria and ataxia; wide-based stance; intention tremors of the head and the body
B. Palpation
C. Postural reactions

---

*0, Absent; +1, decreased; +2, normal; +3, exaggerated; +4, very exaggerated or clonus; *PL*, pelvic limb; *TL*, thoracic limb.

Left	Reactions	Right
	Proprioceptive positioning	
+2	PL	+2
+2	TL	+2
Dysmetric	Wheelbarrowing	Dysmetric
	Hopping	
+2	PL	+2
+2	TL	+2
+2	Extensor postural thrust	+2
+1 to +2	Hemistand-hemiwalk	+1 to +2
	Placing, tactile	
Hypermetric	PL	Hypermetric
Hypermetric	TL	Hypermetric
	Placing, visual	
Hypermetric	TL	Hypermetric

D. Spinal reflexes

Left	Reflex (Spinal Segment)	Right
	Quadriceps (L4-L6)	
+2 to +3		+2 to +3
	Extensor carpi radialis (C7-T1)	
+2		+2
	Triceps (C7-T1)	
+2		+2
	Flexion, PL (L5-S1)	
+2		+2
	Flexion, TL (C6-T1)	
+2		+2
+0	Crossed extensor	+0
	Perineal (S1-S2)	
+2		+2

E. Cranial nerves

Left	Nerve—Function (Response, Test)	Right
+2	CN II—vision (menace)	+2
Normal	CN II, III—pupil size	Normal
+2	(Stimulus left eye)	+2
+2	(Stimulus right eye)	+2
Normal	CN II—fundus	Normal
	CN III, IV, VI	
+0	(Strabismus)	+0
+0	(Nystagmus)	+0
Normal	CN V—sensation	Normal

Left		Right
Normal	CN V—mastication	Normal
Normal	CN VII—facial muscles	Normal
+2	(Palpebral)	+2
Normal	CN IX, X—swallowing	Normal
Normal	CN XII—tongue	Normal

F. Sensation: Location
Hyperesthesia: None
Superficial pain: Normal
Deep pain: Normal

Complete sections G and H before reviewing the case summary.

G. Assessment (anatomic diagnosis and estimation of prognosis)

H. Plan (diagnostic)

Rule-outs	Procedure
1.	
2.	
3.	
4.	

CASE HISTORY 8B

Signalment
Canine, Pekingese, male, 2 years old.

History
Progressive lack of coordination and falling from side to side in past 72 hours. The head swings from side to side and bobs up and down. No history of trauma exists, and no other signs are present.

Physical Examination
Normal except for the neurologic problem.

Neurologic Examination*
A. Observation
   1. Mental status: Alert, hyperventilating
   2. Posture: Sternal recumbency, rolls to right, extreme head tilt to right
   3. Gait: Cannot stand; moderate truncal and severe head ataxia; head drop is present; severe dysmetria of limbs
B. Palpation: Negative
C. Postural reactions

Left	Reactions	Right
	Proprioceptive positioning	
+1 to +2	PL	+1
+0 to +1	TL +0 to	+1
+2	Wheelbarrowing	+1
	Hopping	
+1	PL	+0
+1 to+2	TL	+1

*0, Absent; +1, decreased; +2, normal; +3, exaggerated; +4, very exaggerated or clonus; *PL*, pelvic limb; *TL*, thoracic limb.

Left	Reactions	Right
+1	Extensor postural thrust	+0
+0	Hemistand-hemiwalk	+0
	Placing, tactile	
+0	PL	+0
+1	TL	+0 to +1
	Placing, visual	
+1	TL	+0 to +1

D. Spinal reflexes

Left	Reflex (Spinal Segment)	Right
+3	Quadriceps (L4-L6)	+4
+3	Extensor carpi radialis (C7-T1)	+3
+3	Triceps (C7-T1)	+3
+3	Flexion, PL (L5-S1)	+3
+2	Flexion, TL (C6-T1)	+2
+0	Crossed extensor	Present
+2	Perineal (S1-S2)	+2

E. Cranial nerves

Left	Nerve—Function (Response, Test)	Right
+2	CN II—vision (menace)	+2
Normal	CN II, III—pupil size	Normal
+2	(Stimulus left eye)	+2
+2	(Stimulus right eye)	+2
Normal	CN II—fundus	Normal
+0	CN III, IV, VI	+0
Positional-fast phase to left	(Strabismus) (Nystagmus)	Positional-left
Normal	CN V—sensation	Normal
Normal	CN V—mastication	Normal
Normal	CN VII—facial muscles	Normal
+2	(Palpebral)	+2
Normal	CN IX, X—swallowing	Normal
Normal	CN XII—tongue	Normal

F. Sensation: Location
Hyperesthesia: None
Superficial pain: Good perception
Deep pain: Good perception

Complete sections G and H before reviewing the case summary

G. Assessment (anatomic diagnosis and estimation of prognosis)

H. Plan (diagnostic)

Rule-outs	*Procedure*
1.	
2.	
3.	
4.	

CASE HISTORY 8C

Signalment
Feline, domestic, male, 6 months old.

History
The cat has been ill for 10 days. He is depressed, confused, ataxic, and sleeps most of the time. He has gotten progressively worse.

Physical Examination
The cat is dehydrated, thin, and extremely depressed. His temperature is 102.5° F.

Neurologic Examination*
A. Observation
   1. Mental status: Depressed, stuporous; grinds teeth when aroused
   2. Posture: Recumbent, slight head tilt
   3. Gait: Tetraparesis; falls to left and right when forced to stand; thoracic limbs are extended
B. Palpation: Hypertonus of thoracic limbs
C. Postural reactions

Left	Reactions	Right
	Proprioceptive positioning	
+1	PL	+1
+0 to +1	TL	+0 to +1
+1	Wheelbarrowing	+1
	Hopping	
+1	PL	+1
+1	TL	+1
+1	Extensor postural thrust	+1
+0	Hemistand-hemiwalk	+0
	Placing, tactile	
+1 to +2	PL	+1 to +2
+1	TL	+1
	Placing, visual	
+1	TL	+1

*0, Absent; +1, decreased; +2, normal; +3, exaggerated; +4, very exaggerated or clonus; *PL*, pelvic limb; *TL*, thoracic limb.

D. Spinal reflexes

Left	Reflex (Spinal Segment)	Right
+3	Quadriceps (L4-6)	+3
+2	Extensor carpi radialis (C7-T1)	+2
+2	Triceps (C7-T1)	+2
+3	Flexion, PL (L5-S1)	+3
+3	Flexion, TL (C6-T1)	+3
Present	Crossed extensor	+0
+2	Perineal (S1-S2)	+2

E. Cranial nerves

Left	Nerve—Function (Response, Test)	Right
+2	CN II—vision (menace)	+2
Normal +2 +2	CN II, III—pupil size (Stimulus left eye) (Stimulus right eye)	Normal +2 +2
Normal	CN II—fundus	Normal
+0 Rotatory	CN III, IV, VI (Strabismus) (Nystagmus)	+0 Rotatory
Normal	CN V—sensation	Normal
Normal	CN V—mastication	Normal
Normal +2	CN VII—facial muscles (Palpebral)	Normal +2
Normal	CN IX, X—swallowing	Normal
Normal	CN XII—tongue	Normal

F. Sensation: Location
    Hyperesthesia: None
    Superficial pain: Good
    Deep pain: Good
Complete sections G and H before reviewing the case summary
G. Assessment (anatomic diagnosis and estimation of
    prognosis)
H. Plan (diagnostic)

   Rule-outs   *Procedure*
   1.
   2.
   3.
   4.

CASE HISTORY 8D

Signalment
Feline, domestic, female, 2 years old.

History
The cat developed acute ataxia and lack of coordination. The head tilts to the right and the cat circles right. Her appetite is good. No history of previous ear infection exists.

Physical Examination
Otic examination is negative.

Neurologic Examination[*]
A. Observation
    1. Mental status: Alert
    2. Posture: Circles to the right; head tilts to the right; falls
       to the right
    3. Gait: Asymmetric ataxia; the cat drifts and falls to the
       right
B. Palpation: Negative
C. Postural reactions

Left	Reactions	Right
	Proprioceptive positioning	
+2	PL	+2
+2	TL	+2
+2	Wheelbarrowing	Dysmetria
+2	Hopping, PL	+2
+2	Extensor postural thrust	+2
Ataxia	Hemistand-hemiwalk	Ataxia
	Placing, tactile	
+2	PL	+2
+2	TL	+2
	Placing, visual	
+2	TL	+2

D. Spinal reflexes

Left	Reflex (Spinal Segment)	Right
+2	Quadriceps (L4-6)	+2
+2	Extensor carpi radialis (C7-T1)	+2
+2	Triceps (C7-T1)	+2
+2	Flexion, PL (L5-S1)	+2

---

[*]*0*, Absent; *+1*, decreased; *+2*, normal; *+3*, exaggerated; *+4*, very exaggerated or clonus; *PL*, pelvic limb; *TL*, thoracic limb.

	Flexion, TL	
+2	(C6-T1)	+2
+0	Crossed extensor	+0
+2	Perineal (S1-2)	+2

E. Cranial nerves

Left	Nerve—Function (Response, Test)	Right
+2	CN II—vision (menace)	+2
Normal	CN II, III—pupil size	Normal
+2	(Stimulus left eye)	+2
+2	(Stimulus right eye)	+2
Normal	CN II—fundus	Normal
+0	CN III, IV, VI (Strabismus)	Ventrolateral when head is elevated
Horizontal-fast phase to left	(Nystagmus)	Horizontal-fast phase to left
Normal	CN V—sensation	Normal
Normal	CN V—mastication	Normal
Normal	CN VII—facial muscles	Normal
+2	(Palpebral)	+2
Normal	CN IX, X—swallowing	Normal
Normal	CN XII—tongue	Normal

F. Sensation: Location
   Hyperesthesia: None
   Superficial pain: Normal
   Deep pain: Normal
Complete sections G and H before reviewing the case summary.
G. Assessment (anatomic diagnosis and estimation of prognosis)
H. Plan (diagnostic)

Rule-outs	Procedure
1.	
2.	
3.	
4.	

CASE HISTORY 8E

Signalment
14-year-old female spayed border collie.

History
Three days ago, this dog developed acute nonprogressive tetraparesis, severe ataxia, right head tilt, and falling to the right. The dog has a long-standing history or pelvic limb lameness

and hormone-responsive urinary incontinence and has been receiving diethylstilbesterone, phenylpropanolamine, and nonsteroidal antiinflammatory agents. Medications were stopped 3 days ago, and the dog has steadily improved.

Physical Examination
No abnormalities were detected.

Neurologic Examination*
A. Observation
   1. Mental status: Alert and responsive
   2. Posture: When supported, dog is very ataxic and has right head tilt.
   3. Gait: Reluctant to walk. Prefers to lie in sternal recumbancy. Base-wide stance and hypermetric in thoracic limbs (worse right compared to left).
B. Palpation: Negative
C. Postural reactions

Left	Reactions	Right
	Proprioceptive positioning	
+1-+2	PL	+1
+1-+2	TL	+1
NE	Wheelbarrowing	NE
	Hopping	
+2	PL	+1
+2	TL	+1
	Extensor postural thrust	
NE	Hemistand-hemiwalk	NE
	Placing-tactile	
NE	PL	NE
NE	TL	NE
	Placing-visual	
NE	TL	NE

D. Spinal reflexes

Left	Reflexes (Spinal Segment)	Right
+2	Quadriceps (L4-6)	+2
NE	Extensor carpi radialis (C7-T1)	NE
NE	Triceps (C7-T1)	NE
+2	Flexion-PL (L5-S1)	+2

*0, Absent; +1, decreased; +2, normal; +3, exaggerated; +4, very exaggerated or clonus; *PL*, pelvic limb; *TL*, thoracic limb.

+2	Flexion-TL (C6-T1)	+2
0	Crossed Extensor	0
+2	Perineal	+2

E. Cranial nerves

Left	Nerve—Function (Response, Test)	Right
+2	CN II—Vision (menace)	+2
Normal +2 +2	CN II, III—pupil size (Stimulate left eye) (Stimulate right eye)	Normal +2 +2
Normal	CN II—fundus	Normal
None	CN III, IV, VI (Strabismus)	Positional-ventrolateral
Rotary to vertical to left	(Nystagmus)	Rotary to vertical to left
+2	CN V—sensation	+2
+2	CN V—mastication	+2
+2	CN VII—facial muscles (Palpebral)	+2
+2	CN IX, X—swallowing	+2
Normal	CN XII—tongue	Normal

F. Sensation: Location
    Hyperesthesia: None
    Superficial pain: +2
    Deep pain: +2
Complete sections G and H before reviewing the case summary.
G. Assessment (anatomic diagnosis and estimation of prognosis)
H. Plan (diagnostic)

Rule-outs	Procedure
1.	
2.	
3.	
4.	

CASE HISTORY 8F

Signalment
14-week-old miniature schnauzer male.

History
Ataxia and mild head tremors developed at 10 to 11 weeks of age and have slowly worsened. Puppy has received all vaccinations at appropriate intervals and is eating and growing normally. Ticks have been found on the puppy during the past 2 to 3 weeks.

Physical Examination
No abnormalities detected.

Neurologic Examination[*]
A. Observation
    1. Mental status: Alert and responsive
    2. Posture: Base wide stance, truncal swaying, and mild head tremor. No head tilt.
    3. Gait: Marked hypermetria of all limbs, marked truncal ataxia, and falls in all directions.
B. Palpation: No abnormalities detected
C. Postural reactions

Left	Reactions Proprioceptive Positioning	Right
+1-+2	PL	+2
0-+1	TL	+2
+1-+2	Wheelbarrowing	+2
	Hopping	
+1-+2	PL	+2
+1	TL	+2
+2	Extensor postural thrust	+2
NE	Hemistand-hemiwalk	NE
	Placing-tactile	
+2	PL	+2
+2	TL	+2
	Placing-visual	
+2	TL	+2

D. Spinal reflexes

Left	Reflexes (Spinal Segment)	Right
+2	Quadriceps (L4-6)	+2
NE	Extensor carpi radialis (C7-T1)	NE
NE	Triceps (C7-T1)	NE
+2	Flexion-PL (L5-S1)	+2
+2	Flexion-TL (C6-T1)	+2
None	Crossed extensor	None
+2	Perineal	+2

[*]*0*, Absent; *+1*, decreased; *+2*, normal; *+3*, exaggerated; *+4*, very exaggerated or clonus; *PL*, pelvic limb; *TL*, thoracic limb.

E. Cranial nerves

Left	Nerve—Function (Response, Test)	Right
0	CN II—Vision (menace)	0
Normal +2 +2	CN II, III—pupil size (Stimulate left eye) (Stimulate right eye)	Normal +2 +2
Normal	CN II—fundus	Normal
0	CN III, IV, VI (Strabismus)	0
0	(Nystagmus)	0
+2	CN V—sensation	+2
+2	CN V—mastication	+2
+2	CN VII—facial muscles (Palpebral)	+2
+2	CN IX, X—swallowing	+2
Normal	CN XII—tongue	Normal

F. Sensation: Location
   Hyperesthesia: None
   Superficial pain: +2
   Deep pain: +2

Complete sections G and H before reviewing the case summary.

G. Assessment (anatomic diagnosis and estimation of prognosis)

H. Plan (diagnostic)

Rule-outs	Procedure
1.	
2.	
3.	
4.	

ASSESSMENT 8A

Anatomic Diagnosis

The dog has generalized symmetric ataxia associated with head tremor and intention tremor. No paresis, cranial nerve dysfunction, or vestibular signs are present. The signs are related to generalized cerebellar disease. A congenital or early postnatal syndrome is suspected because the signs began at an early age. The signs have been nonprogressive, which tends to rule out abiotrophies, storage diseases, and inflammation. A good choice for the diagnosis would be cerebellar hypoplasia. Parvoviral DNA can be amplified from archival brains (cerebellum) of some dogs with cerebellar hypoplasia. This suggests that in utero parvoviral infection might be associated with cerebellar hypoplasia in dogs.[96]

Diagnostic Plan (Rule-outs)

1. Cerebellar hypoplasia: CT and particularly MRI may provide anatomic evidence of hypoplasia
2. Cerebellar abiotrophy: History, histopathology
3. Inflammation: CSF analysis (if early in course); this test probably is not useful at this time

Therapeutic Plan

None. The disease is untreatable.

Client Education

The dog will not improve but can function as a pet in her current condition. The dog should not be bred because the disease may be hereditary.

Case Summary

The presumptive diagnosis was cerebellar hypoplasia. A follow-up was not recorded.

ASSESSMENT 8B

Anatomic Diagnosis

Both cerebellar (head drop, head ataxia, truncal ataxia) and vestibular (head tilt, rolling, nystagmus) signs are present. Because the dog has motor deficits associated with the vestibular signs, central vestibular (brainstem) disease probably is present. A lesion or a disease involving the cerebellomedullary junction could cause both cerebellar and central vestibular signs. The progressive course suggests inflammation, neoplasia, or degeneration.

Diagnostic Plan (Rule-outs)

1. Encephalitis: CSF examination (white blood cells 380, 88% lymphocytes, 12% neutrophils; protein 120 mg/dl), CSF culture (negative), conjunctival smear-fluorescent antibody titer for distemper (negative)
2. Neoplasia: CT (negative)
3. Degeneration: Check complete blood cell (CBC) count and profile (normal) for evidence of polysystemic disease

Therapeutic Plan

Antibiotics, although they are unlikely to be beneficial.

Client Education

The prognosis is guarded because a viral infection is most likely present. Distemper encephalitis is a possibility; however, other potentially treatable or reversible diseases should be considered. CSF titers to different agents should be evaluated.

Case Summary

The diagnosis was nonsuppurative encephalitis of unknown etiology. The dog recovered in 6 weeks.

ASSESSMENT 8C

Anatomic Diagnosis

The predominant signs are those of central vestibular disease (vestibular signs plus postural reaction abnormalities = brainstem disease). The severe depression and altered mental attitude could be of cerebral or brainstem origin. Inflammation or degeneration is most probable.

Diagnostic Plan (Rule-outs)

1. Infectious diseases, including feline infectious peritonitis (FIP), bacterial, fungal, protozoal, or viral agents: CSF analysis (white blood cells 200, 90% segmented neutrophils, 10% lymphocytes; protein 120 mg/dl), electron microscopy (negative), culture (negative), fundus examination (negative)
2. Thiamine deficiency: Response to thiamine therapy

Therapeutic Plan
1. Intramuscular thiamine: No response
2. Antibiotics were given intravenously for 5 days, with continued progression of the disease

Client Education
The prognosis is poor.

Case Summary
Noneffusive FIP was suspected based on CSF analysis results. The diagnosis was confirmed by necropsy evaluation.

ASSESSMENT 8D

Anatomic Diagnosis
The circling, head tilt, asymmetric ataxia, positional strabismus, and spontaneous nystagmus with the quick left phase suggest a right vestibular lesion. The absence of paresis localizes the lesion to the right peripheral vestibular system.

Diagnostic Plan (Rule-outs)
1. Acute bacterial otitis media interna: Otoscopic examination (negative), skull radiography (negative), CBC and chemistries (normal)
2. Trauma: History, physical examination, and radiography
3. Feline vestibular syndrome: Exclude diagnostic plan numbers 1 and 2

Therapeutic Plan
Although otitis media interna is unlikely, one still could choose to treat the cat with the appropriate antibiotics, just to be safe. In this case the cat was treated with a broad-spectrum antibiotic for 10 days.

Client Education
Feline vestibular syndrome is a disease of unknown cause and no specific therapy is known. Recovery usually takes 3 to 6 weeks.

Case Summary
The cat recovered in 3 weeks. The presumptive diagnosis was feline vestibular syndrome.

ASSESSMENT: 8E

Anatomic Diagnosis
The clinical signs are those of an acute vestibular syndrome (peripheral, central, or paradoxical) localized primarily to the right side. The presence of paresis detected on examination of postural reactions strongly suggests a lesion in the right anterior dorsal medulla affecting vestibular nuclei. The marked hypermetria noted in the right thoracic limb suggests involvement of the cerebellum or cerebellar peduncles. The signs had an acute onset and were not progressive. Categories of neurologic disease with these characteristics include trauma, inflammation (may be progressive), and infarction. Given the history, neurologic findings, and improvement without definitive treatment, infarction of the right dorsal anterior medulla and cerebellum is the leading rule-out in this case (see the article by Berg and Joseph, 2003).[57]

Diagnostic Plan (Rule-outs)
1. Infarction of the anterior cerebellar artery or acute hemorrhage associated with neoplasia: MRI of the brain would be the best diagnostic procedure in this case. The owner declined the procedure because the dog was improving.

2. Brainstem inflammation: CSF analysis and serology for rickettsial infection are indicated. CSF analysis was normal, and no titer to *Ehrlichia canis* was detected.
3. Trauma: There is no history of trauma in this case.

Therapeutic Plan
Only supportive therapy was given because there is no definitive treatment for CNS infarction.

Client Education
The owner, a physician, was well informed regarding the prognosis of stroke patients. A guarded prognosis was given for total recovery of neurologic function, but the marked improvement over the last 48 hours provides evidence for a more optimistic prognosis.

Case Summary
The presumptive diagnosis was brainstem and cerebellar infarction secondary to occlusion of the right anterior cerebellar artery. The dog made an excellent recovery. Conditions that might predispose an animal to CNS infarction such as systemic hypertension and hypothyroidism were ruled out. A definitive diagnosis was not made in this case.

ASSESSMENT 8F

Anatomic Diagnosis
The preponderance of clinical signs suggests generalized cerebellar disease; however, upper motor neuron signs are present in the left pelvic and thoracic limbs. A lesion in the left brainstem or cranial cervical spinal cord could explain these findings. The absent menace response could be explained by generalized cerebellar disease, bilateral occipital cortical disease, or just normal behavior in this puppy. The clinical signs are progressive and thus more indicative of inflammatory or degenerative diseases versus congenital disorders.

Diagnostic Plan (Rule-outs)
1. Encephalomyelitis: Toxoplasmosis, neosporosis, distemper including postvaccinal encephalitis and rickettsial diseases should be considered and ruled out: Serology and CSF examination are indicated
2. Cerebellar abiotrophy: Given the age and progressive nature of the disorder, this degenerative disorder should be strongly considered. Definitive diagnosis is histopathology.

Therapeutic Plan
The referring veterinarian placed the dog on doxycycline, and 2 weeks later the dog was worse and definitive tests were performed. Spinal fluid analysis was normal, and serology for rickettsial infections was negative. No abnormalities were detected in CBC, biochemical profile, or urinalysis. Given the likely diagnosis of degenerative CNS disease, the owner elected euthanasia and necropsy. The histopathologic diagnosis was abiotrophy affecting the cerebellum and brainstem.

References

1. Little CJL: Otitis media in the dog: a review, *Vet Annu* 29:183-188, 1989.
2. Holliday T: Clinical signs of acute and chronic experimental lesions of the cerebellum, *Vet Res Commun* 3:259-278, 1980.

3. Schunk KL, Averill DR: Peripheral vestibular syndrome in the dog: a review of 83 cases, *J Am Vet Med Assoc* 182:1354-1357, 1983.

4. Mayhew IG: *Large animal neurology: a handbook for veterinary clinicians.* Philadelphia, 1989, Lea & Febiger.

5. Jensen R, et al: Cause and pathogenesis of middle ear infection in young feedlot cattle, *J Am Vet Med Assoc* 182:967-972, 1983.

6. Olson LD: Gross and microscopic lesions of middle and inner ear infections in swine, *Am J Vet Res* 42:1433-1440, 1981.

7. Geiser DR, Henton JR, Held JP: Tympanic bulla, petrous temporal bone, and hyoid apparatus disease in horses, *Compendium Continuing Educ Pract Vet* 10:740-756, 1988.

8. Power HT, Watrous BJ, de Lahunta A: Facial and vestibulocochlear nerve disease in six horses, *J Am Vet Med Assoc* 183:1076-1080, 1983.

9. Blythe LL, et al: Vestibular syndrome associated with temporohyoid joint fusion and temporal bone fracture in three horses, *J Am Vet Med Assoc* 185:775-781, 1984.

10. Remedios AM, Fowler JD, Pharr JW: A comparison of radiographic versus surgical diagnosis of otitis media, *J Am Anim Hosp Assoc* 27:183-188, 1991.

11. Mansfield PD: Ototoxicity in dogs and cats, *Compendium Continuing Educ Pract Vet* 12:332-337, 1990.

12. Beckman SL, Henry WB, Jr, Cechner P: Total ear canal ablation combining bulla osteotomy and curettage in dogs with chronic otitis externa and media, *J Am Vet Med Assoc* 196:84-90, 1990.

13. Matthiesen DT, Scavelli T: Total ear canal ablation and lateral bulla osteotomy in 38 dogs, *J Am Anim Hosp Assoc* 26:257-267, 1990.

14. Burke EE, Moise NS, de Lahunta A, et al: Review of idiopathic feline vestibular syndrome in 75 cats, *J Am Vet Med Assoc* 187:941-943, 1985.

15. Schunk KL: Diseases of the vestibular system, *Prog Vet Neurol* 1:247-254, 1990.

16. de Lahunta A: *Veterinary neuroanatomy and clinical neurology,* 2nd ed. Philadelphia, WB Saunders, 1983.

17. Chrisman CL: *Problems in small animal neurology,* 2nd ed. Philadelphia, 1991, Lea & Febiger.

18. Lee M: Congenital vestibular disease in a German shepherd dog, *Vet Rec* 113:571, 1983.

19. Forbes S, Cook JR: Congenital peripheral vestibular disease attributed to lymphocytic labyrinthitis in two related litters of Doberman pinscher pups, *J Am Vet Med Assoc* 198:447-449, 1991.

20. Indrieri RJ, Taylor RF: Vestibular dysfunction caused by squamous cell carcinoma involving the middle ear and inner ear in two cats, *J Am Vet Med Assoc* 184:471-473, 1984.

21. Fischer A, Obermaier G: Brainstem auditory–evoked potentials and neuropathologic correlates in 26 dogs with brain tumors, *J Vet Intern Med* 8:363-369, 1994.

22. Kapatkin AS, et al: Results of surgery and long-term follow up in 31 cats with nasopharyngeal polyps, *J Am Anim Hosp Assoc* 26:387-392, 1990.

23. Faulkner JE, Busberg SC: Results of ventral bulla osteotomy for treatment of middle ear polyps in cats, *J Am Anim Hosp Assoc* 26:496-499, 1990.

24. de Lahunta A: Comparative cerebellar disease in domestic animals, *Compendium Continuing Educ Pract Vet* 2:8-19, 1980.

25. Csiza C, et al: Spontaneous feline ataxia, *Cornell Vet* 62:300-322, 1972.

26. Herndon R, Margolis G, Kilham L: The synaptic organization of the malformed cerebellum induced by perinatal infection with the feline panleukopenia virus (PLV), *J Neuropathol Exp Neurol* 30:196-205, 1971.

27. Carpenter M, Harter D: A study of congenital feline cerebellar malformations: an anatomic and physiologic evaluation of agenetic defects, *J Comp Neurol* 105:5194, 1956.

28. Greene CE, Gorgacz EJ, Martin CL: Hydranencephaly associated with feline panleukopenia, *J Am Vet Med Assoc* 180:767-768, 1982.

29. Kornegay JN: Ataxia of the head and limbs: cerebellar diseases in dogs and cats, *Prog Vet Neurol* 1:255-274, 1990.

30. Wilson T, de Lahunta A, Confer L: Cerebellar degeneration in dairy calves: clinical, pathologic, and serologic features of an epizootic caused by bovine viral diarrhea virus, *J Am Vet Med Assoc* 183:544-545, 1983.

31. Kornegay JN: Congenital cerebellar diseases of dogs and cats. In Kirk RW, editor: *Current veterinary therapy X.* Philadelphia, 1989, WB Saunders.

32. Knecht C, et al: Cerebellar hypoplasia in chow chows, *J Am Anim Hosp Assoc* 15:51-53, 1979.

33. O'Sullivan B, McPhee C: Cerebellar hypoplasia of genetic origin in calves, *Aust Vet J* 51:469-471, 1975.

34. Harari J, et al: Cerebellar agenesis in two canine littermates, *J Am Vet Med Assoc* 182:622-623, 1983.

35. Pass DA, Howell JMcC, Thompson RR: Cerebellar malformation in two dogs and a sheep, *Vet Pathol* 18:405-407, 1981.

36. Kornegay J: Cerebellar vermian hypoplasia in dogs, *Vet Pathol* 23:374-379, 1986.

37. Palmer AC, Payne JE, Wallace ME: Hereditary quadriplegia and amblyopia in the Irish Setter, *J Small Anim Pract* 14:343-352, 1973.

38. de Lahunta A: Abiotrophy in domestic animals: a review, *Can J Vet Res* 54:65-76, 1990.

39. de Lahunta A, Averill DR: Hereditary cerebellar cortical and extrapyramidal nuclear abiotrophy in Kerry Blue terriers, *J Am Vet Med Assoc* 168:1119-1124, 1976.

40. Montgomery D, Storts R: Hereditary striatonigral and cerebello-olivary degeneration of the Kerry Blue terrier, II: ultrastructural lesions in the caudate nucleus and cerebellar cortex, *J Neuropathol Exp Neurol* 43:263-275, 1984.

41. Montgomery D, Storts R: Hereditary striatonigral and cerebello-olivary degeneration of the Kerry blue terrier, *Vet Pathol* 20:143-159, 1983.

42. de Lahunta A, et al: Hereditary cerebellar cortical abiotrophy in the Gordon setter, *J Am Vet Med Assoc* 177:538-541, 1980.

43. Cork LC, Troncoso JC, Price DL: Canine inherited ataxia, *Ann Neurol* 9:492-499, 1981.

44. Steinberg S, Troncoso J, Cork L, et al: Clinical features of inherited cerebellar degeneration in Gordon setters, *J Am Vet Med Assoc* 179:886-890, 1981.

45. Hartley WJ, et al: Inherited cerebellar degeneration in the rough coated collie, *Aust Vet Pract* 8:79-85, 1978.

46. White ME, Whitlock RH, de Lahunta A: A cerebellar abiotrophy of calves, *Cornell Vet* 65:476-491, 1975.

47. Clark RG, Hartley WJ, Burgess GS, et al: Suspected neuroaxonal dystrophy in collie sheep dogs, *N Z Vet J* 30:102 103, 1982.

48. Kortz GD, et al: Neuronal vacuolation and spinocerebellar degeneration in young rottweiler dogs, *Vet Pathol* 34:296-302, 1997.

49. van den Ingh TS, Mandigers PJ, van Nes JJ: A neuronal vacuolar disorder in young rottweiler dogs, *Vet Rec* 142:245-247, 1998.

50. Steinberg HS, et al: Cerebellar degeneration in Old English sheepdogs, *J Am Vet Med Assoc* 217:1162-1165, 2000.

51. Dial SM, et al: GM$_1$-Gangliosidosis (Type II) in three cats, *J Am Anim Hosp Assoc* 30:355-359, 1994.

52. Parker AJ, Park RD: Occipital dysplasia in the dog, *J Am Anim Hosp Assoc* 10:520-525, 1974.

53. Bardens JW: Congenital malformations of the foramen magnum in dogs, *Southwest Vet* 18:295-298, 1965.

54. Evans HE, Christensen GC: *Miller's anatomy of the dog.* Philadelphia, WB Saunders, 1979.

55. Watson AG, de Lahunta A, Evans HE: Dorsal notch of foramen magnum due to incomplete ossification of supraoccipital bone in dogs, *J Small Anim Pract* 30:666-673, 1989.

56. Lefbom BK, Parker GA: Ataxia associated with lymphosarcoma in a dog, *J Am Vet Med Assoc* 207:922-923, 1995.

57. Berg JM, Joseph RJ: Cerebellar infarcts in two dogs diagnosed with magnetic resonance imaging, *J Am Anim Hosp* 39:203-207, 2003.

58. Osweiler GD, et al: *Clinical and diagnostic veterinary toxicology,* 3rd ed. Dubuque, IA, Kendall/Hunt Publishing, 1985.

59. Plumlee KH, Galey FD: Neurotoxic mycotoxins: a review of fungal toxins that cause neurological disease in large animals, *J Vet Intern Med* 8:49-54, 1994.

60. Tyler JW, et al: Naturally occurring neurologic disease in calves fed *Claviceps* sp. infected dallis grass hay and pasture, *Prog Vet Neurol* 3:101-106, 1990.

61. Galey FD, et al: Staggers induced by consumption of perennial ryegrass in cattle and sheep from northern California, *J Am Vet Med Assoc* 199:466-470, 1991.

62. Hopper K, Aldrich J, Haskins SC: Ivermecin toxicity in 17 collies, *J Vet Intern Med* 16:89-94, 2002.

63. Nelson OL, et al.: Ivermectin toxicity in an Australian shepherd dog with the MDR1 mutation associated with ivermectin sensitivity in collies, *J Vet Intern Med* 17:354-356, 2003.

64. Oliver JE, Geary JC: Cerebellar anomalies: two cases, *Vet Med Small Anim Clin* 60:697, 1965.

65. Kay WJ, Budelovich GN: Cerebellar hypoplasia and agenesis in the dog, *J Neuropathol Exp Neurol* 29:156, 1970.

66. Regnier AM, et al: Dandy Walker syndrome in a kitten, *J Am Anim Hosp Assoc* 29:514-518, 1993.

67. Thomas JB, Robertson D: Hereditary cerebellar abiotrophy in Australian dogs, *Aust Vet J* 66:301-302, 1989.

68. Carmichael S, Griffiths IR, Harvey MJA: Familial cerebellar ataxia with hydrocephalus in bull mastiffs, *Vet Rec* 112:354-358, 1983.

69. O'Brien D: Hereditary cerebellar ataxia. In *Proceedings of the 11th American College of Veterinary Internal Medicine Forum,* Washington, DC, 1993.

70. Sakai T, et al: Two cases of hereditary quadriplegia and amblyopia in a litter of Irish setters, *J Small Anim Pract* 35:221-223, 1994.

71. Perille AL, et al: Postnatal cerebellar cortical degeneration in Labrador retriever puppies, *Can Vet J* 32:619-621, 1991.

72. Cummings JF, de Lahunta A: A study of cerebellar and cerebral cortical degeneration in miniature poodle pups with emphasis on the ultrastructure of Purkinje cell changes, *Acta Neuropathol (Berl)* 75:261-271, 1988.

73. Inada S, Mochizuki M, Izumo S, et al: Study of hereditary cerebellar degeneration in cats, *Am J Vet Res* 57:296-301, 1996.

74. Cordy DR, Snelbaker HA: Cerebellar hypoplasia and degeneration in a family of Airedale dogs, *J Neuropathol Exp Neurol* 11:324-328, 1952.

75. Yasuba M, et al: Cerebellar cortical degeneration in beagle dogs, *Vet Pathol* 25:315-317, 1988.

76. Gill JM, Hewland ML: Cerebellar degeneration in the border collie, *N Z Vet J* 8:170, 1980.

77. LeCouteur RA, Kornegay JN, Higgins RJ: Late onset progressive cerebellar degeneration of Brittany spaniel dogs. In *Proceedings of the Sixth Annual Veterinary Medical Forum,* Washington, DC, 1988.

78. Tatalick LM, Marks SL, Baszler TV: Cerebellar abiotrophy characterized by granular cell loss in a Brittany, *Vet Pathol* 30:385-388, 1993.

79. Cummings JF, de Lahunta A, Gasteiger EL: Multisystemic chromatolytic neuronal degeneration in Cairn Terriers, *J Vet Intern Med* 5:91-94, 1991.

80. Jaggy A, Vandevelde M: Multisystem neuronal degeneration in cocker spaniels, *J Vet Intern Med* 2:117-120, 1988.

81. Tontitila P, Lindberg LA: ETT fall av cerebellar ataxi hos finsk stovare, *Svoman Elainlaakarilehti* 77:135, 1971.

82. Troncoso JC, Cork LC, Price DL: Canine inherited ataxia: ultrastructural observations, *J Neuropathol Exp Neurol* 44:165-175, 1985.

83. Chrisman CL, Spencer CP, Crane SW, et al: Late onset cerebellar degeneration in a dog, *J Am Vet Med Assoc* 182:717-720, 1983.

84. Chieffo C, et al: Cerebellar Purkinje's cell degeneration and coat color dilution in a family of Rhodesian ridgeback dogs, *J Vet Intern Med* 8:112-116, 1994.

85. Kahrs RF, Scott FW, de Lahunta A: Congenital cerebellar hypoplasia and ocular defects in calves following bovine viral diarrhea-mucosal disease infection in pregnant cattle, *J Am Vet Med Assoc* 156:1443-1450, 1970.

86. Emmerson JL, Delez AL: Cerebellar hypoplasia, hypomyelinogenesis and congenital tremors of pigs associated with prenatal hog cholera vaccination of sows, *J Am Vet Med Assoc* 147:47-54, 1965.

87. Edmonds L, Crenshaw D, Selby LA: Micrognathia and cerebellar hypoplasia in an Aberdeen Angus herd, *J Hered* 64:62-64, 1973.

88. Jeffrey M, Preece BE, Holliman A: Dandy Walker malformation in two calves, *Vet Rec* 126:499-501, 1990.

89. Cudd TA, Mayhew IG, Cotrill CM: Agenesis of the corpus callosum with cerebellar vermian hypoplasia in a foal resembling Dandy Walker syndrome: premortem diagnosis by clinical evaluation and CT scanning, *Equine Vet J* 21:378-381, 1989.

90. Kidd A, et al: A new genetically determined congenital nervous disorder in pigs, *Br Vet J* 142:275-285, 1986.

91. Palmer AC, et al: Cerebellar hypoplasia and degeneration in the young Arab horse: clinical and neuropathological features, *Vet Rec* 93:6266, 1973.

92. Bjorck G, Everz KE, Hansen HJ, et al: Congenital cerebellar ataxia in the Gotland pony breed, *Zentralbl Veterinarmed* 20:341-354, 1973.

93. Poss M, Young S: Dysplastic disease of the cerebellum of an adult horse, *Acta Neuropathol (Berl)* 75:209-211, 1987.

94. Whittington RJ, Morton AG, Kennedy DJ: Cerebellar abiotrophy in crossbred cattle, *Aust Vet J* 66:12-15, 1989.

95. Harper P, Duncan D, Plant J, et al: Cerebellar abiotrophy and segmental axonopathy: two syndromes of progressive ataxia of Merino sheep, *Aust Vet J* 63:18-21, 1986.

96. Schatzberg SJ, Haley NJ, Barr SC, et al: Polymerase chain reaction (PCR) amplification of parvoviral DNA from the brains of dogs and cats with cerebellar hypoplasia. *J Vet Intern Med* 17:538-544, 2003.

Chapter 9

Disorders of the Face, Tongue, Esophagus, Larynx, and Hearing

LESION LOCALIZATION

The problems described in this chapter result from dysfunction of cranial nerves (CNs) V, VII, VIII (cochlear), IX, X, and XII. Disorders of CN VIII (vestibular) are discussed in Chapter 8, and disorders of the cranial nerves associated with vision and the eyes are discussed in Chapter 11. The localization of cranial nerve lesions is presented in Chapters 1 and 2 and is reviewed briefly in this chapter (see Table 2-5 and Figure 1-23).

Injury to cranial nerves may be peripheral (nerve fibers) or central (neurons in the brainstem). Differentiation is based on the results of a careful neurologic examination. Peripheral cranial nerve disorders are characterized by specific nerve deficits with no evidence of appendicular paresis.

Cranial nerve dysfunction resulting from brainstem lesions is characterized by isolated or multiple cranial nerve involvement and, more importantly, by specific brainstem signs such as paresis, central vestibular disease, and depression. Occasionally, the generalized lower motor neuron (LMN) diseases produce cranial nerve signs. These diseases usually are recognized because of LMN signs in the limbs. In some cases, electromyography (EMG) is needed to establish the generalized nature of the neuropathy.

Cranial Nerve V (Trigeminal Nerve)

Anatomy

The motor neurons of CN V are located in the pons near the rostral cerebellar peduncles. The motor fibers are distributed to the muscles of mastication by the mandibular branch of CN V. Sensation to the surface of the head is supplied by CN V through its divisions. The ophthalmic nerve innervates the dorsal eyelids and the cornea, and the maxillary division provides sensation to the ventral eyelids, the face, and the nasal area. The ophthalmic nerve is the sensory arc of the corneal reflex and, together

with the maxillary nerve, the palpebral reflex. The mandibular nerve provides sensation to the lower jaw. Cell bodies of these sensory neurons are located in the trigeminal ganglia. The trigeminal nerve enters the pons just rostral to the origin of the facial and vestibulocochlear nerves. Its sensory axons course caudally through the medulla in the spinal tract of the trigeminal nerve. This tract continues caudally into the first cervical segment. Nerve fibers within this tract synapse on neurons that are located in nuclei distributed along its course.

The anatomic distribution of pain fibers in CN V is of considerable importance in the location of lesions involving the trigeminal nerve. Lesions in the medulla involving the spinal tract of CN V result in ipsilateral loss of facial sensation but no impairment of the masticatory muscles. Loss of both sensory and motor function of the trigeminal nerve usually results from pontine lesions or extramedullary disorders that affect both motor and sensory neurons or fibers. Loss of motor function with no sensory impairment is associated with discrete lesions in the trigeminal motor nucleus in the pons or preferential involvement of the motor nerve fibers.

Clinical Signs

For the reasons just described, sensation may be lost ipsilateral to the lesion. In addition, corneal and palpebral reflexes may be diminished because of interference with the sensory arcs of these reflexes. The pinna of the dog (and probably other species) is innervated by the facial nerve on the concave surface and by branches of C2 on the convex surface, not by the trigeminal nerve (Figure 9-1).[1,2] Diminished conscious reaction to facial stimulation can also be caused by lesions of the somatosensory cerebral cortex. In this case, sensation is decreased but usually not totally absent. Palpebral and corneal reflexes are normal with cortical lesions (Figure 9-2). Bilateral involvement of motor nerves

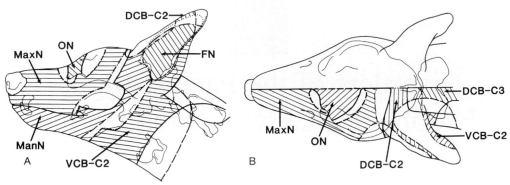

Figure 9-1 Areas of cutaneous innervation of the head that are supplied by one nerve (autonomous zones). **A,** Lateral view. **B,** Dorsal view. *DCB-C2,* Dorsal cutaneous branch of the second cervical nerve; *VCB-C2,* ventral cutaneous branch of the second cervical nerve; *DCB-C3,* dorsal cutaneous branch of the third cervical nerve; *FN,* facial nerve; *MaxN,* maxillary nerve, CN V; *ManN,* mandibular nerve, CN V; *ON,* ophthalmic nerve, CN V. (From Whalen LR, Kitchell RL: Electrophysiologic studies of the cutaneous nerves of the head of the dog, *Am J Vet Res* 44:615, 1983.)

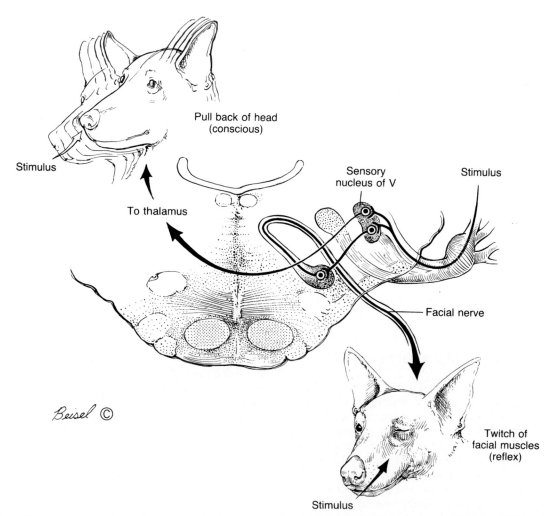

Figure 9-2 Reflex and conscious pain perception pathways of the trigeminal nerve (CN V). (From Greene CE, Oliver JE: Neurologic examination. In Ettinger SJ, editor: *Textbook of veterinary internal medicine,* 2nd ed. Philadelphia, 1983, WB Saunders.)

results in a dropped jaw that cannot be closed voluntarily (mandibular paralysis). The jaw muscles are atonic and become atrophic if the paralysis persists for longer than 7 days. Unilateral motor lesions are difficult to detect until specific muscle atrophy develops.

Cranial Nerve VII (Facial Nerve) Anatomy

The facial nerve innervates the muscles of facial expression. Its neurons are located in the facial nuclei of the rostral medulla (Figure 9-3). Nerve fibers leave the facial nuclei and course dorsomedially and around the abducent nucleus. The fibers leave the ventrolateral surface of the medulla ventral to CN VIII. The facial nerve enters the petrosal bone through the internal acoustic meatus on the dorsal side of CN VIII. The nerve emerges from the skull through the stylomastoid foramen to innervate the muscles of facial expression. A disease involving the inner ear may extend to the facial nerve, resulting in ipsilateral facial palsy. The facial nerve is the main motor pathway for the corneal and palpebral reflexes. Lesions of the upper motor neurons (UMNs) to the facial nucleus may cause abnormal facial expression without loss of facial reflexes.[3]

Clinical Signs

Lesions of CN VII result in ipsilateral facial paresis or paralysis. The lip may droop on the affected side, and food or saliva may fall from that side of the mouth. The nasal philtrum may deviate to the normal side. Drooping of the ear may be observed in animals with erect ears (Figure 9-4). The palpebral fissure may be wider than normal and may fail to close during the palpebral or corneal reflexes. Exposure keratitis is a common sequela of facial nerve injury in dogs, especially in breeds that tend to have ectropion or exophthalmic globes.

Vestibular signs are commonly associated with facial paresis or paralysis because of the close anatomic relationship of the facial and vestibular nerves at the brainstem and in their course through the petrosal bone. These two locations must be differentiated because of the difference in prognosis

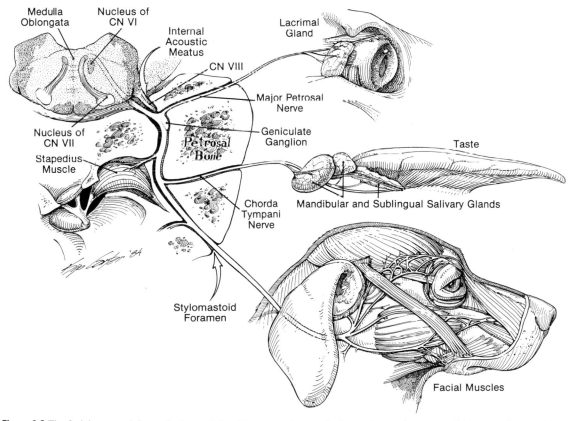

Figure 9-3 The facial nerve originates in the medulla oblongata and enters the internal acoustic meatus of the petrosal bone with the vestibulocochlear nerve (CN VIII). Branches include nerves to the lacrimal glands, stapedius muscle, mandibular and sublingual salivary glands, and sensory fibers for taste. The major component exits the stylomastoid foramen and innervates the muscles of facial expression. Testing for function of the various branches can localize the site of the lesion in facial paralysis.

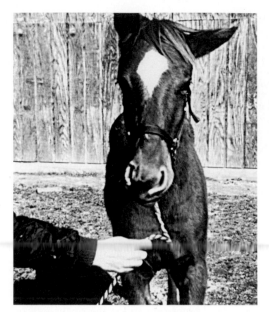

Figure 9-4 A horse with left facial nerve paralysis. Note the drooped ear and deviation of the nose to the right.

and therapy. Lesions at the brainstem result in central vestibular disease, whereas lesions in the petrosal bone cause peripheral vestibular disease. See Chapter 8 for a discussion of these disorders.

Cranial Nerve VIII (Cochlear Nerve)

Anatomy

The vestibular branch of CN VIII is discussed in Chapter 8. The tympanic membrane separates the external ear from the middle ear. Auditory ossicles transmit vibrations from air entering the external ear across the middle ear to the oval window of the inner ear. The waveform is transmitted to the perilymph in the inner ear, moving the basilar membrane containing the hair cells of the spiral organ. Movement of the hair cells causes release of transmitter, activating the cochlear nerve. The bipolar cell bodies of the cochlear nerve form the spiral ganglion in the petrosal bone. Axons extend proximally to join the vestibular neurons in the internal acoustic meatus. They enter the brainstem at the junction of the medulla and pons, terminating on the cochlear nuclei. The central pathway is bilateral and multisynaptic, projecting to the medial geniculate nuclei of the thalamus. Other axons project to several brainstem nuclei and the caudal colliculi in the midbrain. Conscious perception of sound is served by the projection from the geniculate nuclei to the temporal lobes of the cerebral cortex. Although the pathway has significant bilateral

components, the cortical projection is largely from the contralateral ear.[4]

Clinical Signs

Deafness can be classified as either conductive or sensorineural.[5] Conductive deafness occurs due to lesions of the external or middle ear cavities, whereas inner ear lesions lead to sensorineural deafness. Chronic otitis externa or media is the most common cause of conductive deafness. In sensorineural deafness, receptor cells generally fail to develop or are damaged by toxins. Conductive deafness typically causes partial hearing loss and only rarely total loss. Lesions of the cochlear nerve or the receptors cause complete deafness. Unilateral deafness is difficult to recognize clinically without electrophysiologic tests. Central lesions rarely cause clinically detectable hearing loss. Tests for hearing are discussed in Chapters 1 and 4.

Cranial Nerve IX (Glossopharyngeal Nerve), Cranial Nerve X (Vagus Nerve), and Cranial Nerve XI (Accessory Nerve)

Anatomy

These cranial nerves are discussed as a group because their nerve fibers originate from the same medullary nuclei and because they interact to control pharyngeal and laryngeal motor activity. They originate in the nucleus ambiguus in the medulla. The rostral two thirds of this nucleus is involved in swallowing by means of motor impulses through the glossopharyngeal and vagus nerves. The caudal nucleus ambiguus controls the laryngeal and esophageal muscles through the accessory and vagus nerves and branches of the vagus nerves (recurrent laryngeal nerves).

Clinical Signs

Dysphagia is the primary clinical sign of lesions involving the rostral nucleus ambiguus or its nerves (glossopharyngeal, vagus). The gag reflex is absent or depressed. Inspiratory dyspnea from laryngeal paralysis is the primary clinical sign of lesions involving the caudal nucleus ambiguus or its nerves (vagus, recurrent laryngeal). Regurgitation may occur as a result of megaesophagus.

Cranial Nerve XII (Hypoglossal Nerve)

Anatomy

This nerve originates from cell bodies in the medulla, exits the medulla just caudal to the accessory nerve, and innervates the muscles of the tongue.

Clinical Signs

Paresis or paralysis of the tongue is the main clinical sign of bilateral lesions. Affected animals cannot grasp or hold food or water. With unilateral lesions, the tongue, when protruded, tends to deviate toward the side of the lesion. Atrophy of the tongue may be severe (Figure 9-5).

DISEASES

Idiopathic Bilateral Mandibular Nerve Paralysis

Idiopathic trigeminal neuritis that results in sudden bilateral paralysis of the masticatory muscles has been observed in dogs and cats.[4,6] Most dogs and cats recover in 2 to 3 weeks. Extensive bilateral, nonsuppurative inflammation, demyelination, and some axonal degeneration of all portions of the trigeminal nerve and the ganglion, with no brainstem lesions, have been observed at necropsy.[1] More recently, Panciera[7] and colleagues reported a case of polyradiculoganglioneuritis in a 9-year-old Airedale terrier with left-sided Horner's syndrome and left-sided atrophy of the masticatory muscles. Extensive nonsuppurative inflammation was identified in the pre- and post-ganglionic trigeminal nerve trunks. The lesions were more severe on the left side. The Horner's syndrome likely occurred because of the close proximity of ocular sympathetic nerve fibers and the inflamed left trigeminal nerve. In addition, less intense inflammatory lesions were identified in spinal nerve roots and in sciatic and radial nerves. The nature of the inflammatory response supports the notion that the lesions are immune mediated.

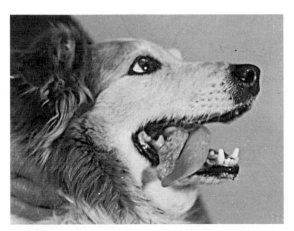

Figure 9-5 A right hypoglossal nerve injury in a dog hit by a car 4 years before. Notice the atrophy of the right side of the tongue. When it is protruded, the tongue deviates to the injured side. The dog submerges its muzzle to drink.

Clinical Signs

The onset of clinical signs is acute or subacute. The jaw hangs open, and the mouth cannot be closed voluntarily. The dog cannot grasp food and has difficulty drinking water. Mild dysphagia may be present. Dehydration and drooling saliva are associated signs. Horner's syndrome is seen in some dogs. Affected dogs are alert and responsive and have no other detectable neurologic deficits. Facial sensation appears normal. The clinical signs are suggestive of bulbar paralysis, which is observed with rabies. Until sufficient evidence has been found to exclude rabies, clinicians should be extremely cautious about examining these dogs. A diagnosis is based on the clinical signs and the absence of other brainstem signs. The disease should not be confused with masticatory myositis. In the latter disease, the mouth is closed, and the animal resents having its jaw moved or manipulated. Pain may be associated with muscle palpation.

Treatment

No definitive treatment is available. Affected animals should be given fluid therapy and enteral caloric support. Pharyngostomy or gastrotomy tubes may be beneficial. The clinician should exercise caution to avoid aspiration pneumonia, especially in dysphagic animals. Performing frequent physical therapy by opening and closing the mouth helps to delay muscle atrophy. Recovery is usually complete in 2 to 3 weeks. Multiple episodes may occur in the same dog. The prognosis is good.

Unilateral Mandibular Neuronopathy

Neoplasia of the mandibular nerve produces chronic progressive unilateral atrophy of the masticatory muscles.[8] Ipsilateral alterations in facial sensation may also be present. Affected dogs tend to be older and are usually presented for examination because of profound unilateral atrophy of the temporalis muscle. Skull radiographs are usually normal, but lesions can be detected by using computed tomography (CT) or magnetic resonance imaging (MRI). Lesions most commonly are found in the proximal trigeminal nerve near the brainstem or in the trigeminal ganglion. Nerve sheath tumors and meningiomas are the most common tumors causing this syndrome. Surgical resection of the neoplastic process has been reported.[8]

Abnormal Facial Sensation

Hyperesthesia of the face is a common problem in humans but is rarely observed in animals. We have seen one cat with unilateral facial hyperesthesia.

Apparently self-inflicted excoriations were on the face. Nonsuppurative meningoencephalitis that involved the trigeminal nerve and ganglion was found on necropsy.

Hypesthesia is seen with many causes of trigeminal nerve damage. One case of bilateral sensory loss with normal motor function in a dog has been reported.[9] The condition did not progress for 18 months. Neuronal loss in the ganglia and axonal loss in the nerve and spinal tract of CN V occurred. No cause could be found. Decreased facial sensation with normal palpebral reflexes indicates a lesion of the sensory cortex or in the pathways from the sensory nucleus of CN V to the cerebrum.

Facial Paralysis

The most common disease that produces facial nerve injury is otitis media interna (see Chapter 8). Polyneuropathies also can affect the facial nerve (see Chapter 7).

Idiopathic Facial Paralysis

This idiopathic disease occurs in the absence of otitis media interna. The clinical signs are similar to those of human facial neuritis (Bell's palsy), the cause of which is not known.[10] Undoubtedly, many cases are caused by viral inflammation, with herpes zoster and herpes simplex viruses suspected.[11] Swelling of the nerve in the petrosal bone causes compression and ischemia, presumably leading to degenerative change.

In a study of 95 cases of facial paralysis in dogs and cats, the condition was judged idiopathic because of lack of any other findings in 74.7% of dogs and 25% of cats.[11] Otitis media interna was the most frequently associated disease in dogs. Hypothyroidism was found in some.[13] In dogs, the cocker spaniel has an increased incidence of facial paralysis.[11,12] Cocker spaniels are also at greater risk of otitis media interna than is the general canine population. Biopsy of facial nerves in two cases showed nerve fiber degeneration and loss of large-diameter myelinated fibers.[12]

Clinical Signs. Facial paralysis usually occurs acutely, is unilateral, and is not associated with vestibular disease or otitis media interna. Affected animals are afebrile and have no polysystemic signs. The course is variable; however, the clinical signs are maximal in 7 days. Recovery takes 3 to 6 weeks. Exposure keratitis occurs commonly because of improper lubrication of the cornea. The contralateral nerve may become involved subsequently.

Diagnosis. All possible causes should be excluded before the diagnosis of idiopathic facial paralysis is made. Otitis media interna is the most common

problem; therefore, a thorough otoscopic examination and imaging of the bulla should be performed. Because hypothyroidism may be associated with facial paralysis,[11] thyroid function should be critically evaluated. EMG of the face and other muscles helps to exclude polyneuropathy.

Treatment. No specific treatment is known. The treatment of Bell's palsy in humans is controversial. Corticosteroids are beneficial if given early.[8] The prognosis for recovery, with or without therapy, is good. If tear production is decreased, artificial tears should be prescribed.

Hemifacial Spasm

This syndrome is rarely observed in dogs or cats. In humans, pressure on the nerve by tortuous vessels in the caudal fossa is the most common cause.[10] A similar syndrome has been reported in dogs with otitis media and presumed facial neuritis and a degenerative lesion of the medulla.[12,13,15] Signs include blepharospasm, elevation of the ear, deviation of the nose to the affected side, and wrinkling or displacement of the upper lip (Figure 9-6). Ipsilateral Horner's syndrome has been reported.[14] This condition may precede signs of facial paralysis. Spasm must be differentiated from contractures secondary to denervation. Muscular contractures result from denervation atrophy and fibrosis. Hemifacial spasm also may occur as a sign of UMN dysfunction. Lesions that isolate the facial nuclear motor neurons from UMN control can result in hemifacial spasm as a result of the loss of

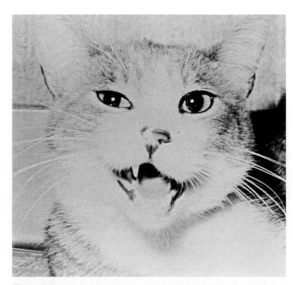

Figure 9-6 A cat with right hemifacial spasm. Note the deviation of the nose and the wrinkling of the right upper lip. Narrowing of the right palpebral fissure is present. The right pupil is smaller than the left, suggesting right-sided Horner's syndrome.

inhibitory interneuronal activity. The palpebral reflex may be hyperactive in that spasm of the eyelids may be observed when the reflex is elicited. This form of hemifacial spasm is associated with other signs of brainstem dysfunction.[4] The diagnosis and treatment are the same as described for facial nerve paralysis.

Facial Nerve Trauma

Injury to one or more branches of the facial nerve can occur in all species. The most common causes are recumbency and tight halters in large animals.[3,16] Closed injury to the facial nerve causes varying degrees of neurapraxia and axonotmesis. Clinical signs caused by neurapraxia usually improve in 2 weeks or less. Axonotmesis requires regrowth of the axon from the site of injury at an approximate rate of 1 inch per month.

Deafness

Most of the information on deafness in animals relates to cats and dogs. Deafness can be acquired or congenital.

Acquired Deafness

Older animals often have some degree of hearing loss. Loss of cells in the spiral ganglion appears to be the primary cause.[17] Attempts have been made to fit dogs with hearing aids, but training dogs to wear them is difficult.

Some polyneuropathies, especially that of hypothyroidism, affect the cochlear nerve.[13] Severe hypoxia may also cause damage to the cochlear nerve or receptors. Neoplasms and trauma may cause deafness in rare cases. Toxic agents and drugs cause progressive cochlear damage (see Table 8-1). Common agents include aminoglycoside antibiotics, salicylates, loop diuretics such as furosemide, and topically applied antiseptics such as chlorhexidine and cetrimide.[5,18] Severe middle ear infections may cause conduction problems, but toxins that reach the inner ear may produce receptor or nerve degeneration.

Congenital Deafness

Animals with congenital deafness have different degrees of abnormal development of the spiral organ of the cochlea.[19] Congenital deafness in large animals has been recognized infrequently, but Mayhew[3] describes a Paint gelding with blanched brown patches that was deaf. Small animals with reported hereditary deafness are listed in Table 9-1. These animals are deaf at birth, but the owner usually does not notice until the animal is 8 to 10 weeks of age. Animals with a known predisposition for congenital deafness, such as the Dalmatian, may be

Table 9-1 Hereditary Deafness in Dogs and Cats: Sources of Additional Information

Breed	Reference
Canine*	
Akita	81
American Staffordshire terrier	81
Australian heeler	82
Australian shepherd	82,83
Beagle	4
Border collie	83
Boston terrier	82
Boxer	82
Bull terrier	83
Catahoula	81
Cocker spaniel	82
Collie	84,85
Dalmatian	84,86,89
Dappled dachshund	81
Doberman pinscher	90
Dogo Argentino	81
English bulldog	82
English setter	82,91
Fox terrier	92
Great Dane	85
Great Pyrenees	81
Maltese	81
Miniature poodle	81
Mongrel	81
Norwegian Dunkerhound	4,86
Old English sheepdog	82
Papillon	81
Pointer	93
Rhodesian ridgeback	81
Scottish terrier	92
Sealyham terrier	92
Shetland sheepdog	82
Shropshire terrier	83
Walker foxhound	94
West Highland white terrier	81
Feline	
White, blue eyes	75-80

*Associated with white or merle color gene.

From Oliver JE: Deafness. In Lorenz MD, Cornelius LM, editors: *Small animal medical diagnosis,* 2nd ed. Philadelphia, 1993, JB Lippincott.

tested with brainstem auditory-evoked potentials (BAER) at about 5 to 6 weeks of age. The BAER is absent in affected dogs. Use of this test to identify unilateral deafness in potential breeding animals is particularly helpful. The BAER is normally not present until 3 weeks of age. Some of the breed groups are actively promoting auditory testing in an effort to reduce the incidence of this hereditary condition. Deafness has been linked to other breed characteristics.[20-22] Dalmatians with incomplete iris pigmentation (heterochromia iridis) are at increased risk of deafness. Absence of patch also correlated with deafness in one study. Lack of eye rim, nose, and ear pigmentation and the size and density of spots were not associated with deafness. These data did not support a definite link between deafness and pigmentation. No treatment for congenital deafness is available.

Laryngeal Paralysis

Unilateral and bilateral paresis or paralysis of the laryngeal muscles has been reported in dogs, cats, and horses. Unilateral paralysis results in moderate inspiratory dyspnea and inspiratory noise. Bilateral paralysis leads to episodes of gagging, cyanosis, severe inspiratory dyspnea, and collapse. The intrinsic muscles of the larynx are innervated by the recurrent laryngeal nerves, which are branches of the vagus nerve. Injury to these nerve fibers or their cell bodies in the caudal nucleus ambiguus results in the clinical signs. Laryngeal paralysis may be acquired or congenital. Congenital causes accounted for 21% to 30% of the cases reported in two studies.[23,24] Laryngeal paralysis is inherited in Bouvier des Flandres and Siberian huskies. Idiopathic laryngeal paralysis occurs frequently in horses.

Hereditary Laryngeal Paralysis in the Bouvier des Flandres

Laryngeal paralysis in Bouvier des Flandres dogs is inherited as an autosomal dominant trait and results in bilateral partial denervation of the larynx.[25,26] The disease results from progressive degeneration of neurons within the nucleus ambiguus, with subsequent wallerian degeneration of the laryngeal nerves. A similar syndrome has been identified in Siberian huskies and Husky crosses.[27]

Clinical Signs. Clinical signs occur at 4 to 6 months of age and include decreasing endurance and noisy breathing. Severe respiratory distress associated with cyanosis or regurgitation occurs in more severely affected dogs. Signs are progressive. Laryngeal stridor, pharyngitis, and tonsillitis are consistent physical findings. Some dogs have bilateral pelvic limb "foot drop" as a result of cranial tibial muscle paralysis.[25]

Diagnosis. Laryngoscopy usually reveals unilateral or bilateral immobility of the vocal folds. In a study of 105 affected Bouvier des Flandres, 28 had bilateral immobility, 71 had immobility of the left vocal fold and moderate abduction of the right on inspiration, 3 had slight motion of both vocal folds, and 3 had abduction of both vocal folds on inspiration.[25]

Electromyographic examination reveals bilateral denervation of the abductor muscles of differing severity. The EMG and laryngoscopic findings usually correlate. Normal motor unit potentials frequently are found in muscles with denervation activity. Histologic examination of the affected muscles reveals characteristic changes of denervation atrophy.

Evidence of laryngeal dysfunction can be established when the animal is as young as 12 weeks with laryngoscopy or, more specifically, with EMG. Normal abduction or adduction or both can be observed even though EMG findings clearly indicate denervation.

Treatment. No cure exists, but surgery may relieve airway obstruction.[23,24,28-30] In a recent study of 140 dogs that underwent various surgical procedures for laryngeal paralysis, postoperative complications were documented in 48 (34.3%), and 20 dogs died.[31] Aspiration pneumonia was the most common complication. Dogs undergoing bilateral arytenoid lateralization had a greater incidence of complications and mortality than dogs that underwent unilateral arytenoid lateralization or partial laryngectomy. Dogs may have a lifelong risk for respiratory complications. Because the disease is inherited as an autosomal dominant trait, it can be eradicated through selective breeding.

Acquired Laryngeal Paralysis in Dogs and Cats

Laryngeal paralysis has been associated with chronic polyneuropathy (see Chapter 7), injury to the vagus nerve during neck surgery, lead and organophosphate toxicity, and retropharyngeal infection (discussed with dysphagia, below).[3,24,27,32-35]

Middle-aged to older large-breed dogs are most commonly affected. Males may be predisposed. Hypothyroidism may cause polyneuropathy with concurrent laryngeal paralysis.[13] Laryngeal paralysis also is infrequently associated with polyradiculoneuritis (coonhound paralysis). Other animals with chronic progressive neuropathy often have laryngeal paralysis. EMG confirms the involvement of laryngeal muscles and establishes the involvement of other muscles.[26,33]

Underlying causes of neuropathy, such as hypothyroidism, should be treated. Many animals require surgical correction of the obstructed airway because of severe inspiratory dyspnea. Several surgical techniques are used.[23,24,28-31]

In recent study of 16 cats with laryngeal paralysis, no breed or sex predilection was found.[36] The clinical signs were similar to those previously described for dogs, and 12 of 16 cats had bilateral disease. Concurrent disease was documented in seven cats. All four cats with unilateral disease were successfully treated with exercise restriction in an indoor environment. Of the 12 cats with bilateral disease, five were treated medically because of concurrent dysphagia, megaesophagus, or laryngeal cancer. Of the seven cats treated surgically, two died within 3 days after surgery, four had long-term successful outcomes, and one was lost to follow-up.[36]

Laryngeal Paralysis in Rottweilers

A progressive degenerative disease characterized by neuronal vacuolation and axonal degeneration has been described in young Rottweiler dogs. Ataxia, paresis, head and muscle tremors, and inspiratory dyspnea have been described (see also Chapter 8). The disease has been reported in dogs from the United States, Europe, and Australia.[37-39]

Laryngeal paralysis associated with polyneuropathy has been reported in five Rottweiler puppies from three unrelated litters.[40] Respiratory signs developed at 11 to 13 weeks of age, and all dogs had tetraparesis and four of five had bilateral lenticular cataracts. The disease is characterized by neurogenic atrophy of distal limb and laryngeal muscles. All dogs were euthanized because of the progressive nature of the laryngeal paralysis and polyneuropathy.

Equine Laryngeal Paralysis

Idiopathic laryngeal paralysis occurs frequently in young, mature, Thoroughbred, hunter types, and draft horses.[41-43] Males are predisposed. Long necks and larger size may correlate with laryngeal paralysis. Hereditability has not been substantiated, but evidence of pathologic changes in foals supports a hereditary basis.[44] Laryngospasm and pharyngospasm also may occur in foals with hyperkalemic periodic paralysis (also see Chapter 7).[45,46]

Because of paralysis of the muscles innervated by the left recurrent laryngeal nerve, the vocal fold cannot be abducted during inspiration and an audible sound ("roaring") is produced. Axonal degeneration with demyelination and regeneration are noted pathologically in the left and, to a lesser degree, right recurrent laryngeal nerves. The disease has been characterized as a distal axonopathy that preferentially affects the longest and largest fibers. Nerves of the limbs and axons of the long fiber tracts of the central nervous system (CNS) are involved in some animals.[41,47] Causes of distal axonopathy include energy-dependent metabolic disorders, antioxidant deficiency at the cell membrane, and filamentous neuropathies.[29] Neuronal metabolic dysfunction would presumably place distal axons of longer nerves at greater risk and also explain the fact that larger horses are predisposed.

Diagnosis is by endoscopic examination of the paralyzed vocal folds. The "slap test" reveals poor adduction of the vocal fold. Slapping the horse behind the withers on the right side should cause adduction of the left arytenoid cartilage.[3] Unilateral atrophy of the muscles of the larynx may be detected on palpation.[48] EMG is also useful.[49] Surgical treatment usually is effective.[3,50-52] In thoroughbred racing horses, performance following surgery improves but not necessarily to pre-disease status in older animals.[53]

Dysphagia

Ingestion of food includes prehension, bolus formation, initiation of swallowing reflex contractions of the pharynx to propel food aborally, relaxation of the upper esophageal sphincter, passage of the bolus into the esophagus, closure of the sphincter, passage of the food down the esophagus, and relaxation of the lower esophageal sphincter.[4] Prehension includes the function of the lips (CN VII), jaw (CN V), and tongue (CN XII). Normal swallowing is coordinated by CNs V, IX, X, and XII and their nuclei in the brainstem.[54,55] Brainstem nuclei are, in turn, controlled by areas of the reticular formation referred to as the *swallowing center.*[55]

Swallowing disorders (dysphagias) can be classified as problems of (1) bolus formation and passage from the mouth to the cranial esophagus (oropharyngeal dysphagia), (2) passage of the bolus from the cranial esophagus to the gastroesophageal junction, (3) disturbances in passage of the bolus from the esophagus into the stomach, and (4) mixed swallowing problems.[55]

Oropharyngeal swallowing disorders are further subdivided into (1) disorders of the initiation of swallowing (oral-stage deficits), (2) disorders in the propulsion of the bolus across the pharynx (pharyngeal phase deficits), (3) failure of relaxation (achalasia) or closure (chalasia) of the cricopharyngeal sphincter between the pharynx and the esophagus, and (4) lack of coordination of cricopharyngeal sphincter relaxation with pharyngeal or esophageal contraction (also see discussion of megaesophagus to follow).

Clinical signs of swallowing disorders of dogs include gagging, difficulty in drinking water or forming a solid bolus, excessive mandibular or head motion, persistent forceful ineffective swallowing efforts, foaming from the mouth, salivation, nasal regurgitation, dropping food from the mouth, coughing, failure to thrive, aspiration pneumonia, and reluctance to eat.[55] Dogs with oral-stage deficits commonly have a reduced ability to hold food in the mouth or transport food to the base of the tongue, whereas dogs with pharyngeal and cricopharyngeal dysfunction more commonly cough, have aspiration pneumonia, and make repeated unsuccessful attempts to swallow.

These forms of dysphagia can best be distinguished by specialized radiographic techniques such as cinefluorography or videofluorography.[55,56] Most dogs with functional swallowing disorders have either multiple cranial nerve dysfunction causing oral or pharyngeal stage deficits[55] or cricopharyngeal achalasia (see following discussion).[56] Myasthenia gravis also may selectively affect the pharyngeal muscles and the esophagus.[55,57] The general underlying cause must be differentiated because although cricopharyngeal myotomy may alleviate dysphagia because of cricopharyngeal achalasia, other swallowing disorders are not helped (oral deficits) or may even be aggravated (pharyngeal deficits).

Dysphagia is a common problem in large animals and frequently results from nonneurologic disorders such as pharyngitis, obstructive choke in the esophagus, and abscesses.[3,58,59] Inability to grasp food or to propel food or water into the pharynx with the tongue may be confused with the inability to swallow. Prehension and bolus formation are functions of the facial muscles (CN VII) and the tongue (CN XII). These functions may be altered with forebrain diseases. Neurologic causes of dysphagia include polyneuropathies (see Chapter 7), botulism (see Chapter 7), rabies (see Chapter 15), other infectious diseases such as listeriosis and protozoal encephalitis (see Chapter 15), guttural pouch infections in horses, nigropallidal encephalomalacia in horses, and idiopathic cricopharyngeal achalasia in dogs.

Guttural Pouch Infections

Infections of the guttural pouch, usually by *Aspergillus* spp. or *Streptococcus equi*, may cause dysphagia, epistaxis, nasal discharge, and pain. Horner's syndrome and laryngeal and facial paresis may be present. The infection tends to localize in the dorsal wall of the guttural pouch close to the course of the glossopharyngeal nerve, the pharyngeal branch of the vagus nerve, and the internal carotid artery and closely associated sympathetic nerves.[3,4]

Diagnosis is made by endoscopy, radiography, and culture of material from the pouch. Treatment with topical antifungal agents has not been successful. Surgical removal or cauterization of lesions may be effective. Occlusion of the internal carotid artery may lessen or prevent epistaxis. Mycotic infections have a poorer prognosis than do bacterial infections.[3,4]

Nigropallidal Encephalomalacia

This disease is characterized by acute dysfunction of muscles innervated by the motor fibers of CNs V, VII, and XII. It was first described in horses from northern California and southern Oregon that grazed on pastures containing large quantities of yellow star thistle.[60] Because of the typical clinical signs and the association with yellow star thistle, the disease also is called *chewing disease* and *yellow star thistle poisoning*. This condition also has been reported in horses from Colorado and Utah that grazed on pastures containing abundant Russian knapweed, a plant related to yellow star thistle.[61,62]

Although the specific factor or toxin has not been identified, necrosis develops in the brainstem in the region of the globus pallidus and the substantia nigra, both components of the extrapyramidal system. The disease occurs in the western United States and in Australia, where the offending plants are endemic. Bilateral symmetric necrosis of the substantia nigra and pallidum occurs.

Clinical Signs. Affected horses range in age from 4 months to 10 years. In general, younger horses are affected more often. Foals that are nursed by clinically normal mares have been affected. Conversely, foals of affected mares have remained normal. Affected horses are acutely unable to grasp food or drink water. The mouth is held partially open, the lips are retracted, and rhythmic tongue movements and purposeless chewing motions are apparent. Lip and tongue movements are similar to "pill-rolling" movements of humans with Parkinson's disease. Affected horses are drowsy and have a fixed facial expression. The facial muscles are hypertonic. Facial muscle flaccidity and gait impairment do not develop. Food or water placed in the caudal pharynx can be swallowed. The clinical signs suggest specific UMN dysfunction of CNs V, VII, and XII. Some horses may improve, but complete recovery has not been reported. Most horses die of starvation or aspiration pneumonia.

Diagnosis. Because no specific tests are available, the diagnosis is based on history and clinical signs. The facial hypertonicity and the lack of ataxia or paresis differentiate nigropallidal encephalomalacia from other diseases.

Treatment. No specific treatment is known. Feeding affected horses by tube prolongs life, allowing time for clinical improvement. The prognosis is poor. Horses should not be allowed to graze on pastures where the offending plants are abundant.

Glossopharyngeal Neuralgia

A brainstem tumor causing a sensory and autonomic syndrome associated with the glossopharyngeal nerve has been reported.[63] A 7-year-old male miniature poodle had cervical pain that was unresponsive to confinement and medication. Episodes of syncope and seizures were associated with pharyngeal stimulation, including palpation. Bradycardia, cyanosis, weak pulse pressure, and miotic pupils were observed. Dysphagia was observed with eating, but not with drinking. No EMG or cerebrospinal fluid (CSF) abnormalities were present. CT demonstrated a mass in the brainstem, presumed to be a tumor. Necropsy was not performed. The syndrome is apparently caused by activation of the brainstem cardiovascular centers.

Cricopharyngeal Achalasia

The cricopharyngeal muscle forms a sphincter around the proximal esophagus. Relaxation of this muscle is part of the swallowing reflex. Failure of relaxation is seen as an acquired or congenital condition, especially in cocker spaniels and springer spaniels. Attempts to swallow result in gagging, coughing, and sneezing. The diagnosis is made by barium swallow examination. Treatment entails resection of the dorsal portion of the cricopharyngeus muscle.[64]

Megaesophagus

Megaesophagus is common in dogs, infrequent in cats, and rare in large animals. The canine esophagus has striated muscle innervated by the vagus nerve throughout its length. Esophageal paralysis and dilatation are common in generalized neuropathies and myopathies, including myasthenia gravis and hypothyroidism (see Chapter 7). Megaesophagus may occur alone, without generalized weakness, in dogs with myasthenia gravis.[57] Diagnosis is made by identifying serum antibodies to acetylcholine receptors. Megaesophagus is reported as an inherited disease in miniature schnauzers and wire fox terriers.[65,66] An increased prevalence is reported in great Danes, German shepherd dogs, and Irish setters.[67] Congenital megaesophagus has been reported in litters of Newfoundlands, shar-peis, and Siamese cats.[68-70]

Regurgitation is the primary sign of megaesophagus. The diagnosis is made radiographically. EMG of the esophageal muscles can be done by passing a stomach tube to define the cervical esophageal wall. The examination should include representative muscles of the limbs and face to rule out neuropathies and myopathies. Primary diseases are treated appropriately. Symptomatic management of megaesophagus entails feeding the animal with the head elevated. Aspiration pneumonia is a common complication. The prognosis for functional recovery is poor in many cases. Megaesophagus that is due to myasthenia gravis, however, resolves in some dogs in association with decreasing antibody titers either spontaneously or subsequent to treatment with pyridostigmine (see Chapter 7).

Hypoglossal Paralysis

Paralysis of the tongue usually results from neoplastic and inflammatory diseases affecting the medulla. Hypoglossal paralysis is a common sign in rabies. The tongue is often affected in generalized neuropathies (see Chapter 7). Specific inflammatory disease of the hypoglossal nerve has not been reported. Bilateral sectioning of the hypoglossal nerves causes oral dysphagia (see preceding discussion).[55]

Dysautonomia

Dysautonomia, also called the *Key Gaskell syndrome*, affects cats worldwide and dogs in midwestern United States. Except for isolated cases, most feline reports are from the United Kingdom and Scandinavia.[71,72] The clinical signs include depression, anorexia, reduced production of tears and saliva, bradycardia, dilated pupils with normal vision, megaesophagus, and, less commonly, fecal and urinary incontinence. Most of the signs can be attributed to loss of parasympathetic innervation, but some sympathetic dysfunction is also seen. Somatic innervation may be affected (e.g., anal sphincter function), but paresis is not a feature of the disease.

The cause of this condition is unknown. Pathologically, both the sympathetic and parasympathetic neurons are vacuolated, both centrally and in the ganglia. Ultrastructurally, the rough endoplasmic reticulum and the Golgi apparatus are disrupted. The incidence peaked in the United Kingdom between 1982 and 1984 and seems to be decreasing in recent years. Several of the feline cases reported in the United States were imported from the United Kingdom. A similar condition in horses, called *grass sickness*,[73] is also prevalent in the United Kingdom, but it has been seen in various European countries. More recently, an analogous condition has been characterized in dogs in the midwestern United States.[74] The diagnosis and treatment of dysautonomia are described in Chapter 11.

Unilateral Cranial Polyneuropathy

Unilateral tumors expanding along the floor of the brainstem may produce chronic compressive polyneuropathy that affects primarily CN III, V, VII, and VIII. Animals are usually presented because of unilateral facial nerve paralysis, unilateral masticatory muscle atrophy, or vestibular signs. Sometimes animals are presented for unilateral pupillary dilation or ventrolateral strabismus. Examination of cranial nerve reflexes reveals multiple cranial nerve involvement and decreased facial sensation ipsilateral to the lesion. CT or MRI reveals a mass lesion that extends along the floor of the brainstem. In our experience, meningioma and lymphosarcoma are the most common tumors producing this syndrome. In some cases, compression of the brainstem may result in paresis and ataxia. Because of the extensive nature of the tumor, the prognosis is poor for most dogs. Radiation treatment may be beneficial.

Case Histories

CASE HISTORY 9A

Signalment
Canine, poodle, male, 8 years old.

History
Right head tilt of 10 days' duration. The dog fell down stairs 1 week before developing signs. A severe ocular discharge is present in the right eye.

Physical Examination
Exposure keratitis of the right eye.

Neurologic Examination*
A. Observation
   1. Mental status: Alert
   2. Posture: Right head tilt
   3. Gait: The dog drifts to the right and falls if he turns quickly
B. Palpation: Negative
C. Postural reactions

Left	Reactions	Right
	Proprioceptive positioning	
+2	PL	+2
+2	TL	+2
+2	Wheelbarrowing	+2
	Hopping	
+2	PL	+2
+2	TL	+2
+2	Extensor postural thrust	+2
+2	Hemistand-hemiwalk	+2
	Placing, tactile	
+2	PL	+2
+2	TL	+2
	Placing, visual	
+2	TL	+2

*0, Absent; +1, decreased; +2, normal; +3, exaggerated; +4, very exaggerated or clonus; PL, pelvic limb; TL, thoracic limb.

D. Spinal reflexes

Left	Reflex (Spinal Segment)	Right
+2	Quadriceps (L4-6)	+2
+2	Extensor carpi radialis (C7-T1)	+2
+2	Triceps (C7-T1)	+2
+2	Flexion, PL (L5-S1)	+2
+2	Flexion, TL (C6-T1)	+2
+0	Crossed extensor	+0
+2	Perineal (S1-S2)	+2

E. Cranial nerves

Left	Nerve—Function (Response, Test)	Right
+2	CN II—vision (menace)	+2
Normal +2 +2	CN II, III—pupil size (Stimulus left eye) (Stimulus right eye)	Normal +2 +2
Normal	CN II—fundus	Normal
+0 Present	CN III, IV, VI (Strabismus) (Nystagmus)	Positional, ventral Present
+2	CN V—sensation	+2
+2	CN V—mastication	+2
Normal +2	CN VII—facial muscles (Palpebral)	Paralyzed +0
Normal	CN IX, X—swallowing	Normal
Normal	CN XII—tongue	Normal

F. Sensation: Location
   Hyperesthesia: None
   Superficial pain: +2
   Deep pain: +2
Complete sections G and H before reviewing the case summary.
G. Assessment (anatomic diagnosis and estimation of prognosis)
H. Plan (diagnostic)

   Rule-outs   *Procedure*
   1.
   2.
   3.
   4.

CASE HISTORY 9B

Signalment
Canine, English setter, female, 7 years old.

History
In the last week, the dog has been "throwing up" shortly after eating. The owner reports that the dog will not run with her anymore.

Physical Examination
The dog is very thin and is mildly dehydrated.

Neurologic Examination*
A. Observation
   1. Mental status: Alert
   2. Posture: Pelvic limbs seem slightly more flexed than usual, especially at hocks
   3. Gait: Slight tendency to sway a little on turns
B. Palpation: Some generalized loss of muscle mass and body fat
C. Postural reactions

Left	Reactions	Right
	Proprioceptive positioning	
+2	PL	+2
+2	TL	+2
+2	Wheelbarrowing	+2
	Hopping	
+2	PL	+2
+2	TL	+2
+2	Extensor postural thrust	+2
+2	Hemistand-hemiwalk	+2
	Placing, tactile	
+2	PL	+2
+2	TL	+2
	Placing, visual	
+2	TL	+2

D. Spinal reflexes

Left	Reflex (Spinal Segment)	Right
+1	Quadriceps (L4-6)	+1
+2	Extensor carpi radialis (C7-T1)	+2
+1	Flexion, PL (L5-S1)	+1
+2	Flexion, TL (C6-T1)	+2
+0	Crossed extensor	+0
+2	Perineal (S1-2)	+2

E. Cranial nerves

Left	Nerve—Function (Response, Test)	Right
+2	CN II—vision (menace)	+0
Normal +2 +2	CN II, III—pupil size Stimulus left eye Stimulus right eye	Normal +2 +2
Normal	CN II—fundus	Normal
+0 +0	CN III, IV, VI (Strabismus) (Nystagmus)	+0 +0
+2	CN V—sensation	+2
+2	CN V—mastication	+2
+1 +1	CN VII—facial muscles (Palpebral)	+1 +1
+2	CN IX, X—swallowing	+2
+2	CN XII—tongue	+2

F. Sensation: Location
   Hyperesthesia: None
   Superficial pain: +2
   Deep pain: +2
Complete sections G and H before reviewing the case summary.
G. Assessment (anatomic diagnosis and estimation of prognosis)
H. Plan (diagnostic)

Rule-outs	Procedure
1.	
2.	
3.	
4.	

CASE HISTORY 9C

Signalment
Canine, poodle, male, 6 years old.

History
Sudden onset of inability to close the mouth. The jaw hangs open. The dog cannot prehend food but can lap water. No other signs have been observed.

Physical Examination
Negative except for the neurologic signs.

*0, Absent; +1, decreased; +2, normal; +3, exaggerated; +4, very exaggerated or clonus; *PL*, pelvic limb; *TL*, thoracic limb.

Neurologic Examination*
A. Observation
  1. Mental status: Alert
  2. Posture: Normal
  3. Gait: Normal
B. Palpation: Lower jaw hangs open; hypotonus of masticatory muscles
C. Postural reactions

Left	Reactions	Right
	Proprioceptive positioning	
+2	PL	+2
+2	TL	+2
+2	Wheelbarrowing	+2
	Hopping	
+2	PL	+2
+2	TL	+2
+2	Extensor postural thrust	+2
+2	Hemistand-hemiwalk	+2
	Placing, tactile	
+2	PL	+2
+2	TL	+2
	Placing, visual	
+2	TL	+2

D. Spinal reflexes

Left	Reflex (Spinal Segment)	Right
+2	Quadriceps (L4-6)	+2
+2	Extensor carpi radialis (C7-T1)	+2
+2	Triceps (C7-T1)	+2
+2	Flexion, PL (L5-S1)	+2
+2	Flexion, TL (C6-T1)	+2
+2	Crossed extensor	+2
+2	Perineal (S1-S2)	+2

E. Cranial nerves

Left	Nerve—Function (Response, Test)	Right
+2	CN II—vision (menace)	+2
+2	CN II, III—pupil size	+2
+2	(Stimulus left eye)	+2
+2	(Stimulus right eye)	+2
Normal	CN II—fundus	Normal
	CN III, IV, VI	
+0	(Strabismus)	+0
+0	(Nystagmus)	+0
+2	CN V—sensation	+2
Paralysis	CN V—mastication	Paralysis
+2	CN VII—facial muscles	+2
+2	(Palpebral)	+2
+2	CN IX, X—swallowing	+2
+2	CN XII—tongue	+2

F. Sensation: Location
  Hyperesthesia: None
  Superficial pain: +2
  Deep pain: +2
Complete sections G and H before reviewing the case summary.
G. Assessment (anatomic diagnosis and estimation of prognosis)
H. Plan (diagnostic)

  Rule-outs   *Procedure*
  1.
  2.
  3.
  4.

CASE HISTORY 9D

Signalment
8-year-old male Doberman pinscher.

History
The dog was presented to referring veterinarian for atrophy of the left temporalis muscle. A muscle biopsy revealed neurogenic muscle atrophy. The dog has no difficulty eating or drinking. The muscle atrophy is progressively worsening.

Physical Examination
See neurologic examination.

Neurologic Examination*
A. Observation
  1. Mental status: Alert and responsive
  2. Posture: Normal
  3. Gait: Normal

---

*0, Absent; +1, decreased; +2, normal; +3, exaggerated; +4, very exaggerated or clonus; *PL,* pelvic limb; *TL,* thoracic limb.

*0, Absent; +1, decreased; +2, normal; +3, exaggerated; +4, very exaggerated or clonus; *PL,* pelvic limb; *TL,* thoracic limb.

B. Palpation: Severe atrophy of left muscles of mastication.
C. Postural reactions

Left	Reactions	Right
	Proprioceptive Positioning	
+2	PL	+2
+2	TL	+2
+2	Wheelbarrowing	+2
	Hopping	
+2	PL	+2
+2	TL	+2
NE	Extensor postural thrust	NE
+2	Hemistand-hemiwalk	+2
NE	Placing tactile PL TL	NE
NE	Placing-visual TL	NE

D. Spinal reflexes

Left	Reflexes (Spinal Segment)	Right
+2	Quadriceps (L4-6)	+2
NE	Extensor carpi radialis (C7-11)	NE
+2	Triceps (C7-T1)	+2
+2	Flexion-PL (L5-S1)	+2
+2	Flexion-TL (C6-T1)	+2
0	Crossed extensor	0
+2	Perineal	+2

E. Cranial nerves

Left	Nerve—function (Response, Test)	Right
+2	CN II—vision (menace)	+2
Small	CN II, III—pupil size	Normal
+2	(Stimulate left eye)	+2
+2	(Stimulate right eye)	+2
NE	CN II—fundus	NE
0	CN III, IV, VI (Strabismus)	0
0	(Nystagmus)	0
0-+1	CN V—sensation	+2
Atrophy	CN V—mastication	Normal
+2	CN VII—facial muscles (Palpebral)	+2
+2	CN IX, X—swallowing	+2
Normal	CN XII—tongue	Normal

F. Sensation: Location
   Hyperesthesia: None
   Superficial pain: +2 in all areas except the left facial area, which is decreased.
   Deep pain: +2
Complete sections G and H before reviewing the case summary.
G. Assessment (anatomic diagnosis and estimation of prognosis)
H. Plan (diagnostic)

   Rule-outs   *Procedure*
   1.
   2.
   3.
   4.

CASE HISTORY 9E

Signalment
12-year-old male-neutered Labrador retriever.

History
The dog presented for cough, regurgitation, dysphagia, and ocular discharge of 1 month's duration. Horner's syndrome was diagnosed 3 months ago. Mild atrophy of left temporalis muscle was noticed recently.

Physical Examination
Dog has problem grasping food.

Neurologic Examination*
A. Observation
   1. Mental status: Alert and responsive
   2. Posture: Normal
   3. Gait: Normal
B. Palpation: Atrophy of left temporalis muscle
C. Postural reactions

Left	Reactions	Right
	Proprioceptive Positioning	
+2	PL	+2
+2	TL	+2
+2	Wheelbarrowing	+2

*0, Absent; +1, decreased; +2, normal; +3, exaggerated; +4, very exaggerated or clonus; *PL,* pelvic limb; *TL,* thoracic limb.

	Hopping	
+2	PL	+2
+2	TL	+2

NE	Extensor postural thrust	NE

+2	Hemistand-hemiwalk	+2

	Placing-tactile	
NE	PL	NE
	TL	

	Placing-visual	
NE	TL	NE

D. Spinal reflexes

Left	Reflexes (Spinal Segment)	Right
+2	Quadriceps (L4-6)	+2
+2	Extensor carpi radialis (C7-T1)	+2
+2	Triceps (C7-T1)	+2
+2	Flexion-PL (L5-S1)	+2
+2	Flexion-TL (C6-T1)	+2
0	Crossed extensor	0
+2	Perineal	+2

E. Cranial nerves

Left	(Response, Test) Nerve—Function	Right
+1 - +2	CN II—vision (menace)	+2
Large	CN II, III—pupil size	Normal
+1	(Stimulate left eye)	+2
+1	(Stimulate right eye)	+2
Normal	CN II—fundus	Normal
	CN III, IV, VI	
0	(Strabismus)	0
0	(Nystagmus)	0
0	CN V—sensation	+2
Atrophy	CN V—mastication	Normal
Weak	CN VII—facial muscles	Normal
+1	(Palpebral)	+2
0	CN IX, X—swallowing	+1
Normal	CN XII—tongue	Normal

F. Sensation: Location
   Hyperesthesia: None
   Superficial pain: +2 in all areas except left facial area, which is decreased
   Deep pain: +2

Complete sections G and H before reviewing the case summary.

G. Assessment (anatomic diagnosis and estimation of prognosis)
H. Plan (diagnostic)

Rule-outs	Procedure
1.	
2.	
3.	
4.	

ASSESSMENT 9A

Anatomic Diagnosis

Two major findings are important in the localization of this lesion. Vestibular signs with no paresis strongly suggest a right peripheral vestibular disease. Facial paralysis on the right side probably has occurred secondary to the peripheral vestibular disorder.

Diagnostic Plan (Rule-outs)

1. Otitis media interna: Otoscopic examination (negative), skull radiography (negative)
2. Geriatric vestibular syndrome: Diagnosis of exclusion
3. Facial nerve paralysis: EMG

Therapeutic Plan

1. Treatment of the exposure keratitis of the right eye
2. Chloramphenicol, 50 mg/kg three times daily for 10 days

Client Education

The prognosis is good.

Case Summary

Otitis media interna with facial paralysis was suspected. The dog recovered from otitis media interna after therapy. The facial paralysis persisted.

ASSESSMENT 9B

Anatomic Diagnosis

"Throwing up" may be either vomiting or regurgitation. Careful questioning reveals that it occurs within a few minutes of eating and that the food is an undigested bolus. These findings suggest regurgitation. A major cause of regurgitation is megaesophagus. Other findings indicate slightly reduced strength in the limbs and reduced flexion reflexes. Reduced facial nerve function is also present. No single lesion could account for these signs. The likely explanation is polyneuropathy or polymyopathy.

Diagnostic Plan (Rule-outs)

1. Polymyopathy: Creatine kinase (normal), EMG (see below)
2. Polyneuropathy: Definitive diagnosis requires EMG and biopsy. The EMG revealed fibrillations and positive waves in all distal muscles of the limbs and face and some areas of abnormality in the paravertebral muscles. Radiography of the chest revealed

megaesophagus with no evidence of pneumonia or metastases. Causes of polyneuropathy include endocrine, toxic, and immune diseases. No history of toxic exposure was present. Thyroxine (T_4) values were 1.0 mg/dl and 1.4 mg/dl before and after thyroid-stimulating hormone stimulation. A presumptive diagnosis of polyneuropathy secondary to hypothyroidism was made.

Therapeutic Plan
Levothyroxine was prescribed. The dog was fed soft food in an elevated position and was monitored carefully for signs of pneumonia.

Client Education
The prognosis is guarded because of the megaesophagus.

Case Summary
The dog began to improve after 3 weeks of treatment. At a recheck 6 months later, the megaesophagus could not be seen on radiographs.

ASSESSMENT 9C

Anatomic Diagnosis
The neurologic findings localize the lesion to bilateral involvement of the motor division of CN V. (Normal facial sensation and palpebral reflexes suggest clinically normal function of the sensory fibers of CN V.) Strict motor involvement is suggestive of idiopathic mandibular nerve paralysis.

Diagnostic Plan (Rule-outs)
1. Mandibular nerve paralysis: EMG of masticatory muscles (diffuse evidence of denervation 7 days after the onset of the signs)
2. Temporal, masseter myositis: History and physical examination (negative for pain; the jaw is open rather than closed; the muscles are hypotonic rather than firm), muscle biopsy (not done in this case)
3. Rabies: Clinical history and course of the disease; rabies always is considered when bulbar signs are present
4. Trauma: Skull radiography (negative)

Therapeutic Plan
Support hydration and nutrition with tube feedings.

Client Education
The disease is of unknown cause. Recovery takes 3 to 6 weeks and is usually complete. No specific therapy is known.

Case Summary
An uneventful recovery occurred in 4 weeks. A second episode was recorded 6 months later. A complete recovery again occurred in 4 weeks.

ASSESSMENT 9D

Anatomic Diagnosis
Trigeminal nerve lesion on the left side with involvement of sympathetic innervation to the left pupil. Given the chronic progressive course and unilateral lesion, neoplasia or granuloma of the trigeminal nerve should be suspected.

Diagnostic Plan (Rule-outs)
1. Neoplasia: MRI or CT of the skull
2. Granulomatous disease: MRI or CT of skull
   CT revealed a mass lesion affecting the left trigeminal nerve and ganglion. A nerve sheath tumor was suspected.

Therapeutic Plan
Owner refused referral for radiation therapy.

Case Summary
The presumptive diagnosis is nerve sheath tumor affecting the left trigeminal nerve and sympathetic innervation to the left pupil.

ASSESSMENT 9E

Anatomic Diagnosis
Multiple cranial nerves are affected on the left side, including CN III, V, VII, IX, and X. Because there is no paresis or ataxia, the lesion must not involve the brainstem at this time. Neoplastic or granulomatous disease extending along the floor of the brainstem can create these neurologic signs.

Diagnostic Plan (Rule-outs)
1. Neoplasia: CT or MRI of skull
2. Granulomatous disease: CT or MRI of skull and CSF
   The CSF examination was negative. CT revealed a large linear mass on the ventrolateral floor of the brainstem.

Therapeutic Plan
The owner declined biopsy and possible radiation therapy.

Case Summary
The dog was euthanized, and no necropsy was permitted.

References

1. Whalen LR, Kitchell RL: Electrophysiologic studies of the cutaneous nerves of the head of the dog, *Am J Vet Res* 44:615-627, 1983.
2. Whalen LR, Kitchell RL: Electrophysiologic and behavioral studies of the cutaneous nerves of the concave surface of the pinna and the external ear canal of the dog, *Am J Vet Res* 44:628-634, 1983.
3. Mayhew IG: *Large animal neurology: a handbook for veterinary clinicians.* Philadelphia, 1989, Lea & Febiger.
4. de Lahunta A: *Veterinary neuroanatomy and clinical neurology,* 2nd ed. Philadelphia, 1983, WB Saunders.
5. Sims MH: Hearing loss in small animals: occurrence and diagnosis. In Kirk RW, editor: *Current veterinary therapy, X.* Philadelphia, 1989, WB Saunders.
6. Hoelzle RJ: Idiopathic trigeminal neuropathy in a dog, *Vet Med Small Anim Clin* 58:345, 1983.
7. Panciera RJ, et al: Trigeminal and polyradiculoneuritis in a dog presenting with masticatory muscle atrophy and Horner's syndrome, *Vet Pathol* 30:146-149, 2002.
8. Bagley RS, Wheeler SJ, Klopp L, et al: Trigeminal nerve sheath tumor in 10 dogs, *J Am Anim Hosp Assoc* 34:19-25, 1998.
9. Carmichael S, Griffiths IR: Case of isolated sensory trigeminal neuropathy in a dog, *Vet Rec* 109:280-282, 1981.
10. Asbury AK, McKhann GM, McDonald WI: *Diseases of the nervous system.* Philadelphia, 1986, Ardmore Medical Books.
11. Kern TJ, Erb HN: Facial neuropathy in dogs and cats: 95 cases (1975-1985), *J Am Vet Med Assoc* 191:1604-1609, 1987.
12. Braund KG, et al: Idiopathic facial paralysis in the dog, *Vet Rec* 105:297-299, 1979.
13. Jaggy A, et al: Neurological manifestations of hypothyroidism: a retrospective study of 29 dogs, *J Vet Intern Med* 8:328-336, 1994.
14. Roberts SR, Vainisi SJ: Hemifacial spasm in dogs, *J Am Vet Med Assoc* 150:381-385, 1967.

15. Parker AJ, et al: Hemifacial spasm in a dog, *Vet Rec* 93:514-516, 1973.

16. Renegar WR: Auriculopalpebral nerve paralysis following prolonged anesthesia in a dog, *J Am Vet Med Assoc* 174:1007-1009, 1979.

17. Knowles K: Reduction of spiral ganglion neurons in the aging canine with hearing loss. In *Proceedings of the Eighth Annual Veterinary Medical Forum*. Washington, DC, 1990, American College of Veterinary Internal Medicine.

18. Mansfield PD: Ototoxicity in dogs and cats, *Compend Cont Educ Pract Vet* 12:332-337, 1990.

19. Oliver JE: Deafness. In Lorenz MD, Cornelius LM, editors: *Small animal medical diagnosis,* 2nd ed. Philadelphia, 1993, JB Lippincott.

20. Holliday TA, et al: Unilateral and bilateral brainstem auditory-evoked response abnormalities in 900 Dalmatian dogs, *J Vet Intern Med* 6:166-174, 1992.

21. Strain GM, et al: Brainstem auditory-evoked potential assessment of congenital deafness in Dalmatians: associations with phenotypic markers, *J Vet Intern Med* 6:175-182, 1992.

22. Greibrokk T: Hereditary deafness in the Dalmatian: relationship to eye and coat color, *J Am Anim Hosp Assoc* 30:170-176, 1994.

23. Harvey CI, O'Brien JA: Treatment of laryngeal paralysis in dogs by partial laryngectomy, *J Am Anim Hosp Assoc* 18:551-556, 1982.

24. Greenfield CL: Canine laryngeal paralysis, *Compend Cont Educ Pract Vet* 10:1011-1020, 1987.

25. Venker van Haagen AJ, Hartman W, Goedegebuure SA: Spontaneous laryngeal paralysis in young Bouviers, *J Am Anim Hosp Assoc* 14:714-720, 1978.

26. Venker van Haagen AJ, Bouw J, Hartman W: Hereditary transmission of laryngeal paralysis in young Bouviers, *J Am Anim Hosp Assoc* 17:75-76, 1981.

27. Hendricks JC, O'Brien JA: Inherited laryngeal paralysis in Siberian husky crosses. In *Proceedings of the Third Annual Veterinary Medical Forum*. San Diego, 1985, American College of Veterinary Internal Medicine.

28. Smith M, et al: Evaluation of a modified castellated laryngofissure for alleviation of upper airway obstruction in dogs with laryngeal paralysis, *J Am Vet Med Assoc* 188:1279-1283, 1986.

29. Greenfield CL, et al: Neuromuscular pedicle graft for restoration of arytenoid abductor function in dogs with experimentally induced laryngeal hemiplegia, *Am J Vet Res* 49:1360-1366, 1988.

30. Payne JT, Martin RA, Rigg DL: Abductor muscle prosthesis for correction of laryngeal paralysis in 10 dogs and one cat, *J Am Anim Hosp Assoc* 26:599-604, 1990.

31. MacPhail CM, Monnet E: Outcome of and postoperative complications in dogs undergoing surgical treatment of laryngeal paralysis: 140 cases (1985-1998), *J Am Vet Med Assoc* 218:1949-1956, 2001.

32. Gaber CE, Amis TC, LeCouteur RA: Laryngeal paralysis in dogs: a review of 23 cases, *J Am Vet Med Assoc* 186:377-380, 1985.

33. Braund KG, et al: Laryngeal paralysis in immature and mature dogs as one sign of a diffuse polyneuropathy, *J Am Vet Med Assoc* 194:1735-1740, 1989.

34. Hardie EM, et al: Laryngeal paralysis in three cats, *J Am Vet Med Assoc* 179:879-882, 1981.

35. O'Brien JA, et al: Neurogenic atrophy of the laryngeal muscles of the dog, *J Small Anim Pract* 14:521-532, 1973.

36. Schachter S, Norris CR: Laryngeal paralysis in cats: 16 cases (1990-1999), *J Am Vet Med Assoc* 216:1100-1103, 2000.

37. Kortz GD, et al: Neuronal vacuolation and spinocerebellar degeneration in young rottweiler dogs, *Vet Pathol* 34:296-302, 1997.

38. van den Ingh TS, Mandigers PJ, van Nes JJ: A neuronal vacuolar disorder in young rottweiler dogs, *Vet Rec* 142:245-247, 1998.

39. Eger CE, Huxtable CR, Chester ZC, Summers BA: Progressive tetraparesis and laryngeal paralysis in a young rottweiler with neuronal vacuolation and axonal degeneration: an Australian case, *Aust Vet J* 76:733-737, 1998.

40. Mahoney OM, et al: Laryngeal paralysis-polyneuropathy complex in young Rottweilers, *J Vet Intern Med* 12:330-337, 1998.

41. Cahill JI, Goulden B: The pathogenesis of equine laryngeal hemiplegia: a review. *N Z Vet J* 35:82-90, 1987.

42. Bohanon TC, Beard WL, Robertson JT: Laryngeal hemiplegia in draft horses: a review of 27 cases, *Vet Surg* 19:456-459, 1990.

43. Goulden BE, Anderson LJ, Cahill JI: Roaring in Clydesdales, *N Z Vet J* 33:73-76, 1985.

44. Duncan ID: Determination of the early age of onset of equine recurrent laryngeal neuropathy, *Acta Neuropathol (Berl)* 84:316-321, 1992.

45. Traub-Dargatz JL, et al: Respiratory stridor associated with polymyopathy suspected to be hyperkalemic periodic paralysis in four Quarter Horse foals, *J Am Vet Med Assoc* 201:85-89, 1992.

46. Guglick MA, MacAllister CG, Breazile JE: Laryngospasm, dysphagia, and emaciation associated with hyperkalemic periodic paralysis in a horse, *J Am Vet Med Assoc* 209:115-117, 1996.

47. Cahill JI, Goulden B: Equine laryngeal hemiplegia, Part I: A light microscopic study of peripheral nerves, *N Z Vet J* 34:161-169, 1986.

48. Cook WR: Diagnosis and grading of hereditary recurrent laryngeal neuropathy in the horse, *Equine Vet Sci* 8:432-455, 1988.

49. Moore MP, et al: Electromyographic evaluation of horses with laryngeal hemiplegia, *Equine Vet Sci* 8:424-427, 1988.

50. Ducharme NG, et al: Attempts to restore abduction of the paralyzed equine arytenoid cartilage, I: Nerve-muscle pedicle transplants, *Can J Vet Res* 53:202-209, 1989.

51. Fulton IC, et al: Treatment of left laryngeal hemiplegia in standardbreds, using a nerve muscle pedicle graft, *Am J Vet Res* 52:1461-1467, 1991.

52. Tulleners EP, Harrison IW, Raker CW: Management of arytenoid chondropathy and failed laryngoplasty in horses: 75 cases (1879-1985), *J Am Vet Med Assoc* 192:670-675, 1988.

53. Strand E, et al: Career racing performance in Thoroughbreds treated with prosthetic laryngoplasty for laryngeal neuropathy: 52 cases (1981-1989), *J Am Vet Med Assoc* 217:1689-1696, 2000.

54. Venker van Haagen A, Hartman W, Wolvekamp W: Contributions of the glossopharyngeal nerve and the pharyngeal branch of the vagus nerve to the swallowing process in dogs, *Am J Vet Res* 47:1300-1307, 1986.

55. Suter PF, Watrous BJ: Oropharyngeal dysphagias in the dog: a cinefluorographic analysis of experimentally induced and spontaneously occurring swallowing disorders, *Vet Radiol* 21:24-39, 1980.

56. Watrous BJ, Suter PF: Oropharyngeal dysphagias in the dog: A cinefluorographic analysis of experimentally induced and spontaneously occurring swallowing disorders, II: Cricopharyngeal stage and mixed oropharyngeal dysphagias, *Vet Radiol* 24:11-24, 1983.

57. Shelton GD, et al: Acquired myasthenia gravis: selective involvement of esophageal, pharyngeal, and facial muscles, *J Vet Intern Med* 4:281-284, 1990.
58. Greet T: Dysphagia in the horse, *In Practice* 11:256-262, 1989.
59. Baum KH, et al: Dysphagia in horses: the differential diagnosis, Part II, *Compend Cont Educ Pract Vet* 10:1405-1410, 1988.
60. Fowler ME: Nigropallidal encephalomalacia in the horse, *J Am Vet Med Assoc* 147:607-616, 1965.
61. Young S, Brown WW, Klinger B: Nigropallidal encephalomalacia in horses caused by ingestion of weeds of the genus Centaurea, *J Am Vet Med Assoc* 157:1602-1605, 1970.
62. Larson KA, Young S: Nigropallidal encephalomalacia in horses in Colorado, *J Am Vet Med Assoc* 156:626-628, 1970.
63. Shores A, et al: Glossopharyngeal neuralgia syndrome in a dog, *J Am Anim Hosp Assoc* 27:101-104, 1991.
64. Morgan RV: *Handbook of small animal practice.* New York, 1988, Churchill Livingstone.
65. Osborne CA, Clifford DH, Jessen C: Hereditary esophageal achalasia in dogs, *J Am Vet Med Assoc* 151:572-581, 1967.
66. Cox VS, Wallace LJ, Anderson VE, et al: Hereditary esophageal dysfunction in the miniature schnauzer dog, *Am J Vet Res* 41:326-330, 1980.
67. Strombeck DR: Pathophysiology of esophageal motility disorders in the dog and cat, *Vet Clin North Am* 8:229-244, 1978.
68. Guilford WG: Megaesophagus in the dog and cat, *Semin Vet Med Surg* 5:37-45, 1990.
69. Knowles KE, O'Brien DP, Amann JF: Congenital idiopathic megaesophagus in a litter of Chinese shar-peis: Clinical, electrodiagnostic, and pathological findings, *J Am Anim Hosp Assoc* 26:313-318, 1990.
70. Schwartz A, et al: Congenital neuromuscular esophageal disease in a litter of Newfoundland puppies, *J Vet Radiol* 17:101-105, 1976.
71. Sharp NJH: Feline dysautonomia, *Semin Vet Med Surg* 5:67-71, 1990.
72. Edney ATB, Gaskell CJ, Sharp NJH: Feline dysautonomia, *J Small Anim Pract* 28:333-416, 1987.
73. Pollin MM, Griffiths IR: A review of the primary dysautonomias of domestic animals, *J Comp Pathol* 106:99-119, 1992.
74. Longshore RC, et al: Dysautonomia in dogs: a retrospective study, *J Vet Intern Med* 10:103-109, 1996.
75. Creel D, Conlee JW, Parks TN: Auditory brainstem anomalies in albino cats, I: Evoked potential studies, *Brain Res* 260:1-9, 1983.
76. Delack JB: Hereditary deafness in the white cat, *Compend Cont Educ Pract Vet* 6:609-616, 1984.
77. Elverland HH, Mair IWS: Hereditary deafness in the cat, *Acta Otolaryngol* 90:360-369, 1980.
78. Rebillard G, et al: Histophysiological relationships in the deaf white cat auditory system, *Acta Otolaryngol* 82:48-56, 1976.
79. Bosher SK, Hallpike CS: Observations on the histologic features, development, and pathogenesis of the inner ear degeneration of the deaf white cat, *Proc R Soc Lond Biol Sci (Series B)* 162:147-170, 1965.
80. Wolff D: Three generations of deaf white cats, *J Hered* 33:39-43, 1942.
81. Strain GM: Congenital deafness in dogs and cats, *Compend Cont Educ Pract Vet* 13:245-253, 1991.
82. Hayes HM, Wilson GP, Fenner WR, et al: Canine congenital deafness: epidemiologic study of 272 cases, *J Am Anim Hosp Assoc* 17:473, 1981.
83. Igarashi M, Alford B, Cohn A, et al: Inner ear anomalies in dogs, *Ann Otol Rhinol Laryngol* 81:249-255, 1972.
84. Lurie M: The membranous labyrinth in the congenitally deaf Collie and Dalmatian dog, *Laryngoscope* 58:279-287, 1948.
85. Gwin RM, et al: Multiple ocular defects associated with partial albinism and deafness in the dog, *J Am Anim Hosp Assoc* 17:401-408, 1981.
86. Hudson W, Ruben R: Hereditary deafness in the Dalmatian dog, *Arch Otolaryngol* 75:213-219, 1962.
87. Johnsson L, et al: Vascular anatomy and pathology of the cochlea in Dalmatian dogs. In Darin de Lorenzo AJ, editor: *Vascular disorders and hearing defects.* University Park, MD, 1973, University Park Press.
88. Suga F, Hattler K: Physiological and histopathological correlates of hereditary deafness in animals, *Laryngoscope* 80:80-104, 1970.
89. Marshall A: Use of brain stem auditory-evoked response to evaluate deafness in a group of Dalmatian dogs, *J Am Vet Med Assoc* 188:718-722, 1986.
90. Wilkes M, Palmer A: Congenital deafness in Dobermans, *Vet Rec* 118:218, 1986.
91. Sims MH, Shull Selcer E: Electrodiagnostic evaluation of deafness in two English Setter littermates, *J Am Vet Med Assoc* 187:398-404, 1985.
92. Erickson F, Leipold HW, McKinley J: Congenital defects in dogs, Part 2. *Canine Pract* 14:51-61, 1977.
93. Steinberg SA, et al: Inherited deafness among nervous pointer dogs. In *Proceedings of the Seventh Annual Veterinary Medicine Forum,* San Diego, 1989, American College of Veterinary Internal Medicine.
94. Adams EW: Hereditary deafness in a family of foxhounds, *J Am Vet Med Assoc* 128:302-303, 1956.

Chapter 10

Disorders of Involuntary Movement

Involuntary movement disorders are of two kinds: those with negative defects and those with positive defects (Table 10-1).[1] A *negative defect* refers to a movement that cannot be performed, as in paresis or paralysis; these are discussed in Chapters 5 to 7.

A *positive defect* is an involuntary movement such as seizure, ataxia, tremor, or abnormal posture. Seizures are discussed in Chapter 13, and ataxia is discussed in Chapter 8.

Disorders of involuntary movement can be further classified as those characterized by increased muscle tone as the primary defect and those characterized by repetitive movements.

Movement disorders in which muscle tone is increased include tetanus and tetany, spasticity, myotonia, and opisthotonos. Those characterized by repetitive movements include tremor, myoclonus, and several abnormal movements seen primarily in nonhuman primates and humans, such as athetosis, chorea, and ballismus.

Tetanus is "a state of sustained muscular contraction without periods of relaxation caused by repetitive stimulation of the motor nerve trunk at frequencies so high that individual muscle twitches are fused and cannot be distinguished from one another, called also tonic spasm and tetany."[2] In clinical medicine, the term *tetanus* is generally reserved for the disease caused by *Clostridium tetani* toxin. *Tetany* is generally used to describe a condition that is similar but characterized by intermittent tonic muscular contractions. Tetany is frequently caused by hypocalcemia but may be seen in a variety of conditions.

Spasticity is a motor disorder characterized by a velocity-dependent increase in tonic stretch reflexes ("muscle tone") with exaggerated myotatic reflexes resulting from hyperexcitability of the stretch reflex.[2] It is often associated with damage to the upper motor neurons. *Opisthotonos* is a posture with the head and neck severely extended and the back arched in an exaggerated lordotic position. The posture is generally accompanied by increased extensor tone in the limbs.

Myotonia is a sustained contraction of muscles caused by a primary defect in the muscle membrane. Both congenital and acquired forms are described in animals.

Tremor is an involuntary trembling or quivering that may occur at rest or during movement. Resting tremors are unusual in domestic animals. Most tremors occurring with movement are associated with diseases of the cerebellum and its related pathways. Intention tremors occur with purposeful movements such as movement of the head when an animal attempts to eat or drink. Intention tremors are most often associated with cerebellar disorders and are described in Chapter 8.

Myoclonus denotes repetitive, rhythmic contractions of a portion of a muscle, an entire muscle, or a group of muscles. Myoclonus may be restricted to one area or may occur synchronously or asynchronously in several areas.[2] The primary example is canine myoclonus associated with canine distemper viral infection.

Numerous other involuntary movement disorders are described in humans and nonhuman primates. Most of these disorders have not been reproduced in quadrupeds, even with experimental lesions in areas thought to cause the disorder in primates. *Chorea* is the contraction of random muscles throughout the body, occurring at random times and for random durations.[3] Canine distemper myoclonus was called *chorea* for many years, but it does not fit the definition. *Dystonia* is contraction of muscles, either focal or generalized, often including antagonist muscles that contract simultaneously. The movements in humans are frequently described as twisting on the long axis of the body part. *Athetosis* is a slow, writhing movement of the fingers, sometimes described as pill-rolling movements in humans. The movements of the lips in horses with nigropallidal encephalomalacia caused by a plant toxin have been compared with athetosis.

Table 10-1   **Disorders of Movement**[*]

Negative Defects
Paresis-paralysis (5-7, 9)
Cataplexy (13)

Positive Defects
Gait abnormalities
    Ataxia, dysmetria (7, 8)
    Circling, compulsive walking (8, 12, 15)
Seizures (13)
Involuntary movements
    Increased muscle tone
        Tetanus, tetany (10)
        Spasticity, opisthotonos (6-8, 10, 12)
    Repetitive movements
        Tremor (8, 10)
        Myoclonus (10)
        Other adventitious movements (10)

[*]Numbers in parentheses refer to chapters in which the disorders are discussed.

The comparison is interesting because the fingers of primates are the primary prehensile organ, with fine motor control, as are the lips of horses. A related movement disorder has been produced in cats with lesions in the caudate nucleus. The cats had slow kneading movements of the paws of the thoracic limb.[4] *Ballismus* denotes wild, large-amplitude, irregular limb movements. It frequently occurs on one side of the body and is then referred to as *hemiballismus*. Ballismus is apparently related to chorea because human patients often have ballismus after a stroke, which then gradually changes to chorea over days.[3] Some of the movements seen in dogs with hypomyelination are almost suggestive of ballismus, but they tend to be more rhythmic and are called *myoclonus* or *tremor,* depending on frequency and amplitude.

LESION LOCALIZATION

Increased Muscle Tone

The disorders of increased muscle tone, including tetanus, tetany, and spasticity, are caused by an imbalance of facilitation and inhibition on the lower motor neuron (LMN). The firing pattern of an individual LMN is determined by synaptic connections from the primary peripheral afferents, descending pathways from the brain, and local interneuron connections. Loss of adequate facilitation causes decreased muscle tone and reflexes. Loss of inhibitory control causes increased firing of the LMN and intermittent or continuous contraction of the muscles it innervates. Each of the disorders of importance has a specific pathogenesis.

Tetanus and Tetany

Tetanus is caused by the toxin produced by *Clostridium tetani.* The bacterial spores are resistant and can persist in the environment for long periods. Bacteria gain access to the animal's tissues through open wounds, proliferate, and produce the toxin. The toxin ascends to the spinal cord through the axons of peripheral nerves. From the LMN, the toxin invades the inhibitory interneurons and blocks the release of the inhibitory neurotransmitters glycine and γ-aminobutyric acid (GABA).[5] Glycine is the transmitter for primary inhibitory interneurons and for the Renshaw cells, which mediate recurrent inhibition; GABA is the inhibitory transmitter for descending pathways. The result is an uninhibited firing of the LMN, a decrease in long-latency reflexes, and an increase in short-latency reflexes.

Tetany is generally similar to tetanus, but with intermittent relaxation of the muscles. The most common forms are caused by abnormalities in electrolytes, principally decreased serum calcium or magnesium levels. The blood calcium level may vary considerably because the abnormality is specifically related to a decrease in ionized calcium below 2.5 mg/dl.[7] For example, in hypoproteinemia, low total calcium levels are associated with hypoalbuminemia because albumin is the primary binding protein for calcium. Ionized calcium levels may be normal, and clinical signs of hypocalcemia do not occur. Calcium is necessary for the release of neurotransmitters and for excitation contraction coupling in muscle. Magnesium has the opposite effect on the synapse, blocking release of the transmitter. Hypocalcemia and hypomagnesemia can cause either tetany or weakness, apparently depending on the degree and rate of development of the decrease in the ionic form. Hypocalcemia is caused by (1) increased loss of calcium in milk, (2) decreased absorption from the intestinal tract in renal disease and in the presence of oxalates and ethylene glycol, and (3) saponification of fat in acute pancreatitis. *Hypoparathyroidism* (decreased parathormone production) causes decreased calcium by increased renal excretion and urinary loss, reducing gastrointestinal absorption and decreased reabsorption of calcium from the bones.

Hypomagnesemia is caused by inadequate intake, usually in large animals feeding on fresh green pastures that are low in magnesium content.

Strychnine causes tetany by blocking glycine, but it differs from tetanus in that it acts at the receptor.[6] Restrictions on the use of strychnine as a pesticide have reduced the frequency of problems, but accidental or malicious poisonings of dogs still occur.

Myotonia

Myotonia is characterized by sustained contraction of muscle fibers caused by repetitive depolarization of their cell membranes. Muscle relaxation is delayed after a voluntary or evoked contraction.[8] The congenital myotonia of goats has been studied most extensively. The defect is a lowered muscle membrane permeability to chloride and sodium. One of the characteristic clinical signs is "dimpling" of the muscle after percussion, which reflects the prolonged contraction of the small group of muscle fibers excited by the stimulus. No evidence of LMN or upper motor neuron (UMN) involvement exists in these animals. They have normal postural reactions within the limitations of the prolonged contractions of the muscles.

Spasticity and Opisthotonos

Spasticity is generally related to UMN deficits, with reduced inhibition of the extensor motor neurons. The term is also used for some poorly defined syndromes, such as spastic paresis of cattle and Scotty cramp in dogs. These diseases may result from a primary defect in neurotransmitters. With UMN disease, paresis or paralysis, increased myotatic reflexes, and sometimes abnormal reflexes such as crossed extensor and extensor toe reflexes occur. Lesion localization for UMN disease is described in Chapter 2.

Lesions of the rostral brainstem (midbrain, rostral pons) produce a posture called *decerebrate rigidity*. All four limbs are extended with increased extensor tone. Forced flexion of the limb causes increased resistance to a point, then abrupt loss of resistance and flexion, called the *clasp-knife reflex*. If the rostral lobe of the cerebellum is also damaged, the head and neck are extended dorsally in a posture called *opisthotonos*.[9] Acute lesions of the cerebellum without damage to the brainstem cause a posture termed *decerebellate rigidity* that is similar to decerebrate posture, but the pelvic limbs are flexed and uncoordinated movements occur.

Repetitive Movements

Tremor

Tremor may occur with movement or at rest. Most of the tremor syndromes in domestic animals are associated with movement. The lesion causing the tremor is usually in the cerebellum or is associated with a diffuse abnormality of myelin. Tremors may also be a component of tetany. The classic tremor syndromes of humans associated with an abnormality of the extrapyramidal system (Parkinson's disease) have not been reported in domestic animals.

Cerebellar tremor is called an *intention tremor* because it progresses in severity as the animal initiates movement. The tremor subsides as the animal relaxes. Tremor is one manifestation of the abnormal control of the rate, range, and force of the movements. Dysmetria is similar, but the movement is of greater amplitude. The head must be affected to localize the lesion to the cerebellum because similar signs in the limbs can be caused by lesions in the pathways that mediate these functions. A simple test entails giving the animal food or water. The animal with cerebellar disease shows tremors or dysmetria of the head as it tries to eat or drink.

Tremor in animals with myelin disease is usually worse than in those with cerebellar disease. The tremor is often accompanied by movements of greater amplitude resembling myoclonus, is more persistent at rest, and may even be present during light sleep.

Tremors may also be associated with mycotoxins, some poisonous plants, several chemical poisons, and diffuse nonsuppurative encephalitis. The tremor is similar to that seen with cerebellar disease in most cases, and the diagnosis must depend on other signs and the history.

Myoclonus

The most common cause of myoclonus in domestic animals is canine distemper. Synonyms include flexor spasm, canine chorea, and tremor. The myoclonus is characterized by a repetitive contraction of a muscle or group of muscles at rates up to 60 per minute. The contractions may occur in more than one muscle group in a dog, and different groups may be affected as the disease progresses. At any one time, the myoclonus is constant in the same groups of muscles. The myoclonus may persist during sleep. Any muscle group can be affected, but the condition is most frequent in the appendicular or masticatory muscles. The cause is unknown, but once established, the LMN and interneuron pool of the affected segment are sufficient for the movement. Transection of the spinal cord cranial and caudal to the affected segment and sectioning of the dorsal root afferents do not abolish the movement. Ventral root section stops the myoclonus. Minimal histologic changes are seen in the affected segments. Distemper myoclonus may occur during the acute phase of the disease, but more frequently it occurs in the chronic phases. The myoclonus may persist for years after the animal recovers from the initial disease. Spontaneous remission is sometimes seen. Inherited myoclonus of cattle is caused by a deficit of glycine/strychnine receptors in the spinal cord.

DISEASES

Tetanus and Tetany

Tetanus

Tetanus is caused by the toxin (tetanospasmin) produced by the bacterium *Clostridium tetani*, a spore-bearing anaerobic bacillus.[5] The spores are resistant to most sporicidal agents and can remain viable for years.[10] The organisms may be found in soil and are common in the feces of many species. Infection usually occurs through contamination of wounds. Deep wounds with poor oxygenation are most susceptible. Once tetanus toxin is liberated in tissues, it binds to gangliosides in nerves and travels to the spinal cord by retrograde axonal transport. In the spinal cord, the toxin passes transsynaptically to inhibitory interneurons. It specifically blocks the release of the inhibitory neurotransmitters glycine and GABA.[5,6] Tetanus toxin can block sympathetic preganglionic neurons, resulting in autonomic dysfunction. Finally, tetanus toxin may bind directly at neuromuscular junctions and directly cause neuromuscular facilitation.

If the toxin ascends in a nerve of a limb, that limb shows tetanus first, followed by the opposite limb and eventually the entire body. If the toxin circulates in the blood, signs of tetanus start in the head. Prolapse of the nictitating membrane and contraction of the facial muscles and mastication muscles are seen before development of tetanus in the rest of the body.[10]

All domestic animals are susceptible to tetanus. The ruminants and canines are more resistant than the horse. Birds are naturally resistant.

The clinical signs of tetanus occur 5 to 10 days after infection but may be delayed for up to 3 weeks in dogs and cats. Generalized signs include increased muscle tone and stiffness, usually in all the limbs and in the muscles of the head. In the early stages, the prolapsed nictitating membrane, contraction of the muscles of facial expression, and contraction of the muscles of mastication are characteristic. The lips are drawn in an exaggerated "grin"; in erect-eared breeds, the ears are drawn toward each other and the jaws are tightly closed. Other early signs are a stiff gait and tail elevation. In the later stages the animal is recumbent with extension of all four limbs and opisthotonos. Signs are enhanced by stimulation. Death may occur from respiratory paralysis.

Localized tetanus is more common in dogs and cats than in horses and humans because of the increased resistance of carnivores to tetanus toxin.

Clinical signs develop in the limb or region of the body closest to the wound. Signs may progress to the opposite limb, and with time they may generalize. In some cases, signs may stay localized to one limb, which may confuse the diagnosis.

Autonomic effects may also be present. Bradycardia, because of increased parasympathetic activity, has been reported in dogs.[11] Increased sympathetic activity has been demonstrated experimentally and in human patients.[5]

The diagnosis is based on the characteristic clinical signs and evidence of infection. The source of infection is not always evident, especially in dogs and cats, in whom the onset of signs may be delayed for up to 3 weeks. Intraabdominal infections, such as metritis, enteritis, and abscesses, may be a cause. Infection of the reproductive tract may cause tetanus localized to the pelvic limbs. Serum antibody titers to tetanus toxin can be used to confirm the diagnosis, but they are rarely used in clinical practice.

Treatment includes wound debridement, systemic administration of antibiotics to kill vegetative organisms, and antitoxin to neutralize unbound toxin. Penicillin G (20,000 to 100,000 IU per kilogram of body weight, administered intravenously, intramuscularly, or subcutaneously, every 6 to 8 hours), tetracycline (22 mg per kilogram, administered orally or intravenously every 8 hours), metronidazole (10 mg per kilogram of body weight, administered orally every 8 hours), and clindamycin (3 to 10 mg per kilogram of body weight, administered orally, intravenously, or intramuscularly every 8 to 12 hours) are effective. Although penicillin G has been the drug of choice for several years, metronidazole may be superior because it is bactericidal against *C. tetani* and is effective in anaerobic tissues. Antibiotics should be administered for 10 days.

Tetanus antitoxin is available as antitetanus equine serum (ATS) or human tetanus immune globulin (TIG). ATS can be given intramuscularly or intravenously, whereas TIG is licensed for intramuscular use only. Intravenous administration of ATS gives a rapid increase in circulating antitoxin and is the preferred route of administration. It neutralizes any toxin not bound to the central nervous system (CNS). A dose of 100 to 1000 IU per kilogram is recommended for dogs and 10,000 IU for horses. Intravenous ATS is associated with a high incidence of anaphylaxis. Pretreatment with antihistamines and glucocorticoid steroids is recommended. Intravenous epinephrine (0.1 ml/kg of 1:10,000 dilution) is the treatment of choice for anaphylactic reactions.

Sedation may be required to control severe muscle spasms, hyperexcitable states, and seizures.

Phenothiazine tranquilizers such as chlorpromazine depress descending excitatory neurons in the brainstem. Unlike other seizure disorders, phenothiazines are not contraindicated in animals with tetanus-induced seizures. Phenobarbital is used to control seizures. It can be combined with the phenothiazines, but its dose should be reduced. Glycopyrrolate can be used to treat bradycardia. The benzodiazepines, such as diazepam or clonazepam, may be helpful because they block polysynaptic reflexes in the medulla and spinal cord.

Nursing care must include a quiet environment, frequent turning if the animal is recumbent, and skin cleanliness. Oral intake may be impossible; hence, parenteral fluids and nutrients may be needed. Nasogastric or pharyngostomy tubes may be used. Respiratory assistance may be required.

Abdominal distention should be monitored in ruminants and breeds of dogs susceptible to bloat. The prognosis is usually good for dogs and cats unless respiratory problems occur. Horses or cows that become recumbent have poor prognoses. In young animals, before epiphysial closure is complete, tetanus may cause a variety of growth abnormalities in long bones.

Immunization with toxoid is recommended in horses. It is given to newborn foals and boosters are given every few years. Toxoid is given at the time of injury or surgery or before parturition.[12]

Metabolic Causes of Tetany

Hypocalcemia. Hypocalcemia results in tetany when serum calcium concentrations drop below 6 mg per deciliter. Calcium ion concentrations control neuronal membrane permeability; however, both protein-bound and ionized calcium are measured when serum calcium levels are quantitated. Thus, in hypoproteinemic conditions, low total serum calcium levels may be encountered without concomitant tetany. In dogs, cats, and horses, hypocalcemic tetany may result from hypoparathyroidism, postparturient eclampsia (rare in cats), terminal renal failure, protein-losing enteropathy, or severe alkalosis. Hypocalcemia in cows usually causes weakness, sometimes with tremor.

Postparturient eclampsia (puerperal tetany) in the bitch usually occurs within 3 weeks after whelping. Small-breed dogs with nervous temperaments are more susceptible to this disorder. The exact mechanism of postparturient hypocalcemia in the bitch is not known; however, calcium losses from fetal ossification and lactation combined with deficient osteoclastic activity or calcium absorption are probably responsible for altered calcium homeostasis. Although some bitches may become hypoglycemic during puerperal tetany, lowered blood glucose values probably are not important in the production of tetany. Some believe that nervous dogs are predisposed to puerperal tetany because they hyperventilate during parturition, inducing respiratory alkalosis. Alkalosis favors protein binding of calcium, thus lowering the concentrations of ionized calcium. Because ionized calcium is biologically active, alkalosis enhances the development of tetany.

Early clinical signs include nervousness, pacing, whining, and panting. Muscle spasm and ataxia are subsequent signs. These early manifestations usually progress to tonic–clonic tetanic spasms. Dogs are often febrile and, in severe cases, major motor seizures may be encountered.

Diagnosis of puerperal tetany is based on clinical signs and low blood calcium concentrations. On presentation, a blood sample should be collected for calcium analysis. Five to 10 ml of 10% calcium gluconate is given slowly, administered intravenously; heart rate and rhythm are monitored simultaneously. Ten-percent calcium gluconate, 2 to 5 ml, diluted with equal volumes of normal saline, can be given intramuscularly to prolong the calcium effect. Severely hyperthermic patients (body temperature greater than 105° F) are cooled with ice packs or alcohol soaks. Animals that continue to have seizures or that remain excessively irritable or restless are mildly sedated with diazepam or phenobarbital. For maintenance therapy, puppies are separated from the bitch for 24 hours and supplemented with bitch's milk formula. Full nursing is restricted for an additional 48 hours. Calcium lactate is given in oral dosages of 0.5 to 2.0 g per day.

Eclampsia of mares is rarely encountered except in draft horses. Most cases reportedly occur in lactating mares near the 10th day after parturition or 1 to 2 days after weaning. Factors that may predispose the animal to eclampsia in mares include grazing on a lush pasture, strenuous work, and prolonged transport. Affected mares tend to sweat profusely, develop muscle spasticity of the limbs, and become ataxic. Rapid respiration, muscular fibrillation, and trismus are evident, but no protrusion of the nictitating membrane occurs. The rectal temperature is normal or mildly elevated, and the pulse may be rapid and irregular. Swallowing may be impeded, and urination and defecation may cease. The diagnosis is based on clinical signs and the presence of reduced serum calcium concentrations (4 to 6 mg/dl). Treatment with intravenous calcium solutions produces rapid, complete recovery. Otherwise, within 24 hours tetanic convulsions develop, followed by death within an additional 24 hours.

Hypoparathyroidism results in decreased secretion of parathormone (PTH) with subsequent hypocalcemia and hyperphosphatemia. This condition has been recognized and studied most frequently in dogs, but it also occurs in cats. Although the exact cause is unknown, most dogs have histologic parathyroid changes indicative of a primary autoimmune disease (lymphocytic plasmacytic cellular infiltration). Parathyroid deficiency also may occur after thyroid gland surgery. An acute form of the disease is characterized by a sudden onset of tetany or convulsions or both. A chronic form of the disease is associated with recurrent depression, lethargy, anorexia, vomiting, intermittent facial and thoracic limb spasm, and latent tetany. Primary hypoparathyroidism is suspected in a dog with persistent hypocalcemia and hyperphosphatemia in the presence of normal renal function. Decreased concentrations of PTH in the presence of hypocalcemia substantiate the diagnosis.

Primary hypoparathyroidism is treated with drugs to overcome the PTH deficiency. Dihydrotachysterol, ergocalciferol (vitamin D_2), and calcitriol (1,25 dihydroxycholecalciferol) are frequently recommended. The clinician must individualize the dosage by monitoring the serum calcium levels of each patient twice a week. Approximate initial dosages of these drugs are dihydrotachysterol, 0.01 mg per kilogram of body weight daily; ergocalciferol, 1000 to 2000 U per kilogram of body weight daily; and calcitriol, 0.25 µg once a day. The clinician should monitor the serum calcium concentrations carefully to prevent hypercalcemia. The effect of vitamin D therapy may be delayed for 2 to 3 weeks. Calcium supplementation must be administered with caution because its use with vitamin D increases the probability of hypercalcemic toxicity.

Hypomagnesemic Tetanies. These syndromes occur primarily in ruminants. Several hypomagnesemic conditions have been described, including grass tetany, wheat pasture poisoning, milk tetany of calves, and transport tetany. The basic pathophysiology of each is similar and probably is related to decreased dietary intake and mobilization or increased excretion of magnesium.

Grass tetany occurs in lactating cattle that graze in a lush pasture. This tetany also occurs in pregnant and lactating ewes and occasionally in feeder cattle. Lush pastures are low in magnesium, and when magnesium requirements are increased, as in the case of lactating cattle, clinical signs are likely to occur. Early signs include restlessness, extreme alertness, and muscular twitching. Animals may become excitable, belligerent, and even aggressive. Stimulation may induce severe signs of tetany, ataxia, and bellowing. Animals may become recumbent with opisthotonos and paddling movements. The diagnosis of grass tetany is supported by laboratory findings of hypomagnesemia (<1 mg/dl), hypocalcemia (<7 mg/dl), and high normal levels of potassium. Therapy should correct the immediate ionic imbalance and should supplement the dietary intake of magnesium. Magnesium lactate in a 3.3% solution (2.2 ml/kg), magnesium gluconate in a 15% solution (0.44 ml/kg), and magnesium sulfate in a 20% solution (0.44 ml/kg) can be given slowly by the intravenous route or subcutaneously. Commercial combination solutions may also be used effectively. Magnesium oxide, 1 g/45 kg daily, should be force fed or supplied in blocks containing protein supplements and molasses. Animals on high-risk pastures should be given magnesium oxide or chloride supplements.

Wheat pasture poisoning is similar to grass tetany, except it occurs in cattle and sheep that graze on a cereal grain pasture during its early growth. Diagnosis and treatment are the same as those for grass tetany.

Milk tetany occurs in 2- to 4-month-old calves that are fed only milk. Signs may occur after episodes of diarrhea. Digestive disorders may decrease magnesium absorption, thus complicating the magnesium deficiency. Clinical signs include hyperesthesia, nervousness, recumbency, and seizures. Repeated attacks may occur. Diagnosis is based on the history, clinical signs, and serum magnesium concentrations below 0.7 mg/dl. Calves respond to parenteral magnesium ionic therapy. Susceptible calves should be given magnesium oxide supplements, 1 g per day.

Transport tetany occurs after stressful events such as transportation, vaccination, deworming, adverse weather, and marked dietary changes. Transport tetany occurs in both cattle and sheep. Dietary reduction in calcium, magnesium, and potassium coupled with stress produces ionic imbalances that result in a wide range of clinical signs, from spastic to flaccid paralysis. The signs usually begin within 24 hours of the stress but may be delayed for 72 hours. Early manifestations include restlessness, anorexia, and excitement. These signs progress to muscular trembling, teeth grinding, ataxia, and recumbency. Opisthotonos, paddling, and coma may develop. Treatment consists of parenteral administration of polyionic glucose solutions and attentive nursing care.

Renal Disease. Terminal stages of renal failure may cause tetany or seizures. Chronic renal disease may be associated with muscle wasting and weakness. Encephalopathy, polyneuropathy, and polymyopathy occur in humans with chronic renal disease, especially those receiving hemodialysis, but are not well documented in animals. Alterations in electrolyte metabolism, especially calcium metabolism, may cause signs related to the nervous system, as already discussed.

Toxicoses

Strychnine. Strychnine is a rodenticide that is sometimes used in malicious poisonings of small animals. It produces tetanic spasms that are exacerbated by auditory or tactile stimuli. The animal is fully conscious. The signs may appear within 10 minutes to 2 hours after ingestion.[13] The clinical signs are strongly suggestive of the diagnosis. Tetanus is not as acute in onset. Hypocalcemia can be quickly ruled out by finding normal serum calcium concentrations in affected dogs. Other toxins cause signs other than tetany. Metaldehyde causes tetany that progresses rapidly to seizures. Organophosphates cause muscle fasciculations, tremor, seizures, and autonomic signs. Chemical analysis of the stomach contents may confirm the diagnosis.

Treatment is directed at limiting absorption and controlling the tetany. Induction of vomiting or gastric lavage with activated charcoal is used to reduce the absorption. Tetany is controlled with pentobarbital sodium given intravenously to effect. Caution must be used to avoid overdosing. Endotracheal intubation and maintenance of respiration are mandatory. Inhalation anesthesia may be used to avoid large doses of barbiturates for prolonged periods. Diuresis is established with intravenous fluids. Acidification of the urine is recommended to enhance elimination, which should be completed in 24 to 48 hours.

Spasticity

Anomalous and Hereditary

Hereditary Myotonia. Myotonic myopathy, a condition of sustained contractions of the muscles, is an inherited disorder in dogs, goats, and horses. Table 10-2 lists the heredity and muscular changes

in these animals. In the goat, signs are noticed shortly after birth, whereas signs in the dog are usually not noticed until 6 weeks to 3 months of age. This difference probably reflects the degree of mobility at these ages in the species affected. The horse has a much milder form that is usually not recognized until the animal is about 6 months of age.

The signs are a progressive stiffening of the gait with exercise. The muscles maintain contraction after a normal contraction is elicited. The limbs become stiff and abducted in a sawhorse-like posture. With time, the muscles become hypertrophied, especially in the proximal parts of the limbs and in the neck. Percussion of a muscle causes a prolonged contraction of that part of the muscle, with a resultant dimple or bulge. In long-haired animals, the dimple is easily seen on the tongue. Electromyography (EMG) is useful to detect the characteristic "myotonic" discharge—a high-frequency, waxing–waning series of potentials. It sounds like a dive bomber or a motorcycle engine. Similar potentials called *complex repetitive discharges,* without the waxing–waning character, are found with many other forms of myopathy, such as inflammatory myositis. Both forms may be found in myotonias from increased adrenocortical hormones, whether acquired or iatrogenic.

Dogs and horses with myotonia may live a reasonable life. Cell membrane–stabilizing drugs have been used to provide some relief. Procainamide (500 mg given orally four times a day for dogs) has been recommended.[14]

Acquired Myotonia. Several forms of myopathy may have myotonic features. Inflammatory myopathy, whether immune mediated or caused by an infectious agent such as toxoplasmosis, may have myotonic discharges on the EMG and some increased contraction of the muscles. Endocrine myopathy, notably that caused by increased circulating corticosteroids, frequently has some myotonia associated with the degenerative changes.

Table 10-2 **Myotonia**

Species/Breed	Heredity	Dystrophic Changes	References
Canine			
Chow chow	Autosomal recessive (?)	Minimal	63-69
Staffordshire terrier	Unknown	Minimal	67, 70
Rhodesian ridgeback	Unknown	Moderate	71
Cavalier King Charles spaniel	Unknown	Minimal	72
Great Dane	Unknown	Minimal	73
Golden retriever	Unknown	Marked	14, 16, 64
Irish terrier	X-linked autosomal recessive	Marked	16, 74
Caprine	Autosomal dominant or recessive	Minimal	75-77
Equine	Unknown	Unknown	78

Hyperadrenocorticism (Cushing's syndrome) may be caused by adrenal tumors, pituitary tumors, or exogenous administration of corticosteroids. The myopathic changes occur late in the course of the syndrome when polyuria, polydipsia, abdominal distention, and cutaneous changes are usually evident. A stiff gait or weakness on exercise may be recognized. Clinical signs generally improve dramatically with appropriate therapy for the hyperadrenocorticism. Myotonic discharges may persist for weeks to months, even with resolution of the other signs of Cushing's syndrome.

Spastic Paresis. Spastic paresis, also called *Elso heel* and *spastic paralysis,* occurs in young cattle of many breeds. Although it is thought to be heritable, the evidence is not clear.

Affected calves are recognized between the ages of 1 week and 12 months. The signs are usually bilateral, but one side is often worse. The pelvic limbs are straight, especially at the hock. The limb is advanced like a pendulum and may be held caudally in extension. Some improvement occurs with walking, but movement never becomes normal. Forceful attempts to flex the limb cause increased tone and clonic contractions of the extensors.[15] The pathogenesis appears to be an increase in the activity of the gamma efferent system. Section of the dorsal roots or blocking of the small gamma motor neurons reduces the clinical signs.[16] Lowered levels of homovanillic acid, the main metabolite of dopamine, were found in the cerebrospinal fluid (CSF) of affected calves, suggesting a primary defect in dopamine metabolism.[17] Surgical management by sectioning the tibial nerve or severance of all or part of the gastrocnemius and flexor tendons allows the cattle to reach market age.[15] A genetic basis is suspected.

Spastic Syndrome. Periodic spasticity, crampiness, stretches, or Standing disease are names given a syndrome that affects the extensor muscles of the lumbar region and pelvic limbs. The condition is similar to spastic paresis except that it occurs in older animals and is more episodic. Episodes of muscle spasm are induced by movement and are not seen at rest. Spastic syndrome may occur in one limb or in both; in the latter case the movements alternate from side to side. The affected limb is raised and extended caudally or forcefully flexed. With time the episodes increase in severity. One study of the nerves and muscles of an affected bull failed to reveal any significant changes.[18] Evidence for an autosomal dominant inheritance is reported.[12]

Shivering. A syndrome of spasms of the pelvic limbs that includes flexion, abduction, and shaking when the limb is moved has been called *shivering.* The tail may also show tremors and it may be held elevated. The thigh muscles atrophy. The disorder is seen most often in draft horses. No lesion or treatment has been described.[16,19]

Stringhalt. Two forms of stringhalt are described. The gait is characterized by hyperflexion of one or both pelvic limbs during movement. Australian stringhalt occurs in epidemics and may involve the thoracic limbs. Degeneration is reported in the distal sciatic nerve. A toxic factor is postulated, especially for the epidemic form. Several plants have been investigated, but no clear cause is known.[20] Many horses improve slowly over a time span of weeks to a year. Affected animals should be removed from access to toxic plants and rested. Tenectomy of the lateral digital extensor tendon may help in severe cases.[12]

Scotty Cramp. Scottish terriers are affected by an inherited disorder characterized by episodic hypertonus of the muscles. The syndrome is inherited as a recessive trait.[21,22] The clinical signs are similar to those described for myotonia. Episodes are precipitated by exercise, fear, excitement, and some drugs. The limbs gradually become stiff, the back is arched, and the animal becomes reluctant to move. The thoracic limbs initially tend to abduct. The pelvic limbs often have both flexor and extensor hypertonus, resulting in a high-stepping, dysmetric gait. The animal becomes so stiff after a time that it falls down. Facial muscles may be involved. The severity is variable between dogs, some being only mildly affected, others incapacitated.

No gross or histologic lesions of the nervous system or muscles are present. The cause is believed to be an alteration in serotonin metabolism. The signs are made worse by the administration of agents that decrease serotonin levels in the CNS, such as methysergide (Sansert). Drugs that increase serotonin levels, such as monoamine oxidase inhibitors, provide a beneficial effect. Methysergide can be used to help confirm the diagnosis. A dose of 0.3 mg per kilogram administered orally increases the signs in most cases. A maximum dose of 0.6 mg per kilogram is recommended.[22] Diazepam is recommended at a dose of 0.5 to 1.5 mg per kilogram every 8 hours to reduce the clinical signs. Vitamin E, 125 IU per kilogram once a day, has been effective in reducing the frequency, but not the severity, of episodes.

Muscle Spasms

Metabolic

Exertional Myopathy. Exertional myopathy may occur in any species but is most common in athletic animals after exercise. Racing or working horses and racing greyhounds are frequently affected.

Exertional myopathy is also seen in newly captured wild animals. Working horses tend to have the problem shortly after exercise following several days of rest.

The signs are stiffness and extension of the limbs, distress, and pain and swelling of the muscles. The pathogenesis is thought to be metabolic acidosis in the muscle, swelling, local ischemia, muscle cell necrosis, and myoglobinuria. The myoglobinuria may be severe enough to cause nephropathy. Elevated serum levels of muscle enzymes (creatinine kinase [CK], lactate dehydrogenase [LDH], and aspartate aminotransferase [AST]) aid in the diagnosis. Type II muscle fibers are affected to a greater extent, but not exclusively, in horses.[23] Renal failure may occur in severe cases, resulting in the death of the animal.

Treatment entails administration of intravenous fluids to maintain renal function and bicarbonate to correct the acidosis, cooling the animal, and rest.[16,24] Dantrolene and phenytoin may help alleviate attacks but are still considered experimental.[12]

Tremor

Cerebellar Diseases

The primary cerebellar degenerations, anomalies, malformations, viral degenerations, toxic syndromes, steroid-responsive tremor syndrome (SRTS), and miscellaneous causes of cerebellar disease are discussed in Chapter 8.

These diseases produce all the signs of cerebellar disease, including tremor (Table 10-3).
Steroid-responsive Tremor Syndrome (Idiopathic Cerebellitis, Idiopathic Tremors, Little White Shakers). An acute tremor syndrome responsive to glucocorticoid steroids has been reported in young small-breed adult dogs. Initially, the syndrome was observed most frequently in small white breeds, such as Maltese, poodles, and West Highland white terriers. Hence the term *little white shakers* was used to describe the syndrome. An identical condition occurs in other small breeds that are not white.[25,93,94] In a recent study, 22 of 24 dogs with generalized tremors were diagnosed with SRTS based on excellent and rapid response to treatment with prednisone.[94] Most of these dogs were 1 to 5 years of age, and all weighed less than 15 kg. More than 50% of these dogs were nonwhite mixed breeds.

The tremor worsens with movement, an intention tremor, and it decreases at rest. Concurrent clinical signs include opsoclonus, head tilt, hypermetria, and decreased menace response. Although paresis is not a common finding, Bagley reported

tetraparesis in two of seven and paraparesis in one of seven affected Maltese.[93] The disease is nonprogressive after the first 2 to 3 days. Spontaneous remission may occur. The tremor is worse than usually expected with cerebellar disease, and the ataxia is less. In the few cases in which dogs were necropsied, mild nonsuppurative inflammation of the nervous system, not confined to the cerebellum, was found.[16] About 50% of affected dogs have mild to moderate mixed or mononuclear inflammatory changes in the CSF.[94]

Speculated causes include viral or immune-mediated inflammatory disease. The relation to white coat color has led to hypotheses involving a relation to tyrosine metabolism; however, as Parker points out, these are not albino animals.[26] Treatment is with immunosuppressive doses of corticosteroids, diazepam, or both.[93,94] Propranolol, a ß-adrenergic blocker, was effective in one of two dogs described by Bagley. The corticosteroids should be given in decreasing doses for 8 to 12 weeks. Stopping therapy early may lead to relapse. Clinical improvement is expected in 2 to 3 days. The response to treatment is usually dramatic, but some dogs are less responsive. Relapses after recovery have been seen.

Head Tremor. A coarse tremor, often called a "head bob," has been recognized, most often in the Doberman pinscher.[95] Similar movements were reported in a Shetland sheepdog.[96] Parker suggests that it is an anxiety or habit syndrome.[99] One Doberman that we observed over a number of years had a head tremor that waxed and waned at various times. Diagnostic test results, which were all negative, included those of hematology and blood chemistries, thyroxine and thyroid-stimulating hormone stimulation tests, computed tomography scan, CSF analysis, EMG and nerve-conduction studies, and myelography. The tremor usually consists of up and down movements of the head; these movements disappear at rest. We could not identify any precipitating factors in the periods when it was worse. The tremor usually appears in the first year of life and may persist for many years.

Demyelinating Diseases

Primary demyelinating diseases such as globoid cell leukodystrophy and those secondary to systemic diseases such as canine distemper frequently cause cerebellar signs, including tremor. These diseases are discussed in Chapter 15.

Anomalous or Hereditary

Hypomyelination. Hypomyelination is a developmental disorder of normal myelin causing thinly myelinated and some nonmyelinated axons.

Table 10-3   Tremor Syndromes Categorized by Time of Disease Onset

Species	At or Within a Few Days of Birth	A Few Weeks/Months to Adult	Adult	Any Age
Dogs	1. Inherited hypomyelination/ dysmyelination 2. Central axonopathy	1. Inadequate glycogen stores 2. Glycogen storage disease	1. Metabolic diseases (hypocalcemia, hypoglycemia, hypoadrenocorticism, hyperthyroidism) 2. Steroid-responsive tremor syndrome	Hexachlorophene toxicity
Pigs	1. Congenital hypomyelinogenesis (type A-I to A-V,B)	1. Encephalomyocarditis virus disease 2. Pseudorabies 3. Talfan/Teschen disease 4. Inadequate glycogen stores		1. Organic arsenical toxicity 2. Organic mercurial toxicity
Cattle	1. Shaker calf syndrome 2. Inherited congenital myoclonus 3. Maple syrup urine disease 4. Citrullinemia 5. Hereditary hypomyelinogenesis 6. Bovine viral diarrhea	1. Milk tetany 2. Polioencephalo-malacia 3. Glycogen storage disease 4. White muscle disease	Metabolic diseases (hypocalcemia, hypomagnesemia, hypoglycemia/ketosis)	1. Monensin toxicity 2. Urea toxicity 3. Organic mercurial toxicity 4. Hexachlorophene toxicity 5. Tremorogenic pasture grasses 6. Louping ill (rare)
Sheep and goats	1. Border disease (sheep) 2. Congenital swayback (goats)	1. Systemic neuraxial dystrophy (sheep) 2. Polioencephalo-malacia 3. Glycogen storage disease (sheep) 4. White muscle disease (sheep)	1. Metabolic diseases, sheep (see cattle, above) 2. Visna (sheep) 3. Scrapie	1. Louping ill (sheep) 2. Tremorogenic pasture grasses 3. Urea toxicity (sheep) 4. Hexachlorophene toxicity
Horses		1. Shaker foal syndrome (botulism) 2. Inadequate glycogen stores 3. White muscle disease	Hyperkalemic periodic paralysis	1. Yellow star thistle poisoning 2. Tremorogenic pasture grasses
Cats		Glycogen storage disease	Hyperthyroidism	Hexachlorophene toxicity
All species		1. Lysosomal storage disease 2. Hepatic encephalopathy		1. End-stage liver failure 2. Poisoning: orga-nophosphate/ carbamate, metaldehyde, chlorinated hydrocarbons, strychnine, lead 3. Botulism

From Cuddon PA: Tremor syndromes. *Prog Vet Neurol* 1:285-299, 1990.

Dysmyelination is similar, but with predominantly abnormal myelin.[27] Both terms have been used in describing these diseases. Hypomyelination is an inherited defect in some species and breeds. It also occurs secondary to in utero infection with several viral agents.[28] The disorder is distinct from demyelinating disease, in which the myelin develops normally and is later destroyed by external agents (e.g., canine distemper) and from metabolic storage disease (e.g., globoid cell leukodystrophy). Table 10-4 lists the primary disorders of myelin development.

Table 10-4 Disorders of Abnormal Myelin Development

Species/Breed	Inherited	References
Canine		
Springer spaniel	Yes	27, 28, 79, 80
Chow chow	Probably	27, 28, 81-84
Samoyed	Probably	27, 28, 85
Weimaraner	Probably	27, 28, 86-88
Bernese mountain dog	Probably	89
Lurcher	Unknown	27, 28, 90
Dalmatian	Unknown	91
Spaniel	Unknown	27
Australian silky terrier	Unknown	16
Porcine		
Type A-I	No, hog cholera virus	30-32
Type A-II	No, unknown virus	30-32
Type A-III Landrace	Yes	29, 33-35
Type A-IV Saddleback	Yes	29, 31, 36, 37
Type A-V	No, toxic	30
Type B	Unknown	30
Ovine		
Border disease	No, virus (BVD?)	38, 39
Bovine		
Jersey	?	32, 40
Shorthorn	?	32, 41
Angus shorthorn	?	32, 92
Hereford	?	32, 41, 53

The clinical signs of these syndromes are usually noticed in the first few weeks of life. The signs are similar to those of cerebellar disease (see Chapter 8), with ataxia, tremor, dysmetria, and pendular nystagmus being common in most animals. The primary difference is that most of the myelin disorders have a larger-amplitude movement disorder in addition to the fine tremor. In fact, one of the original names for the condition in pigs was myoclonia congenita.[29] In the chow chows that we have evaluated in our clinic, a large-amplitude, repetitive clonic movement is present in most of the affected animals.

The diagnosis in dogs is based on the history, presenting signs, and lack of positive findings on any diagnostic test. Generally more than one pup in a litter is affected. Distinguishing hypomyelination from other causes of cerebellar disease or demyelination is difficult. Most of the demyelinating diseases are not apparent at such an early age.

Six different myelin disorders have been defined in pigs (see Table 10-4).[29-37] Only two of these—type A-III, which is sex-linked in Landrace, and type A-IV, which is an autosomal recessive trait in Saddlebacks—are inherited. Affected pigs develop signs at 2 to 3 days of age. Myelin is abnormal in the Saddlebacks, and oligodendrocytes are reduced in the Landrace and in some dogs. No treatment for the inherited forms is known.

Sheep with border disease have a hairy fleece that is characteristic and are often called *hairy shakers*.[38,39] Border disease is caused by a virus that is transmitted to the lamb in utero. Affected lambs are often stunted and may have skeletal deformities. Hereford calves have a rare degenerative disorder characterized by neurofilament accumulation in neurons. Tremor is a prominent sign seen hours after birth. Bovine diarrhea virus has been implicated in hypomyelination in other cattle.[12,32,40-42]

Many animals that are not severely affected improve with age, but assistance with feeding is usually necessary because they cannot nurse properly. In springer spaniels, males do not show much improvement, but the carrier females are less severely affected and improve considerably with maturation. Chow chows and weimaraners improve to near-normal behavior with maturity. Sheep and pigs may recover if assisted with nutrition. Cattle may also improve, but the degenerative disease in Herefords is progressive and fatal. No treatment exists.

Central Axonopathy. A generalized axonopathy occurred in three Scottish terriers with generalized tremor and ataxia.[98] The dogs were from different locations but had a common sire. Age at presentation was 4 to 5 months, and all were euthanized within 2 months. The axonal degeneration differed from that seen in other breeds in that few axonal spheroids were present. The primary lesion was an increase in the diameter of axons with secondary changes of decreased myelin, spongy state, and gliosis.

Toxicoses

Mycotoxicoses. A mycotoxin, penitrem A, may cause severe generalized tremors, opsoclonus, and seizures in dogs.[43,94] Tremor syndromes followed the ingestion of moldy foods. The tremors lessened in severity with intravenous administration of diazepam. All dogs recovered quickly.[94] Mycotoxins associated with plants in large animals are discussed in the next section and are listed in Chapter 15.

Poisonous Plants. Plant toxicoses causing tremors usually affect multiple animals in a group, are seasonal, and often occur late in the growth period of the plants.[12] Food animals are affected more frequently than horses. Tremors are often associated with ataxia, dysmetria, and in some cases seizures.

Dallis grass and some other similar grasses are infested with *Claviceps paspali*, which produces a neurotoxin. *Phalaris* neurotoxicity is caused by alkaloids that interfere with serotonin release. Perennial ryegrass is infested with mycotoxins, and annual ryegrass has a toxin produced by a *Corynebacterium*.[25] See Table 15-17 for details.

Heavy-metal Poisoning. Lead is the most common heavy metal causing toxicosis in animals. Gastrointestinal and CNS signs dominate the clinical picture in most cases. Horses seem to be more resistant and generally have peripheral neuropathies and respiratory problems.[44] In cats and dogs, vomiting and diarrhea may occur, especially with acute poisoning. Cattle may bloat and have diarrhea. CNS signs include seizures, blindness, abnormal behavior, and tremors.[13,45,46] Tremors are usually associated with chronic low-grade poisoning and probably are caused by the demyelinating effects of lead. The acute cases often have laminar cerebrocortical necrosis accounting for the predominance of cerebral signs. Lead poisoning and other heavy-metal toxicities, including diagnosis and management, are discussed in Chapter 15.

Hexachlorophene. Hexachlorophene, an ingredient in antiseptic soaps, may cause generalized tremors, especially in young animals. Oral administration of hexachlorophene in an attempt to reproduce the clinical syndrome caused vomiting and diarrhea, salivation, tachypnea, and depression.[47] Clinical cases of hexachlorophene toxicity have resulted from both topical and oral contact. Examples include puppies exposed to nursing mammary glands that were washed daily with hexachlorophene soap, a cat with a skin lesion near the mouth that was washed with undiluted hexachlorophene soap, and a dog that ingested a bar of hexachlorophene soap.[48-50] Lesions are primarily vacuolation of the white matter. Treatment is eliminating exposure and supportive care. Acute intoxication may be helped by osmotic diuresis.[48] Dogs often recover with time.

Organophosphates and Chlorinated Hydrocarbons. Organophosphate compounds may cause tremor in some cases of chronic intoxication. The tremor usually precedes the more common findings of seizures and neuromuscular weakness. Chlorinated hydrocarbons often produce tremor as a major component of toxicity. Fine tremor or fasciculation of the muscles may be accompanied by seizures, tonic spasms, and autonomic manifestations. These toxicities are discussed in Chapter 15.

Other Tremorogenic Agents. Carbamates, pyrethrins, pyrethroids, ivermectin, bromethalin, and theobromine may cause tremors.[94]

Myoclonus

Anomalous or Hereditary

Inherited Congenital Myoclonus. This syndrome is also described as neuraxial edema in the literature (Table 10-5). Healy and colleagues differentiated two syndromes found in Hereford and Polled Hereford cattle.[51] Congenital myoclonus occurs primarily in Polled Herefords and their crossbreeds. It is inherited as an autosomal recessive trait with onset before birth. No histologic lesions are present in these animals, but they have a deficit of glycine/strychnine receptors in the spinal cord.[52] The clinical syndrome is characterized by a stimulus-responsive myoclonic spasm. Many of the calves have traumatic lesions of the hip joints. The second disease was found in Polled Herefords and Herefords. Clinical signs developed after birth and consisted of dullness, opisthotonos, and recumbency. The animals had a characteristic status spongiosus of the nervous system. Ketone concentrations were high in the urine, with a distinct aroma of burnt sugar. Healy and colleagues compared this syndrome with maple syrup urine disease in humans, one of several disorders of amino acid metabolism. The disease appears to be inherited as an autosomal recessive trait. The exact nature of the amino acid abnormality is not known. Neuraxial edema has also been reported in conjunction with hypomyelinogenesis in Hereford calves, but subsequent studies demonstrated that this was only hypomyelinogenesis.[42,53]

Spongy Degeneration. A group of diseases characterized by intracellular and extracellular vacuoles in either gray matter, white matter, or both produce a variety of signs, including ataxia and tremor, spasticity, opisthotonos, and myoclonus. Table 10-5 lists the diseases described in dogs, cats, and cattle.[42,51,52,54-58] All these syndromes occur in neonatal animals except the one described in Labrador retrievers. Congenital, infantile, and juvenile forms are described in humans.[55] Some of these diseases, such as maple syrup urine disease, are related to abnormal amino acid metabolism and can be managed in a limited way by controlling dietary intake of certain amino acids. All these syndromes are rare.

Familial Reflex Myoclonus in Labrador Retrievers and Dalmatians. A myoclonic syndrome of a group of Labrador retrievers has many characteristics of the congenital myoclonus of Hereford cattle.[59] The abnormality was recognized

Table 10-5 **Spongy Degenerations**

Species/Breed	Signs	Age	Lesion	References
Canine				
Labrador retriever	Ataxia, extensor rigidity, tremor	4-6 mo	Intramyelin, astrocytes	54, 55
Saluki	Seizures, behavioral change	3 mo	Gray and white matter	56
Samoyed	Tremors	12 d	White matter	57
Silky terrier	Myoclonus of paravertebral muscles			57
Feline				
Egyptian mau	Ataxia	7 wk	Intramyelin	58
Bovine				
Hereford, Polled Hereford	Recumbency, dullness, opisthotonus	1-3 d	Gray and white matter, maple syrup urine	42, 51
Polled Hereford*	Myoclonus	Birth	No lesion; deficiency of glycine, strychnine receptors	51, 52

*"Neuraxial edema," not spongiform degeneration

at 3 weeks of age. Clinical, laboratory, electrophysiologic, and tissue evaluations were done at 6 weeks of age. The pups were unable to rise without assistance. Extensor muscle tone was increased, but the neurologic examination was normal otherwise. Resistance to manipulation of the limbs or neck was increased. Muscles were of normal size with no dimpling on percussion. The characteristic finding was increased muscle contraction with any tactile or auditory stimulus or with voluntary activity. The muscle activity included all four limbs, opisthotonos, and contractures of the muscles of facial expression and the muscles of mastication.

Laboratory values were normal. EMG showed large motor-unit potentials (up to 5000 μV) and a stereotyped set of three evoked compound muscle-action potentials in response to a tactile stimulus. Normal dogs had no response to the same stimulus. Muscle biopsies were normal. Necropsy revealed mild esophageal dilatation, but no other gross or histologic lesions. A similarity was suggested to the spastic mutant mouse that has a deficiency in glycine receptors.[59]

We have examined one Labrador pup with a similar clinical presentation. Clorazepate may be beneficial in some cases. No gross or histologic lesions were seen at necropsy. Two unrelated Dalmatian dogs had a similar syndrome, although Woods[97] thought it resembled Scotty cramp. These dogs were somewhat responsive to acetylpromazine treatment. Dalmatians we have seen appeared to have the same syndrome as the Labrador retrievers.

Idiopathic

Tic in a Horse. A myoclonic twitch in the thoracic limb of a horse occurred after an unknown traumatic accident.[60] The limb was stiff and lame and had swelling and abrasions of the distal portions. A week after the injury, a twitch developed in the triceps and latissimus dorsi muscles. The contractions were at a relatively constant rate of about 30 to 60 per minute. All test findings were negative. A large number of drugs were tried, with no improvement. The twitch resolved in 11 weeks.

Inflammation

Canine Distemper Myoclonus. This syndrome was recognized and described as early as 1862.[61] The disorder has been called *chorea* and the *flexor spasm syndrome.* Chorea is continual, irregular, rapid, jerky movements of varying groups of muscles. Myoclonus is repetitive, rhythmic contractions of the same group of muscles.[3] The more appropriate term for the syndrome that follows distemper virus infection is *myoclonus.* Any group of muscles may be affected. Frequently myoclonus is confined to the flexor group in one limb, but myoclonus of combinations of muscle groups in more than one limb, the facial muscles, or the muscles of mastication are also seen. The syndrome may occur before, during, or after the overt encephalitis typical of distemper. The myoclonus often continues during sleep and light anesthesia. Most often it is a later developing sequela that may persist after all other clinical signs have resolved.[61]

Experimental studies have demonstrated that the abnormality lies in the spinal cord or brainstem within intrinsic neural circuits.[62] Sectioning the spinal cord cranial and caudal to the segments containing the LMN to the affected muscle groups does not abolish the response, nor does sectioning the dorsal roots. Sectioning the ventral roots does eliminate it.[62] No effective pharmacologic treatment exists. Anticonvulsants have no benefit.

Fortunately, the decreased incidence of canine distemper with modern vaccination programs makes this syndrome a relatively rare occurrence. Some individual animals seem to improve with time. If the myoclonus does not interfere with eating or locomotion, the dog can live with it.

Case Histories

CASE HISTORY 10A

Signalment
Canine, miniature pinscher, female, 2.5 years old.

History
Owner noticed shaking 7 to 8 days ago. The shaking markedly decreases when the dog sleeps or is resting. Shaking greatly intensifies with exercise or purposeful movements. The dog seems to feel good otherwise, and appetite and urinary and fecal continence are normal. The dog has received yearly immunizations and has recently tested positive for *Dirofilaria immitis* via heartworm antigen test. The dog has controlled access to outdoors. The owner recently sprayed nitrogen on her garden, and the walls of the home were sprayed for ants within the past 2 weeks.

Physical Examination
Temperature 103° F, heart rate 108, respiratory rate 30. The physical examination is normal except for neurologic findings.

Neurologic Examination
The dog is alert and responsive. Severe tremors (shaking) affect the head and body and are much worse with activity. The tremors lessen when the dog is held or the head is elevated. At gait, moderate hypermetria is present in all limbs but is more pronounced in the thoracic limbs. Postural reactions are normal, and extensor spinal reflexes cannot be evaluated because of intense shaking. Flexor reflexes are normal. Cranial nerves are normal, and the dog develops normal conjugate eye movements.

Complete the following sections before reviewing the case summary.

Assessment (Anatomic Diagnosis and Estimation of Prognosis)

Plan (Diagnostic)

Rule-outs   Procedure
1.
2.
3.
4.

CASE HISTORY 10B

Signalment
Bovine, Holstein Friesian, female, 9 months old.

History
Lameness developed in the right pelvic limb when the animal was 6 months of age and has gradually progressed.

Physical Examination
The animal is normal except for lameness in the right pelvic limb. The gait is hindered by inability to flex the limb. The stifle and hock are extended and do not flex at gait. The joints are normal on palpation.

Neurologic Examination
Normal except for the right pelvic limb. Increased tone is present in the gastrocnemius muscle. The limb cannot be flexed. Sensation to the limb is normal.

Complete the following sections before reviewing the case summary.

Assessment (Anatomic Diagnosis and Estimation of Prognosis)

Plan (Diagnostic)

Rule-outs   Procedure
1.
2.
3.
4.

CASE HISTORY 10C

Signalment
Canine, chow chow, female, 3 months old.

History
The puppy has a lameness of several weeks' duration. The owners report that the puppy seems to tire easily. She is one of five in a litter; the others are normal.

Physical Examination
All systems are normal except the puppy is unusually well muscled.

Neurologic Examination

Observation
1. Mental status: Alert.
2. Posture: The limbs are abducted and the joints are straighter than normal.
3. Gait: The pup has some difficulty getting up. The gait is stiff. The thoracic limbs are abducted and rotated medially. The pelvic limbs are dragged the first few steps and then are abducted. After a few steps the gait improves.

The remainder of the neurologic examination is normal.

Assessment (Anatomic Diagnosis and Estimation of Prognosis)

Plan (Diagnostic)

Rule-outs   Procedure
1.
2.
3.
4.

ASSESSMENT 10A

Anatomic Diagnosis
The tremors and hypermetria in association with normal postural reactions are characteristic of generalized cerebellar disease. Given the history in this case, the following rule-outs were considered:
1. Steroid-responsive tremor syndrome (SRST): The age, breed, history and clinical signs are very suggestive of this disorder.

2. Toxicity: Lead, organophosphate/carbamate, ivermectin, hexachlorophene, and moldy food intoxication were considered. There were no other clinical signs suggestive of these toxins. The dog had no access to moldy foods.
3. Cerebellitis: Consideration was given to infectious/inflammatory diseases such as canine distemper encephalitis, protozoal encephalitis, and granulomatous meningoencephalitis. The absence of other neurologic signs plus the excellent vaccination history made these conditions unlikely.

Diagnostic Plan

The owner was given the option of complete diagnostic evaluation, including complete blood count (CBC), urinalysis (UA), biochemical profile, CSF analysis, CSF serology, toxicologic tests, and CT of skull. The CBC, biochemical profile, and blood-lead analysis were all normal. The owner then elected treatment.

Therapeutic Plan

Prednisone, 7.5 mg (2.2 mg/kg twice daily), was given every 12 hours for 3 days and the dose then reduced to 5.0 mg every 12 hours for 3 additional days. Following a quick and complete recovery, prednisone was continued at 5 mg once a day for 10 days. After 16 days of prednisone therapy, the dog was clinically normal. Prednisone was continued at 2.5 mg once a day for 2 additional weeks.

Case Summary

The decision to pursue aggressive diagnostic procedures should be made by the owner. The possibility of exacerbating an infectious disease with corticosteroids must be considered when a therapeutic trial is considered. SRST responds to treatment, but relapses can occur. SRST has been reported in miniature pinchers.[94]

ASSESSMENT 10B

Anatomic Diagnosis

The lack of neurologic deficits other than increased tone in the gastrocnemius muscle is significant. Other diseases that must be considered are arthropathies, including infections and arthrogryposis, and upward fixation of the patella.

1. Spastic paresis: Local anesthetic block of the tibial nerve should relieve the lameness temporarily, as it did in this case. The other diseases would not be improved with this procedure.

Therapeutic Plan

Tibial neurectomy, either partial or total, provides relief of the signs. The primary branches supplying the gastrocnemius muscle were transected. These were identified by electrical stimulation during surgery.

Case Summary

The calf had a relatively normal gait in 5 days. (Case from Yamada H et al: A successful case of spastic paresis in a calf by partial tibial neurectomy, *Jpn J Vet Sci* 51:213-214, 1989.)

ASSESSMENT 10C

Anatomic Diagnosis

The increased tone in all muscles of the limbs with no neurologic deficits suggests a muscle disease. Muscle hypertrophy, some improvement after moving, and the breed should suggest congenital myotonia. Other possibilities include myositis and other myopathies.

1. Muscle disease: CK is increased. Other laboratory values are normal. EMG discloses prolonged insertion activity that increases and then decreases in amplitude and frequency. Percussion of muscles, including the tongue, causes prolonged contraction, producing a dimple. Nerve-conduction velocities are normal. Muscle biopsies show hypertrophy and a few atrophic fibers. These findings are consistent with myotonia.

Therapeutic Plan

The pup was treated with procainamide, which partially relieved the signs. A trial with phenytoin resulted in no improvement.

Case Summary

Congenital myotonia is an inherited disease in chow chows. Treatment relieves the signs to some degree, but a cure is not available. (Case from Amann JF, Tomlinson J, Hankison JK: Myotonia in a chow chow. *J Am Vet Med Assoc* 187:415-417, 1985.)

References

1. Thach WT, Montgomery EB: Motor system. In Pearlman AL, Collins RC, editors: *Neurological pathophysiology*. New York, 1984, Oxford University Press.
2. Taylor EJ: *Dorland's illustrated medical dictionary*. Philadelphia, 1988, WB Saunders. 1988.
3. Hallett M, Ravits J: Involuntary movements. In Asbury AK, McKhann GM, McDonald WI, editors: *Diseases of the nervous system*. Philadelphia, 1986, Ardmore Medical Books.
4. Liles SL, Davis GD: Athetoid and choreiform hyperkinesias produced by caudate lesions in the cat. *Science* 164:195-197, 1969.
5. Bleck T: Pharmacology of tetanus. *Clin Neuropharmacol* 9:103-120, 1986.
6. Luttgen PJ: An outline of neurotransmitters and neurotransmission, Part II. Function and dysfunction. *J Am Anim Hosp Assoc* 23:663-673, 1987.
7. Kornegay JN, Mayhew IG: Metabolic, toxic, and nutritional diseases of the nervous system. In Oliver JE, Hoerlein BF, Mayhew IG, editors: *Veterinary neurology*. Philadelphia, 1987, WB Saunders.
8. Furman RE, Barchi RL: Pathophysiology of myotonia and periodic paralysis. In Asbury AK, McKhann GM, McDonald WI, editors: *Diseases of the nervous system*. Philadelphia, 1986, Ardmore Medical Books.
9. Roberts TDM: *Neurophysiology of postural mechanisms*. New York, 1967, Plenum Press.
10. Timoney JF, Gillespie JH, Scott FW, et al: *Hagan and Bruner's microbiology and infectious diseases of domestic animals*. Ithaca, NY, 1988, Comstock Publishing Associates.
11. Panciera DL, Baldwin CJ, Keene BW: Electrocardiographic abnormalities associated with tetanus in two dogs. *J Am Vet Med Assoc* 192:225-227, 1988.
12. Mayhew IG: *Large animal neurology: a handbook for veterinary clinicians*. Philadelphia, 1989, Lea & Febiger.
13. Grauer GF, Hjelle JJ: Toxicology. In Morgan RV, editor: *Handbook of small animal practice*. New York, 1988, Churchill Livingstone.
14. Duncan ID, Griffiths I: Neuromuscular diseases. In Kornegay JN, editor: *Neurologic disorders*. New York, 1986, Churchill Livingstone.

15. Denniston JC, Shive RJ, Friedli U, et al: Spastic paresis syndrome in calves. *J Am Vet Med Assoc* 152:1138-1149, 1968.

16. de Lahunta A: *Veterinary neuroanatomy and clinical neurology,* 2nd ed. Philadelphia, 1983, WB Saunders.

17. DeLey G, DeMoor A: Bovine spastic paralysis: cerebrospinal fluid concentrations of homovanillic acid and 5-hydroxyindoleacetic acid in normal and spastic calves. *Am J Vet Res* 36:227-228, 1975.

18. Wells GAH, Hawkins SAC, O'Toole DT, et al: Spastic syndrome in a Holstein bull: a histologic study. *Vet Pathol* 24:345-353, 1987.

19. Palmer AC: *Introduction to animal neurology,* 2nd ed. Oxford, England, 1976, Blackwell Scientific Publishing.

20. Cahill JI, Goulden BE, Pearce HG: A review and some observations on stringhalt. *N Z Vet J* 33:101-104, 1985.

21. Meyers KM, Padgett GA, Dickson WM: The genetic basis of a kinetic disorder of Scottish terrier dogs. *J Hered* 61:189-192, 1970.

22. Clemmons RM, Peters RI, Meyers KM: Scotty cramp: a review of cause, characteristics, diagnosis and treatment. *Compend Cont Educ Pract Vet* 2:385-390, 1980.

23. McEwen S, Hulland T: Histochemical and morphometric evaluation of skeletal muscle from horses with exertional rhabdomyolysis (tying-up). *Vet Pathol* 23:400-410, 1986.

24. Braund KG: Diseases of peripheral nerves, cranial nerves, and muscle. In Oliver JE, Hoerlein BF, Mayhew IG, editors: *Veterinary neurology.* Philadelphia, 1987, WB Saunders.

25. Cuddon PA: Tremor syndromes. *Prog Vet Neurol* 1:285-299, 1990.

26. Parker AJ: How do I treat? "Little white shakers." *Prog Vet Neurol* 2:151, 1991.

27. Duncan I: Abnormalities of myelination of the central nervous system associated with congenital tremor. *J Vet Intern Med* 1:10-23, 1987.

28. Duncan I: Congenital tremor and abnormalities of myelination. In *Proceedings of the American College of Veterinary Internal Medicine Forum,* San Diego, 1987.

29. Done J: The congenital tremor syndrome in pigs. *Vet Annu* 16:98-102, 1975.

30. Done JT, Bradley R: Nervous and muscular system. In Leman AD, editor: *Diseases of swine.* Ames, Iowa, 1985, Iowa State University Press.

31. Emmerson JL, Delez AL: Cerebellar hypoplasia, hypomyelinogenesis and congenital tremors of pigs associated with prenatal hog cholera vaccination of sows. *J Am Vet Med Assoc* 147:47-54, 1965.

32. Braund KG: Degenerative and developmental diseases. In Oliver JE, Hoerlein BF, Mayhew IG, editors: *Veterinary neurology.* Philadelphia, 1987, WB Saunders 1987.

33. Foulkes JA: Myelin and dysmyelination in domestic animals. *Vet Bull* 8:441-450, 1974.

34. Done JT: Congenital nervous diseases of pigs: a review. *Lab Anim* 2:207-217, 1968.

35. Done J, Woolley J, Upcott D, et al: Porcine congenital tremor AII: spinal cord morphometry. *Br Vet J* 142:145, 1986.

36. Harding JDJ, Done JT, Harbourne JF, et al: Congenital tremor type A III in pigs: a hereditary sex linked cerebrospinal hypomyelinogenesis. *Vet Rec* 92:527-529, 1973.

37. Patterson DSP, Sweasey D, Brush PJ, et al: Neurochemistry of the spinal cord in British saddleback piglets affected with congenital tremor type A IV, a second form of hereditary cerebrospinal hypomyelinogenesis. *J Neurochem* 21:397-406, 1973.

38. Saperstein G, Leipold HW, Dennis SM: Congenital defects in sheep. *J Am Vet Med Assoc* 167:314-322, 1974.

39. Clarke GL, Osburn BI: Transmissible congenital demyelinating encephalopathy of lambs. *Vet Pathol* 15:68-82, 1978.

40. Saunders LZ, Sweet JD, Martin SM, et al: Hereditary congenital ataxia in Jersey calves. *Cornell Vet* 42:559-591, 1952.

41. Hulland TJ: Cerebellar ataxia in calves. *Can J Comp Med* 21:72-76, 1957.

42. Duffell S: Neuraxial oedema of Hereford calves with and without hypomyelinogenesis. *Vet Rec* 117:95-98, 1986.

43. Hocking AD: Intoxication by tremorgenic mycotoxin (penitrem A) in a dog. *Aust Vet J* 65:82-85, 1988.

44. Dollahite JW, Younger RL, Crookshank HR, et al: Chronic lead poisoning in horses. *Am J Vet Res* 39:961-964, 1978.

45. Zook BC, Carpenter JL, Leeds EB: Lead poisoning in dogs. *J Am Vet Med Assoc* 155:1329-1342, 1969.

46. Knecht CD, Crabtree J, Katherman A: Clinical, clinicopathologic, and electroencephalographic features of lead poisoning in dogs. *J Am Vet Med Assoc* 175:196-201, 1979.

47. Scott DW, Bolton GR, Lorenz MD: Hexachlorophene toxicosis in dogs. *J Am Vet Med Assoc* 162:947-949, 1973.

48. Thompson J, Senior D, Pinson D, et al: Neurotoxicosis associated with the use of hexachlorophene in a cat. *J Am Vet Med Assoc* 190:1311-1312, 1987.

49. Ward BC, Jones BD, Rubin GJ: Hexachlorophene toxicity in dogs. *J Am Anim Hosp Assoc* 9:167-169, 1973.

50. Bath ML: Hexachlorophene toxicity in dogs. *J Small Anim Pract* 19:241-244, 1978.

51. Healy P, Harper P, Dennis J: Diagnosis of neuraxial oedema in calves. *Aust Vet J* 63:95-96, 1986.

52. Gundlach AL, Dodd PR, Grabara CSG, et al: Deficit of spinal cord glycine/strychnine receptors in inherited myoclonus of Poll Hereford calves. *Science* 241:1807-1810, 1988.

53. Duffell SA, Harper PAW, Healy PJ, et al: Congenital hypomyelinogenesis of Hereford calves. *Vet Rec* 123:423-424, 1988.

54. O'Brien DP, Zachary JF: Clinical features of spongy degeneration of the central nervous system in two Labrador retriever littermates. *J Am Vet Med Assoc* 186:1207-1210, 1985.

55. Zachary JF, O'Brien DP: Spongy degeneration of the central nervous system in two canine littermates. *Vet Pathol* 22:561-571, 1985.

56. Luttgen PJ, Storts RW: Central nervous system status spongiosus. In *Proceedings of the American College of Veterinary Internal Medicine Forum.* San Diego, 1987, p 841.

57. Braund K: *Clinical syndromes in veterinary neurology.* Baltimore, 1986, Williams & Wilkins.

58. Kelly DF, Gaskell CJ: Spongy degeneration of the central nervous system in kittens. *Acta Neuropathol* 35:151-158, 1976.

59. Fox JG, Averill DR, Hallett M, et al: Familial reflex myoclonus in Labrador retrievers. *Am J Vet Res* 45:2367-2370, 1984.

60. Beech J: Forelimb tic in a horse. *J Am Vet Med Assoc* 180:258-260, 1982.

61. Whittier JW: Flexor spasm syndrome in the carnivore. *Am J Vet Res* 17:720-732, 1956.

62. Breazile JE, Blaugh BS, Nail N: Experimental study of canine distemper myoclonus. *Am J Vet Res* 27:1375-1379, 1966.

63. Shores A, Redding RW, Braund KG, et al: Myotonia congenita in a chow chow pup. *J Am Vet Med Assoc* 188:532-533, 1986.

64. Braund KG: Identifying degenerative and developmental myopathies. *Vet Med* 81:713-718, 1986.

65. Shelton G, Cardinet H: Pathophysiologic basis of canine muscle disorders. *J Vet Intern Med* 1:36-44, 1987.

66. Farrow BRH: Canine myotonia. In *Proceedings of the Sixth Annual Veterinary Medical Forum,* 1988.

67. Nafe LA, Shires P: Myotonia in the dog. In *Proceedings of the American College of Veterinary Internal Medicine Forum,* 1984, pp 191-192.

68. Jones BR, Anderson LJ, Barnes GRG, et al: Myotonia in related chow chow dogs. *N Z Vet J* 25:217-220, 1977.

69. Farrow BRH, Malik R: Hereditary myotonia in the chow chow. *J Small Anim Pract* 22:451-465, 1981.

70. Shires PK, Nafe LA, Hulse DA: Myotonia in a Staffordshire terrier. *J Am Vet Med Assoc* 183:229-232, 1983.

71. Simpson ST, Braund KG: Myotonic dystrophy like disease in a dog. *J Am Vet Med Assoc* 186:495-498, 1985.

72. Wright JA, Smyth JBA, Brownlie SE, et al: A myopathy associated with muscle hypertonicity in the cavalier King Charles spaniel. *J Comp Pathol* 97:559-565, 1987.

73. Honhold N, Smith DA: Myotonia in the Great Dane. *Vet Rec* 119:162, 1986.

74. Wentink GH, van der Linde-Sipman JS, Meijer AEF, et al: Myopathy with a possible recessive X-linked inheritance in a litter of Irish terriers. *Vet Pathol* 9:328-349, 1972.

75. Bryant SH: Altered membrane potentials in myotonia. In Bolis L, Hoffman LA, editors: *Membranes and diseases.* New York, 1976, Raven Press.

76. Bryant SH: Myotonia in the goat. *Ann N Y Acad Sci* 317:314-325, 1979.

77. Atkinson JB, LeQuire VS: Myotonia congenita. *Comp Pathol Bull* 17:3-4, 1985.

78. Steinberg S, Bothelo S: Myotonia in a horse. *Science* 137:979, 1962.

79. Griffiths IR, Duncan ID, McCulloch M, et al: Shaking pups: a disorder of central myelination in the spaniel dog, Part 1: Clinical, genetic, and light microscopical observations. *J Neurol Sci* 50:423-433, 1981.

80. Farrow BRH: Tremor syndromes in dogs. In *Proceedings of the Sixth Annual Veterinary Medical Forum.* Washington, DC, 1988.

81. Vandevelde M, Braund K, Luttgen PJ, et al: Dysmyelination in chow chow dogs: Further studies in older dogs. *Acta Neuropathol* 55:81-87, 1981.

82. Vandevelde M, Braund KG, Walker T, et al: Dysmyelination of the central nervous system in the chow-chow dog. *Acta Neuropathol* 42:211-215, 1978.

83. Duncan I: Congenital tremor and abnormalities of myelination. In *Proceedings of the Fifth Annual Veterinary Medical Forum.* San Diego, 1987.

84. Farrow B: Generalized tremor syndrome. In Kirk RW, editor: *Current veterinary therapy IX.* Philadelphia, WB Saunders, 1986.

85. Cummings J, Summers B, de Lahunta A, et al: Tremors in Samoyed pups with oligodendrocyte deficiencies and hypomyelination. *Acta Neuropathol* 71:267-277, 1986.

86. Kornegay J: Hypomyelination in Weimaraner dogs. *Acta Neuropathol* 72:394-401, 1987.

87. Comont PSV, Palmer AC, Williams AE: Weakness associated with myelopathy in a Weimaraner puppy. *J Small Anim Pract* 29:367-372, 1988.

88. Kornegay JN: Dysmyelinogenesis in dogs. In *Proceedings of the Third Annual Medical Forum,* American College of Veterinary Internal Medicine. San Diego, 1985.

89. Palmer A, Blakemore W, Wallace M, et al: Recognition of 'trembler,' a hypomyelination condition in the Bernese mountain dog. *Vet Rec* 120:609-612, 1987.

90. Mayhew IG, Blakemore WF, Palmer AC, et al: Tremor syndromes and hypomyelination in Lurcher pups. *J Small Anim Pract* 25:551-559, 1984.

91. Greene CE, Vandevelde M, Hoff EJ: Congenital cerebrospinal hypomyelinogenesis in a pup. *J Am Vet Med Assoc* 171:534-536, 1977.

92. Young S: Hypomyelinogenesis congenita (cerebellar ataxia) in Angus Shorthorn calves. *Cornell Vet* 52:84-93, 1962.

93. Bagley RS, Kornegay JN, Wheeler SJ, et al: Generalized tremors in Maltese: clinical findings in seven cases. *J Am Anim Hosp Assoc* 29:141-145, 1993.

94. Wagner SO, Podell M, Fenner WR: Generalized tremors in dogs: 24 cases (1984-1995). *J Am Vet Med Assoc* 211:731-735, 1997.

95. Bagley RS: Tremor syndromes in dogs: diagnosis and treatment. *J Small Anim Pract* 33:485-490, 1991.

96. Nakahata K, Uzuka Y, Matsumoto H, et al: Hyperkinetic involuntary movements in a young Shetland sheepdog. *J Am Anim Hosp Assoc* 28:347-348, 1992.

97. Woods CB: Hyperkinetic episodes in two Dalmatian dogs. *J Am Anim Hosp Assoc* 13:254-257, 1977.

98. Van Ham L, Vandevelde M, Desmidt M, et al: A tremor syndrome with a central axonopathy in Scottish terriers. *J Vet Intern Med* 8:290-292, 1994.

99. Parker AJ: Some unusual motor activities in dogs and cats. *Prog Vet Neurol* 7:20-24, 1996.

Chapter 11

Blindness, Anisocoria, and Abnormal Eye Movements

Problems related to abnormalities of the eyes and the visual pathways are important to the formulation of a neurologic diagnosis.[1] The retina and the optic nerve are the only sensory receptors and the only nerve that can be examined directly. The sensory and motor pathways of vision and eye movements traverse the brain from the orbit to the occipital region of the cerebral cortex and the medulla oblongata, so that diseases affecting the brain are likely affecting some portion of the visual system. Systemic diseases often affect the retina.

LESION LOCALIZATION

The visual system is considered in three parts: (1) vision, (2) pupillary light reflexes, and (3) movements of the eye. Combinations of abnormal signs should lead to an anatomic diagnosis.

Vision

The visual pathways are presented in Figures 11-1 and 11-2. Methods of testing vision are discussed in Chapter 1. Lesions of the lateral geniculate nucleus of the thalamus, the optic radiation (fiber tracts), or the occipital cortex cause loss of sight without affecting pupillary reflexes (Table 11-1). Many of these lesions are unilateral, resulting in a loss of vision in the contralateral field. Bilateral lesions such as those that can occur with encephalitis or hydrocephalus cause complete blindness. Lesions of the retina, the optic nerve, the optic chiasm, or the optic tracts cause blindness and pupillary abnormalities (see Figure 11-1). Optic chiasm lesions almost always cause bilateral blindness. Retinal and optic nerve lesions are frequently bilateral (e.g., retinal atrophy, optic neuritis) but may be unilateral (e.g., trauma, neoplasia). Optic tract lesions causing clinical signs are rare.

The degree of decussation of optic nerve fibers at the optic chiasm varies in different species. As a rule, the more lateral the eyes are placed in the skull, the greater the degree of decussation and the less binocular vision. In primates, essentially all the fibers from the nasal half of the retina cross, whereas all the fibers from the temporal half of the retina remain ipsilateral. In carnivores, about half the fibers of the temporal retina cross, and all the nasal retinal fibers cross. In most herbivores, 80% or more of the fibers cross. In horses, about 17% of fibers cross.[2] Rabbits have almost all crossed fibers. Visual field testing may be of importance for lesion localization in dogs and cats, but each eye can be considered to have an independent pathway in other domestic animals.

Assessment of the visual field is difficult. The usual methods of the menace and visual placing reactions test the lateral field, nasal retina, and crossing fibers. Deficits in these responses that are central to the optic chiasm are usually on the contralateral side of the brain.

Caution must be exercised in the interpretation of visual deficits. Because the examiner must rely on motor or behavioral reactions, he or she should use several tests to confirm an impression that the animal does not see. See Chapter 1 for details.

Pupillary Light Reflexes

The pathway for pupillary light reflexes is outlined and illustrated in Figures 11-1 to 11-3 and in Table 11-1. The methods of testing pupillary reflexes are described in Chapter 1.

Lesions of cranial nerve III (CN III), (the oculomotor nerve, including the ciliary ganglion and the short ciliary nerves) or of the constrictor muscle of the pupil cause loss of pupillary constriction in response to light on the involved side without affecting vision. Bilateral lesions are unusual except in lesions of the brainstem. Lesions of the pretectal nucleus or the parasympathetic nucleus of CN III cause loss of pupillary constriction. Usually both eyes are affected because the nuclei are

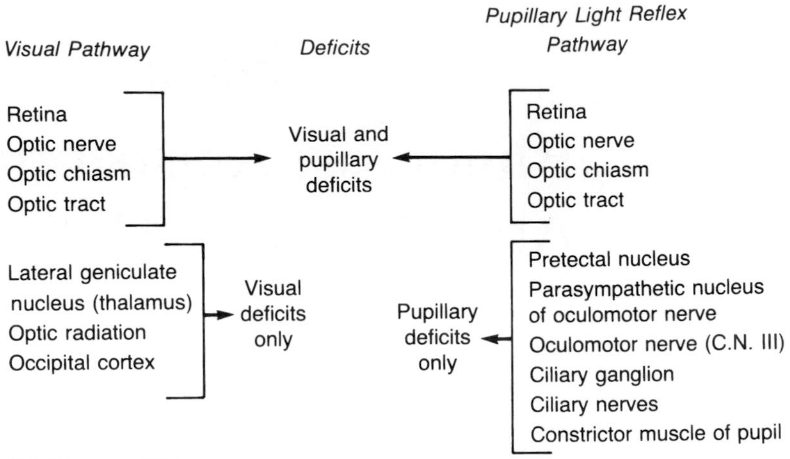

*Pupillary Light Reflex
Pathway*

Visual Pathway   *Deficits*

Retina	Visual and	Retina
Optic nerve	pupillary	Optic nerve
Optic chiasm	deficits	Optic chiasm
Optic tract		Optic tract

Figure 11-1 Deficits from lesions of the visual and pupillary light reflex pathways.

Lateral geniculate	Visual	Pretectal nucleus
nucleus (thalamus)	deficits	Parasympathetic nucleus
Optic radiation	only	of oculomotor nerve
Occipital cortex	Pupillary	Oculomotor nerve (C.N. III)
	deficits	Ciliary ganglion
	only	Ciliary nerves
		Constrictor muscle of pupil

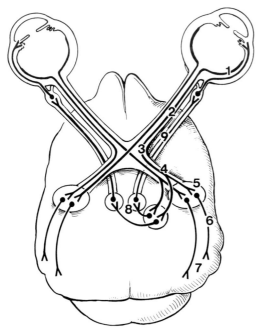

Figure 11-2 Pathways for vision and the pupillary light reflex pathway. *1,* Retina/optic nerve; *2,* orbit (cranial nerve [CN] II, III); *3,* optic chiasma; *4,* optic tract; *5,* lateral geniculate nucleus (thalamus); *6,* optic radiation; *7,* occipital cortex; *8,* parasympathetic nucleus of CN III (midbrain); *9,* CN III (oculomotor).

anatomically close together in the midbrain. Lesions of the retina, the optic nerve, or the optic chiasm cause loss of constriction of the pupil on the affected side in response to direct stimulation, but the pupil reacts to light shined in the opposite eye. Vision is impaired in the affected eye (see Table 11-1).

Sympathetic control of the dilator muscle of the pupil is illustrated in Figure 11-3. Note that these pathways originate in the midbrain, and nerve

fibers course down the brainstem and cervical spinal cord to synapse on lower motor neurons located in spinal cord segments T1 through T3. Second-order fibers leave the spinal cord with roots of the brachial plexus. In the thorax, fibers compose the cranial sympathetic nerve, which courses rostrally with the vagus nerve synapsing in the cranial cervical ganglion located near the tympanic bulla. Third-order sympathetic fibers then follow other cranial nerves to innervate structures in the head. Sympathetic activation is produced by emotional reactions such as fear and rage. Sympathetic nerves also innervate smooth muscle in the periorbital fascia and the eyelids, including the third eyelid in some species. Lesions of this pathway cause a constricted pupil *(miosis)*, slight retraction of the globe because of loss of tone in the periorbita *(enophthalmos)*, narrowing of the palpebral fissure *(ptosis)*, and extrusion of the third eyelid.[3] Sweating of the ipsilateral face occurs in horses.[4] This cluster of signs is called Horner's syndrome.

Horner's syndrome usually is not associated with visual deficits. Localization is dependent on associated clinical signs. For example, avulsion of the brachial plexus may cause monoparesis and Horner's syndrome on the same side. T1-3 spinal cord lesions cause upper motor neuron (UMN) signs in the pelvic limb, lower motor neuron (LMN) signs in the thoracic limb, and Horner's syndrome. Middle-ear disease is frequently associated with Horner's syndrome in dogs because the sympathetic fibers pass through the tympanic bulla. Guttural pouch infections may cause Horner's syndrome in horses. In dogs and cats, the most common causes of Horner's syndrome include head, neck, or chest trauma; chronic otitis media/interna; brachial plexus avulsion; intracranial and intrathoracic neoplasia; and vigorous ear cleaning.[5,6]

Table 11-1 **Signs of Lesions in the Visual and Pupillary Light Reflex Pathways**

Lesion Location	Vision/Menace Response	Pupil Size	Pupillary Light Reflexes
Retina/optic nerve (unilateral lesion)	Absent on affected side Normal on opposite side	Usually normal but may be slightly dilated on affected side	Direct and consensual response absent when testing affected side Normal when testing opposite side
Bilateral retina/optic nerve/optic chiasm	Absent in both eyes	Bilaterally dilated	Absent in both eyes
Unilateral optic tract, lateral geniculate nucleus, optic radiation, occipital cortex	Absent in contralateral eye* Normal in ipsilateral eye	Normal in both eyes	Normal in both eyes
Midbrain (bilateral) parasympathetic nucleus of CN III	Normal in both eyes	Bilaterally dilated	Absent in both eyes
Unilateral CN III	Normal in both eyes	Dilated on affected side, normal in contralateral eye	Negative direct response on affected side but positive in contralateral eye Positive direct response in contralateral eye but negative consensual response on affected side
Sympathetic nerve	Normal in both eyes	Constricted on affected side and does not dilate in dark Normal on contralateral side and dilates in dark	Positive in both eyes

*Depending on how menace response is tested, loss of vision occurs in nasal retina (temporal field) with partial sparing in temporal retina (nasal field). See Figure 11-2.
CN, cranial nerve.

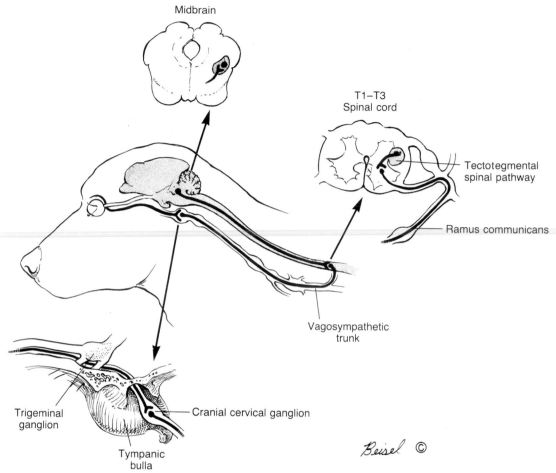

Midbrain

T1–T3
Spinal cord

Tectotegmental
spinal pathway

Ramus communicans

Vagosympathetic
trunk

Trigeminal
ganglion

Cranial cervical ganglion

Tympanic
bulla

Beisel ©

Figure 11-3 Pathway of sympathetic innervation of the eye. (From Greene CE, Oliver JE Jr: Neurologic examination. In Ettinger SE, editor: *Textbook of veterinary internal medicine,* ed 2. Philadelphia, 1982, WB Saunders.)

The condition is thought to be idiopathic in 42% to 55% of cases. Horner's syndrome spontaneously resolves in a large percentage of cases.[5]

Differentiation of preganglionic and postganglionic lesions can be determined in the first few weeks of Horner's syndrome. Denervation hypersensitivity causes exaggerated responses when the postganglionic neuron is involved and stimulated with direct-acting agents. Indirect-acting agents require an intact postganglionic neuron for an effect. Instillation of 1% hydroxyamphetamine, an indirect-acting agent, causes good dilation of a normal eye, one with a preganglionic lesion, or one with a central pathway lesion; but it causes minimal dilation of an eye with a postganglionic lesion. Instillation of 1% phenylephrine causes minimal dilation of a normal eye or one with a presynaptic lesion but good dilation of an eye with a postganglionic lesion.[1,3] Topical testing with adrenergic agents is inconclusive in many cases, however.[6]

Anisocoria or unequal pupils may be caused by ocular or neurologic disorders. Ocular diseases include abnormalities of the iris, cornea, lens, or retina. Ocular pain, especially if uveitis is present, causes miosis. Atrophy of the iris results in a dilated pupil. Increased intraocular pressure causes a dilated pupil. Unilateral retinal blindness causes a mild dilation of the affected eye in dogs and cats because of weaker consensual stimulation. Moving the stimulating light from eye to eye *(the swinging light test)* causes a noticeable shift in the size of the pupil in the affected eye.

Eye Movements

The extraocular eye muscles are innervated by CN III (oculomotor), CN IV (trochlear), and CN VI (abducent) (Figure 11-4). Eye movements are controlled by UMNs from the cerebral cortex and through brainstem vestibular reflexes. The eye muscles normally act in a synergistic or antagonistic manner to provide coordinated conjugate movements. Testing of eye movements is discussed in Chapter 1. Abnormalities of eye movements include paralysis of gaze in a direction related to a muscle or a group of muscles, strabismus or globe deviation, loss of conjugate movements, and nystagmus.

When the globe is fixed, regardless of head position, a lesion of CN III, IV, or VI is suspected. Lesions of the trochlear nerve (CN IV) may cause slight rotation of the globe, which is difficult to evaluate in animals that have a round pupil (see Figure 11-4).[7] Lesions of CN III cause ventrolateral strabismus, and lesions of CN VI cause medial strabismus. Several weeks after an injury, the globe may return to its normal midposition, but loss of movement occurs dorsally, medially, and ventrally with a lesion of CN III and laterally with a lesion of CN VI (see Figure 11-4). Positional strabismus

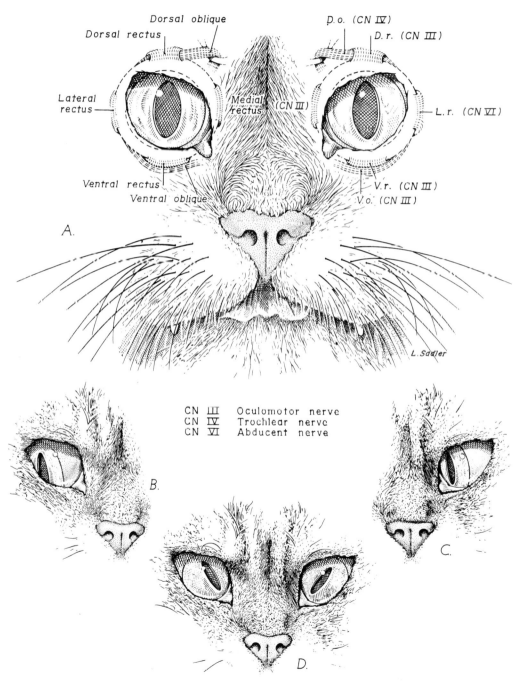

Figure 11-4 **A**, Functional anatomy of the extraocular muscles. Direction of strabismus after paralysis of the oculomotor **(B)**, abducent **(C)**, and trochlear **(D)** nerves. (From de Lahunta A: *Veterinary neuroanatomy and clinical neurology.* Philadelphia, 1977, WB Saunders.)

(disconjugate deviation of the eye in certain head positions) is characteristic of lesions of the vestibular system. Typically, the eye ipsilateral to the vestibular abnormality is ventral in the palpebral fissure when the nose is elevated. In this case, eye movements can be elicited in all directions by appropriate movements of the head, demonstrating that all extraocular muscles are functional (see Chapter 8). Both eyes tend to maintain a horizontal position in large animals; therefore, they are ventrally placed when the head is elevated, although the affected side may be deviated relative to the normal side.

The function of the extraocular muscles has not been established in large animals. Presumably the movements and the physiologic deficits produced by lesions of the cranial nerves are similar to those in other species.[8]

Conjugate eye movements require coordination of the three cranial nerves and their muscles. The pathway responsible for this coordination is the medial longitudinal fasciculus (MLF), which runs in the center of the brainstem from the vestibular nuclei to the nuclei of CN III, CN IV, and CN VI. Lesions of the MLF may cause disconjugate movements or, more commonly, a lack of eye movements in response to moving the head (internuclear ophthalmoplegia). Lesions of the MLF are seen most commonly after an acute head injury that produces hemorrhage in the center of the brainstem (see Chapter 12). Ophthalmoplegia has also been reported from thyroid adenocarcinoma invading the cavernous sinus intracranially and affecting the three cranial nerves.[9]

Nystagmus is involuntary rhythmic movement of the eyes. Normal nystagmus may be visual in origin (for example, watching telephone poles go by from a moving car), or it may be vestibular in origin (e.g., turning the head rapidly). The visual and vestibular types are called *jerk nystagmus* because of the slow phase to one side followed by the rapid recovery movement *(jerk)*. The direction of the nystagmus is classified according to the jerk component. Nystagmus also is categorized by the direction of the movement (horizontal, vertical, or rotatory) and by any change in direction with varying head positions. Jerk nystagmus that is horizontal or rotatory and that does not change direction with varying head positions is indicative of peripheral vestibular disease but may be seen in central disease. Vertical jerk nystagmus or nystagmus that changes direction with varying head positions is associated with central vestibular brainstem lesions (including lesions of the flocculonodular lobe of the cerebellum) (Figure 11-5; see also Chapter 8).

A less frequent form called *pendular nystagmus* consists of small oscillations of the eye that do not have fast and slow components. Pendular nystagmus usually occurs with cerebellar disease and is most pronounced during fixation of the gaze. It may also be seen in animals with visual deficits.

Except for lesions of the globe and the orbit, most diseases affecting the visual system produce other clinical signs that are related to abnormal function of surrounding structures. For example, masses affecting the optic chiasm or the optic tracts usually affect hypothalamic function. Lesions of CN III, CN IV, or CN VI cause other brainstem signs. Lesions of the occipital cortex affect other cerebral functions. The combination of signs defines the location of the lesion (see Chapter 2).

DISEASES

Diseases causing blindness, pupillary abnormalities, and ocular movement disorders are listed in Tables 11-2 through 11-4. Many diseases cause abnormalities in more than one of these functions.

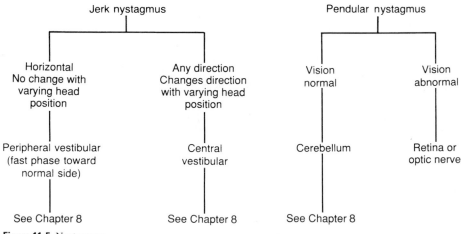

Figure 11-5 Nystagmus.

The history and the physical and neurologic examinations should provide the clinician with a list of the most probable diseases to be considered. Most of the diseases presented in the figures are also discussed in other chapters. Only those that are related primarily to the visual system are discussed here.

Degenerative Diseases

An abnormality of the intracellular enzyme systems causes an accumulation of the products of metabolism in the neurons (neuronal storage diseases). Affected neurons function abnormally and eventually die. This group of diseases is listed in Figures 11-2 through 11-4 as storage diseases (see Chapter 15). Because neurons are affected, the retina, the lateral geniculate nucleus, and the occipital cortex are the most common targets in the visual system. Cranial nerve nuclei usually are not affected until late in the disease. The diseases are hereditary, progressive, and invariably fatal. Diagnosis is difficult except by assessment of the history, knowledge of the breed selectivity, and exclusion of other diagnoses. Brain biopsy can confirm a diagnosis. Biopsy of tissues other than brain may provide a diagnosis in some of the systemic storage diseases.

Demyelinating diseases also are considered degenerative diseases; for example, one type, globoid cell leukodystrophy, is caused by an abnormal enzyme system similar to that of the neuronal storage diseases. Signs of cerebellar and spinal cord tract involvement (UMN signs, proprioceptive deficits) are characteristic of the clinical syndrome. Visual pathways (optic nerve, optic tract, optic radiation) may be affected. Demyelination also may occur secondary to inflammatory diseases, especially canine distemper. The visual pathways are often affected, but other signs predominate.

Primary retinal degenerations are common causes of blindness, especially in dogs. Some dogs with severe retinal degeneration and functional blindness may still have intact pupillary light reflexes. These degenerations are generally called *progressive retinal atrophy,* with several variants, such as central progressive retinal atrophy. Numerous breeds of dogs and a few breeds of cats are affected. The affected breeds are listed in several textbooks of veterinary ophthalmology and in a comprehensive review by Whitley.[10-12]

Anomalies

Hydrocephalus, which may be the result of a congenital anomaly or may be secondary to mass lesions or inflammation, involves primarily the optic radiations and the occipital cortex through enlargement of the lateral ventricles. Hydrocephalus should always be considered in a blind animal that has intact pupillary light reflexes. A diagnosis of hydrocephalus requires computed tomography, ventricular tap, pneumoventriculography, or electroencephalography (see Chapter 12).

Primary retinal anomalies are relatively common in dogs but are less common in other species. Anomalies include coloboma, optic nerve hypoplasia, the collie eye anomaly, and various forms of retinal dysplasia. As with the retinal degenerations, numerous breeds of dogs, a few breeds of cats, and large animals are affected. The types of anomaly and the breeds affected are listed in the references.[10-12] These diseases cause blindness and in some cases nystagmus and pupillary abnormalities.

Cats with visual pathway abnormalities, primarily Siamese and white cats, often have medial strabismus and pendular nystagmus but good vestibular eye movements. Pendular nystagmus is also seen in dairy cows. One survey of 2932 cows in New York State reported an incidence of 0.51% in several breeds. It has also been reported as a familial problem in Ayrshire bulls.[13,14] Medial strabismus has been reported in several breeds of cattle, apparently as an inherited trait in some.[15]

Metabolic Diseases

A disease that alters the normal biochemical processes of the eye or the central nervous system (CNS) may produce signs of abnormal vision, although other signs usually are more apparent. Diabetes mellitus may cause vascular changes, including retinal hemorrhage. Cataracts are common and make retinal examination difficult.

Diseases that affect cortical function may produce blindness with intact pupillary light reflexes. Examples include hypoglycemia, hepatic encephalopathy, and uremia. Acute metabolic problems such as hypoxia and hyperthermia usually affect the cerebral cortex most severely. Cortical blindness frequently follows severe hypoxic episodes such as cardiac arrest (see Chapters 12 and 15).

Neoplasms

Visual pathway abnormalities are often helpful for localizing intracranial tumors. Primary tumors of the globe are apparent on physical examination.[10]

Tumors of the pituitary gland can cause visual-field deficits from compression of the optic chiasm; however, most pituitary tumors grow dorsally into the hypothalamus instead of spreading out rostrally and caudally. Visual signs are therefore seen very late in the development of the mass.[16]

Table 11-2   **Etiology of Blindness***

Disease Category	Nonprogressive	Acute Progressive	Chronic Progressive
Degenerative			Storage diseases (R, C) (15) Retinal degenerations (R) Demyelinating diseases (O, C) (15)
Anomalous	Optic nerve hypoplasia (O) Coloboma (O) Retinal dysplasia (R) Collie eye syndrome (R) Cerebral malformations (C) (12)		Hydrocephalus (C) (12)
Metabolic	Hyperthermia (C) (15) Hypoxia (C) (12)	Hypoglycemia (C) (12) Hepatic encephalopathy (C) (12)	Hypoglycemia (C) (12) Hepatic encephalopathy (C) (12)

Neoplastic (15)		Lymphosarcoma (R)
		Malignant melanoma (R)
			1. Primary (15)
			  a. Pituitary adenoma (O, X, C)
			  b. Meningioma (O, X, C)
			  c. Gliomas (O, X, C)
			  d. Ependymoma (C)
			  e. Choroid plexus papilloma (C)
			2. Metastatic (R, O, X, C)
			3. Lymphoreticular (R, O, X, C)
			4. Skull origin (C)

Nutritional		Thiamine deficiency—ruminants (O) (12)	Hypovitaminosis A (R, O) Taurine deficiency—cats (R)
Inflammatory (15)		Canine distemper (R, O, X, C) Feline infectious peritonitis (R, O, X, C) Toxoplasmosis (R, C) Thromboembolic meningoencephalitis—bovine (R, C) Bovine virus diarrhea (R, O) Systemic mycoses (O, X, C) Bacterial infections (O, X, C)	Canine distemper (R, O, X, C) Feline infectious peritonitis (R, O, X, C) Toxoplasmosis (R, C) Systemic mycoses (O, X, C) Bacterial infections (O, X, C) GME—dogs (O, X, C) Prototheocosis (C) Immune mediated (O)
Toxic (15)		Lead and other heavy metals (C) Hexachlorophene (C)	Lead and other heavy metals (C) Hexachlorophene (C)
Traumatic	Retinal detachment Retinal hemorrhage Edema (O, X, C) Hemorrhage (O, X, C)	Edema (O, X, C) Hemorrhage (O, X, C)	
Vascular	Infarcts (R, C) Hemorrhage (R, O, X, C)		

*Numbers in parentheses refer to chapters in which entities are discussed.
R, Retina; *O*, optic nerve; *X*, optic chiasm; *C*, optic tract and cerebral cortex.

Table 11-3 **Etiology of Pupillary Abnormalities***

Disease Category	Nonprogressive	Acute Progressive	Chronic Progressive
Degenerative	Hypoplasia of optic nerve (O) Coloboma (O) Retinal dysplasia (R) Collie eye syndrome (R)		Retinal degenerations (R) Hydrocephalus[†] (12)
Neoplastic			Rostrotentorial tumor[†] (15)
Nutritional		Thiamine deficiency— dogs and cats (15)	
Idiopathic	Pupillotonia Anisocoria—cats	Dysautonomia	
Inflammatory		Retrobulbar abscess Several infectious diseases (15) Middle ear infections (8)	
Toxic	Organophosphates	Lead[†] (15)	
Traumatic	Brainstem hemorrhage Brachial plexus lesions (5)	Hematoma[†]	Cerebral edema[†]

*Numbers in parentheses refer to chapters in which entities are discussed.
[†]Oculomotor signs secondary to tentorial herniation.
R, Retina; *O*, optic nerve; *FeLV,* feline leukemia virus.

Table 11-4 **Etiology of Ocular Movement Disorders***

Disease Category	Nonprogressive	Acute Progressive	Chronic Progressive
Degenerative			Storage diseases (R, C) (15) Demyelinating diseases (O, C) (15) Hydrocephalus (C) (12)
Anomalous	Strabismus with optic pathway anomalies—cats		Hydrocephalus (C) (12)
Neoplastic			Any tumor affecting the brainstem, cerebellum, vestibular system, or CN III, IV, VI (15)
Nutritional		Thiamine deficiency— dogs and cats (15)	
Inflammatory		Any disease affecting the brainstem, cerebellum, vestibular system, or CN III, IV, VI (8, 15)	
Toxic		Hexachlorophene (15)	
Traumatic (12)	Lesions of the brainstem, cerebellum, vestibular system, or CN III, IV, VI		
Vascular (12)	Lesions of the brainstem, cerebellum, vestibular system, or CN III, IV, VI		

*Numbers in parentheses refer to chapters in which entities are discussed.
CN, Cranial nerve.

A lymphosarcoma may infiltrate all portions of the globe. Involvement of the orbit may cause exophthalmos, especially in cattle. Compression of the optic nerves may cause papilledema or atrophy of the optic disk.

Granulomatous encephalomyelitis (GME), a suspected immune-mediated inflammatory disease, may have clinical signs suggestive of neoplasia. Lesions may infiltrate or compress the optic nerves and cause atrophy or swelling of the optic disk, depending on the degree of involvement.

Neoplasia of the CNS is discussed in Chapter 15.

Nutritional Deficiencies

Animals that are fed normal commercial rations rarely have nutritional deficiencies severe enough to cause CNS abnormality. Hypovitaminosis A causes abnormal bone growth with stenosis of the optic foramen that secondarily constricts the optic nerve, producing papilledema in the early stages followed eventually by retinal degeneration. This syndrome is seen more commonly in calves than in companion animals.[17]

Feline central retinal degeneration (FCRD) can be produced by diets that are deficient in the amino acid taurine. Cats that are exclusively fed commercial dogfood develop FCRD.[17]

Polioencephalomalacia of ruminants is characterized by cerebral necrosis and edema. Signs of cerebral dysfunction, including blindness, are noted. The pupillary light reflexes are usually normal, unless edema has caused tentorial herniation with compression of the oculomotor nerves. Extorsion of the globe, supposedly from damage to the trochlear nucleus (CN IV), is seen in this syndrome, but the pathogenesis is not clear. An excess of thiaminase in the rumen, producing an acute thiamine deficiency, causes this condition. Thiamine deficiency in small animals, primarily in cats, causes hemorrhages and malacia in the brainstem. Eye movements and pupillary reflexes may be affected (see Chapter 15).

Idiopathic

Several diseases are currently of unknown cause and are included here.

Dysautonomia, also called the *Key Gaskell syndrome* in cats, is a diffuse degeneration of the autonomic nervous system; its cause is unknown.[18-23] It has been reported in several countries, including the United States. In the United States, the disease has been reported most frequently in dogs living in Missouri and Kansas.[22,23] Clusters of affected animals have been reported.[23] Risk factors

for canine dysautonomia include young to middle-aged and predominately medium- to large-breed dogs of either sex that inhabit rural environments. The clinical signs include dysuria, bladder distention, decreased anal tone, mydriasis with absent pupillary light reflexes, elevated membrane nictitans, intestinal ileus, vomiting or regurgitation, xerostomia, decreased tear production, and dry nose. Animals are visual, and the menace response is normal. Megaesophagus and aspiration pneumonia are common findings. Chromatolytic degeneration of autonomic ganglia, brainstem nuclei, and lateral and ventral horns of the spinal cord are the most common histopathologic lesions.

Denervation of the iris muscle can be detected in many dogs by instilling 0.1% pilocarpine in one eye and observing for miosis in the treated eye. The test is positive in 85% to 100% of affected dogs.[22,23] Intradermal histamine (0.05 ml of 1:10,000 histamine) produces a wheal, but the expected flare response is often blunted in affected dogs.[23] Administration of atropine (0.02 mg/kg administered intravenously) is not predictable for increasing heart rate.[23] Schirmer tear testing may detect decreased tear production in many affected dogs.

The prognosis for recovery is poor. Although the cause is unknown, toxic or infectious etiologies are suspected. *Clostridium botulinum* toxin may create similar histologic changes and clinical signs. Studies linking botulinum toxin with dysautonomia have not been reported in animals.

Pupillotonia is a pupil that is slow to react to light, both on direct and consensual responses. It is thought to be immune system mediated. Primary abnormalities of the visual and oculomotor pathways must be excluded. Only one case has been reported.[26]

Horner's syndrome with no detectable cause was found in 62 golden retrievers in a 6-year period.[24] The lesion was of the preganglionic neuron based on pharmacologic testing. The investigators reported only 25 cases of Horner's syndrome in other breeds in the same period. Of those, 20 had specific diseases causing the signs. Horner's syndrome was reported in 10 horses.[25] Most of the cases resulted from surgical or external trauma.

Inflammations

Systemic infectious diseases with CNS involvement frequently affect the visual system. Retinal lesions are common in canine distemper, feline infectious peritonitis, toxoplasmosis, rickettsial disease, systemic mycosis, GME, and thromboembolic meningoencephalitis.[17,27-29] A fundic examination may help to confirm the diagnosis.

Optic neuropathy includes degenerative, compressive, ischemic, and inflammatory conditions of the optic nerve. Optic neuritis is inflammation of the optic nerve. Sudden blindness may be noticed if both eyes are affected. Papilledema and vascular congestion are seen on fundic examination if that portion of the nerve is affected. Atrophy of the disk is noted as the process resolves. The electroretinogram (ERG) can help to differentiate primary retinal disease from optic nerve disease.

Sudden acquired retinal degeneration (SARD) also causes acute blindness, and the fundus may appear normal. The ERG is abnormal in SARD. Canine distemper, toxoplasmosis, and cryptococcosis are among the infectious diseases that cause optic neuritis. Granulomatous meningoencephalitis frequently affects the optic nerve.[30] Some of the diseases causing optic neuropathy are not treatable and may lead to death; however, many cases occur without evidence of systemic disease. Edema and inflammation may lead to loss of function of the nerve, regardless of the outcome of the primary disease. Early treatment therefore should include antiedema doses of corticosteroids. Other supportive or antibiotic therapy is given as indicated by the animal's condition. Prognosis is guarded to poor. In one report of 12 dogs with optic neuropathy, seven remained alive, five were permanently blind, and two had partial vision.[31]

Toxic Disorders

Heavy-metal poisoning, especially lead poisoning, may produce cortical blindness. Toxins that affect the brainstem or cerebellum, such as hexachlorophene, may cause nystagmus (see Chapter 15).

Trauma

Any portion of the visual system can be affected by trauma. Assessing the function of the oculomotor nerve is of primary importance in evaluating a patient with head injury. Brain swelling that leads to tentorial herniation compresses the oculomotor nerve at the tentorium cerebelli. One of the earliest signs of tentorial herniation is a fixed, dilated pupil usually ipsilateral to the herniation (if it is unilateral). A paralysis of the extraocular muscles that produces a ventrolateral strabismus follows the mydriasis. Hemorrhage in the brainstem also produces abnormal pupils. Hemorrhage rostral or caudal to the oculomotor nucleus (midbrain) may destroy the UMN to the sympathetic pathway, producing small but responsive pupils. Midbrain hemorrhage may cause fixed, dilated pupils if the oculomotor nucleus is destroyed with the sympathetic pathway intact, but in most cases the pupils are fixed and midposition because both pathways are affected. Serial assessment of pupillary function, together with mental status, motor function, and other cranial nerve signs, is important for evaluation of patients with head trauma. Bilateral, fixed, dilated, or midposition pupils from the time of injury strongly suggest brainstem hemorrhage that is often irreversible, and progressive dilation of the pupils suggests a developing tentorial herniation that may be treatable (see Chapter 12). Traumatic injuries of the eye can cause abnormal vision or pupillary responses.

Vascular

Cerebral infarction, primarily in the cat, may cause contralateral vision loss (see Chapter 12).

Case Histories

The case histories in this chapter emphasize localization of the lesion. Only the pertinent neuroophthalmologic findings are given. Make your decision before reading the assessment.

CASE HISTORY 11A

Neurologic Examination[*]
 Vision: Normal.
 Pupillary Light Reflexes (PLR): The right pupil is dilated.

Shine light	Reaction	
	OS	OD
OS	+	−
OD	+	−

Eye Position and Movement: Left eye is normal; fixed ventrolateral strabismus in right eye.

CASE HISTORY 11B

Neurologic Examination
 Vision: Normal in left eye; absent in right eye.
 PLR: The right pupil is larger than the left.

Shine light	Reaction	
	OS	OD
OS	+	+
OD	−	−

Eye Position and Movement: Normal.

---

[*]*OS,* Left; *OD,* right

CASE HISTORY 11C

Neurologic Examination
Vision: Absent in both eyes.
PLR: The pupil size is normal; the pupils are symmetric.

	Reaction	
Shine light	OS	OD
OS	+	+
OD	+	+

Eye Position and Movement: The vestibular eye movements are normal. No strabismus, but the animal does not follow moving objects.

CASE HISTORY 11D

Neurologic Examination
Vision: Normal in both eyes.
PLR: The pupil size is normal; the pupils are symmetric.

	Reaction	
Shine light	OS	OD
OS	+	+
OD	+	+

Eye Position and Movement: Medial strabismus of the left eye. Dorsal and ventral movements can be elicited by moving the head. The right eye is normal.

CASE HISTORY 11E

Neurologic Examination
Vision: Absent in both eyes.
PLR: The pupils are dilated bilaterally.

	Reaction	
Shine light	OS	OD
OS	−	−
OD	−	−

Eye Position and Movement: Normal eye position and normal vestibular eye movements, but the animal does not follow moving objects.

CASE HISTORY 11F

Neurologic Examination
Vision: Normal in both eyes.
PLR: The pupil size is normal.

	Reaction	
Shine light	OS	OD
OS	+	+
OD	+	+

Eye Position and Movement: The eyes are in the normal midposition, but no vestibular eye movements can be elicited.

ASSESSMENT 11A

Right oculomotor nerve (CN III) lesion. The unilateral lesion suggests a lesion after the nerve leaves the brainstem. The nuclei are only millimeters apart, and lesions at this level usually affect both sides.

ASSESSMENT 11B

Right optic nerve or retinal lesion. A funduscopic examination is likely to differentiate between these two disorders. An electroretinogram may be necessary if no retinal lesions are visible.

ASSESSMENT 11C

The finding of bilateral occipital cortex or optic radiation lesions suggests a diffuse lesion such as hydrocephalus, encephalitis, or increased intracranial pressure.

ASSESSMENT 11D

Left abducent nerve (CN VI) lesion. Isolated lesions of CN VI are rare. In a clinical case, other signs of brainstem disease may be present.

ASSESSMENT 11E

Optic chiasm, bilateral optic nerve, or bilateral retinal lesions. This situation is one in which two lesions (actually a diffuse disease) are more common than a single chiasmatic lesion. Retinopathies and optic neuropathies are seen more often than are primary lesions of the optic chiasm.

ASSESSMENT 11F

This MLF lesion is in the tract connecting the vestibular nuclei to the nuclei of CN III, IV, and VI. Alternatively, a lesion could exist of CN III, IV, and VI bilaterally, but pupillary abnormalities should occur with oculomotor involvement. In either case, other signs probably would predominate. MLF lesions usually are associated with severe brainstem lesions (hemorrhage, tumor), and the animal is often comatose when these disorders are present.

References

1. Neer TM: Horner's syndrome: anatomy, diagnosis, and causes, *Compend Cont Educ Pract Vet* 6:740-747, 1984.
2. Tinney B, Macuda T: Vision and hearing in horses, *J Am Vet Med Assoc* 218:1567-1574, 2001.
3. Van Den Broek A: Horner's syndrome in cats and dogs: a review, *J Small Anim Pract* 28:929-940, 1987.
4. Sweeney RW, Sweeney CR: Transient Horner's syndrome following intravenous injections in two horses, *J Am Vet Med Assoc* 185:802-803, 1984.
5. Morgan RV, Zanotti SW: Horner's syndrome in dogs and cats: 49 cases (1980-1986), *J Am Vet Med Assoc* 194:1096-1099, 1989.
6. Kern TJ, Aromando MC, Erb HN: Horner's syndrome in dogs and cats: 100 cases (1975-1985), *J Am Vet Med Assoc* 195:369-372, 1989.
7. de Lahunta A: *Veterinary neuroanatomy and clinical neurology,* ed 2. Philadelphia, 1983, WB Saunders.

8. Mayhew IG: *Large animal neurology: a handbook for veterinary clinicians.* Philadelphia, 1989, Lea & Febiger.

9. Lewis GT, Blanchard GL, Trapp AL, et al: Ophthalmoplegia caused by thyroid adenocarcinoma invasion of the cavernous sinuses in the dog, *J Am Anim Hosp Assoc* 20:805- 812, 1984.

10. Slatter D: *Fundamentals of veterinary ophthalmology.* Philadelphia, 1981, WB Saunders.

11. Whitley RD: Focusing on eye disorders among purebred dogs, *Vet Med* 83:50-63, 1988.

12. Barnett KC: Inherited eye disease in the dog and cat, *J Small Anim Pract* 29:462-475, 1988.

13. Nurmio P, Remes E, Talanti S, et al: Familial undulatory nystagmus in Ayrshire bulls in Finland, *Nord Vet Med* 34:130-132, 1982.

14. McConnon JM, White ME, Smith MC, et al: Pendular nystagmus in dairy cattle, *J Am Vet Med Assoc* 182:812-813, 1983.

15. Power EP: Bilateral convergent strabismus in two Friesian cows, *Ir Vet* 41:357-358, 1987.

16. Davidson MG, Nasisse MP, Breitschwerdt EB, et al: Acute blindness associated with intracranial tumors in dogs and cats: eight cases (1984-1989), *J Am Vet Med Assoc* 199:755-758, 1991.

17. Aguirre GD, Gross SL: Ocular manifestations of selected systemic diseases, *Compend Cont Educ Pract Vet* 2:144-153, 1980.

18. Edney A, Gaskell C, Sharp N: Feline dysautonomia—an emerging disease, *J Small Anim Pract* 28:333-416, 1987.

19. Guilford WG, O'Brien DP, Allert A, et al: Diagnosis of dysautonomia in a cat by autonomic nervous system function testing, *J Am Vet Med Assoc* 193:823-828, 1988.

20. Pollin M, Sullivan M: A canine dysautonomia resembling the Key Gaskell syndrome, *Vet Rec* 118:402-403, 1986.

21. Presthus J, Bjerkas I: Canine dysautonomia in Norway, *Vet Rec* 120:463-464, 1987.

22. Longshore RC, O'Brien DP, Johnson GC, et al: Dysautonomia in dogs: a retrospective study, *J Vet Intern Med* 10:103-109, 1996.

23. Harkin KR, Andrews GA, Nietfield JC: Dysautonomia in dogs: 65 cases (1993-2000), *J Am Vet Med Assoc* 220:633-639, 2002.

24. Boydell P: Idiopathic Horner's syndrome in the golden retriever, *J Small Anim Pract* 36:382-384, 1995.

25. Green SL, Cochrane SM, Smith-Maxie L: Horner's syndrome in ten horses, *Can Vet J* 33:330-333, 1992.

26. Gerding PA, Brightman AH, Brogdon J: Pupillotonia in a dog, *J Am Vet Med Assoc* 189:1477-1478, 1986.

27. Martin CL: Retinopathies of food animals. In Howard JL, editor: *Current veterinary therapy: food animal practice.* Philadelphia, 1981, WB Saunders.

28. Gelatt KN, Whitley RD, Samuelson DA, et al: Ocular manifestations of viral disease in small animals, *Compend Cont Educ Pract Vet* 7:968-978, 1985.

29. Ellett EW, Playter RF, Pierce KR: Retinal lesions associated with induced canine ehrlichiosis: a preliminary report, *J Am Anim Hosp Assoc* 9:214-218, 1973.

30. Nafe LA, Carter JD: Canine optic neuritis, *Compend Cont Educ Pract Vet* 3:978-984, 1981.

31. Fischer CA, Jones GT: Optic neuritis in dogs, *J Am Vet Med Assoc* 160:68-79, 1972.

Chapter 12

Stupor or Coma

Altered states of consciousness are always related to abnormal brain function. The nomenclature of these disorders is often confusing because the terms extend beyond simple medical analysis and encompass psychology, philosophy, and other disciplines. Applying the terminology used in human medicine to animals is difficult because we must interpret behavior to assess mental status. For purposes of the clinician, the following definitions are adequate:

Normal: The animal is alert, responds to external stimuli, is aware of its surroundings, and responds to commands as expected.

Depressed: The animal is lethargic and less responsive to its environment but still has the capability to become responsive in a normal manner. Most sick animals are depressed.

Disoriented, confused: Although the animal can respond to its environment, it may do so in an inappropriate manner.

Stuporous: The animal appears to be asleep when undisturbed but can be aroused by strong stimulation, especially noxious stimuli. No clear boundary separates depression and stupor.

Comatose: The animal is unconscious and does not respond to any stimulus except by reflex activity. For example, a strong toe pinch may elicit a flexion reflex or may increase extensor posturing but does not cause a behavioral reaction such as crying, biting, or turning the head.

Vegetative: The animal lacks awareness of the environment but shows arousal. Brainstem function is present, but cortical responses are absent.[1]

Brain dead: The animal is in a coma, is apneic, lacks all brainstem reflexes, and has electrocerebral silence. Currently, in human medicine, electrocerebral silence includes absence of all evoked responses as well as a flat electroencephalogram (EEG).

LESION LOCALIZATION

Consciousness is maintained by sensory stimuli that act through the *ascending reticular activating system* (ARAS) on the cerebral cortex (Figure 12-1). The ARAS is located in the midbrain. Decreasing levels of consciousness indicate abnormal function of the cerebral cortex or interference with cortical activation by the ARAS.

All sensory pathways have collateral input to the reticular formation of the pons and the midbrain. The reticular formation projects diffusely to the cerebral cortex, maintaining a background of activity through cholinergic synapses on cortical neurons. A balance is maintained between the ARAS and an adrenergic system that projects from nuclei in the midbrain and the diencephalon, which may be considered the sleep system.[2-4] Alterations in the balance of these two systems can produce signs ranging from hyperexcitability to coma. Narcolepsy, a syndrome of sleep attacks, is discussed in Chapter 13.

Stupor and coma are caused by (1) diffuse, bilateral cerebral disease; (2) metabolic or toxic encephalopathies; (3) compression of the rostral brainstem (midbrain, pons); or (4) destructive lesions of the rostral brainstem.

An anatomic diagnosis can be made on the basis of mental status, motor function, and neuroophthalmologic signs (vision, pupils, and eye movements) (see Chapter 11 and Table 12-1). Alterations in the respiratory pattern may be correlated with levels of brainstem abnormalities, but they are less reliable than the other signs.

Diffuse cerebral disease usually does not produce localizing signs, although some inflammatory processes may be somewhat asymmetric. Voluntary motor activity and postural reactions are absent or severely depressed. Rhythmic walking movements, reflecting brainstem and spinal cord activity, may be elicited if the animal is suspended in a normal standing posture. Vision and the menace response are absent, although the pupillary light reflexes are normal. Vestibular (conjugate) eye movements are normal, but the animal does not follow moving objects. Normal pupils and vestibular eye movements indicate an intact brainstem, whereas loss of vision and voluntary motor activity indicates an abnormal cerebral cortex.

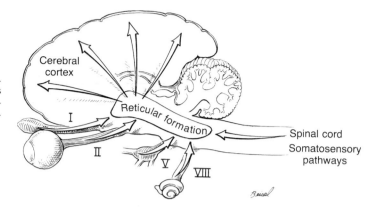

Figure 12-1 Reticular activating system (RAS). The reticular system of the brainstem receives input from most sensory systems. Diffuse projections from the RAS to the cerebral cortex maintain consciousness.

In its most severe form, diffuse cerebral involvement produces the chronic vegetative state wherein the animal has brainstem reflexes but no behavioral reactions. Signs of meningeal inflammation include pain on palpation of the head and the neck, rigidity of the neck muscles, and resistance to flexion of the neck. Infection, immune reactions, or blood in the subarachnoid space can cause meningeal inflammation.

Metabolic or toxic encephalopathies usually depress higher (cortical) functions early and affect brainstem functions later. They do not produce focal localizing signs. The signs are generally the same as those of diffuse cortical lesions but may have other components, depending on the cause. For example, barbiturates can cause depression of the spinal reflexes, organophosphate insecticides can cause muscle fasciculation and autonomic signs, and a number of toxins can cause seizures. Specific entities are discussed in Chapter 15.

Compression of the brainstem can be caused by a mass (tumor, abscess) adjacent to the brainstem or by herniation of the cerebral cortex under the tentorium cerebelli; this secondarily compresses the brainstem.[5]

The skull forms an inelastic case around the brain. Any developing mass (tumor, abscess, hematoma), increase in the volume of the brain (cerebral edema), or deformation of the skull must displace cerebrospinal fluid (CSF), blood, or nervous tissue. An increase in brain bulk can come from changes in any of the three compartments: *vascular*, *cellular*, and *extracellular* (Table 12-2).[6] In addition, many disease processes cause increased brain volume by multiple mechanisms. For example, trauma can cause vasogenic edema, venous obstruction, and osmotic edema. Tumors can cause vasogenic, compressive, and hydrocephalic changes. The average dog has approximately 7 ml of CSF. Blood volume

is maintained nearly constant up to pressures equal to arterial pressures.

Increased pressure causes displacement of the cerebral hemispheres caudally under the tentorium cerebelli, resulting in compression of the brainstem (Figures 12-2 and 12-3). Unilateral masses cause a herniation on the same side, whereas cerebral edema usually causes a bilateral herniation. This may differ depending on the specific cause.

If the pressure continues to rise, or if the mass starts in the caudotentorial compartment, the cerebellum may herniate through the foramen magnum, compressing the medulla oblongata. The respiratory pathways are blocked, resulting in death.

The signs of brainstem compression from tentorial herniation are outlined in Tables 12-3 and 12-4. Masses that compress the brainstem usually cause similar signs, although the animal's mental status is not altered as severely because the cerebral cortex is not directly affected. The involvement of cranial nerve (CN) III is particularly important to the clinician because it is one of the earliest detectable signs of herniation. In some cases, pupillary dilation is preceded by a slight pupillary constriction. Either of these signs indicates impending deterioration of the patient, and treatment must be instituted quickly.

Destructive lesions of the brainstem are most frequently parenchymal hemorrhages after head injury. Neoplasia and inflammation also may produce a destructive lesion. Table 12-5 lists the signs of a focal lesion at various levels of the brainstem.

DISEASES

The causes of stupor and coma are classified in Table 12-6 according to the presence or absence of focal, lateralizing, or meningeal signs and the onset and progression of the signs.

Text continued on p. 303

Table 12-1 **Signs of Lesions Causing Stupor and Coma**

Lesion	Motor Function	Vision	Pupils	Eye Movements
Severe diffuse cerebral cortex	Tetraparesis; postural reactions absent	Absent	Normal	Normal; no visual following
Metabolic or toxic encephalopathy	Tetraparesis; reflexes may be depressed	Absent	Usually normal	Normal but no following; absent in deep coma
Bilateral compression of rostral brainstem	Tetraparesis; increased extensor tone (decerebrate rigidity)	Absent in herniation; present in primary brainstem lesions	Dilated or midposition, absent PLRs	Ventrolateral strabismus; poor vestibular eye movements
Unilateral compression of rostral brainstem	Hemiparesis or tetraparesis; increased extensor tone on affected side	Present; may be contralateral loss in herniation	Dilated, ipsilateral	Ipsilateral ventrolateral strabismus, poor vestibular eye movements
Destructive lesion of rostral brainstem	Decerebrate rigidity	Present if not comatose	Midposition, no PLRs	No vestibular eye movements, ventrolateral strabismus +/–

PLR, Pupillary light reflex.

Table 12-2 **Classification of Brain Swelling**

Increased Vascular Volume	Cellular Swelling	Interstitial Eedma
Arterial dilation	Cytotoxic	Vasogenic
Venous obstruction	Metabolic	Osmotic
		Compressive
		Hydrocephalic

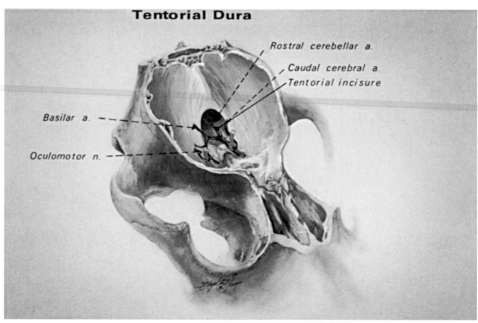

Figure 12-2 Increased pressure rostral to the tentorium cerebelli causes herniation of the cerebral cortex under the tentorium, resulting in compression of the brainstem. *a*, artery; *n*, nerve.

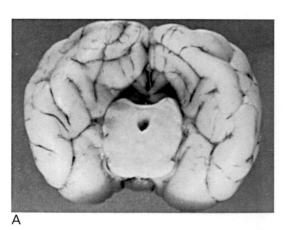
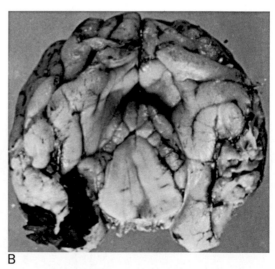

A B

Figure 12-3 Caudal view of the brain, transected at the midbrain. **A,** Normal brain. Note the open mesencephalic aqueduct. **B,** Severe cerebral edema has caused herniation of the cerebrum under the tentorium cerebelli, resulting in compression and distortion of the brainstem. The mesencephalic aqueduct is closed, causing further increases in intracranial pressure. (From Oliver JE Jr: Neurologic emergencies in small animals, *Vet Clin North Am* 2:341-357, 1972.)

Table 12-3 Signs of Progressive Bilateral Tentorial Herniation

Level	Consciousness	Pupils	Eye Movements	Motor Function	Autonomic Responses
Cerebral	Apathy	Small, reactive	Normal	Hemiparesis	Normal to irregular
Late diencephalon	Stupor	Small, reactive	Normal	Hemiparesis to tetraparesis	Cheyne-Stokes respiration
Midbrain	Coma	Dilated	Poor	Decerebrate rigidity	Hyperventilation
Pons	Coma	Midposition and unresponsive	Absent	Tetraparesis; decreased muscle tone	Rapid shallow respirations
Medulla	Coma	Midposition, dilated terminally	Absent	Same as pons	Irregular to apnea, slow pulse

Modified from Oliver JE Jr: Neurologic emergencies in small animals. *Vet Clin North Am* 2:341-357, 1972.

Table 12-4 Signs Characteristic of Progressive Unilateral Tentorial Herniation

Level	Consciousness	Pupils	Eye Movements	Motor Function	Autonomic Responses
CN III	Normal to stupor	Ipsilateral dilation	Normal to slight lateral strabismus	Normal to hemiparesis	Normal
Early midbrain	Stupor	Ipsilateral to bilateral dilation	Ipsilateral ventrolateral strabismus	Hemiparesis, ipsilateral or contralateral	Normal
Late midbrain	Coma	Dilated bilaterally to fixed midposition	Ventrolateral strabismus to fixed midposition	Decerebrate rigidity	Hyperventilation
Pons	Coma	Midposition, no PLRs	Absent	Tetraparesis; ↓ muscle tone	Rapid, shallow respirations
Medulla	Coma	Midposition, dilate terminally	Absent	Same as pons	Irregular to apnea, slow pulse

Modified from Oliver JE Jr: Neurologic emergencies in small animals. *Vet Clin North Am* 2:341-357, 1972.

Table 12-5 **Signs Characteristic of Focal Brainstem Hemorrhage at One Level**[*]

Level	Consciousness	Pupils	Eye Movements	Motor Function	Autonomic Functions
Diencephalon	Apathy to stupor	Small; reactive	Normal	Hemiparesis to tetraparesis	Normal to Cheyne-Stokes respiration
Midbrain	Stupor to coma	Dilated or midpoint, no PLRs	Ventrolateral strabismus	Decerebrate rigidity	Hyperventilation
Pons	Coma	Midpoint, no PLRs	Absent	Decerebrate tetraparesis or ↓ muscle tone	Rapid, shallow respirations; loss of micturition reflex
Medulla	Coma	Midpoint	Absent	Same as pons	Apnea, slow pulse

Modified from Oliver JE Jr: Neurologic emergencies in small animals, *Vet Clin North Am* 2:341-357, 1972.
[*]Assuming a large intramedullary hemorrhage confined primarily to one level. The most frequent is in the caudal midbrain and the pons after acute head injury. Asymmetric or smaller lesions produce less severe signs.
PLR, Pupillary light reflex.

Table 12-6 **Etiology of Stupor and Coma**[*]

Condition	Acute Nonprogressive	Acute Progressive	Chronic Progressive
Focal or Lateralizing Signs			
Neoplastic (15)		Metastatic	Primary Gliomas Meningiomas
Traumatic (12)	*Parenchymal hemorrhage*	Epidural, subdural hematoma; intracarotid injections in large animals	Subdural hematoma
Vascular (12)	Hemorrhage, infarction		
No Focal or Lateralizing Signs But Meningeal Signs Present			
Inflammatory (15)		*Meningitis* *Meningoencephalitis*	
Traumatic (12)	Subarachnoid hemorrhage		
No Focal, Lateralizing or Meningeal Signs			
Degenerative (15)			Storage diseases
Anomalous	Brain malformations		*Hydrocephalus*
Metabolic (15)		*Hypoglycemia* Liver failure Renal failure Diabetic coma Hypothyroid coma Heat stroke Hypoxia	
Nutritional (15)		*Thiamine deficiency*	
Idiopathic (12, 13)		Postictal seizure Narcolepsy	*Equine peripartum asphyxia*
Inflammatory (15)		Encephalitis	Encephalitis
Toxic (15)		Heavy metals Barbiturates Carbon monoxide	Water intoxication Plants Salt poisoning Enterotoxemia
Traumatic		Cerebral edema	

[*]*Italics* indicate most common diseases clinically. Numbers in parentheses refer to chapters in which conditions are discussed.

Focal or Lateralizing Signs

Acute Progressive

Craniocerebral Trauma (CCT). Head injuries in dogs and cats are most often the result of motor vehicle accidents.[7] In horses, direct blows to the frontal region, collision with a solid object, or impact to the poll when a horse flips over backward are the most common causes of brain injury.[8] Most of the available information concerns dogs, but other species respond similarly to injuries of the brain.[7,8] Primary events occur at the time of injury. The terms that are commonly used in describing head injury are defined in Table 12-7. The clinical differentiation of concussion from contusion is not clear and has no significance for clinical management. Concussions represent reversible physiologic disruptions of cells and are completely reversible. Contusions cause mechanical disruption of cells and tracts and may not be reversible. The most common types of intracranial hemorrhage are subarachnoid and intramedullary. Surgical treatment is of no benefit in either case.

Secondary events develop quickly following brain injury and cause irreversible central nervous system (CNS) pathology. Medical treatment is directed at preventing or decreasing the severity of these events. Increased intracranial pressure (ICP) occurs in most patients with CCT. The most common causes are brain edema, hemorrhage, and depressed skull fractures. Increased ICP decreases cerebral blood flow and leads to hypoxia and brain herniation.

Two types of brain edema may occur: cytotoxic or vasogenic. Cytotoxic edema results from fluid accumulation in neurons and astrocytes secondary to cellular hypoxia that disrupts cell membrane function. Vasogenic edema results from damage to the blood-brain barrier (BBB), and the fluid accumulation is extracellular. Cerebral edema can be assumed to exist in any patient with neurologic signs after head injury.

Table 12-7 **Terminology of Head Injury**

Concussion: Transient loss of consciousness without structural lesions

Contusion: Pathologic alterations in the brain including edema, petechial hemorrhage, disruption of nerve fibers, and so forth

Coup and Contrecoup: Injuries at the point of impact (coup) and at the opposite pole of the brain (contrecoup)

Cerebral Edema: An increase in intracellular (gray matter) and extracellular (white matter) fluid, present in most head injuries

Hemorrhage:

Epidural: Bleeding between the dura and the calvaria, usually caused by a skull fracture with laceration of a meningeal artery; relatively rare in animals

Subdural: Bleeding between the dura and the arachnoid, usually caused by disruption of the bridging veins, so it develops slowly; relatively rare in animals

Subarachnoid: Bleeding into the subarachnoid space, usually caused by disruption of the veins or the arteries of the arachnoid; relatively common in animals

Intramedullary (intracerebral): Bleeding into the tissue of the brain, usually caused by disruption of the intramedullary vessels; relatively common in animals

Skull Fractures:

Linear: Fractures of the calvaria that are not displaced

Depressed: Fractures of the calvaria that encroach on the brain

Compound (open): Fractures of the calvaria that have a laceration of the skin

Other possible biochemical events include increases in intracellular calcium concentrations, free radical production, and endorphin-associated ischemia. Hyperglycemia, a sympathoadrenal response, may occur in dogs and cats following CCT.[9] The degree of hyperglycemia may be associated with increased mortality rates or decreased prognosis, but the exact relationship is not known. Hyperglycemia may potentiate neurologic injury by increasing free radical production, cerebral edema, excitatory amino acid release, and cerebral acidosis.[9]

Differentiation of the signs of diffuse cerebral and focal brainstem lesions from the signs of tentorial herniation is discussed earlier and is summarized in Table 12-8.

Shores[10,11] modified the coma scales used in assessing human patients for use in animals (Table 12-9). The patient's status in each of three categories—motor activity, brainstem reflexes, and level of consciousness—is assessed. Total scores of 3 to 8 indicate a grave prognosis, scores of 9 to 14 indicate a poor to guarded prognosis, and scores of 15 to 18 indicate a good prognosis. The scale has not been evaluated on large numbers of patients to assess its reliability, but it emphasizes the importance of these clinical parameters. Serial evaluations are important to determine whether improvement is occurring.

Treatment. The treatment of head injury cannot be separated from the management of the whole patient because multiple system injuries are common in animals injured by motor vehicles. The owner should be instructed by telephone to establish a patent airway by extending the animal's head and pulling the tongue forward if the animal is unconscious. The animal should be carried on a piece of plywood or some similar rigid support to avoid displacement of the vertebral column.[12]

The priorities for management on presentation of the animal to the veterinary clinic are (1) maintenance of adequate ventilation by endotracheal catheter or tracheostomy if necessary, (2) treatment of shock, (3) assessment for multisystemic injuries, (4) neurologic examination and lesion localization, (5) medical or surgical treatment for neurologic injury, and (6) monitor patient for worsening signs (Table 12-10).

Table 12-8 **Comparison of Acute Brainstem Hemorrhage with Tentorial Herniation After Head Injury**

Feature Compared	Brainstem Hemorrhage	Tentorial Herniation
Onset	Early	Delayed
Course	Usually static	Progressive
Mental status	Coma, stupor if small lesion	Depressed, progressing to coma
Pupils	Fixed midposition, may be dilated if a small lesion	Miosis, progressing to fixed
Eye movements	Absent	Normal progressing to fixed
Motor function	Decerebrate posture	Normal or hemiparesis, progressing to decerebrate posture
Respiration	Hyperventilation or cluster breathing	Normal or Cheyne-Stokes

Table 12-9 **Small Animal Coma Scale**[*]

Neurologic Function Assessed	Score
Motor Activity	
Normal gait, normal spinal reflexes	6
Hemiparesis, tetraparesis, or decerebrate activity	5
Recumbent, intermittent extensor rigidity	4
Recumbent, constant extensor rigidity	3
Recumbent, constant extensor rigidity with opisthotonus	2
Recumbent, hypotonia of muscles, depressed or absent spinal reflexes	1
Brainstem Reflexes	
Normal pupillary light reflexes and oculocephalic reflexes	6
Slow pupillary light reflexes and normal to reduced oculocephalic reflexes	5
Bilateral unresponsive miosis with normal to reduced oculocephalic reflexes	4
Pinpoint pupils with reduced to absent oculocephalic reflexes	3
Unilateral unresponsive mydriasis with reduced to absent oculocephalic reflexes	2
Bilateral, unresponsive mydriasis with reduced to absent oculocephalic reflexes	1
Level of Consciousness	
Occasional periods of alertness, responsive to environment	6
Depression or delirium, capable of responding to environment but response may be inappropriate	5
Stupor, responsive to visual stimuli	4
Stupor, responsive to auditory stimuli	3
Stupor, responsive only to repeated noxious stimuli	2
Coma, unresponsive to repeated noxious stimuli	1
Assessment	
Good prognosis	15-18
Guarded prognosis	9-14
Grave prognosis	3-8

[*]Neurologic function is assessed for each of the three categories and a grade of 1 to 6 is assigned according to the descriptions for each grade. The total score is the sum of the three category scores.
Modified from Shores A: Craniocerebral trauma. In Kirk RW, editor: *Current veterinary therapy X.* Philadelphia, 1989, WB Saunders.

Hypoventilation causes hypercapnia, which leads to vasodilatation and increased ICP. Elevating the head facilitates emptying of venous sinuses and prevents excessive cerebral blood flow. Oxygen should be administered via oxygen chamber, nasal O_2 line, or intubation (if the patient is comatose). Hyperventilation and O_2 therapy lowers CO_2, reduces the risk of hypoxia, and helps prevent cerebral edema.

Standard protocols for treating shock are recommended. Fluid therapy should be vigorous if shock is present, but excessive fluid therapy should be avoided because it contributes to cerebral edema. Methylprednisolone sodium succinate (MPSS) may be indicated in the treatment of shock and is used in the treatment of CCT.

The patient should be appropriately evaluated for thoracic and abdominal injuries. Radiography and ultrasonography are useful aids in the diagnosis of a variety of thoracic and abdominal injuries. The extent of the injury must be determined quickly. Cardiopulmonary function, internal hemorrhage, and fractures of the limbs or the spinal column should be evaluated.[7]

The nervous system should then be evaluated as described previously. Evaluations of the level of consciousness, pupillary function and eye movements, dysfunction of other CNs, and motor function are adequate for the assessment of the level and the extent of damage to the CNS. Neurologic examination and lesion localization have been previously discussed.

Methylprednisolone sodium succinate is used in the medical treatment for CCT. Corticosteroids decrease edema, stabilize cell membranes and the BBB, and decrease the secondary biochemical events previously described. They should not be administered for longer than 3 to 5 days because they inhibit remyelination, suppress the immune system, and induce gastrointestinal ulceration. The efficacy of corticosteroids in trauma-induced edema has been questioned, but several studies have provided objective evidence of reduced ICP with high doses.[13] Several studies of spinal cord trauma also indicate their efficacy.[13-15] Because spinal cord and brain tissue respond to injury in a similar manner, we assume that similar treatments would be effective in brain injury. The two key factors appear to be adequate dose and early administration. MPSS is given at a dose of 30 mg/kg administered intravenously, and the same dose is repeated 2 and 6 hours later. Then MPSS is given by continuous infusion at a rate of 2.5 to 5.0 mg/kg per hour for 48 hours. The treatment must be given as early as possible, preferably within the first hour after injury, and should be maintained for up to 48 hours. Within 6 hours of injury, irreversible neuronal and axonal loss occurs. One study indicated that patients with spinal cord injury who receive a first dose more than 8 hours after injury have less recovery of function than those who receive placebo treatment.[14]

Furosemide decreases the production of CSF and facilitates resorption of edematous fluid. An intravenous dose of 0.6 to 1.0 mg per kilogram of body weight is given every 4 hours for 12 to 24 hours.

Table 12-10 **Management of Intracranial Injury**[*]

| Assessment[†] | Level and Type of Injury | | | |
	Cerebral Nonprogressive	Cerebral Progressive	Brainstem Progressive	Brainstem Nonprogressive
Coma scale score	15-18	9-14	3-8	3-8
Management	Corticosteroids, monitor	Corticosteroids, mannitol, furosemide, DMSO,[‡] monitor	CT, skull radiography, corticosteroids, mannitol, furosemide, DMSO, surgical decompression	Corticosteroids, mannitol, DMSO, monitor
Prognosis	Usually good	Guarded	Poor unless reverses	Poor

[*]Emergency management: Treat shock, maintain airway, stop bleeding, provide cardiopulmonary resuscitation.
Evaluate: History, physical examination, neurologic examination
[†]For assessment, see Tables 12-1 to 12-5. Progressive signs frequently follow the pattern from left to right in the table.
[‡]DMSO is not licensed for systemic use, but is frequently recommended for large animals.
DMSO, Dimethyl sulfoxide; *CT,* computed tomography.

Mannitol, a nonmetabolizable 6-carbon polyalcohol, is an osmotic diuretic that can lower ICP by decreasing CSF production and CSF volume in traumatic brain injuries.[16,17] It may also act as an oxygen free radical scavenger and reduce ischemic damage to the brain.[17] We use mannitol in comatose patients following the administration of fluids, MPSS, and furosemide. Its use is contraindicated in hypovolemia, anuria, and hyperosmolality.[17] It is used with caution in patients with concurrent heart failure. Twenty-percent mannitol solution is administered at a dosage of 1.0 g per kilogram of body weight, administered intravenously over 20 to 30 minutes. It can be repeated every 4 to 6 hours. Brain hemorrhage may be exacerbated by mannitol through its ability to decrease ICP.

Seizures may occur anytime following CCT. Seizures should be controlled with intravenous diazepam at a dose of 0.5 to 1.0 mg per kilogram of body weight. It can be repeated at 5- to 10-minute intervals for three or four doses. If seizures continue, diazepam can be constantly infused at a dose of 5 to 10 mg per hour. Injectable phenobarbital may be required in some cases, but it will increase depression. See Chapter 13 for additional information on seizure management.

After the patient is stabilized, frequent monitoring of the severity of signs is imperative. The coma scale is useful for comparison between examinations. Magnetic resonance imaging (MRI) or computed tomography (CT) scan, if available, or radiography should be performed on a patient that has minimal deficits (alert or depressed) to detect skull fractures. The animal should be observed closely for 24 to 48 hours for progressive signs. Depressed skull fractures in conscious patients are elevated surgically when the patients are stable. Animals with linear fractures do not need surgery unless progressive signs indicate continuing intracranial hemorrhage. Open fractures are debrided and closed as early as possible.

Stuporous or comatose patients require more critical assessment and care and have a poorer prognosis. Brainstem hemorrhage usually can be differentiated from tentorial herniation from the time course of the neurologic signs (Figure 12-4; see Table 12-8). Intramedullary brainstem hemorrhage, which usually occurs in the midbrain or the pons, produces coma immediately after the trauma. Little or no improvement occurs in this case (Figure 12-5). Tentorial herniation may develop from cerebral edema (usually bilateral) or from rostrotentorial hemorrhage (epidural, subdural). The progression of signs is usually characteristic (see Tables 12-3 and 12-4). Animals with brainstem hemorrhage rarely recover, and those that do

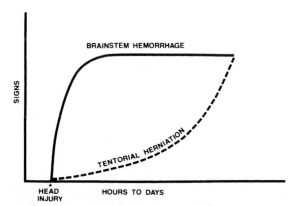

Figure 12-4 Sign-time graph of head injury. Tentorial herniation and brainstem hemorrhage may be differentiated by the clinical course. (From Oliver JE Jr: Neurologic emergencies in small animals, *Vet Clin North Am* 2:341-357, 1972.)

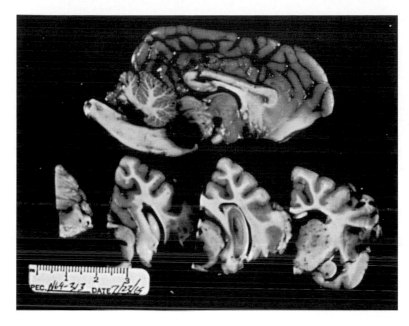

Figure 12-5 Brainstem hemorrhage in a Boxer dog that was hit by a car. The hemorrhage extends from the caudal midbrain into the middle of the pons. The sulci and the gyri of the cortex are prominent, indicating minimal brain swelling. No evidence of tentorial herniation is present. (Compare the brainstem section second from the right with that in Figure12-3.) (From Oliver JE Jr: Neurologic examination, *Vet Med Small Anim Clin* 67:654-659, 1972.)

usually have severe neurologic deficits. Tentorial herniation must be managed early for the treatment to be successful. Severe tentorial herniation with compression and distortion of the brainstem produces secondary brain hemorrhages that are irreversible. In addition, increased pressure transmitted to the caudotentorial compartment produces cerebellar herniation through the foramen magnum, causing death by interference with the medullary respiratory centers (Figure 12-6).

Brainstem hemorrhage and tentorial herniation are treated as previously described. If the signs do not improve or if progression is observed in the first few hours, craniotomy for evacuation of the hematoma and relief of increased ICP may be indicated.[18]

Management of the comatose patient must include maintaining hydration and nutrition; regulating body temperature; providing adequate ventilation (including hyperventilation in the early stages); preventing decubital ulcers by frequent turning, meticulous cleaning of the skin, and cushioning with sponge rubber or fleece pads; and maintaining urinary and fecal elimination. Management of the comatose patient can be time-consuming and expensive but is rewarding when successful.

Equine Head Trauma. Two types of skull fractures in horses result in serious brain injury.[8] Frontal bone fractures result from direct impact and are often open, depressed fractures with direct cerebral laceration and hemorrhage from the fracture fragments. Neurologic signs include contralateral cortical

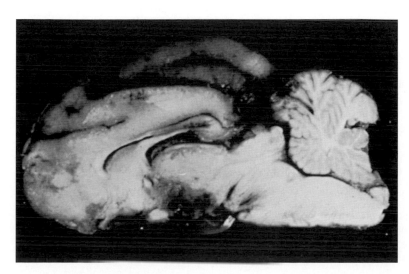

Figure 12-6 Brain of a cat with head trauma. Tentorial herniation with compression of the rostral cerebellum and foramen magnum herniation with compression of the caudal cerebellum and the brainstem are present. (Courtesy Joe N. Kornegay, DVM.)

blindness, decreased facial sensation, depression, compulsive wandering toward the side of the lesion, and generalized seizures. Development of anisocoria or mydriasis with slow pupillary light reflexes indicates increasing ICP and risk of caudal cerebral herniation. Loss of consciousness and development of mydriatic, unresponsive pupils indicate herniation of the occipital lobes of the cerebral cortex under the tentorium cerebelli.

Basilar skull fractures occur when horses flip over backwards and strike the poll. These fractures result in compression and hemorrhage of the brainstem. Occipital bone fractures may lacerate the basilar artery and venous sinuses and produce massive hemorrhage into the calvaria, guttural pouch, or inner ear. Neurologic signs include coma that lasts from minutes to days. Horses that regain consciousness demonstrate depression, vestibular dysfunction, facial nerve paralysis, tetraparesis, and hemorrhage from the nostrils and ear. Leakage of CSF or blood from the external ear canal is evidence of petrous temporal bone fracture. Epistaxis may result from fracture of the cribriform plate, basisphenoid/basioccipital bones, or hemorrhage into the guttural pouch.

In some cases, trauma to the poll or frontal area may cause bilateral blindness with mydriatic, unresponsive pupils. This injury results from damage to the optic nerves or optic chiasm. The prognosis for recovery of vision is poor.

Skull radiographs are required to determine the type, location, and displacement of fractures and fracture fragments. Depressed, comminuted fractures of the frontal and parietal bones are readily identified radiographically. Petrous temporal bone fractures are difficult to identify, and multiple oblique views are necessary to identify the fracture line. Absence of an obvious fracture line does not preclude a diagnosis of basilar skull fracture. Hemorrhage from the guttural pouch, nose, or external ear canal following a traumatic poll injury is presumptive evidence of a basilar skull fracture.

Medical treatment includes intravenous fluids, corticosteroids (usually dexamethasone because of the expense of MPSS in large animals), furosemide, mannitol, and dimethyl sulfoxide (DMSO). Broad-spectrum antibiotics that penetrate into the CSF are indicated for basilar skull fractures, petrosal bone fractures, and open frontal bone fractures. Cefotaxime is bactericidal, has broad-spectrum antibacterial activity, and penetrates into the CSF in good concentrations (see Chapter 15).

Surgical therapy is indicated for horses with depressed frontal fractures that penetrate nervous tissue and open fractures that communicate with nervous tissue. Animals that have deterioration of neurologic status despite medical therapy also need surgery. Burr holes placed in the frontal or parietal bone may relieve ICP. Horses that are comatose and fail to respond to therapy within 36 hours are unlikely to recover. Response to therapy within 6 to 8 hours indicates a favorable prognosis for life; however, the ultimate usefulness of the horse is not apparent for weeks to months after the injury.

Acute Nonprogressive

Vascular Diseases. *Vascular diseases* include occlusions causing infarctions and disruption of vessels causing hemorrhage.[19] Primary vascular changes, such as arteriosclerosis, are rare in animals.[20,21] Atherosclerosis can be produced with atherogenic diets and may be more common in animals with hypothyroidism.[22] Most vascular lesions are caused by emboli from sepsis or neoplasia. Fibrocartilaginous emboli from degenerating disks cause infarction in the spinal cord (see Chapter 6). The causes of vascular diseases are listed in Table 12-11.

A *stroke*, or a *cerebrovascular accident* (CVA), is an acute onset of neurologic deficit from spontaneous intracranial hemorrhage or occlusion of an intracranial blood vessel by a thrombus or an embolus. *Cerebral vasospasm* is a temporary constriction of an intracranial artery, producing transient ischemia. Vasospasm is difficult to document clinically. Transient loss of consciousness *(syncope)* is usually caused by a cardiac arrhythmia, not by vasospasm (see Chapter 13).

Table 12-11 Etiology of Vascular Disease in the Brain*

Hemorrhage
Trauma
Infectious disease (rickettsial, FIP septicemia, infectious canine hepatitis) (15)
Toxins (warfarin) (15)
Neoplasia (15)
Disseminated intravascular coagulopathy
Idiopathic thrombocytopenic purpura
Intracarotid injections (equine)
Peripartum asphyxia
Vascular anomalies

Infarction
Septic emboli (endocarditis, septicemia, thromboembolic meningoencephalitis) (15)
Neoplasia (metastases) (15)
Parasites *(Dirofilaria)* (15)
Idiopathic feline cerebral infarction
Vasospasm, vascular insufficiency, heart failure
Emboli secondary to surgery (air, fat, clot)

---

*Numbers in parentheses refer to chapters in which the conditions are discussed.
FIP, Feline infectious peritonitis.

Hemorrhage in the brain is usually due to trauma. All other causes of hemorrhage combined have a much lower incidence. Small hemorrhages *(petechiae)* are seen on examination of the brain, with inflammation as the primary problem, but other changes predominate.[23] The exceptions are infections, such as Rocky Mountain spotted fever, that cause thrombocytopenia and vasculitis.[24] Hemorrhage-producing stroke syndromes are seen most often with neoplasms that have compromised an artery (Figure 12-7). Systemic coagulation disorders such as disseminated intravascular coagulopathy (DIC) and idiopathic thrombocytopenic purpura (ITP) usually are recognized by systemic signs.[25]

Infarcts are usually the result of septic emboli, frequently in association with endocarditis (Figure 12-8). Cardiomyopathy should be considered in small animals with suspected cerebral infarctions. Thromboembolic meningoencephalitis (TEME) is an acute disease of cattle that is characterized by infarcts produced by septic emboli. Disseminated coagulopathy may develop subsequently. The disease is caused by *Haemophilus somnus* and usually is seen in feedlot cattle. Cerebral signs predominate, but brainstem infarcts may produce focal signs (see Chapter 15). Metastatic neoplasia or parasites, including the microfilaria of *Dirofilaria immitis*, are less common causes of vascular occlusion.[26,27] Air, fat, or blood clots may be introduced into the circulation during surgical procedures. Air emboli are of particular concern during vascular surgery of the head and the neck.

Idiopathic feline cerebral infarction has been described as a distinct syndrome associated with vasculitis and thrombosis.[28,29] No breed, sex, or age predilection occurs. Idiopathic feline cerebral

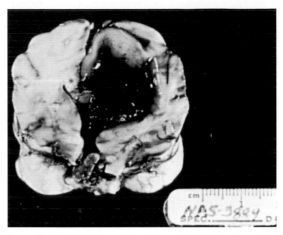

Figure 12-7 Massive hemorrhage in an oligodendroglioma in a Samoyed. No clinical signs were present before an acute episode related to the hemorrhage.

infarction has not been correlated with feline cardiomyopathy but an association with CNS *Cuterebra* larvae myiasis has been reported.[30,31] Young to middle-aged indoor–outdoor domestic short-haired cats developed acute neurologic signs from July to September.[31] Eighty percent of affected cats had cerebral infarction.[30] It is postulated that a toxin elaborated by the fly larvae induces vascular compromise and eventual infarction. Furthermore, feline cerebral infarction has not been reported in regions of the world devoid of the *Cuterebra* fly.[30]

The lesions are often confined to the distribution of the middle cerebral artery (Figure 12-9). The rostral and caudal cerebral arteries are affected less often, possibly because they anastomose with each other, offering a source of collateral circulation, except in their terminal branches (Figure 12-10).[32]

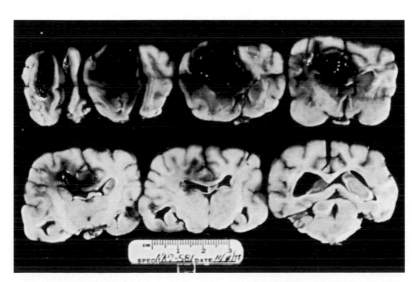

Figure 12-8 Hemorrhagic infarct in a dog with endocarditis. A cingulate herniation is present across the midline.

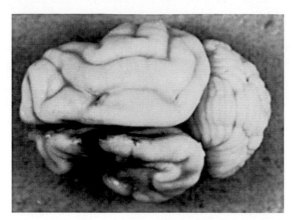

Figure 12-9 Infarction of the left cerebral hemisphere of a cat.

severe or are confined entirely to one side. Diffuse cerebral or rostral brainstem lesions may cause a loss of consciousness, which may persist (coma) or may be transient. Hemiparesis is frequent, and behavioral changes may be present.

Management of the unconscious patient is discussed in the section on trauma in this chapter. Less severe lesions are usually not life threatening; however, the amount of residual damage often depends on the adequacy of therapy. Although their efficacy is still disputed, corticosteroids should be given in antiedema doses (30 mg/kg of methylprednisolone sodium succinate) to control edema.[33] Adequate ventilation must be ensured if respiration is compromised. Anticoagulants generally are not given unless a clotting problem is known to exist (e.g., DIC). If the source of the problem (e.g., bacterial endocarditis) can be identified, specific antibiotic therapy is instituted.

Most animals that are diagnosed clinically as likely to have had CVAs recover. Unless the lesion is large or involves the brainstem, neurologic function is adequate for survival. Idiopathic feline cerebral infarction is characterized by massive cortical damage that causes seizures or behavioral disorders, which often are unacceptable in a pet.

Clinical signs of hemorrhage and infarction depend on the location and extent of the involvement. In all cases of vascular occlusion or hemorrhage, a sudden onset with little or no progression is characteristic. Depending on the state of oxygenation and other factors, neuronal death begins in 3 to 10 minutes. Because most vascular lesions are unilateral, clinical signs are frequently more

Figure 12-10 Areas of the brain supplied by the cerebral arteries. *a*, artery. (From Evans HE, Christensen GC: *Miller's anatomy of the dog,* 2nd ed. Philadelphia, 1979, WB Saunders.)

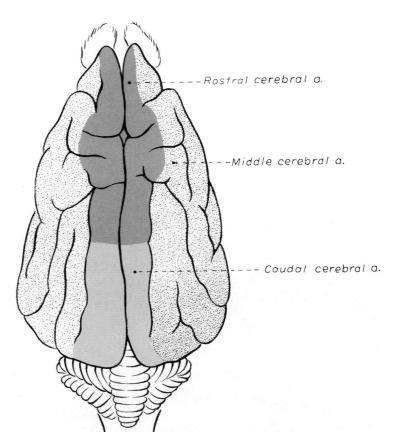

Rostral cerebral a.

Middle cerebral a.

Caudal cerebral a.

Chronic Progressive

Neoplasia. Neoplasms of the brain may cause stupor and coma, depending on location, rate of growth, development of cerebral edema, and alterations in circulation. A sudden onset of stupor or coma has occurred in cases of acute hemorrhage into a cerebral tumor. The signs were attributed to an acute increase in ICP (see Figure 12-7). Neoplasia is discussed in Chapter 15.

No Focal or Lateralizing Signs, But Evidence of Meningitis Present

Acute Progressive

Inflammation. Inflammatory diseases of the CNS may affect both the nervous tissue and the meninges, although one of these entities may be more severely involved than the other one. Stupor or coma results from a direct effect on neurons, cerebral edema, increased ICP from hydrocephalus, hypoxia from vasculitis, or systemic metabolic abnormalities.

Viral agents tend to have a greater effect on the nervous tissue, with only minimal involvement of the meninges. Vasculitis is common with rickettsial and some viral infections. Bacterial and fungal agents produce a greater meningeal reaction. Formulation of a diagnosis requires analysis of CSF for cells, protein content, and antibody titers (see Chapter 4).

The management of patients with stupor or coma secondary to inflammatory disease includes treatment of the primary disease, if possible, management of increased ICP, and suppression of the inflammatory response. Increased ICP from cerebral edema and CNS inflammation should be treated with corticosteroids. Whereas suppression of the immune system by corticosteroids may occur in a patient with an infectious disease, the consequences of not treating the increased ICP and CNS inflammation are worse, namely, death. Initially, the patient is treated with MPSS (see previous sections) and then maintained on antiinflammatory doses of prednisone once the patient improves. See Chapter 15 for a complete discussion of inflammatory diseases.

No Focal or Lateralizing Signs

Acute Progressive

Inflammation. Many of the viral encephalitides cause depression, stupor, or coma. They are discussed in Chapter 15.

Metabolic Diseases. Nervous tissue depends on a continuous supply of glucose and oxygen for normal function. It is protected from toxic substances by the BBB. Alterations in brain metabolism can cause severe clinical signs ranging from depression to coma and from tremors to seizures. The most common metabolic problems causing stupor or coma are listed in Table 12-6. Hypoglycemia is discussed in Chapter 15. Hepatic encephalopathy, uremic encephalopathy, and diabetic coma are discussed in Chapter 15.

Heat stroke is an acute failure of the heat-regulating mechanisms of the body that results in a body temperature exceeding 40° C (105° F).[34,35] High ambient temperature, high humidity, and poor ventilation are the inciting factors. Brachycephalic breeds of dogs are especially susceptible. A long haired coat, obesity, and high fever may also predispose the animal to heat stroke.

The primary mechanism for dissipation of heat in dogs and cats is panting. The airflow is unidirectional—in through the nose and out through the mouth.[36] The large surface area of the nasal turbinates promotes heat exchange. Prolonged panting causes respiratory alkalosis that later is modified by metabolic acidosis, presumably from increased muscular activity. If hyperthermia continues, cerebral edema and DIC occur frequently, either of which can cause death. Although all of the CNS is involved, the neurons of the cerebral cortex and the cerebellum seem most susceptible to permanent damage.[37,38] The diagnosis of heat stroke is based on the clinical signs and elevation of the body temperature.

The three major objectives of treatment are to reduce body temperature, prevent cerebral edema, and manage DIC if it develops. Antiedema doses of MPSS should be given. The body temperature is decreased by immersing the animal in cold or iced water. The rectal temperature should be monitored continuously by thermistor or at 10-minute intervals. To prevent hypothermia, cooling is stopped when the rectal temperature reaches 39.5° C (103° F). Iced-water enemas may be used in refractory cases, but they prevent accurate monitoring of body temperature unless an esophageal thermistor is available. If shivering interferes with the cooling process, a tranquilizer (acetylpromazine, 0.1 mg/kg) may be given.

If the animal shows evidence of cerebral edema, especially if signs of tentorial herniation are present (see Table 12-3), mannitol (0.25 to 1 g/kg) should be administered intravenously. If serious blood loss or DIC is a complication, mannitol should not be given. Fluids should be given intravenously to maintain cardiac output and renal function. Overhydration must be avoided.

Hemorrhagic diarrhea, petechiae, or excessive bleeding from venipuncture sites signifies the onset of DIC. Intravenous heparin (250 to 300 IU/kg every 8 hours) therapy should be instituted immediately. Coagulation studies can confirm the presence of DIC.[25,35]

The patient should be monitored carefully for at least 24 hours after normothermia is achieved so that recurrences can be avoided. The prognosis for patients with heat stroke is relatively good if they are treated early (i.e., before signs of cerebral edema or DIC develop).

Hypoxia is an inadequate supply of oxygen for normal brain function. Arterial oxygen tension levels below 50 mm Hg are detrimental to brain function. Increased levels of carbon dioxide have a profound effect on cerebral blood flow. Because no oxygen reserves are present in the brain, merely a few minutes of hypoxia can cause irreversible damage. More than 10 minutes of hypoxia will produce neuronal death. The cerebral cortex and cerebellum are most susceptible to hypoxic damage, and the lower brainstem is most resistant.

The most frequent causes of hypoxia in animals are anesthesia accidents, cardiopulmonary failure, suffocation, smoke inhalation, paralysis of respiration, carbon monoxide poisoning, cyanide poisoning, and near drowning.

Despite the almost universal use of inhalation anesthesia with controlled ventilation, complications of anesthesia are common. Cardiac arrhythmias, overdoses of the anesthetic agent, improper intubations, and faulty apparatuses are but a few of the problems encountered. Meticulous attention to detail in the administration and the monitoring of anesthesia is essential.

Heart, lung, and peripheral circulatory failure rival anesthesia as the most common cause of hypoxia. Heart and lung disease may cause a mild to severe hypoxemia. If the condition does not cause unconsciousness, the danger of cerebral damage is low. Shock may cause profound cerebral hypoxia and irreversible damage to the brain. A primary concern in the management of shock is maintenance of adequate ventilation. Management of the various forms of cardiopulmonary failure, however, is beyond the scope of this text.[25]

Suffocation is a less frequent problem in animals. Examples of causes are aspiration of vomitus, especially in injured or anesthetized animals; aspiration of foreign bodies; and near drowning.

Paralysis of respiration may occur with lesions of the CNS between the medullary respiratory centers and the origin of the phrenic nerve at C5-7 (sometimes C4). The lesion may affect the respiratory center directly, or it may interrupt the descending pathway in the cervical spinal cord and produce the same effect: apnea. Lesions in the lower cervical (C7) or the upper thoracic region may block motor pathways to the intercostal lower motor neurons, but the intact phrenic pathway allows diaphragmatic ("abdominal") breathing to occur. The most common cause of this lesion is trauma. If the damage to the CNS is irreversible, life can be maintained only by use of a respirator. Generalized lower motor neuron (LMN) disease also may cause respiratory paralysis through its effect on both the intercostal and phrenic nerves (see Chapter 7).

Carbon monoxide poisoning occurs occasionally in animals that have been transported in a car trunk. Carbon monoxide combines with hemoglobin, preventing the formation of oxyhemoglobin. The animal typically has bright red mucous membranes and rapid, shallow respiration. Transfusion of fresh (not stored) whole blood and administration of oxygen may be effective if hypoxia has not persisted too long.

Cyanide poisoning is rare, except in ruminants that eat plants containing hydrocyanic acid (cherry trees, sorghum grasses, and others). Cyanide interferes with the cellular utilization of oxygen through blockage of the cytochrome system.[39] Treatment is with sodium nitrite and sodium thiosulfate.

Equine peripartum asphyxia syndrome (PAS) has been recognized for many years in newborn foals. Ischemic or hypoxic damage of many organs is the suspected cause.[40] Neurologic abnormalities usually develop within 24 hours after birth. The severity of neurologic signs depends on the degree and duration of hypoxia. Mild signs include jitteriness and hyperalertness. More severe signs include irregular respirations, apnea, random intermittent tongue protrusions and sucking behavior, drooling, strabismus, and nystagmus. Foals may show stiff, rhythmic marching behavior; others may wander aimlessly, may be depressed or stuporous, and may circle in one direction.[40]

Tonic-clonic seizures are common findings. Severely affected foals may bark like dogs (barker foals), and this sign is often accompanied by clonic seizures. The most severely affected foals may be comatose and completely hypotonic, showing seizures and apnea.[40]

In addition to the CNS signs, other signs of systemic organ failure may be present. Renal hypoxia produces elevated serum creatinine levels, oliguria, hypocalcemia, hyponatremia, and hypochloremia. Gastrointestinal signs include colic, ileus, bloody diarrhea, and gastric reflux. Cardiac signs include arrhythmia, tachycardia, murmur, hypotension, and generalized edema. Icterus may develop in foals with hypoxic liver injury.

The diagnosis of PAS is based on the characteristic clinical signs of multiple organ dysfunction occurring within 24 to 48 hours of birth. Septic meningitis (see Chapter 15) may cause similar neurologic signs. CSF is normal in foals with PAS, and neutrophilic pleocytosis and elevated protein concentrations are typical CSF findings in foals with septic meningitis.

Treatment is supportive. Phenobarbital and diazepam may be used to control seizures. The prognosis is poor for severely affected foals. Less severely affected foals that survive the first few days may regain vision and suckling ability, and some make complete recoveries.[40]

Nutritional Diseases. Thiamine deficiency may cause stupor or coma, especially in ruminants. Polioencephalomalacia, a symmetric laminar necrosis of the cerebral cortex, occurs in cattle, sheep, and goats. Increased ICP is common. Thiamine deficiency is discussed in Chapter 15.

Chronic Progressive

Toxic Disorders. A large number of toxic agents may produce stupor and coma, especially in the terminal stages (see Chapter 15). An overdose of certain drugs, including barbiturates, tranquilizers, or narcotics, may produce stupor or coma as a primary effect.[39] The drugs may have been given deliberately or may have been ingested accidentally. Historical information may be clear ("he ate my bottle of pills") or misleading ("we never have anything like that around"). A comparison of the signs of coma caused by drugs with those of coma caused by structural changes in the brain is provided in Table 12-1. Spinal reflexes and respirations are depressed more severely by sedative drugs than by most structural lesions, whereas pupillary responses are less affected.

Most patients that are toxic from CNS depressants can be saved with proper management. If the animal is not in coma, attentive nursing is usually all that is necessary. Gastric lavage and activated charcoal are useful if the drug was ingested recently. Maintenance of adequate respiration is the most important consideration for a patient in coma. Controlled respiration through an endotracheal catheter is essential.

Diuresis is promoted by the intravenous administration of glucose or mannitol. Urine output must be monitored through an indwelling urethral catheter. The excretion of many agents (e.g., barbiturates) is dependent on the rate of urine formation. Hydration and acid-base balance must be maintained. Periodic evaluation of serum electrolytes and blood gases is of great benefit in the management of persistent coma. Stimulants have been used in the past but appear to be of little benefit because they do not affect the rate of metabolism or excretion of most drugs.

Degenerative Diseases. *Storage diseases*, which are inherited degenerative diseases with accumulation of metabolic products in neurons, can cause depression or stupor. The animal may be in a coma

terminally. Other signs, such as ataxia or seizures, are more common in the early stages of the disease (see Chapter 15).

Anomalies. *Hydrocephalus* is an enlargement of the cerebral ventricular system secondary to an increased amount of CSF. Excessive CSF may be the result of obstruction to flow (noncommunicating or obstructive hydrocephalus), poor absorption, or increased production (communicating hydrocephalus). Hydrocephalus may be seen in any species and is more often congenital than acquired.

Most of the CSF is produced by the choroid plexus in the lateral, third, and fourth ventricles, but a substantial portion travels through the ependyma lining the ventricles and the subarachnoid space around the brain and spinal cord. CSF flows from the lateral ventricles through the interventricular foramina to the third ventricle. It continues caudally through the mesencephalic aqueduct to the fourth ventricle and into the subarachnoid space through the lateral apertures of the fourth ventricle. In the subarachnoid space, most of the fluid moves around the brainstem into the rostrotentorial compartment. Most of the absorption occurs through the arachnoid villi in the dorsal sagittal sinus (Figure 12-11).

Overproduction of CSF by a choroid plexus papilloma is rare. Communicating hydrocephalus from decreased absorption of CSF is usually the result of inflammation of the meninges. Inflammation is usually caused by infectious diseases such as canine distemper but may be secondary to subarachnoid hemorrhage or to the presence of foreign materials such as radiographic contrast materials that are injected in the subarachnoid space.[41] Obstruction of the flow of CSF occurs most commonly at the mesencephalic aqueduct. Malformations of the aqueduct range from complete absence to stenosis. Obstruction of the aqueduct also can be secondary to inflammation or compression by a mass. For example, brainstem tumors that cause obstruction of the aqueduct produce hydrocephalus.[42,43] Most cases of hydrocephalus that are seen in veterinary practice are congenital. The disorder may be caused by environmental or genetic factors. In calves, vitamin A deficiency can result in altered bone growth that can affect the skull. Deformities of the temporal bone can obstruct CSF flow, producing hydrocephalus. Hereditary hydrocephalus has been reported in Hereford cattle.[44]

Too few studies of the lesion of congenital hydrocephalus in the dog have been performed to determine the primary defect. Some patients have stenosis or atresia of the mesencephalic aqueduct, but others do not. Multiple branching of the aqueduct, called *forking*, has been reported in both dogs and humans.[45,46] The formation of diverticula, clefts, and tears is prevalent in periventricular white

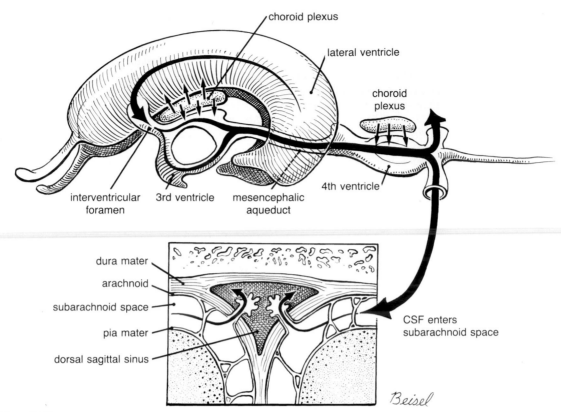

Figure 12-11 Cerebrospinal fluid is produced in all areas of the central nervous system. The bulk of the fluid flows from the lateral ventricles to the third ventricle to the mesencephalic aqueduct and continues from the fourth ventricle to the lateral apertures and then to the subarachnoid space, where it is absorbed.

matter.[47] Tearing may be associated with sudden decline in neurologic status or may exhibit a chronicity of several days.[47] A statistically significant correlation between small body size and hydrocephalus has been demonstrated in dogs (Table 12-12).[46]

Ventricular enlargement without clinical signs is a common finding in some toy breeds, especially

Table 12-12 **Breeds of Dogs at Increased Risk of Hydrocephalus**

Maltese
Yorkshire terrier
English bulldog
Chihuahua
Lhasa apso
Pomeranian
Toy poodle
Cairn terrier
Boston terrier
Pug
Pekingese

Data from Selby LA, Hayes HM, Becker SV: Epizootiologic features of canine hydrocephalus, *Am J Vet Res* 40:411-414, 1979.

Chihuahuas, Yorkshire terriers, and Maltese dogs. A kennel of Chihuahuas was studied by Redding.[48] Subclinical hydrocephalus was common. Behavioral changes could be correlated with abnormal EEGs in many instances. A selective breeding program in which the EEG was used to screen breeding animals reduced the incidence of hydrocephalus. Redding concluded that the dogs had a compensated hydrocephalus (a balance between production and absorption of CSF) that could be decompensated by relatively mild changes such as trauma or infection. These observations correlate with our clinical impression. Redding also observed a high incidence of enlargement of the foramen magnum (occipital dysplasia) (see Chapter 8) in these dogs. Whether this abnormality is related to the cause of hydrocephalus or whether it is secondary to increased pressure is still debated. The clinical signs are related to the (1) age at onset, (2) degree of imbalance between production and absorption of CSF, and (3) location of the defect (communicating or noncommunicating).

Simpson[45] studied a series of hydrocephalic Maltese dogs. Fewer than 20% had seizures, with most seizures occurring during the first year of life.

Behavioral problems were the most frequent complaints. Learned responses such as house training were difficult or impossible to achieve in 75% of the dogs.

Bull terriers affected with complex partial seizures have a high incidence of moderate to severe hydrocephalus.[49] It is unlikely that the behavioral signs in these dogs are directly related to the concurrent hydrocephalus.

In foals, a variety of neurologic signs may be seen.[50] Some foals may be normal behaviorally and neurologically. Typically depression, dementia, and seizures are observed. Exophthalmos and ventrolateral strabismus may also occur.

Congenital hydrocephalus is usually recognized in the very young animal. The increase in intracranial volume occurs before the sutures of the skull have closed, allowing for enlargement of the calvaria. In most animal species, the enlargement of the head, the open sutures and fontanelles, and the poor development of the animal may be recognized shortly after birth.

Affected dogs are usually taken to the veterinarian when they are between 2 and 3 months of age, sometimes when they are older. Palpation of the skull may reveal the persistent sutures and fontanelles. In compensated hydrocephalus, the fontanelle may be open, but no tension is present as the brain is palpated. Active hydrocephalus with increased pressure often causes bulging of the soft tissue through the fontanelle, and palpation reveals the increased tension. The prominent frontal areas encroach on the orbits, causing ventrolateral deviation of the eyes (Figure 12-12). Oculomotor nerve function (pupils and eye movements) (see Chapter 11) is usually normal, indicating that the eye deviation is mechanical, not neurologic, in origin. The widening of the skull is detected by palpation of the parietal area, where the

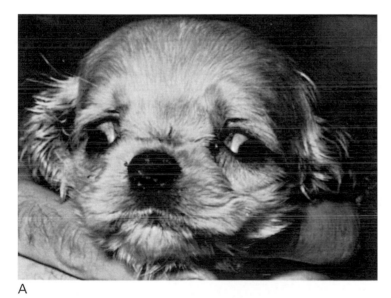

A

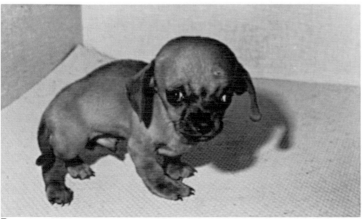

B

Figure 12-12 Cocker spaniel **(A)** and Dachshund **(B)** puppies with hydrocephalus. The large, rounded head and the ventrolateral deviation of the eyes are characteristic.

space between the skull and the zygomatic arch is narrowed. Head pain may be evident in some animals when the skull is palpated.

Young animals with hydrocephalus usually are smaller and less developed than their littermates. They are often depressed, have episodic behavioral changes such as aggression or confusion, and frequently have seizures (see Chapter 13). Because their mental development is retarded, they do not learn as readily as their littermates. Visual deficits with normal pupillary responses are common because of damage to the optic radiation and the occipital cortex (see Chapter 11). Motor function may range from an almost normal gait to severe tetraparesis. Papilledema may be seen on fundic examination in a small percentage of cases.

Hydrocephalus in the adult animal is more difficult to recognize. The skull is normal because the sutures have fused before the increase in pressure. The clinical signs develop more rapidly and are more severe, but they are dependent on the relative balance of production and absorption of CSF. Seizures are a frequent sign in the early stages. Depression, which may progress to stupor or coma, is common. Because hydrocephalus in the adult is usually secondary to inflammation or a mass, signs of the primary problem may predominate early in the course of the disease. Complete obstruction of the CSF causes a rapidly progressive hydrocephalus, which may cause tentorial herniation, cerebellar herniation, or both.

The diagnosis of hydrocephalus in the young animal is relatively certain if the characteristic signs are present. Although the clinical signs of severe hydrocephalus are typical, less severe involvement may produce a more subtle picture. Behavioral changes or seizures may be the only complaint. In these cases, ancillary studies are necessary to confirm the diagnosis.

In these cases, EEG may be useful because it is noninvasive and the recordings are usually suggestive of the diagnosis (Figure 12-13). High-voltage, slow-wave activity (25 to 200 mV, 1 to 6 Hz) that is hypersynchronous (similar in all leads) may be seen both in dogs that are awake and in those that are anesthetized. A fast component (10 to 12 Hz) often is superimposed on the slow waves. In severe hydrocephalus, in which the large slow waves (1 to 4 Hz) predominate, the EEG results are sufficient for diagnosis. Earlier forms, in which faster activity is more prominent, may be confused with inflammatory disease. Adult dogs may have faster activity also.[43] Because many veterinary practices do not have EEG capabilities, the diagnosis must be confirmed by other procedures.

Two procedures, CT and ultrasonography (US) through the open fontanelles, are the most accurate and least invasive methods of diagnosis (Figure 12-14).[45] If CT and US are not available, radiographs of the skull may demonstrate changes that are compatible with hydrocephalus. The diagnosis can also be confirmed by ventricular tap.

Skull radiographs can confirm persistent suture lines and fontanelles. Increased ICP for an extended period causes thinning of the skull with loss of the normal digitate impressions on the inner surface of the calvaria. The cranium has a ground glass-like appearance (Figure 12-15, *A*). Rostral displacement and thinning of the wing of the sphenoid bone and loss of the osseous tentorium cerebelli also may be seen.

The diagnosis can be confirmed in severe cases by a ventricular tap using general anesthesia. A spinal needle is inserted directly into the ventricle.

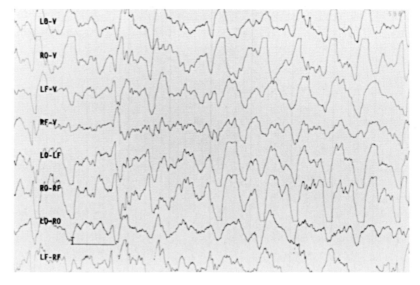

Figure 12-13 Electroencephalogram of a hydrocephalic dog. The recording is characterized by low-frequency, high-voltage activity that is synchronized, generalized, and symmetric. *L*, Left; *R*, right; *O*, occipital; *F*, frontal; *V*, vertex. Calibration markers: *horizontal bar*, 1 second; *vertical bar*, 50 mV.

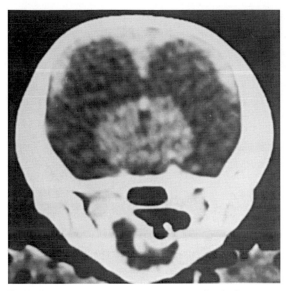

Figure 12-14 Computed tomography scan of a hydrocephalic Chihuahua dog, female, 10 months old, with a history of seizures, progressive dementia, and postural reaction deficits. The ventricles are the dark areas occupying most of the cranial vault.

The depth that is necessary to obtain fluid provides an estimate of the thickness of the cerebral cortex. Normal animals have a lateral ventricle that is only a few millimeters thick. Careful needle placement is required to obtain fluid. Severe hydrocephalus causes thinning of the cerebral cortex (Figure 12-16) so that fluid may be obtained within 0.5 to 1.0 cm of the inner surface of the skull. If it is necessary to go deeper than 1.0 to 1.5 cm to obtain fluid, pneumoventriculography is performed to confirm the ventricular enlargement (Figure 12-15, *B*). The distances given are primarily for toy breed dogs or cats. Those for larger animals of any species may vary somewhat.

Never aspirate fluid using a syringe because the cerebral cortex may collapse, causing a subdural hematoma (Figure 12-17). Fluid may be allowed to escape under its own pressure, providing some therapeutic benefit in addition to establishing the diagnosis. Analysis of the CSF may be useful for formulating an etiologic diagnosis (see Chapter 4). In a potentially hydrocephalic animal with an open fontanelle, less risk exists in obtaining the CSF for analysis from the ventricle than from the cerebellomedullary cistern.

If the results of the ventricular tap are not diagnostic, pneumoventriculography is performed (see Figure 12-15, *B*). Positive-contrast ventriculography may be necessary to determine whether the hydrocephalus is communicating or noncommunicating. Because therapy generally is the same in either case, the increased risk involved in the use of positive contrast material usually is not justified.

In summary, CT and US are the best diagnostic tests that are not invasive. If either one is available, the other tests are not necessary. Ventricular tap may be needed for therapeutic benefit in acute cases. It is the safest method for obtaining CSF if it is needed to substantiate a diagnosis.

The treatment of hydrocephalus depends on the cause of the disorder and the status of the animal. Acquired hydrocephalus in the adult animal requires resolution of the inciting factor. Neoplasia is discussed in Chapter 15. An inflammatory disease may cause permanent reduction of absorptive capacity, and the hydrocephalus must be managed separately. Hydrocephalic cases usually are in one of the following three categories: (1) acute with rapidly progressive signs (in an animal that was previously normal or previously static), (2) chronic progressive deterioration, and (3) mild to severe static signs.

Acute progressive signs indicate a poor prognosis and the need for vigorous treatment. A ventricular tap should be done, and fluid should be allowed to flow under its own pressure with the animal in sternal recumbency and the head elevated slightly above the shoulders. Fluid should not be aspirated. An osmotic diuretic (mannitol, 1 g/kg) should be given slowly by intravenous drip to reduce cerebral edema. A corticosteroid (methylprednisolone, 30 mg/kg administered intravenously) and diuretic (furosemide) should be given to reduce CSF production and edema. The dose of mannitol should be repeated twice at 6-hour intervals. Methylprednisolone may be continued as for brain trauma (5 mg/kg/per hour administered intravenously). If the animal is stable, the glucocorticoid can be given in antiinflammatory doses. Anticonvulsants should be used if needed. If the animal survives and the neurologic status permits, the same long-term treatment should be provided as for chronic progressive cases.

Animals with chronic progressive deterioration of hydrocephalus, as indicated by the history and serial neurologic examinations, may be treated medically or surgically. Progression should be stopped, and some clinical improvement should be seen as a result of treatment. The owner must be made aware, however, that the animal will not be totally normal. If the neurologic status is too poor for the animal to function as a pet, treatment should not be continued. Medical treatment usually is tried first.[45] Dexamethasone, 0.25 mg/5 kg twice daily, or prednisone, 0.25 to 0.5 mg/kg twice daily, should be given orally concurrently with furosemide. Clinical improvement is expected within 3 days. If improvement is seen, the dosage should be reduced by half after

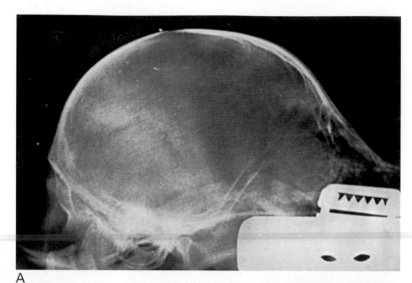

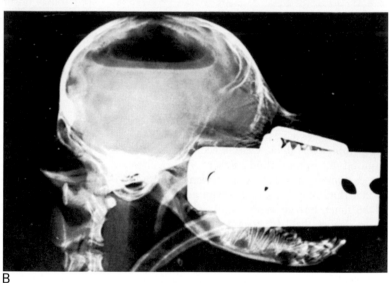

Figure 12-15 A, Radiograph of a hydrocephalic dog. Notice the "ground-glass" appearance of the calvaria, caused by a loss of the digital impressions because of chronic increased pressure. The fontanelle is open on the dorsum of the skull and the osseous tentorium is absent. **B,** Pneumoventriculogram of a dog with hydrocephalus.

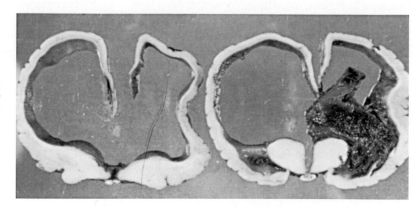

Figure 12-16 Severe hydrocephalus in a Chihuahua. Notice the thinning of the cerebral cortex. An intraventricular hematoma is present.

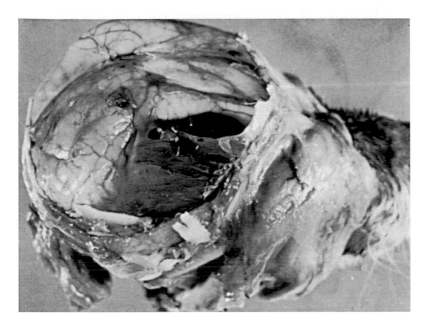

Figure 12-17 A dog with hydrocephalus and a large subdural hematoma that resulted when too much fluid was aspirated from the lateral ventricle. (From Oliver JE Jr, Knecht CD: Diseases of the brain. In Ettinger SJ, editor: *Textbook of veterinary internal medicine,* ed 1. Philadelphia, WD Saunders, 1975.)

1 week. After another week, glucocorticoids are given once every other day. If signs are stable, medication may be discontinued and repeated only as signs develop. Many animals stabilize in remission and only occasionally require medication. Others require continuous medication, in which case signs of Cushing's disease may appear. The objective of medical treatment is to provide remission of signs with the least possible amount of medication. Low dose, alternate-day therapy can be used for extended periods without problems.

Surgical treatment is reserved for animals that cannot be stabilized medically. Surgical treatment entails placement of a drainage tube from the lateral ventricle through a one-way valve to the right atrium or the peritoneal cavity. The major disadvantages of surgery are the expense and the postoperative complications. The complications include the necessity of replacing the tubing as the animal grows, occlusion of the tubes by fibrous tissue or clots, and sepsis. The shunts can be very effective and have functioned well in some dogs for up to 8 years.[18]

Other anomalies of the brain may cause alterations in mental status (see Table 12-5). Some are so grossly abnormal that they are not usually compatible with life, such as hydranencephaly and otocephaly. Others are more typically characterized by seizures and are discussed in Chapter 13.

Case Histories

The cases in this chapter have the common sign of alteration in mental status. After reading the history and the results of the examination, make a problem list, localize the lesion, list the rule-outs, formulate a plan for the diagnosis of each, and make a prognosis. Then read the assessment section and the results of the diagnostic procedures.

CASE HISTORY 12A

Signalment
Canine, boxer, female, 6 months old.

History
The dog was hit by a car 6 hours before examination and has remained unconscious since being injured.

Physical Examination
The dog is unconscious and in lateral recumbency. The temperature is 100.6° F, the pulse is 75 beats per minute, and the respirations are 25 per minute and shallow. The color of the membranes is good, and the capillary refill time is rapid. A small abrasion is on the muzzle on the left side. No fractures or luxations are palpable. Heart and lung sounds are normal.

Neurologic Examination
The dog is unconscious and does not respond to painful stimuli, except for showing withdrawal reflexes. All four limbs are in rigid extension. When the dog is forced to flex the limbs, resistance is considerable to a point, and then the limbs collapse. The postural reactions are absent. When the animal is moved into an erect position, the head and the neck arch dorsally. The myotatic reflexes cannot be evaluated because of the rigid extension of the limbs. Strong stimuli cause an increase in extension followed by a brief partial flexion that reverts to extension almost immediately. Tests for vision are negative. The pupils are small, symmetric, and slightly reactive. In a darkened room, they dilate only slightly (about 2 to 3 mm). Vestibular eye movements are absent. The globes are in the center of the palpebral fissure. The palpebral reflex is present but weak. No evidence of conscious perception of pain from a pinch of the face or a stimulation of the nasal mucosa is present. The gag reflex is present. The tongue retracts symmetrically, but no licking movements occur.

CASE HISTORY 12B

Signalment
Canine, Samoyed, male, 4 years old.

History
The dog has hip dysplasia but no other significant medical problems. At 8:00 AM the dog started walking aimlessly, bumping into walls and doors. Within 30 minutes the rear limbs began to abduct, and the dog fell. When the owner picked him up, he growled. At 9:00 AM the dog was examined by the referring veterinarian, who reported the following:

    Mental Status: The dog is depressed.

    Posture and Gait: The dog is unable to walk and falls to the right side.

    Postural Reactions: Very poor to absent in the right front and the right rear limbs; normal in the left front and the left rear limbs.

    Spinal Reflexes: Normal.

    Cranial Nerves: The menace reaction is poor bilaterally; otherwise, the reactions are normal.

    The dog was referred to our clinic at 6:00 PM, 10 hours after the onset of the signs.

Neurologic Examination
The dog is in a coma. The temperature is 105° F. Mild increased extensor tone of the limbs is noted. The postural reactions are absent. The spinal reflexes are normal. The menace reaction is absent. The pupils are widely dilated and unresponsive to light. The eyes are deviated ventrolaterally and do not respond to head movements. The palpebral reflex is present, but no behavioral response occurs to a pinch of the face or a touch of the nasal mucosa. A weak gag reflex and good retraction of the tongue are present.

CASE HISTORY 12C

Signalment
Canine, Chihuahua, male, 3 months old.

History
Lack of coordination and intermittent depression began at age 2 months. The dog has had no known illness, and his vaccinations have been given on schedule.

Physical Examination
The head is dome shaped with a large, persistent fontanelle. The only other abnormalities appear on the neurologic examination.

Neurologic Examination
The dog is depressed and confused. Loud noises produce a startle reaction, but the response is not oriented toward the sound. The dog can walk but is reluctant to do so. Once he starts walking, he progresses to a wall and then stands with his head against the wall. Some dysmetria and mild ataxia are present. The postural reactions are depressed in all four limbs and are worse in the pelvic limbs than in the thoracic limbs. The spinal reflexes are normal. No menace reaction is present, and the dog does not appear to be able to see. The visual placing reaction is absent, although the tactile placing reaction is present but slow. The pupillary reflexes are normal. The eyes appear deviated ventrolaterally, although vestibular eye movements are present in all directions. Other CNs are normal. Sensation is intact, although reactions to painful stimuli are slow and poorly directed.

ASSESSMENT 12A

The dog is in coma and exhibits decerebrate rigidity. Decerebrate rigidity is caused by loss of the voluntary UMN pathways with retention of the reticulospinal and vestibulospinal pathways, which are facilitatory to the extensor motor neurons. The loss of postural reactions confirms the absence of voluntary UMN pathways. The arching of the head and the neck is opisthotonos. The spinal reflexes are difficult to assess when the limbs are in extensor rigidity, but it is apparent that the extensor neurons are intact. The visual tests are negative in an unconscious animal because we depend on behavioral responses for our assessment. The pupillary reactions indicate that the oculomotor nerve is intact bilaterally. The small size of the pupil suggests a loss of sympathetic input or irritation of the oculomotor nerve. The symmetry suggests a loss of sympathetic tone. The absent eye movements indicate paralysis of CNs III, IV, and VI or a lesion of the medial longitudinal fasciculus (MLF) connecting those nuclei with the vestibular nucleus. Because the parasympathetic component of CN III is functional, a lesion of the MLF is more likely. Other CNs appear relatively normal, considering the level of consciousness.

Localization
The lesion is localized to the brainstem, caudal to CN III (midbrain), rostral to CN VII (rostral medulla), including the midline MLF and a large portion of the reticular activating system (coma). Therefore, it probably is a large intramedullary lesion of the pons.

Rule-outs
Trauma is known. An acute onset of coma without improvement for 6 hours suggests brainstem hemorrhage rather than tentorial herniation. The clinical signs are consistent with this hypothesis. Tentorial herniation usually affects CN III early. The signs indicate a lesion of the pons rather than the midbrain, which is compressed by tentorial herniation. No simple diagnostic tests can confirm intramedullary hemorrhage of the brainstem. The alternatives are to treat and observe for change or to use other tests to rule out epidural or subdural hemorrhage absolutely. Radiographs would demonstrate a skull fracture, but this finding probably would not alter the plan. MRI might show the parenchymal hemorrhage.

    Skull radiographs were taken, revealing a linear fracture extending across the floor of the cranial vault, a basilar fracture. Basilar fractures have been associated with severe brain lesions in cases we have seen.

Prognosis
Poor.

Plan
Treat medically (corticosteroids, mannitol, furosemide, intravenous fluids, nursing care) and observe for 48 hours.

Results
The dog's neurologic status did not change in 48 hours. The owners requested euthanasia. The brain is shown in Figure 12-5.

ASSESSMENT 12B

Localization
The lesion involves the brainstem. Dilated pupils (CN III) and coma (reticular activating system) indicate midbrain involvement. CNs V and VII are intact (palpebral reflex), indicating that the pons and the medulla (also CNs IX, X, XII) are intact.

The progression of signs from the cerebrum (pacing, blindness, postural reaction deficits) to the midbrain suggests tentorial herniation. The early signs were unilateral, indicating a left cerebral lesion with rapid progression to bilateral tentorial herniation.

Rule-outs
The sudden onset of severe signs usually indicates trauma or vascular lesions. The dog was in the house and had not been out since the night before, making trauma unlikely. Severe cerebral vascular lesions in dogs are unusual, but this hypothesis seems most likely. Vascular lesions may be associated with other pathologic conditions such as parasites or neoplasia.

Rule out (1) vascular lesion and (2) trauma.

Plan
Spontaneous epidural or subdural hemorrhages have not been reported in dogs. Parenchymal hemorrhages are not likely to be helped by surgery. These factors, plus the severity of the signs, made the prognosis very poor. The only useful diagnostic test is CT, but it was not available. The animal was given intensive medical treatment (mannitol, corticosteroids, fluids) and was monitored carefully until the next day. The temperature cycled frequently, varying from 101° to 107° F. No change occurred in the neurologic status after 18 hours, and the owner requested euthanasia.

Necropsy
The dog had an oligodendroglioma of the left cerebrum with a massive hemorrhage (see Figure 12-7).

ASSESSMENT 12C

The primary problems are depression, loss of vision, and postural reaction deficits with a reasonably normal gait. All these findings are compatible with forebrain lesions. Postural reaction deficits without significant gait deficits usually are caused by cerebral or diencephalic lesions. Loss of vision with intact pupillary light reflexes indicates that the pathways from the eye to the midbrain and CN III are intact, but bilateral damage exists to the lateral geniculate nucleus, the optic radiations, or the cerebral cortex. Intact vestibular eye movements indicate that the brainstem pathways (MLF) and CN III, IV, and VI are intact. The deviation of the eyes must have another cause. Depression is not localizing but is compatible with diffuse cerebral or diencephalic disease.

Localization
Cerebrum or diencephalon, diffuse.

Rule-outs
The clinical signs are slowly progressive, with an onset at an early age. Inflammation, neurodegenerative disease(s), metabolic disorders, chronic toxicity, and hydrocephalus should be considered. The inherited neurodegenerative diseases have not been reported in the Chihuahua, but hydrocephalus is commonly seen in this breed. The signs are usually cortical in origin. Blindness is frequent. The dog has a dome-shaped head with a persistent fontanelle, which is typical of congenital hydrocephalus. Many Chihuahuas have these skull changes without enlarged ventricles, however. The deviation of the eyes is seen in hydrocephalics because of the malformation of the bones of the orbit (see Figure 12-12). Hydrocephalus must be our first choice until the presence of another condition is proved.

Rule out (1) hydrocephalus, (2) inflammation, and (3) degenerative disease.

Plan
Skull radiographs will not reveal much more than we already can see and feel (shape and open fontanelle). An EEG may be useful but probably will not be absolutely diagnostic because the dog is immature, and we can expect high-voltage slow waves in a normal 3-month-old dog. The best diagnostic test is CT, but it was not available. The next most direct diagnostic test for hydrocephalus is a ventricular tap with a pneumoventriculogram if the tap is not diagnostic. The tap can be made through the lateral margin of the open fontanelle. If fluid is obtained with the needle inserted less than 2 cm, then the ventricles are enlarged. If there is doubt, 2 ml of air can be injected and a radiograph made to confirm the size of the ventricles. The CSF that is obtained can be analyzed. A cisterna magna tap is contraindicated because it may cause cerebral herniation if hydrocephalus is present. Degenerative diseases cannot be diagnosed except by biopsy or necropsy in most cases.

Prognosis
Guarded.

Plan
1. Rule out hydrocephalus: Ventricular tap, CSF analysis, pneumoventriculogram
2. Rule out inflammation: CSF analysis
3. Rule out degenerative diseases: Exclusion

Results
A ventricular tap was performed using general anesthesia. Fluid was obtained with the needle only 1 cm below the scalp. The owners refused treatment for the dog, and he was euthanized.

Many dogs with this degree of abnormality improve with treatment, however, vision may be permanently lost. If vision is present, the prognosis is much better.

Also review Case History E in Chapters 1, 2, and 4.

References

1. Cartlidge NEF: States of altered consciousness. In Swash M, Kennard C, editors: *Scientific basis of clinical neurology*. Edinburgh, 1985, Churchill Livingstone.
2. Hendricks JC, Morrison AR: Normal and abnormal sleep in mammals, *J Am Vet Med Assoc* 178:121-126, 1981.
3. Siegel J, Tomaszewski K, Nienhuis R: Behavioral states in the chronic medullary and midpontine cat, *Electroencephalogr Clin Neurophysiol* 63:274-288, 1986.
4. Kaitin KI, Kilduff TS, Dement WC: Evidence for excessive sleepiness in canine narcoleptics, *Electroencephalogr Clin Neurophysiol* 65:447-454, 1986.
5. Kornegay JN, Oliver JE Jr, Gorgacz EJ: Clinicopathologic features of brain herniation in animals, *J Am Vet Med Assoc* 182:1111-1116, 1983.
6. Milhorat TH: *Cerebrospinal fluid and the brain edemas*. New York, 1987, Neuroscience Society of New York.
7. Griffiths IR: Central nervous system trauma. In Oliver JE, Hoerlein BF, Mayhew IG, editors: *Veterinary neurology*. Philadelphia, 1987, WB Saunders.
8. Moore BR: Central nervous system trauma. In Robinson NE, editor: *Current therapy in equine medicine*, ed 3. Philadelphia, 1992, WB Saunders.
9. Syring R, Otto C, Drobatz K: Hyperglycemia in dogs and cats with head trauma: 122 cases (1997-1999), *J Am Vet Med Assoc* 218:1124-1129, 2001.

10. Shores A: Development of a coma scale for dogs: prognostic value in craniocerebral trauma. In *Proceedings of the Sixth Annual Veterinary Medical Forum,* Washington, DC, 1988, pp 251-253.

11. Shores A: Craniocerebral trauma. In Kirk RW, editor: *Current veterinary therapy X.* Philadelphia, 1989, WB Saunders.

12. Oliver JE: Neurologic emergencies in small animals, *Vet Clin North Am* 2:341-357, 1972.

13. Bracken MB, Shepard MJ, Collins WF, et al: A randomized, controlled trial of methylprednisolone or naloxone in the treatment of acute spinal cord injury, *N Engl J Med* 322:1405-1411, 1990.

14. Bracken MB, Shepard MJ, Collins WF, et al: Methylprednisolone or naloxone treatment after acute spinal cord injury: 1 year follow up data, *J Neurosurg* 76:23-31, 1992.

15. Olby N: Current concepts in the management of acute spinal cord injury, *J Vet Intern Med* 13:399-407, 1999.

16. Parker AJ: Blood pressure changes and lethality of mannitol infusion in dogs, *Am J Vet Res* 34:1523-1528, 1973.

17. Jandrey KE: Using mannitol to treat traumatic brain injuries, *Vet Med* August:717-725, 1999.

18. Oliver J, Hoerlein B: Cranial surgery. In Oliver JE, Hoerlein BF, Mayhew IG, editors: *Veterinary neurology.* Philadelphia, 1987, WB Saunders.

19. Joseph RJ, Greenlee PG, Carillo JM, et al: Canine cerebrovascular disease: clinical and pathologic findings in 17 cases, *J Am Anim Hosp Assoc* 24:569-576, 1988.

20. Fankhauser R, Luginbuhl H, McGrath JT: Cerebrovascular disease in various animal species, *Ann N Y Acad Sci* 127:817-860, 1965.

21. Detweiler DK, Ratcliffe HL, Luginbuhl H: The significance of naturally occurring coronary and cerebral arterial disease in animals, *Ann N Y Acad Sci* 127:868-881, 1968.

22. Zachary J, Patterson J, Rusley M: Neurologic manifestations of cerebrovascular atherosclerosis associated with primary hypothyroidism in a dog, *J Am Vet Med Assoc* 186:499-503, 1985.

23. Braund KG, Brewer BD, Mayhew IG: Inflammatory, infectious, immune, parasitic, and vascular diseases. In Oliver JE, Hoerlein BF, Mayhew IG, editors: *Veterinary neurology.* Philadelphia, 1987, WB Saunders.

24. Greene CE: Rocky Mountain spotted fever and ehrlichiosis. In Kirk RW, editor: *Current veterinary therapy IX.* Philadelphia, 1986, WB Saunders.

25. Morgan RV: *Handbook of small animal practice.* New York, 1988, Churchill Livingstone.

26. Patton CS, Garner FM: Cerebral infarction caused by heartworms (*Dirofilaria immitis*) in a dog, *J Am Vet Med Assoc* 5:600-605, 1970.

27. Segedy AK, Hayden DW: Cerebral vascular accident caused by *Dirofilaria immitis* in a dog, *J Am Anim Hosp Assoc* 14:752-756, 1978.

28. Bernstein N, Fiske R: Feline ischemic encephalopathy in a cat, *J Am Anim Hosp Assoc* 22:205-206, 1985.

29. de Lahunta A: Feline ischemic encephalopathy: a cerebral infarction syndrome. In Kirk RW, editor: *Current veterinary therapy VI.* Philadelphia, 1977, WB Saunders.

30. Williams KJ, Summers BA, de Lahunta A: Cerebrospinal cuterebriasis in cats and its association with feline ischemic encephalopathy, *Vet Pathol* 35:330-343, 1998.

31. Glass EN, Cornetta AM, deLahunta A, et al: Clinical and clinicopathological features in 11 cats with *Cuterebra* larvae myiasis of the central nervous system, *J Vet Intern Med* 12:365-368, 1998.

32. Rasmessen TB: Experimental ligation of the cerebral arteries of the dog. Thesis, University of Minnesota, St Paul, Minn, 1938.

33. Wimalaratna HSK, Capildeo R: Management of stroke: the place of steroids. In Capildeo R, editor: *Steroids in diseases of the central nervous system.* New York, 1989, John Wiley & Sons.

34. Kornegay JN, Mayhew IG: Metabolic, toxic, and nutritional diseases of the nervous system. In Oliver JE, Hoerlein BF, Mayhew IG, editors: *Veterinary neurology.* Philadelphia, 1987, WB Saunders.

35. Schall WD: Heat stroke. In Kirk RW, editor: *Current veterinary therapy VII.* Philadelphia, 1980, WB Saunders.

36. Schmidt Nielsen K, Bretz WL, Taylor CR: Panting in dogs: unidirectional air flow over evaporative surfaces, *Science* 169:1102-1104, 1970.

37. Mehta AC, Baker RN: Persistent neurological deficits in heat stroke, *Neurology* 20:336-340, 1970.

38. Krum SH, Osborne CA: Heat stroke in the dog: a polysystemic disorder, *J Am Vet Med Assoc* 170:531-535, 1977.

39. Osweiler GD, Carson TL, Buck WB, et al: *Clinical and diagnostic veterinary toxicology,* ed 3. Dubuque, Iowa, 1985, Kendall/Hunt Publishing Co.

40. Vaala WE: Peripartum asphyxia, *Vet Clin North Am Equine Pract* 10:187-205, 1994.

41. Braund KG: Degenerative and developmental diseases. In Oliver JE, Hoerlein BF, Mayhew IG, editors: *Veterinary neurology.* Philadelphia, 1987, WB Saunders.

42. Cox NR, Shores A, McCoy CP, et al: Obstructive hydrocephalus due to neoplasia in a Rottweiler puppy, *J Am Anim Hosp Assoc* 26:335-338, 1990.

43. Russell DS: *Observations on the pathology of hydrocephalus.* Medical Research Council Special Report No. 265. London, 1949, Her Majesty's Stationery Office.

44. Axthelm MK, Leipold HW, Phillips RM: Congenital internal hydrocephalus in polled Hereford cattle, *Vet Med Small Anim Clin* 76:567-570, 1981.

45. Simpson ST: Hydrocephalus. In Kirk RW, editor: *Current veterinary therapy X.* Philadelphia, 1989, WB Saunders.

46. Selby L, Hayes H, Becker S: Epizootiologic features of canine hydrocephalus, *Am J Vet Res* 40:411-413, 1979.

47. Wunschmann A, Oglesbee M: Periventricular changes associated with spontaneous canine hydrocephalus, *Vet Pathol* 38:67-73, 2001.

48. Hoerlein BF: *Canine neurology: diagnosis and treatment,* 3rd ed. Philadelphia, WB Saunders, 1978.

49. Dodman NH, Knowles KE, Shuster L, et al: Behavioral changes associated with suspected complex partial seizures in bull terriers, *J Am Vet Med Assoc* 208:688-691, 1996.

50. DeBowes RM, Gift L: Common malformations and congenital abnormalities of the central nervous system. In Robinson NE, editor*: Current therapy in equine medicine,* ed 3. Philadelphia, 1992, WB Saunders.

51. Mayhew IG: Problems in large animal neurologic patients. In *Large animal neurology.* Philadelphia, 1989, Lea & Febiger.

Chapter 13

Seizures, Narcolepsy, and Cataplexy

Epilepsy is a disorder of the brain that is characterized by recurring seizures. *Seizures, fits,* and *convulsions* are synonymous terms used to describe the manifestations of abnormal brain function that are characterized by paroxysmal stereotyped alterations in behavior. The term *convulsion* is reserved for seizures with a generalized motor component. *Narcolepsy* is a disorder of the brain that is marked by sudden recurring attacks of sleep. Narcolepsy is discussed at the end of this chapter. *Syncope* is transient loss of consciousness caused by ischemia of the brain. The most common cause in animals is cardiac arrhythmia. The history is usually indicative of syncope rather than seizures, but when in doubt careful auscultation of the heart and an electrocardiogram (ECG) may disclose the problem.

A seizure has several components. The actual seizure is called the *ictus.* Before the seizure (pre-ictally), a period of altered behavior may occur, called the *aura.* People with seizures report varying sensation, apprehension, and so forth during the aura. Animals may hide, appear nervous, or seek out their owners at this time. The ictus usually lasts for 1 to 2 minutes, but variation is considerable. After the seizure (*postictal phase*), the animal may return to normal in seconds to minutes or may be restless, lethargic, confused, disoriented, or blind for minutes to hours. The aura and the postictal phase do not have any relationship to the severity or the cause of the seizures.

The behavioral changes of seizures are composed of one or more of the following involuntary phenomena: (1) loss or derangement of consciousness or memory *(amnesia);* (2) alteration of muscle tone or movement; (3) alteration of sensation, including hallucinations of special senses (e.g., visual, auditory, olfactory); (4) disturbance of the autonomic nervous system (e.g., salivation, urination, defecation); and (5) other psychic manifestations, abnormal thought processes, or moods recognized as behavioral changes (e.g., fear, rage, tail-chasing).[1]

One or more of the aforementioned changes are present in a seizure. For example, loss of consciousness is usually associated with a generalized motor seizure but may not be a part of a seizure with behavioral manifestations. Behavioral or psychic changes are not necessarily seizure disorders; however, if the changes are paroxysmal, seizures are strongly considered. Seizures may occur in any animal, but they have been reported more frequently in the dog.

PATHOPHYSIOLOGY

Seizures are always a sign of abnormal forebrain function. The dysfunction may be from a primary lesion in the brain or secondary to a metabolic abnormality (e.g., hypoglycemia, toxicity).

Two main categories of seizures include those in which the seizure discharge originates in a circumscribed area of the brain and those in which the discharge appears to involve the two cerebral hemispheres bilaterally and synchronously from the start. Most of the information on the genesis of seizures is taken from models of focal and partial-onset epilepsy.

At the cellular level, seizures represent abnormal hypersynchronous discharges of cortical neurons.[2] An imbalance exists between excitatory and inhibitory mechanisms that favor the sudden onset of excitation. Several neurotransmitters play fundamental roles in the pathogenesis of seizures. Gamma-aminobutyric acid (GABA) and glutamate are the primary inhibitory and excitatory neurotransmitter agents. Multiple cellular receptors exist for each agent. Defective inhibition of GABA-$_A$ and GABA-$_B$ receptors may play fundamental roles in the pathogenesis of partial-onset epilepsy. In addition, defective activation of GABA neurons and defective intracellular buffering of calcium may play important roles.[2]

Increased excitability of neurons may follow defects in inhibition or result from conditions or factors that directly promote neuronal excitation. For instance, increased activation of N-methyl-D-aspartate (NMDA) receptors by glutamate, increased synchrony between neurons, and recurrent excitatory collaterals likely play important roles.[2] Glutamate activation of NMDA receptors may aid the development of the paroxysmal depolarizing shift (PDS), a fundamental reaction in seizure foci. Inherited epilepsy may involve changes in receptors for or metabolism of glutamate.[3]

Two components are recognized as the basis for focal seizure disorders: the seizure focus and the spread of the abnormal activity to other areas of the brain. The paroxysmal alterations in behavior are associated with synchronous excessive discharge in large aggregates of neurons: the seizure focus.[4] If the activity of the seizure focus spreads to other parts of the brain, a generalized cerebral dysrhythmia results, which produces the behavioral change that is recognized as a seizure (Figure 13-1).

Seizure foci apparently are present in many persons who do not have seizures. Some populations of neurons in the brain (e.g., the hippocampus) are much more likely to develop seizure activity than others. The seizure focus has been studied extensively in a variety of experimental models and in naturally occurring epilepsy. Neurons in seizure foci are characterized by large-amplitude, prolonged membrane depolarizations with associated high-frequency bursts of spikes: the PDS. These changes cause paroxysmal interictal spikes in the electroencephalogram (EEG).[5,6] The number of epileptic neurons correlates with the frequency of seizures.

Generalized seizures may also develop simultaneously in many areas of the brain. The two forms of generalized seizures are tonic-clonic convulsions and absence attacks. The latter types are rarely recognized in animals. Much of the research on generalized seizures has been done in the cat model of generalized penicillin-related seizures. Large doses of parenteral penicillin cause generalized spike-wave discharges on the EEG and behavioral unresponsiveness similar to absence attacks.[4] The cause of the diffuse cortical hyperexcitability is still not clear. Reduction of dendrite inhibition and potentiation of excitation mediated by glutamate and aspartate are suggested mechanisms.[2-4] Alteration of GABA inhibition is likely involved in the transition to generalized convulsions.

Seizures can be generated in any individual by pharmacologic, metabolic, or electrical changes; however, the threshold for stimulation varies widely. Normal individuals may require potent convulsant drugs (e.g., pentylenetetrazol) or electrical shock to exceed the threshold. A lower seizure threshold may allow production of convulsions by conditions such as fever and photic stimulation or minor alterations in body chemistry (e.g., hypoglycemia, hypocalcemia, hyperventilation).

Some individuals have seizures with no apparent stimulus. The range from normal individuals to those who have spontaneous seizures is a continuum without sharply defined boundaries. A lower threshold for seizures may be an inherited trait.

Studies indicate that the expression of individual seizures differs from the development of a lasting seizure-prone state.[7] Antagonists to NMDA

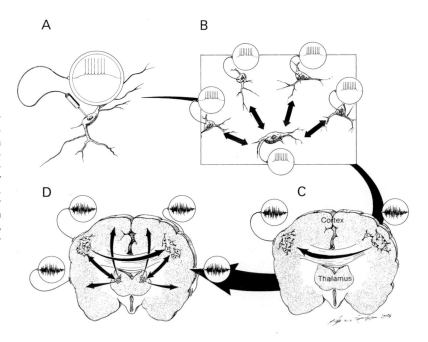

Figure 13-1 Spread of seizure activity from a focal area to the entire cerebrum. **A,** Paroxysmal depolarization shift in a neuron. **B,** Spread of activity to surrounding neurons. **C,** Propagation of seizure activity to other cortical areas by axonal conduction. **D,** Generalization of seizure activity through the diencephalon. (From Oliver JE, Hoerlein BF, Mayhew IG, editors: *Veterinary neurology*. Philadelphia, 1987, WB Saunders.)

prevented the progressive development of seizures but did not block previously induced seizure activity.

CLASSIFICATION

The classification of seizures based on clinical signs is helpful from a descriptive standpoint and may also be helpful in localization (Table 13-1).[8]

Gastaut[9] has proposed that generalized seizures be called *primary generalized epilepsy* if no cause can be ascertained and *secondary generalized epilepsy* if any organic cause can be found. Primary generalized epilepsy includes essential epilepsy, true epilepsy, idiopathic epilepsy, genetic epilepsy, and centrencephalic epilepsy. Partial or focal seizures are usually acquired, thus ruling out primary generalized epilepsy.[10]

Generalized Seizures

Tonic-clonic seizures (grand mal, major motor) are common in animals. The seizure frequently is preceded by an aura. The animal falls and becomes unconscious, the limbs are extended rigidly, opisthotonos is usual, and respiration stops *(apnea)*. The tonic phase is usually brief (10 to 30 seconds) and is rapidly followed by clonic limb movements in the form of running or paddling. Chewing movements of the mouth are common. Autonomic activity may start in the tonic or clonic phase of the ictus and may include pupillary dilation, salivation, urination, defecation, and piloerection. The clonic phase may alternate with tonic activity. The ictus usually lasts 1 to 2 minutes. The postictal phase may be a few minutes of rest followed by normal activity or may include confusion, disorientation, restlessness and pacing, and blindness lasting for minutes to hours.

Generalized tonic-clonic seizures in cats can be violent.[11] Cats may be propelled into the air, and self-inflicted trauma may occur (contusions, excoriations, avulsion of nails, and biting the tongue). Mild generalized seizures in cats are characterized by pupillary dilation, facial twitching, and, less frequently, salivation and urination.

Careful questioning of the owner is required to determine whether the episode described is actually a seizure. Owners frequently confuse syncope or acute vestibular syndromes with seizures. If the event is repetitive and has the same appearance each time, it is likely a seizure. Next the clinician needs to know whether the seizure starts as generalized, symmetric activity or if it has a focal component. The aura should not be confused with focal seizure activity. Any indication of focal motor activity preceding the generalized seizure, such as chewing, forced turning of the head, or clonic jerks of muscle groups, indicates a focal component, even if it generalizes secondarily. Primary generalized seizures cannot be localized anatomically.

Table 13-1 Classification of Seizures: Clinical Signs

Clinical Manifestation	EEG	Etiology	Anatomic Location
Generalized Seizures, Bilateral Symmetric Seizures, or Seizures Without Local Onset			
Primary generalized, tonic-clonic (grand mal, major motor)	Generalized dysrhythmia from onset, symmetric, often normal interictal unless they are activated or have organic or toxic origin	1. Genetic predisposition 2. Diffuse or multiple organic lesions 3. Toxic or metabolic	1. Unlocalized, multifocal 2. Diencephalic
Absences with or without motor phenomena (petit mal) rare or rarely recognized in animals	Generalized; 3 per second spike and wave dysrhythmia, symmetric (human)	Usually genetic predisposition (human)	1. Unlocalized, multifocal 2. Diencephalic
Partial Seizures or Seizures Beginning Locally			
Partial motor (may generalize to tonic-clonic seizure); signs depend on site of discharge	Focal dysrhythmia (spikes, slow waves), may generalize secondarily	Acquired organic lesion (see Tables 13-2 and 13-3)	Focal cortical or subcortical
Psychomotor (may generalize or appear as complex behavioral change: running, fear, aggression)	Dysrhythmia related to temporal lobe	Acquired organic lesion (see Tables 13-2 and 13-3)	Limbic system (hippocampus, temporal or pyriform lobe)

Modified from Oliver JE Jr: Seizure disorders in companion animals. *Compend Cont Educ Pract Vet* 2:77-86, 1980.

Whether the seizure focus is single or multiple, the generalized signs preclude localization.

Absences, or petit mal seizures, either are very uncommon in animals or, more likely, are not easily recognized. They are characterized by a brief (seconds) loss of contact with the environment that occurs without motor activity. Variations in humans include minor motor components such as facial twitching, loss of postural tone, and autonomic activity. Redding[12] reported one dog with absence attacks and characteristic EEG changes (4-Hz spike-wave complexes). Unless these attacks are frequent or the owner is very observant, they are usually not recognized.

Partial Seizures

Partial motor seizures (focal motor, Jacksonian) reflect the activity of a local seizure focus in an area producing motor activity. Movements are restricted to one part of the body, such as the face or one limb. Partial seizures frequently spread, resulting in a generalized convulsion. The focal component of the seizure onset is the key differential diagnosis feature. Because partial seizures are invariably acquired, primary generalized epilepsy is not considered in the differential diagnosis. The true Jacksonian seizure, which includes a focal onset followed by a slow progression of motor activity to adjacent structures, ultimately terminating in a generalized motor seizure, is rare in animals. The motor area of the cerebral cortex of domestic animals is small, allowing seizure activity to generalize rapidly. Patients with partial motor seizures are more likely to have focal EEG abnormalities in interictal periods than are those with generalized seizures. Partial sensory and autonomic seizures are not commonly recognized. Partial motor seizures are presumed to arise from a seizure focus near a primary motor area, usually the frontal cortex. In animals, partial motor seizures are indicative of a lesion in the contralateral cerebral hemisphere (e.g., a left thoracic limb seizure indicates a right cerebral cortex lesion).

Psychomotor seizures may have a predominance of autonomic signs.[1,9,10,13] Animals that have repetitive episodes of "fly biting" may be having focal sensory seizures in the visual cortex; however, psychomotor seizures with a sensory component are the generally accepted explanation.[14]

Psychomotor seizures (complex partial seizures, behavioral seizures) are paroxysmal episodes of abnormal behavior.[13-15] Examples include hysteria, rage, autonomic reactions such as salivation, and hallucinations such as fly biting. Visceral activity such as diarrhea, vomiting, and abdominal discomfort may correlate with lesions of the limbic system.[13] The most frequent locations are probably the hippocampus, the amygdala, and the temporal cortex. These areas commonly are involved in inflammatory diseases such as canine distemper and rabies and are damaged in tentorial herniation of any cause (see Chapters 12 and 15).

Complex partial seizures are recognized in several canine breeds and have been extensively studied in the bull terrier.[16] Behavioral changes such as compulsive tail chasing, rage, trances, preoccupations, fears, hyperactivity, sound sensitivities, and phobias have been described. EEG abnormalities include multiple epileptiform spikes characterized by high-amplitude, low-frequency discharges.

Many affected dogs have concurrent hydrocephalus demonstrated on computed tomography (CT) examination. Clinical signs develop at 6 to 13 months of age and occasionally in older dogs. No abnormalities in zinc, copper, and iron metabolism have been detected. The syndrome in bull terriers may reflect an inherited form of temporal lobe epilepsy similar in many respects to previously described cases of psychomotor epilepsy.

Complex partial seizures occur in cats.[11] They are characterized by lack of response to sensory stimuli and a trance-like state. Unilateral facial twitching, turning the head to one side, and repetitive movements of one limb have been reported. Bizarre behavior, such as inappropriate hissing, growling, and running blindly into objects, and compulsive behavior, such as self-chewing, biting, and circling, have been observed in association with facial twitching and salivation.

Differentiating psychomotor seizures from functional behavioral changes is difficult. Psychomotor seizures are usually preceded by an aura and followed by a postictal phase. The ictus is stereotyped and repetitive. Autonomic components of the ictus are common.

DISEASES

Seizures can be caused by any process that alters normal neuronal function. As with all neurologic diseases, the differential diagnosis is formulated in broad categories. The most likely diseases within each category then are considered. Tables 13-2 and 13-3 outline the major categories of diseases that are likely to produce seizures.

Idiopathic (Genetic)

Primary generalized epilepsy *(idiopathic)* has no demonstrable pathologic cause and may be inherited. Although it may occur in a number of species,[17] the most comprehensive studies have been those of humans and dogs.[17-25] Primary generalized epilepsy is rare in cats.[11]

Table 13-2 Causes of Seizure Disorders of Dogs and Cats*

Classification	Most Frequent Causes	Diagnostic Tests
Degenerative (15)	Storage diseases	Breed, biopsy
Anomalies (12)	Hydrocephalus	PE, CT, EEG, ventriculography
	Lissencephaly	Breed, PE, EEG
Idiopathic (13)	Genetic	Breed, age, history
	Unknown	Absence of other causes
Inflammation/ infectious (15)	Viral: canine distemper, rabies, FIP	History, PE, CSF analysis, CSF titers
	Bacterial: any type	
	Mycotic: cryptococcosis	
	Protozoal: toxoplasmosis, neosporosis	
	Rickettsial: RMSF, ehrlichiosis	
	Granulomatous meningoencephalitis	
	Immune meningoencephalitis	
	Nonsuppurative encephalitis (cats)	
	Aberrant parasites	
Metabolic (15)	Electrolyte: hypocalcemia	CBC, biochemical profile, UA, free bile
	Carbohydrate: hypoglycemia	acids, glucose-insulin pairs, hepatic biopsy
	Renal failure	
	Hepatic failure, portacaval shunt, microvascular dysplasia	
Neoplastic (15)	Primary: gliomas, meningiomas	NE, CT, MRI
	Metastatic	
Nutritional (15)	Thiamine deficiency	History, response to treatment
Toxic (15)	Heavy metal: lead	History, blood lead levels
	Organophosphates	History, NE, cholinesterase levels
	Chlorinated hydrocarbons	History, NE, PE
	Strychnine	
	Tetanus	
	Toad poisoning	
	5-hydroxytryptophan	
Traumatic (13)	Acute: immediately after head injury	History, PE, NE, CT, MRI
	Chronic: weeks to years after head injury	History, EEG, CT, MRI
Vascular (12, 13)	Infarctions	History, NE, CT
	Arrhythmias	Auscultation, ECG

Modified from Oliver JE Jr: Seizure disorders in companion animals, *Compend Cont Educ Pract Vet* 2:77-86, 1980.
*Numbers in parentheses refer to chapters in which disease classes are discussed.
CBC, Complete blood cell count; *CSF,* cerebrospinal fluid; *CT,* computed tomography; *ECG,* electrocardiogram; *EEG,* electroencephalography; *FIP,* feline infectious peritonitis; *MRI,* magnetic resonance imaging; *NE,* neurologic examination; *PE,* physical examination; *RMSF,* Rocky Mountain spotted fever; *UA,* urinalysis.

In animals, primary generalized epilepsy usually occurs in the form of generalized tonic-clonic seizures. Absence attacks are common in humans but are apparently rare in dogs.[23] Breeds of dogs known to have a genetic basis for epilepsy are listed in Table 13-4. Also listed are those breeds reported to have a high incidence of seizure disorders but for which genetic studies have not been documented. Whether these breeds have genetic epilepsy has not been proven. A study at the University of Pennsylvania, School of Veterinary Medicine, found no evidence of an increased incidence of epilepsy in any breed. The incidence of seizures in all breeds closely matched the frequency of admission to the hospital for all problems.[26] The diagnosis of primary generalized epilepsy does not prove inheritance. Only careful breeding studies can prove a genetic trait.

Inherited epilepsy also has been reported in Brown Swiss and Swedish Red cattle.[27] A hereditary syndrome characterized by recurrent seizures and the gradual development of cerebellar ataxia occurs in purebred and crossbred Aberdeen Angus cattle. The seizures start in young calves but decline in frequency in those that survive to approximately 15 months of age. Most cattle are clinically normal by 2 years of age. Pathologic changes have been found in the Purkinje cells of the cerebellum.[28]

The first seizure in a dog with primary generalized epilepsy usually occurs between the ages of 6 months and 5 years.[1] Early onset of seizures in

Table 13-3   **Causes of Seizure Disorders of Large Animals***

Classification	Most Frequent Causes	Diagnostic Tests
Degenerative (15)	Storage diseases (bovine, ovine)	Breed, biopsy
Anomalies (12)	Hydrocephalus	PE, CT, EEG
	Hydranencephaly	
Idiopathic (13)	Genetic (bovine)	Breed, age, history
	Unknown	Absence of other causes
Inflammation (15)	Viral: infectious bovine rhinotracheitis, pseudorabies (bovine, porcine), rabies (all), hog cholera, viral encephalomyelitis (equine)	History, species, PE, CSF analysis, titers
	Bacterial: thromboembolic meningoencephalitis (bovine), any type	
	Aberrant parasites (all)	
Metabolic (15)	Electrolyte: hypocalcemia, hypomagnesemia, water intoxication (porcine)	PE, CBC, biochemical profile, and UA
	Carbohydrate: hypoglycemia, ketosis, pregnancy toxemia (ovine)	
	Renal failure	
	Hepatic failure	
Neoplastic (15)	Primary: gliomas, meningiomas	NE, CSF, CT
	Metastatic	
Nutritional (15)	Thiamine (ruminants)	History, NE, response to treatment
Toxic (15)	Heavy metal: lead, arsenic	History, blood lead levels, tissue levels
	Organophosphates	History, NE, cholinesterase levels
	Chlorinated hydrocarbons	History, NE, tissue levels
	Strychnine	
	Tetanus	
Traumatic (13)	Acute: immediately after head injury	History, PE, NE
Vascular (12)	Infarction	History, NE
	Arrhythmias	Auscultation, ECG

*Numbers in parentheses refer to chapters in which disease classes are discussed.
CBC, Complete blood cell count; *CSF*, cerebrospinal fluid; *CT*, computed tomography; *ECG*, electrocardiogram; *EEG*, electroencephalography; *NE*, neurologic examination; *PE*, physical examination; *UA*, urinalysis.

Table 13-4   **Breeds with Primary Generalized Epilepsy**

Genetic Factor Proved or Highly Suspected
Beagle
Dachshund
German shepherd dog (Alsatian)
Horak's laboratory dog
Keeshond
Belgian tervuren
Aberdeen Angus cattle
Brown Swiss cattle
Swedish Red cattle

High Incidence of Seizure Disorders
Arabian foal
Boxer
Cocker spaniel
Collie
Golden retriever
Irish setter
Labrador retriever
Miniature schnauzer
Poodle
Saint Bernard
Siberian husky
Wire fox terrier

puppies conceived by breeding two epileptic Labrador retrievers has been described.[29] Three puppies of a litter of 10 had seizures beginning at 8 to 9 weeks of age. Eventually, five of eight surviving pups had seizures. In a large beagle colony, 29 dogs had their first seizure at a mean age of 30 months (range, 11 to 70 months).[19] Many dogs with abnormal EEGs did not have seizures by 6 years of age but may have been at risk of future seizures. An incidence of 1% to 2% is reported from two university teaching hospitals.[30,31]

The clinician can make a diagnosis of primary generalized seizures only by excluding other causes. No positive diagnostic findings can substantiate the diagnosis. The breed, the age, and the history may be highly suggestive, especially if a familial history of seizures exists (Tables 13-4 to 13-6). EEG abnormalities are not consistent.

Degenerative

Deficiencies in specific enzymes cause abnormal cellular metabolism with the accumulation of

Table 13-5 **Common Causes of Seizures at Different Ages**

Age/Disease Class	Cause
<1 Yr	
Degenerative	Storage diseases
Developmental	Hydrocephalus
Toxic	Heavy metals: lead, organophosphates, chlorinated hydrocarbons
Infectious	Canine distemper, encephalitis, other infectious diseases
Metabolic	Hypoglycemia: transient, enzyme deficiency, portacaval shunt, hepatic encephalopathy
Nutritional	Thiamine, parasitism
Traumatic	Acute
1-3 Yr	
Genetic	Primary generalized epilepsy (may start at approximately 6 mo)
	Others as above
>4 Yr	
Metabolic	Hypoglycemia: secondary to beta-cell tumor
	Hypocalcemia: hypoparathyroidism
	Hepatic encephalopathy: cirrhosis
Neoplastic	Primary or metastatic brain tumor
Vascular	Cardiovascular: arrhythmia, thromboembolism

Modified from Oliver JE Jr: Seizure disorders in companion animals, *Compend Cont Educ Pract Vet* 2:77-86, 1980.

Table 13-6 **Causes of Seizures by Breed Predisposition**

Breed	Cause
Alsatian (German shepherd dog)	Genetic
Beagle	Genetic
Belgian tervuren	Genetic
Boston terrier	Hydrocephalus, neoplasia
Boxer	Neoplasia
Cairn terrier	Globoid cell leukodystrophy
Chihuahua	Hydrocephalus
English setter	Lipodystrophy
German shepherd (Alsatian)	Genetic
German shorthaired pointer	Lipodystrophy
Irish setter	Genetic (suspected)
Keeshond	Genetic
Lhaso apso	Lissencephaly
Maltese	Portacaval shunts
Miniature pinscher	Hydrocephalus
Miniature schnauzer	Hyperlipoproteinemia, portacaval shunts
Pekingese	Hydrocephalus
Poodle, miniature and standard	Idiopathic
Poodle, toy	Hydrocephalus
Saint Bernard	Idiopathic
West Highland white terrier	Globoid cell leukodystrophy
Yorkshire terrier	Hydrocephalus, portacaval shunts

Modified from Oliver JE Jr: Seizure disorders in companion animals, *Compend Cont Educ Pract Vet* 2:77-86, 1980.

metabolic products within the neurons. These storage diseases may produce seizures as one part of the clinical syndrome (see Chapter 15).

Developmental

Disorders in this group may or may not be inherited but are distinguished from primary generalized (genetic) epilepsy by involving demonstrable pathologic changes in the brain. Hydrocephalus is the most common developmental disorder that causes seizures (see Chapter 12). Other developmental defects that may produce convulsions are lissencephaly and porencephaly (see Tables 13-5 and 13-6).

Lissencephaly is a congenital absence of the convolutions of the cerebral cortex.[32,33] It has been reported in lhasa apso dogs, wire fox terriers, and Irish setters, and in one cat. Affected animals may have behavioral, visual, and slight proprioceptive deficits in addition to seizures.

Porencephaly is a cystic malformation of the cerebrum that usually communicates with the lateral ventricle or the subarachnoid space. It may be congenital or acquired (degenerative).

Inflammatory/Infectious

Any inflammatory or infectious disease has the potential to cause seizures if it invades the forebrain. The most prevalent diseases are listed in Tables 13-2 and 13-3. Canine distemper virus is probably the most common infectious cause of seizures in dogs. Seizures may appear without any noticeable clinical illness or may occur long after a clinical illness has been resolved.

Granulomatous meningoencephalomyelitis (GME) is a common inflammatory cause of seizures in dogs. A nonsuppurative meningoencephalomyelitis was reported as a common cause of seizures in cats from Canada.[11] The diagnosis of inflammatory central nervous system (CNS) disease requires cerebrospinal fluid (CSF) examination, CSF serology, advanced imaging, and in some cases EEG. Inflammatory or infectious diseases are discussed in Chapter 15.

Metabolic

Failure of one of the major organs or of the endocrine glands may produce alterations in the electrolytes or glucose or the accumulation of toxic products, which results in seizures (see Tables 13-2, 13-3, and 13-5).[34] Hypoglycemic syndromes and hepatoencephalopathy are the most common diseases in this category. Some animals have a lower seizure threshold. Relatively minor alterations may cause seizures in these instances. The major metabolic disorders are discussed in Chapter 15.

Neoplastic

Intracranial neoplasia, either primary or metastatic, can cause seizures. The seizure activity is caused by an abnormality in neurons adjacent to the neoplasm that are compressed or distorted or that have an insufficient blood supply. Brain tumors are not electrically active.

Seizures may be the first sign of brain tumor. A neurologic deficit may not be apparent until weeks to months after the onset of seizures, especially if the mass is in the cerebral cortex. Neoplasia as a cause of seizures is relatively common in dogs and cats older than 5 years of age, and the incidence increases as animals age. Older animals with a sudden onset of seizures should be considered to have a tumor until proved otherwise. CT and magnetic resonance imaging (MRI) are the diagnostic procedures of choice. Neoplasia is discussed in Chapter 15.

Nutritional

Seizures may be the terminal manifestation of a number of nutritional disorders. The B complex vitamins are most frequently incriminated. Thiamine deficiency causes polioencephalomalacia in ruminants, which is discussed in Chapter 15. Thiamine deficiency in dogs and cats causes hemorrhage and necrosis in the brainstem.

Animals that are fed most commercial rations do not develop thiamine deficiencies. Dogs that are fed only cooked meat develop paraparesis that progresses to convulsions. Early treatment with thiamine reverses the clinical progression of the disease. Thiamine deficiency in cats has been attributed to fish-based cat foods that contain thiaminase. Supplementation with thiamine eliminates the problem. Cats typically have a seizure syndrome that is characterized by ventroflexion of the head, ataxia, behavioral changes, dilated pupils, and eventually coma. Because thiamine toxicity is unlikely, giving thiamine to cats with seizures is the best treatment. A dose of 50 to 100 mg is given intravenously the first day; thereafter, daily intramuscular injections are given until a response is obtained or another diagnosis is established.[1]

Toxic

Many toxins affect the CNS, and most can cause seizures. The diagnosis usually depends on the history, identification of the toxic substance from analysis of body tissues or intestinal contents, and the response to treatment.

Lead poisoning is a frequent intoxication in animals. Other clinical signs may include depression, tremor, and ataxia, which sometimes are associated with gastrointestinal signs. Seizures are often associated with behavioral signs. Peripheral blood changes may include nucleated erythrocytes (red blood cells [RBCs]) and basophilic stippling of RBCs without anemia. The changes in the RBCs are transient and may not be present in chronic lead poisoning. Blood lead determination is diagnostic. Calcium ethylenediamine tetraacetic acid (CaEDTA) is used in treatment.[35]

Strychnine causes a tonic seizure that is exacerbated by stimulation. The animal remains conscious unless respiration stops. Strychnine blocks inhibitory interneurons in the spinal cord, causing a release of motor neuron activity.

Organophosphate and chlorinated hydrocarbon insecticides are a common cause of seizures.

Seizures induced by the toxin produced by the *Bufo marinus* toad have been reported.[36] Although several species of *Bufo* toads exist worldwide, most reports in the United States are from southern Florida, Colorado, Arizona, Texas, and Hawaii. The incidence was highest during warm months of the year. In addition to seizures, neurologic signs include stupor, ataxia, nystagmus, extensor rigidity, and opisthotonos. Hyperemic oral mucous membranes and ptyalism are common findings. The toxin is released from the toad's parotid glands and is readily absorbed through the oral mucosa. Intoxication may be fatal. The oral cavity should be lavaged with tap water. Diazepam is used to control seizures and extensor rigidity. Intravenous fluids and diuretics are given to promote urinary excretion of the toxin. Overall mortality is low in animals treated within a few hours of intoxication.

In dogs, 5-hydroxytryptophan toxicosis has been reported as a cause of seizures.[37] It is a precursor to serotonin, a common CNS neurotransmitter. The signs in dogs are similar to the "serotonin syndrome" as described in humans. In addition to seizures, neurologic signs include depression, tremors, hyperesthesia, transient blindness, and ataxia. Gastrointestinal signs include vomiting, diarrhea, ptyalism, and abdominal pain Hyperthermia is also a common finding. Signs develop within minutes to hours following accidental ingestion of dietary supplements containing the agent. Most dogs develop signs within 1 hour. Treatment includes decontamination (induction of emesis, gastric lavage, and oral administration of activated charcoal), fluid therapy, thermoregulation, and parenteral administration of anticonvulsant agents (diazepam or phenobarbital). The serotonin antagonist cyproheptadine may be useful as adjunct therapy. A dose of 1.1 mg/kg administered orally or rectally every 1 to 4 hours is suggested.[37]

Toxic disorders are discussed in Chapter 15.

Traumatic

Seizures may be seen immediately after acute head trauma as the result of direct neuronal injury. Posttraumatic seizures may occur many weeks to several years after a head injury. Posttraumatic epilepsy may be focal or generalized, depending on the location of the brain lesion. The focus develops secondary to a scar in the brain at the site of the initial injury. The focal abnormality may be recognized on EEG. The diagnosis is based on the correlation of historical information with the development of seizures and the elimination of other causes. Treatment is directed at controlling the seizures.

PLANS FOR DIAGNOSIS AND MANAGEMENT OF SEIZURE DISORDERS

Most animals with seizures have a similar history of episodic convulsions. Therefore a protocol for diagnosis and a plan for management and treatment that includes a defined database are useful.[8,38]

Database

The recommended database is formulated at two levels to rule out the two major groups of problems causing seizures: (1) extracranial abnormalities

such as metabolic, toxic, and nutritional problems; and (2) intracranial diseases such as encephalitis, brain tumors, anomalies, degenerative diseases, and traumatic injuries. Idiopathic or primary generalized epilepsy is assumed from the history, signalment, and exclusion of other causes (Table 13-7). The minimum database can be obtained at any veterinary clinic with an access to pathology services. The specific serum chemistry analyses can be modified to fit those available in an automated service. The only expense other than the initial examination is the cost of laboratory studies. The risk to the patient is minimal.

The minimum database screens for primary neurologic disease (neurologic examination) and

Table 13-7 Database for Seizure Disorders

Minimum Database
Patient profile
  Species, breed, age, sex
History
  Immunizations: kind, dates, by whom
  Environment
  Age at onset
  Frequency, course
  Description of seizure: general or partial, duration, aura, postictus, time of day, relation to exercise, food, sleep, or stimuli
  Previous or present illness or injury
  Behavioral changes
Physical examination
  Complete examination of systems, including specifically:
    Musculoskeletal: Size, shape of skull, evidence of trauma, atrophy of any muscles
    Cardiovascular: Color of mucous membranes, evidence of arrhythmias, murmurs
    Funduscopic examination
Neurologic examination
  Complete examination: Note time of last seizure; if it was within 24-48 hr and neurologic examination is abnormal, repeat in 24 hr
Clinical pathology
  CBC
  Urinalysis
  BUN, ALT, ALP, calcium, fasting blood glucose levels (GGT, SDH in large animals), free bile acids
  Others as indicated (e.g., blood lead level, Coggin's test)

Complete Database
Computed tomography or magnetic resonance imaging
CSF analysis: Cell count, total and differential; protein levels; pressure
Skull radiographs: Ventrodorsal, lateral, frontal
EEG

ALP, Alkaline phosphatase; *ALT,* serum alanine transaminase; *BUN,* serum urea nitrogen; *CBC,* complete blood cell count; *CSF,* cerebrospinal fluid; *EEG,* electroencephalogram; *GGT,* γ-glutamyltransferase; *SDH,* sorbitol dehydrogenase.

metabolic or systemic disorders (physical examination, laboratory examination).

The more complete database includes CSF analysis, CT, MRI, and EEG (see Table 13-7). CSF analysis can be performed at most clinics. EEG, CT, and MRI usually are not available except at referral centers. CT is available to many veterinarians through local hospitals or mobile units. CT and MRI are the best tests for the detection of organic brain lesions such as neoplasia and infarcts. These tests are performed when the minimum database indicates the presence of neurologic disease, when an older animal experiences a sudden onset of seizures, or if the seizures have not been controlled with medication. These procedures are not recommended as a part of the minimum database in dogs younger than 5 years of age because of the low yield in animals with normal findings, the increased risk of required anesthesia, and the increased cost to the client.

Because cats most commonly have secondary epilepsy, CSF examination and CT or MR imaging are important in determining the cause of seizures in this species. The most common causes of seizures in cats are organic brain diseases such as nonsuppurative meningoencephalitis, feline ischemic encephalopathy, and neoplasia.[11]

In large part, CT and MR imaging have replaced the various contrast-enhanced procedures for evaluating structural alterations in the brain. Arteriography and ventriculography are no longer used because of the risk and poor diagnostic results. Ventriculography may be helpful in the diagnosis of hydrocephalus. CT is helpful. Ultrasonography can be used in animals with persistent fontanelles.[39]

Plan for Management

A minimum database should be completed for every patient that has more than one seizure. Patients that have had only one isolated seizure should be given thorough physical and neurologic examinations. If no abnormalities are found, the owners should be advised to watch for further seizures.

Information from the minimum database yields one of three findings: (1) a definitive diagnosis, (2) a possible cause of the seizures that requires further tests to confirm, or (3) no suggestion of the cause (Figure 13-2).

Seizures occur episodically; therefore, the veterinarian frequently must evaluate an animal without ever seeing the convulsion. The history must be taken carefully and must include a complete description of the seizures and their frequency, duration, and severity. The first goal is to determine that the animal is having convulsions. For example, transient vestibular dysfunction and drug reactions may resemble seizures. The most frequent problem to be confused with seizures is *syncope* (transient loss of consciousness). Syncope is caused by a loss of the blood supply to the brain or hypoglycemia. Cardiac arrhythmia is the most common cause. Acute vestibular episodes may also be mistaken for seizures. Vestibular disease usually causes other deficits, such as a head tilt or ataxia. We encourage all owners to videotape the episodes for our review. This greatly aids in the diagnosis and treatment of seizures, especially those that include complex behavioral signs.

The history also provides information related to the onset and the progression of the disease (see Figure 13-2). Seizures, by definition, are acute in onset; however, the owner may be able to recognize a chronic progression of signs, with seizures being only one component. The diagnostic tests that are most likely to be useful in each disease are listed in Tables 13-2 and 13-3. The minimum database rules out most metabolic diseases. Other diseases may or may not be suggested by the minimum database.

Positive findings include evidence of a metabolic or toxic disease or an abnormal neurologic examination indicating CNS disease. Suggestive findings include some indication of metabolic abnormality that may require further tests. For example, serum albumin and urea nitrogen levels may be low, suggesting liver disease. In the absence of positive or suggestive findings in the minimum database, the animal should be treated with anticonvulsants. Generally, we recommend anticonvulsant therapy in dogs and cats when single seizures occur more than once every 6 weeks and when cluster seizures occur.

Failure to control the seizures after adequate therapy (see Plans for Treatment) warrants a complete database to rule out neurologic disease. Any change in neurologic signs also indicates a complete evaluation. Dogs older than 5 years of age or cats of any age most likely have an acquired disease. Brain tumors must be high on the list of rule-outs in all older animals, even when no neurologic signs are present. The safest and most accurate method of diagnosis is CT or MRI. Therefore, we recommend a scan for all these animals. If the findings are negative, CSF analysis and EEG should be done (see Table 13-7).

Some breeds have primary generalized epilepsy that is difficult to control. The most common examples are German shepherd dogs, Saint Bernards, Labrador retrievers, and Irish setters.[1,10] Negative findings on the complete database for an animal that has been poorly controlled with adequate anticonvulsant medication suggest a poor prognosis.

Minimum Database

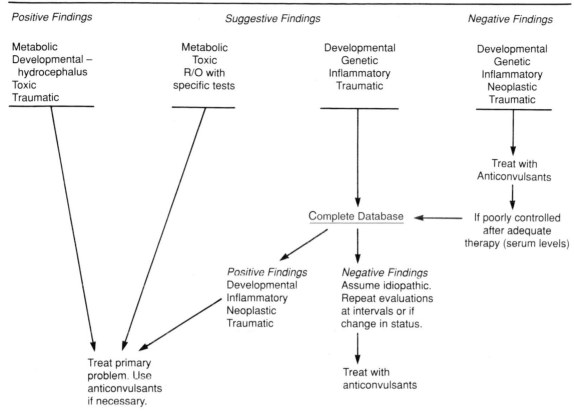

Figure 13-2 Plan for the diagnosis and management of seizures. Positive findings confirm the diagnosis, negative findings eliminate the diagnosis. *R/O*, Rule out. (Modified from Oliver JE Jr: Protocol for diagnosis of seizure disorders in companion animals, *J Am Vet Med Assoc* 172:824, 1978.)

The treatment can be altered by changing the dosage or the drugs, by combining drugs, or by changing the schedule of administration. Periodic reevaluation may reveal a progressive disease that was missed originally.

Plans for Treatment

Successful treatment depends heavily on client education and cooperation. Treatment failures are usually the result of (1) progressive disease, (2) refractory epilepsy, or (3) inadequate client education or poor client compliance leading to subtherapeutic drug concentrations. Clients need to understand the importance of therapeutic drug monitoring to successful seizure management. A progressive disease is identified by repeated examinations. Refractory epilepsy is expected in the breeds that have been listed previously.

The client should understand that successful treatment may be manifested by (1) a reduction in the frequency of seizures, (2) a reduction in the duration of seizures, or (3) a reduction in the severity of seizures. Although complete elimination of seizures is certainly a goal, it is not a realistic expectation for most animals.

The client should be given the following basic rules for treating epileptic animals:

1. Do not judge the efficacy of the medication for at least 2 weeks. Give the medication a chance.
2. Do not change or discontinue the medication suddenly. Status epilepticus (SE) may follow.
3. Phenothiazine tranquilizers are *contraindicated* in epileptics because they lower the threshold for seizure activity.
4. Allow for changes in the animal's environment (e.g., give more medication when increased excitement is expected).
5. Medication may be required for life. Do not decrease dosages rapidly or too soon after seizure control is achieved.
6. No single drug or combination works in all cases. Adjustments in the dosage, the schedule, or the combination of drugs probably will be required. Finding the right combination usually

occurs by trial and error, but monitoring therapeutic serum levels helps to eliminate the guesswork.

7. Good seizure control is more difficult to achieve in certain large-breed dogs.
8. The severity of seizure disorder in cats is not a good predictor of outcome.

We usually do not recommend treatment for animals that have had only one seizure. Knowing the frequency and severity of the seizures is useful in assessing the response to treatment. We usually do not treat animals while we are establishing a diagnosis unless the seizures are frequent or severe or occur in clusters.

We do recommend treating seizures if they are recurrent or intense, especially if they tend to cluster. Our general guidelines are to treat all animals that experience single seizures more frequently than once every 6 weeks. Dogs, especially large-breed dogs, with cluster seizures are at increased risk for developing SE, and we usually initiate anticonvulsant therapy in these cases. Owners should be advised that each time a seizure discharge spreads, it increases the probability that it will spread again. This phenomenon is called *kindling* and can be suppressed with appropriate anticonvulsant therapy.

The final decision about treatment must be made by the client. In essence, if the client feels that the seizures are more of a problem than is giving the medication, treatment is in order.

Antiepileptic Drug Therapy

The strategies of antiepileptic drug therapy have been described by Podell.[40] These strategies include:

1. Modulate membrane action of GABA
2. Reduce excitatory transmission
3. Modulate membrane cation conductance.

Most of the commonly used anticonvulsant agents (phenobarbital, potassium bromide, and diazepam) increase GABA-activated Cl^- conductance, which enhances the inhibitory action of GABA. Several new anticonvulsant agents used in people act to modulate sodium or calcium channels or reduce glutamate-mediated excitation.[40] The ideal anticonvulsant should suppress seizures completely without side effects or toxicity and be reasonable in cost because life-long therapy is usually required. Unfortunately, such a drug is not known.

Phenobarbital

Phenobarbital is the initial drug of choice for treating seizures in dogs and cats.[41-44] In large-breed dogs, some clinicians prefer to initiate treatment with potassium bromide. Phenobarbital is effective, inexpensive, and convenient for administration. The usual starting dosage is 2.5 mg/kg orally twice daily. Some dogs require 5 mg/kg orally twice a day to achieve therapeutic blood levels. Absorption and excretion differ considerably between individuals, and this is especially important in cats. The lower dosage is used if seizures are infrequent and occur as single episodes. Higher dosages are recommended if seizures are frequent or tend to cluster. The dosage is adjusted according to seizure control, side effects, and serum concentrations.

Sedation may occur but usually disappears in the first week. Polyphagia, polydipsia, and polyuria may be seen in some patients. Hepatotoxicity occurs in a small number of cases, but it is less frequent than with most other anticonvulsants.[45]

The peak concentrations of phenobarbital occur 2 to 3 hours after oral administration, and the lowest (trough) concentrations occur just before the next dose. Generally, phenobarbital reaches steady-state concentrations in 2 weeks. Assessing trough concentrations of phenobarbital once every 2 to 3 weeks until serum concentrations are in the therapeutic range of 15 to 45 µg/ml is considered ideal for therapeutic drug monitoring.[41-43] Recent studies indicate, however, that timing may not be clinically important. In a study of 33 epileptic dogs treated with twice-daily phenobarbital, 91% of all samples taken at 0 (trough), 3, and 6 hours post treatment were within the therapeutic range.[46] Many dogs need levels near the high end to achieve control. Generally, we try to maintain serum concentrations in the range of 20 to 40 µg/ml. Dosages as high as 10 to 20 mg/kg per day may be needed in some dogs to maintain these therapeutic blood levels. The response to treatment is more important than the blood level, but monitoring serum levels of phenobarbital may help to determine the cause of inadequate seizure control. Monitoring for evidence of hepatotoxicity or other side effects is strongly encouraged. Routine blood counts and serum chemistries are usually recommended at 6-month intervals; however, a report on monitoring of human epileptics indicates that this grants little benefit, except in high-risk patients.[47] High-risk groups include those with known or presumed biochemical disorders, adverse drug reaction histories, or neurodegenerative diseases.

Side Effects. Hepatotoxicity occurs in a small number of dogs treated with phenobarbital.[45] Whether this represents a direct dose-dependent hepatotoxicity or an idiosyncratic drug reaction is still debated among clinicians; however, dogs with serum concentrations above the therapeutic range (>45 µg/ml) are at greatest risk. Several studies in normal and epileptic dogs document that phenobarbital induces hepatic enzyme production in the absence of liver failure.[48,49] When serum levels were maintained in the range of 20 to 40 μg/ml, both alkaline phosphatase (ALP) and alanine aminotransferase (ALT) were increased following 29 weeks of treatment at 5 mg/kg every 12 hours. Concentrations of ALP may be above the normal reference range, whereas ALT levels are usually in the high normal range. Gamma-glutamyl transferase (GGT) may be transiently increased. Aspartate transaminase (AST), free bile acids (fBA), and bilirubin are not affected. Moderate hepatomegaly may be detected on abdominal radiographs, but hepatic ultrasonography is usually normal. Hepatic enzymes return to normal within 6 to 8 weeks following discontinuation of phenobarbital treatment.[49] Hepatic enzyme induction must be considered when dogs are monitored for hepatotoxicity. The presence of bilirubinuria, bilirubinemia, hypoalbuminemia, and increased concentrations of free bile acids are the best indicators of possible hepatotoxicity. Serum ALT concentrations that are consistently above normal ranges are also indicators of possible hepatotoxicity.

Life-threatening neutropenia and thrombocytopenia have been reported in dogs treated with phenobarbital.[50] Clinical signs resolved when the drug was discontinued. Although the exact mechanism is unknown, it is speculated that phenobarbital most likely induces an immune-mediated reaction directed at cells in circulation rather than suppression of hematopoiesis in the bone marrow.[50]

Several studies have demonstrated the effects of long-term phenobarbital treatment on the thyroid and adrenal axis of normal and epileptic dogs.[48-52] Both serum thyroxine (T_4) and free thyroxine (fT_4) are decreased compared with non-treated dogs. Up to 40% of treated dogs have T_4 concentrations below the normal range. Canine thyroid-stimulating hormone (cTSH) concentrations were either not affected or only mildly increased. Serum triiodothyronine (T_3) concentrations were not affected. Phenobarbital may increase hepatic thyroxine metabolism, decrease thyroxine synthesis and secretion, and alter thyroxine protein binding. The effect is dose related because dogs with phenobarbital levels below 15 μg/ml developed few or no changes in T_4 of fT_4 concentrations. Whereas phenobarbital alters dexamethasone suppression testing in humans, studies in dogs generally show little or no effect on adrenal function tests.[48]

Animals that cannot be controlled with adequate levels of phenobarbital may be given combination therapy. It is most commonly combined with potassium bromide in dogs and benzodiazepines in cats. Phenobarbital is continued while other drugs are added to the regimen. Guidelines for use of the few alternative drugs available are not clearly documented by controlled trials in most cases. Because these drugs are not approved for use in animals, owner consent should be obtained.

Potassium Bromide

Potassium bromide (KBr) is a safe and effective anticonvulsant in dogs. It is the first-choice alternate therapy for phenobarbital and is commonly used as the initial anticonvulsant in large-breed dogs.[53-56] Like phenobarbital, it enhances the activity of GABA. KBr was the principal anticonvulsant for humans in the late 1800s until phenobarbital was introduced in the early 1900s. The therapeutic range is not far from the level that produces toxic side effects, such as skin eruptions, sedation, and weakness. These problems rarely have been seen in animals, despite the increased use of KBr. The initial dosage of KBr is 20 to 40 mg/kg per day.[53-56] Chemical-grade KBr can be used in capsules or dissolved in water (100 to 500 mg/ml), which is mixed with food. KBr is slow to reach steady state and has a long half-life (Table 13-8). Higher levels of chloride in the diet, especially one that promotes urolith dissolution, increase the rate of renal excretion of bromide.[55] Bromide toxicity has been reported in an epileptic dog with renal insufficiency.[57] Two to 3 weeks are required to reach therapeutic levels. Steady state is reached in about 4 months.

The KBr levels in the serum should be determined 30 and 120 days after initiating therapy. Therapeutic trough concentrations are 0.8 to 3.0 mg/ml (880 to 3000 μg/ml).[56,58] The time to reach steady-state concentrations can be decreased by giving loading doses of KBr. The loading dose ranges from 450 to 600 mg/kg for a target serum level of 1.0 to 1.5 mg/ml. The loading dose is divided into equal doses given once a day for 5 days. On day 6, serum bromide levels are measured. Smaller loading doses can be continued for 5 days if the KBr concentration is less than 1 mg/ml. Drug concentrations are again assessed.[58] If in the therapeutic range, maintenance doses are administered, and KBr levels are reassessed in 1 month. KBr combined with phenobarbital has controlled seizures in dogs refractory to phenobarbital alone or to other anticonvulsant therapies.[54,56,58] Serum phenobarbital levels should also be monitored every 6 months and the dosage reduced by 25% if toxic levels are found. When combined with phenobarbital, KBr serum levels of 810 to 2400 μg/ml and serum phenobarbital levels of 9 to 36 μg/ml reduced seizures by 50% or greater in 72% of treated dogs. Forty-five percent

Table 13-8　**Anticonvulsant Drugs for Dogs and Cats**

Drug	Dosage (mg/kg)	Therapeutic Serum Concentration (μg/ml)	Half-Life (H ± Se)	Time to Steady State (D)
Phenobarbital[*]	1.5-5 q12h	20-45	70 ± 16	10-18
Potassium bromide[*]	20-60 q24h or divided	1000-1500	25 (days)	4 (mo)
Diazepam (cats)	0.5-1 q12h	200-500 (ng/ml)	1.5-2	
Clonazepam[*]	0.02-0.5 q12h	0.02-0.08	1.4 ± 0.3	
Valproic acid[*]	60 q8h	40-100	1.7 ± 0.4	6-10
Primidone[*]	10-15 q8h (dog)	5-15 (human)	9-12	6-8
Chlorazepate[*40]	2-4 q12h	20-75 μg/L	5-6	1-2
Felbamate[*40]	20 q8h	30-100 mg/L	5-6	1-2
Gabapentin[*40]	30-60 q8-12h	4-16 mg/L	2-4	1
Topiramate[40] (human)	5-10 q12h	2-25 mg/L	12-30	3-4
Zonisamide[*40]	4-8 q12h	ND	15-20	3-4
Levetiracetam[40] (human)	500-4000 mg/day	ND	7-10	2-3

[*]Data for dogs.
q, Every.

of these dogs had no seizures with phenobarbital concentrations below 20 μg/ml.[59]

Benzodiazepines

Diazepam is the most commonly used drug in this class. It is used in the treatment of SE, cluster seizures, and toxic seizures and may be used as an add-on drug in the long-term treatment of epilepsy. The benzodiazepines enhance the activity of GABA. Diazepam has a quick onset of action when given parenterally to both dogs and cats. In the dog, the duration of action is very short, and tolerance can rapidly develop, making it less useful for long-term management of epilepsy in this species. Diazepam has a longer half-life in cats, and tolerance is not common in this species, making it a more effective drug for long-term management of feline epilepsy. In the cat, dosages of 0.5 to 1.0 mg/kg three times daily are effective.[58] Phenobarbital and diazepam are the only anticonvulsants we recommend for cats, although some neurologists report satisfactory results with KBr (Table 13-9). Diazepam can be hepatotoxic, especially in cats.

Clorazepate can be used for monotherapy, but it is most commonly combined with phenobarbital for long-term seizure control in dogs and cats. The dosage is 2.0 to 4.0 mg/kg every 12 hours. Clorazepate may increase phenobarbital concentrations in the serum, usually within 1 month after initiating therapy.[40,58]

Clonazepam, a longer-acting benzodiazepine, is effective for short-term control of refractory seizures. The beneficial effect seems to last for only a few months. Hepatotoxicity can be a problem in dogs receiving clonazepam for longer than a few months. Currently, we use it during the time

that KBr is reaching therapeutic effect (1 to 3 months), and then we stop it. The dosage is 0.5 mg/kg twice daily.

Primidone

Primidone is largely metabolized to phenobarbital, and a small portion is metabolized to phenylethylmalonamide (PEMA). Phenobarbital is the primary component found in the serum and is assumed to be the primary active agent.[41,44,60] Primidone at a dosage of 50 mg/kg daily produces blood levels of

Table 13-9　**Protocol for Anticonvulsant Medication**

Dogs
Phenobarbital, 2.5-5 mg/kg b.i.d.. Reduce dosage after 1 wk if sedation is a problem. Measure serum levels after 2 wk to establish a baseline standard. Increase dosage to maintain control as needed and measure serum levels 2 wk after changes in dosage.

If seizures are not controlled, add *potassium bromide* (KBr) in a dosage of 40 mg/kg once a day in addition to the phenobarbital. Serum levels of KBr (1000-1500 mg/dl) may be reached in about 4 mo. If seizures are frequent or severe, clonazepam (0.5 mg/kg b.i.d.) may be used during the time KBr is reaching therapeutic levels.

See text for other alternatives.

Cats
Phenobarbital as above.
Diazepam, 0.5-1 mg/kg b.i.d. or t.i.d. (may be combined with phenobarbital).

Horses and Food Animals
Phenobarbital as above.
Phenytoin, 20 mg/kg b.i.d., for horses only (not approved or tested).

b.i.d., Twice daily; *t.i.d.,* three times daily.

phenobarbital of 10 µg/ml, which is subtherapeutic. Although primidone and PEMA concentrations are much lower, they may have an additive effect.[60]

The efficacy of primidone for patients with seizures has been demonstrated clinically for years; however, several studies indicate that it has little or no advantage over phenobarbital, and hepatotoxicity is more frequent.[41,61] Side effects include depression, polydipsia, polyphagia, and hepatic necrosis. The side effects may be dramatic, but they are usually transient. One half to twice the recommended dose may be used, depending on the individual animal's response. Larger animals should be started on a lower dose until tolerance is induced. Primidone is not approved for use in food animals or horses because the dosage and the anticonvulsive effects are unknown.

Phenytoin

Phenytoin is frequently used in humans, but its use in animals is limited because of studies showing marked species differences in the metabolism of the drug. The pharmacokinetics vary, depending on the route of administration, pretreatment, and treatment with other drugs. The action of the drug also differs among individuals, even of the same breed.[60] The approximate plasma half-life of phenytoin is 22 to 28 hours in humans, 3 to 4 hours in dogs, and 24 to 108 hours in cats. In addition, blood concentrations of phenytoin in the dog do not reach therapeutic levels (10 µg/ml, based on human clinical and canine research data) at the dosages prescribed for humans.[60,62] Laboratory studies indicate that at least 35 mg/kg three times daily are needed to reach therapeutic levels in the dog.[62] In another study, therapeutic levels were achieved with 3 to 5 mg/lb three times daily, but the reported concentrations were only 1.5 to 3.0 µg/ml.[63] The variability in serum levels and the short half-life make phenytoin of little benefit in most dogs.

Miscellaneous Anticonvulsant Drugs

Mephobarbital is longer acting than phenobarbital and is given once daily. Its efficacy is essentially the same as that of phenobarbital because it is metabolized into two molecules of phenobarbital. Mephobarbital offers a once-a-day medication schedule at a greater expense.

Sodium valproate, in combination with phenobarbital, has been useful in a limited number of cases. The half-life is short, and therapeutic levels are difficult to achieve. Some evidence indicates that brain levels may be higher and that other metabolites may have some effect. Sodium valproate may be tried in combination with phenobarbital at a dose of 60 mg/kg.[42,64]

Paramethadione and related drugs of that group are given primarily for absence seizures in humans. Paramethadione is reportedly effective for tonic-clonic seizures at a dosage of 10 to 60 mg/kg daily.[65]

Nimodipine is a calcium channel antagonist that penetrates the blood–brain barrier. It has anticonvulsant activity in models of experimental epilepsy. Nimodipine was ineffective in controlling seizures in 10 dogs with idiopathic epilepsy when administered at a dose of 2.5 mg/kg every 12 hours.[66]

Several new anticonvulsant drugs are available for use in humans and have been used on a limited basis in dogs (see Table 13-8). These drugs are expensive at present, and no reports of clinical trials in dogs or cats have appeared. The following are the recommendations adapted from Podell[40]:

1. Felbamate enhances sodium channel inactivation, enhances GABA activity, and reduces glutamate-mediated excitation. It is used to treat partial seizures at a dosage of 20 mg/kg every 8 hours. Blood dyscrasias and liver disease are potential side effects.
2. Gabapentin also enhances sodium channel inactivation, enhances GABA activity, and reduces glutamate-mediated excitation. A dosage of 30 to 60 mg/kg every 8 to 12 hours is suggested for generalized and partial seizures. Sedation is the primary side effect.
3. Topiramate has activity similar to felbamate. It is used as an add-on drug for generalized and partial seizures. Gastrointestinal upsets and irritability are the primary side effects. A dosage of 5 to 10 mg/kg every 12 hours has been suggested.
4. Zonisamide primarily reduces current through calcium[2] channels. It is used as an add-on drug for the treatment of generalized and partial seizures. A dosage of 4 to 8 mg/kg every 12 hours has been suggested. Sedation, ataxia, and anorexia are potential side effects.
5. Levetiracetam enhances GABA inhibition and is used as an add-on drug for generalized and partial seizures. The side effects are few, and a dosage of 500 to 4000 mg daily has been suggested.

A protocol for the treatment of seizures is outlined in Table 13-9.

STATUS EPILEPTICUS AND SEVERE CLUSTER SEIZURES

Status epilepticus is the condition of rapidly recurring seizures with incomplete recovery between episodes. This is a serious emergency that can result in death of the patient. Causes of SE include (1) toxicities or metabolic abnormalities, (2) sudden withdrawal of anticonvulsant medications, (3) ineffective anticonvulsant medications, and (4) progressive brain diseases. The risk factors for development of SE have been studied in dogs with primary epilepsy.[67] Dogs weighing 28.9 kg (63.6 lbs) or more were at increased risk compared with dogs weighing 17.4 kg (28.3 lbs) or less. One or more episodes of SE were predictive of future attacks. The mean life span of dogs with SE was 8.3 years compared with 11.3 years in epileptic dogs with no history of SE.[67]

Animals with SE may develop permanent brain damage and become refractory to anticonvulsant drugs. During severe seizures like those that occur in SE, transient brain hypoxia can occur. Hypoxia can produce central laminar necrosis and may result in permanent neurologic signs such as cortical blindness and mental retardation. Hyperthermia, commonly present in dogs with SE, enhances neuronal swelling and cerebral edema. Treatment for cerebral edema with mannitol and glucocorticoid steroids may be useful in some cases.

Cluster seizures represent individual convulsions that occur close together with short periods of normalcy between episodes. Animals experiencing cluster seizures are at increased risk of developing SE. In a study of 156 epileptic dogs, 66% and 16.5% had generalized cluster seizures and SE, respectively.[68] Of the 156 dogs studied, 52 and 68 had primary or secondary epilepsy, respectively.

Fifty dogs had toxic epilepsy, low anticonvulsant drug concentrations, or undetermined causes. A poor prognosis was associated with the diagnosis of GME, loss of seizure control within 6 hours of initiating treatment, or development of SE.

A protocol for the treatment of SE is presented in Table 13-10. The same protocol can be used for treatment of cluster seizures, except pentobarbital is seldom required to control the seizures. Diazepam, administered per rectum, has been used to treat cluster seizures and to prevent the development of SE.[69] Owners are given injectable diazepam (5 mg/ml) to give at a dose of 0.5 mg/kg per rectum. The drug is given after an initial generalized seizure and when a second or third seizure occurs within 24 hours of the first seizure. Diazepam is well absorbed from the rectum within 10 minutes of administration, and the availability is about 65%.[69] This protocol may greatly decrease visits to emergency clinics for treatment of recurrent seizures in dogs receiving adequate doses of anticonvulsants.

NARCOLEPSY AND CATAPLEXY

Narcolepsy is a brain disorder characterized by recurring sudden attacks of sleep.[70] *Cataplexy* (loss of muscle tone) commonly accompanies the attacks and may be the most common feature of attacks. Two other components occurring in humans—sleep paralysis and hallucinations—are difficult to verify in animals because of their subjective nature.[70]

Table 13-10 **Protocol for Treatment of Status Epilepticus**

---

1. Stop the seizure. Administer diazepam, 10-50 mg in 10-mg boluses IV. Diazepam usually gives at least temporary remission, allowing time for succeeding steps. Clonazepam may also be used in a dosage of 0.05-0.2 mg/kg for a longer duration of action. If seizures are not controlled, administer phenobarbital sodium (2-4 mg/kg IV at 30-min intervals). If neither is effective, administer sodium pentobarbital to effect (estimated dosage, 10-15 mg/kg). Pentobarbital must be given cautiously because diazepam and phenobarbital may potentiate its effect. Ultrashortacting barbiturates should not be used because they may potentiate seizure activity.
2. When the seizures have stopped, ensure ventilation of the patient. An endotracheal tube should be placed if the patient is unconscious.
3. Place an IV catheter, draw blood for hematology and chemistry analysis, and start IV fluids. Measure blood glucose levels as soon as possible.
4. Give 50% dextrose IV (2-3 ml for toy breeds, 50 ml for giant breeds). If the seizures are not violent or if interictal quiet periods occur, you may perform steps 3 and 4 first. Hypoglycemia is the one cause of status that can be treated directly.
5. Ruminants and cats should be given thiamine IV in 0.5- to 1-g doses, repeated several times in 24-48 hr.
6. If you suspect hypoglycemia, give an IV calcium preparation. Carefully monitor the heart rate.
7. Once the seizures are under control, evaluate the animal for etiology of seizures. If a cause is found, treat the specific disease.
8. Monitor the body temperature. If it reaches 105° F, cool the animal with ice to a temperature of 103° F. Maintain the temperature in a normal range.
9. Continue to control the seizures. Intravenous or intramuscular phenobarbital should be given until oral medication can be used. The normal movements of anesthetic recovery should not be mistaken for seizures.

IV, Intravenous

Dogs with narcolepsy typically have episodes in which they suddenly collapse, often while excited or during emotional stimulation. Eating is the most common precipitating factor in reported cases. The dog starts to eat and suddenly falls to the ground asleep. Noise, shaking, or other stimuli may arouse the animal, and often it resumes eating only to fall asleep again. Continual stimulation, such as petting or shaking, may prevent the attack. The episodes often are repeated many times a day.[70-73] Narcolepsy also has been reported in ponies, horses, and a Brahman bull.[74,75]

Normal sleep is characterized on the EEG by a change from low-voltage, fast-wave activity in the animal that is awake to high-voltage, slow-wave activity in the animal that is asleep. Rapid eye movement (REM) sleep develops after approximately 90 minutes of slow-wave sleep and may recur intermittently thereafter. REM sleep is associated with dreaming and is characterized by eye movements, occasional facial movements, and desynchronized low-voltage, fast-wave activity of the EEG.[76]

The sleep attacks of narcolepsy are the same as REM sleep with no intervening slow-wave sleep. Partial attacks and cataplectic episodes may occur without EEG changes.[71]

Narcolepsy has occurred in humans after CNS infection or trauma, and an immune mechanism is suspected in some cases.[73] Narcolepsy/cataplexy has been reported in a young dog with distemper encephalitis.[77] We have documented narcoleptic/cataplectic attacks in dogs with ehrlichial encephalitis that resolved with doxycycline therapy. A biochemical alteration of the neuronal membrane is presumed. Studies in dogs with narcolepsy have demonstrated some biochemical abnormalities.[78-81] Numbers of dopamine and muscarinic receptors are increased, but the numbers of benzodiazepine receptors do not change. The reticular activating system of the rostral brainstem presumably is associated with sleep, and the more caudal portions of the reticular formation in the pons are associated with cataplexy.

A genetic basis for narcolepsy in some breeds is suspected. An autosomal recessive inheritance has been demonstrated in Doberman pinschers and Labrador retrievers.[81] Numerous other breeds of dogs have been diagnosed as narcoleptics, but breeding studies have not been done or have been inconclusive.

A diagnosis usually can be made by observation of the characteristic signs if cataplexy is a prominent part of the syndrome. In the absence of cataplexy, the problem probably will not be recognized by the owner. The EEG is the only available diagnostic test. Sleep beginning with REM sleep is characteristic. Polygraphic recording of the EMG, eye movements, and EEG simultaneously for extended periods is the most definitive test.[82]

Anticholinergic compounds increase the frequency and duration of cataplectic attacks in narcoleptic animals but have no effect on normal animals.[82] A dose of physostigmine salicylate (0.025 to 0.1 mg/kg administered intravenously) produces cataplectic attacks in susceptible animals.

Treatment with stimulants is partially effective. Dextroamphetamine (5 to 10 mg three times daily) and methylphenidate (Ritalin, 5 to 10 mg two or three times daily) have stopped the sleep attacks but have produced undesirable behavioral changes in some cases.[70,82] Excessive somnolence is not a significant problem for most dogs; therefore, managing the cataleptic episodes is of more importance. Imipramine at a dosage of 0.5 to 1.0 mg/kg three times daily is more effective in preventing cataplexy.[82] A combination of methylphenidate and imipramine is recommended to control sleep attacks and cataplexy. The medication should be given at a dosage that reduces attacks without completely eliminating them because complete elimination may require dangerously high dosages. Giving the medication intermittently also reduces the development of tolerance. Protriptyline at a dosage of 10 mg once a day was effective in controlling hypersomnia in a dog.[83] This dog did not have cataplexy

Combining amphetamines and imipramine is potentially dangerous because amphetamines cause a release of catecholamines and imipramine blocks their reuptake. Hypertensive episodes can result. A balanced regimen of therapy must therefore be developed for each individual to attain a relatively normal sleep/wakefulness cycle.

Case Histories

Seizures are a common neurologic problem in dogs. Most patients with seizures do not have other neurologic deficits. The following case histories demonstrate the approach to management. Localizing signs of brain disease are not present in these cases because they are discussed in other chapters. After reading the history and the preliminary laboratory data, the student should develop a plan for further diagnosis or treatment of each case and then read our assessment.

CASE HISTORY 13A

Signalment
Canine, miniature poodle, male, 18 months old.

History
The dog has received all vaccinations on schedule and has had no major medical problems. The first seizure occurred 2 months ago. The second seizure was observed last night at approximately 6:00 PM.

The owner describes the seizure as follows: The dog seemed somewhat apprehensive for approximately 30 minutes, seeking attention from the owner. Suddenly he fell down, extended all four limbs, and arched the head and the neck. After about 30 seconds he started making running movements of the limbs with some chewing movements of the mouth. Some salivation occurred, and the dog urinated. The owner tried to hold and rub the dog, and the movements stopped after about 1 minute. In about 2 or 3 minutes, the dog was able to get up. He seemed a little disoriented for a few minutes, and then he seemed normal.

Other than during the two seizures, the dog appeared to be healthy. He is fed a variety of commercial dog foods twice daily. Water consumption and urination are thought normal.

Physical and Neurologic Examinations
No abnormalities are found.

Laboratory Examination
The complete blood cell count (CBC) and the chemistry profile (see Table 13-7) are normal.

CASE HISTORY 13B

Signalment
Canine, cairn terrier, male, 6 years old.

History
The dog has had no serious illnesses and has had booster vaccinations annually. Ten weeks ago the dog had a generalized motor seizure that lasted about 5 minutes. The dog seemed blind and confused for about 4 hours afterward. Two weeks ago, the dog had a second seizure. Since that time he has not acted "right." His appetite is diminished, and he does not play the way that he did, and he has urinated and defecated in the house several times, which he has not done for years. Last night he had another seizure that lasted over 5 minutes. Today he is very depressed.

Physical Examination
No abnormalities are found other than depression.

Neurologic Examination
The dog can be coaxed to walk, but he prefers to lie down. The gait is good, with a suggestion of slight symmetric dysmetria. The limbs seem to be lifted a bit high and to be put down with increased force. No ataxia is present, however. The postural reactions also seem slightly dysmetric. The spinal reflexes are normal, as are the cranial nerves, although the menace reaction seems a little sluggish. This response is considered within normal limits when the depression is taken into account.

CASE HISTORY 13C

Signalment
Canine, German shepherd dog, female, 4 years old.

History
All vaccinations, including annual boosters, have been given. No major illnesses have occurred. Generalized motor seizures started 18 months ago. The first few were 2 to 3 months apart, but recently they have been 2 to 3 weeks apart. Several recent seizures were prolonged (approaching SE) and were controlled with general anesthesia. Several anticonvulsants, including phenobarbital, phenytoin, and primidone in dosages that appear to be adequate, have been used in the last year, with no

apparent control of the seizures. The seizures have occurred at various times of day, including at night when the dog is asleep. Laboratory evaluations performed on several occasions by the referring veterinarian have not revealed any abnormalities. The owner feels that neither he nor the dog can continue to tolerate these seizures.

Physical and Neurologic Examinations
No abnormalities are found.

Laboratory Examination
No abnormalities are found.

CASE HISTORY 13D

Signalment
Feline, domestic short hair, female, approximately 14 months old.

History
The cat took up residence at the owner's home 6 months ago. She was vaccinated for the usual feline diseases, including rabies, at that time. She has not been ill except for seizures, which started 6 weeks ago. The first seizure, which occurred in the evening, was described as a brief period during which the cat suddenly looked "glassy eyed," stiffened all four limbs, and arched the neck. The seizure lasted less than a minute. The second and third seizures were similar and occurred about 1 week apart. In the last 3 weeks, the cat has had at least two seizures per week. The last two were generalized motor seizures. The most recent seizure was described as starting like the first one. The cat then twisted to the right, urinated, and began paddling, first with the right limb and then with all four limbs. The seizure lasted approximately 2 minutes, and the cat acted dazed and depressed for approximately 2 hours.

Physical Examination
No abnormalities are found.

Neurologic Examination
The only abnormality is a slight anisocoria, with the left pupil slightly smaller than the right. Both pupils are reactive to light, although the right seems slightly slower to react than the left. The iris and the fundus appear normal.

CASE HISTORY 13E

Signalment
Canine, dachshund, male, 6 months old.

History
The dog suddenly became lethargic and exhibited a staggering gait. The owners believe that the onset of signs occurred shortly after he was seen eating some unknown substance in the front yard. Observation of the dog for several days revealed the following pattern of behavior: The dog suddenly collapses to the ground while walking. He appears to be asleep for a few seconds and then awakens, gets up, and behaves normally. While eating, the dog collapses with food in his mouth, wakes up in less than a minute, and continues eating. This pattern might be repeated every 2 to 3 minutes during a meal. The dog can be aroused from sleep easily by noise or touch. No other abnormalities are observed. The dog has not been ill previously and has had all vaccinations.

Physical and Neurologic Examinations
Other than the behavior just described, no abnormalities are found.

Laboratory Examination

All tests, including an ECG, are normal.

ASSESSMENT 13A

The seizures are generalized tonic-clonic (grand mal, major motor; see Table 13-1). To the owner's knowledge, they have occurred twice. The seizures are single and are of short duration. No history of illnesses or injuries is present, and the physical, neurologic, and laboratory examinations are normal. Although a genetic basis for epilepsy has not been demonstrated in miniature poodles, hereditary epilepsy is suspected because of the relatively frequent occurrence of seizures in this breed without specific cause.

Nothing in the database justifies further diagnostic tests at this time. We would recommend prophylactic medication to determine if the seizures can be prevented. If the owner feels that giving medication is a serious problem, we would suggest observing the animal closely for further seizures and then starting medication if another seizure occurs. The owner should be warned that the dog probably will have more seizures and that medication is the preferred alternative. The medication of choice is phenobarbital.

ASSESSMENT 13B

A 6-year-old dog with a sudden onset of seizures probably has an acquired brain problem. The disorder appears to be progressive. The depression suggests brain abnormalities, which may be primary or secondary to metabolic or toxic abnormalities. Dysmetria, especially when it is subtle and occurs in a terrier, may or may not be significant. It could indicate a diffuse abnormality with cerebellar involvement. A laboratory profile is indicated.

Laboratory Examination

Packed cell volume	37%
Hemoglobin	14.5 g/dl
White blood cells (WBCs)	10,950/μL
Neutrophils	7400/μL
Lymphocytes	2400/μL
Monocytes	450/μL
Eosinophils	700/μL
Nucleated RBCs	3 per high-power
Some polychromasia	field
Serum plasma protein	6.5 g/dl
Albumin	3.3 g/dl
Serum urea nitrogen	14 mg/dl
Alkaline phosphatase	80 IU/L
Alanine aminotransferase (ALT)	30 IU/L
Calcium	9.9 mg/dl
Glucose	95 mg/dl
Urinalysis	Normal

No evidence indicates systemic infectious disease (normal WBCs and differential). Severe liver disease is unlikely (normal ALT and alkaline phosphatase, serum albumin, and serum urea nitrogen levels). Calcium and glucose levels are normal. The only unusual findings are nucleated RBCs and polychromasia with a normal packed cell volume and hematocrit (no anemia). This finding is suggestive of lead poisoning. A sample of whole blood was submitted, and 65 mg of lead per 100 ml was reported. These results are diagnostic of lead poisoning. Chelation therapy with calcium ethylenediamine tetraacetic acid (EDTA) was successful. The source of the lead was not found for several weeks, until the owners discovered a thoroughly chewed and very old bowling trophy under a bed.

ASSESSMENT 13C

The history is typical of a form of epilepsy, presumably genetic, that is seen in German shepherd dogs and a few other large breeds. The seizures begin in early adult life and are severe. They often are multiple and are refractory to anticonvulsant therapy. CT or MR imaging and CSF analysis should be recommended to rule out causes of secondary epilepsy. If phenobarbital is ineffective, as in this case, KBr in combination with phenobarbital is the best alternative. The prognosis for significant control is poor, but some dogs can be managed effectively. Phenobarbital and bromide plasma concentrations should be monitored.

The owner declined diagnostic evaluation. The dog's seizures were satisfactorily controlled with KBr therapy for a period of 2 years. Then the dog became increasingly refractory to anticonvulsant therapy and the owner elected euthanasia.

ASSESSMENT 13D

Seizures in cats usually are acquired *(secondary epilepsy)*. Unfortunately, most of the causes are diseases with a poor prognosis. The progression from a partial motor seizure to generalized seizures also suggests primary brain disease. Anisocoria frequently occurs in cats that have had positive tests for feline leukemia virus (FeLV). The signs also may be associated with feline infectious peritonitis (FIP, usually the "dry" form). Meningiomas also may cause seizures without other signs in the early stages. The age of the cat is more suggestive of viral diseases than of neoplasia.

Localization

Cerebral or diencephalic. Rule outs are (1) FIP, (2) FeLV, and (3) meningioma.

Plan

Laboratory examination, titers for FeLV and FIP, CSF analysis, EEG. The significant findings are:

WBCs	16,000/μL
Segmented neutrophils	6700/μL
Bands	2500/μL
Lymphocytes	6000/μL
Eosinophils	800/μL
Serum protein	9.0 g/dl
Albumin	3.0 g/dl
Globulin	6.0 g/dl

CSF

Protein	110 mg/dl
Cells (total)	240/mm^3
Neutrophils	130/mm^3
Lymphocytes	110/mm^3

EEG: Generalized high-voltage slow waves with spikes randomly superimposed

FeLV: Positive

FIP titer: Positive at 1:1600

All these findings are characteristic of FIP. If costs are a factor, the laboratory examination (serum protein) and FeLV and FIP tests are adequate for diagnosis. Treatment of the CNS form of FIP has been uniformly unsuccessful. Many of these cats have either uveitis or retinal lesions, or both, and a strong presumptive diagnosis can be made from the clinical examination alone.

ASSESSMENT 13E

The behavior of this dog is typical of narcolepsy/cataplexy. The EEG is useful for documenting the changes. Clinical management requires long-term therapy because the disease is not reversible. A brief trial with therapy at home was unsatisfactory for this client, and euthanasia was performed.

References

1. Oliver JE Jr: Seizure disorders and narcolepsy. In Oliver JE, Hoerlein BF, Mayhew IG, editors: *Veterinary neurology.* Philadelphia, 1987, WB Saunders.
2. Cavazos JE: Pathogenesis of epilepsy. Proceedings of the 19th ACVIM Forum, 2001, American College of Veterinary Internal Medicine, pp 423-426.
3. Platt SR: The role of glutamate in neurologic diseases. Proceedings of the 19th ACVIM Forum, 2001, American College of Veterinary Internal Medicine, pp 427-429.
4. Gloor P, Fariello RG: Generalized epilepsy: some of its cellular mechanisms differ from those of focal epilepsy, *Trends Neurosci* 11:63-68, 1988.
5. Russo ME: The pathophysiology of epilepsy, *Cornell Vet* 71:221-247, 1981.
6. Bleck TP, Klawans HL: Convulsive disorders: mechanisms of epilepsy and anticonvulsant action, *Clin Neuropharmacol* 13:121-128, 1990.
7. Stasheff SF, Anderson WW, Clark S, et al: NMDA antagonists differentiate epileptogenesis from seizure expression in an in vitro model, *Science* 245:648-651, 1989.
8. Oliver JE Jr: Seizure disorders in companion animals, *Compend Cont Educ Pract Vet* 2:77-85, 1980.
9. Gastaut H: Clinical and electroencephalographic classification of epileptic seizures, *Epilepsia* 10(suppl):512-513, 1969.
10. Holliday TA: Seizure disorders, *Vet Clin North Am* 10:3-29, 1980.
11. Quesnel AD, Parent JM, McDonnell W, et al: Diagnostic evaluation of cats with seizure disorders: 30 cases (1991-1993), *J Am Vet Med Assoc* 210:65-71, 1997.
12. Redding RW: Electroencephalography. In Oliver JE, Hoerlein BF, Mayhew IG, editors: *Veterinary neurology.* Philadelphia, 1987, WB Saunders.
13. Breitschwerdt EB, Breazile JE, Broadhurst JJ: Clinical and electroencephalographic findings associated with ten cases of suspected limbic epilepsy in the dog, *J Am Anim Hosp Assoc* 15:27-50, 1979.
14. Crowell Davis SL, Lappin M, Oliver JE: Stimulus responsive psychomotor epilepsy in a Doberman pinscher, *J Am Anim Hosp Assoc* 25:57-60, 1989.
15. Gastaut H, Toga M, Naquet R: Clinical, electrographical and anatomical study of epilepsy induced in dogs by the ingestion of agenized proteins. In Baldwin M, Bailey P, editors: *Temporal lobe epilepsy.* Springfield, Ill, 1958, Charles C Thomas.
16. Dobman NH, Knowles KE, Shuster L, et al: Behavioral changes associated with suspected complex partial seizures in Bull Terriers, *J Am Vet Med Assoc* 208:688-691, 1996.
17. Falco MJ, Barker J, Wallace ME: The genetics of epilepsy in the British Alsatian, *J Small Anim Pract* 15:685-692, 1974.
18. Van der Velden A: Fits in Tervuren shepherd dogs: a presumed hereditary trait, *J Small Anim Pract* 9:63-70, 1968.
19. Biefelt SW, Redman HC, Broadhurst JJ: Sire and sex-related differences in rates of epileptiform seizures in a purebred beagle dog colony, *Am J Vet Res* 32:2039-2048, 1971.
20. Hegreberg GA, Padget GA: Inherited progressive epilepsy of the dog with comparisons to Lafora's disease of man, *FASEB J* 35:1202-1205, 1976.
21. Tomchick T: Familial Lafora's disease in the beagle dog, *FASEB J* 32:8-21, 1973.
22. Wallace ME: Keeshonds: a genetic study of epilepsy and EEG readings, *J Small Anim Pract* 16:1-10, 1975.
23. Holliday TA: Epilepsy in animals. In Frey HH, Janz D, editors: *Handbook of experimental pharmacology,* vol 74. Berlin, 1985, Springer Verlag.
24. Cunningham JG, Farnbach GC: Inheritance and idiopathic canine epilepsy, *J Am Anim Hosp Assoc* 24:421-424, 1988.
25. Borden J, Manuelidis L: Movement of the X chromosome in epilepsy, *Science* 242:1687-1691, 1988.
26. Farnbach GC: Seizures in the dog, Part I: basis, classification, and predilection, *Compend Cont Educ Pract Vet* 6:569-576, 1984.
27. Chrisman CL: Epilepsy and seizures. In Howard JL, editor: *Current veterinary therapy: food animal practice.* Philadelphia, 1981, WB Saunders.
28. Barlow R: Morphogenesis of cerebellar lesions in bovine familial convulsions and ataxia, *Vet Pathol* 18:151-162, 1981.
29. Gerard VA, Conarck CN: Identifying the cause of an early onset of seizures in puppies with epileptic parents, *Vet Med* 86:1060-1061, 1991.
30. Holliday TA, Cunningham JG, Gutnick MJ: Comparative clinical and electroencephalographic studies of canine epilepsy, *Epilepsia* 11:281-292, 1971.
31. Bunch SE: Anticonvulsant drug therapy in companion animals. In Kirk RW, editor: *Current veterinary therapy VIII.* Philadelphia, 1983, WB Saunders.
32. Braund KG: Degenerative and developmental diseases. In Oliver JE, Hoerlein BF, Mayhew IG, editors: *Veterinary neurology.* Philadelphia, 1987, WB Saunders.
33. Greene CE, Vandevelde M, Braund K: Lissencephaly in two lhasa apso dogs, *J Am Vet Med Assoc* 169:405-410, 1976.
34. Oliver JE, Hoerlein BF, Mayhew IG: *Veterinary neurology.* Philadelphia, 1987, WB Saunders.
35. Kornegay JN, Mayhew IG: Metabolic, toxic, and nutritional diseases of the nervous system. In Oliver JE, Hoerlein BF, Mayhew IG, editors: *Veterinary neurology.* Philadelphia, 1987, WB Saunders.
36. Roberts BK, Aronsohn MG, Moses BL, et al: *Bufo marinus* intoxication in dogs: 94 cases (1997-1998), *J Am Vet Med Assoc* 216:1941-1944, 2000.

37. Gwaltney-Brant SM, Albretsen JC, Khan SA: 5-hydroxytryptophan toxicity in dogs: 21 cases (1989-1999), *J Am Vet Med Assoc* 216:1937-1940, 2000.

38. Oliver JE Jr: Protocol for the diagnosis of seizure disorders in companion animals, *J Am Vet Med Assoc* 172:822-824, 1978.

39. Hudson JA, Simpson ST, Buxton DF, et al: Ultrasonographic diagnosis of canine hydrocephalus, *J Vet Radiol* 31:50-58, 1990.

40. Podell M: Strategies of antiepileptic drug therapy. Proceedings of the 19th ACVIM Forum, 2001, American College of Veterinary Internal Medicine, pp 430-432.

41. Schwartz Porsche D, Loscher W, Frey HH: Therapeutic efficacy of phenobarbital and primidone in canine epilepsy: a comparison, *J Vet Pharmacol Ther* 8:113-119, 1985.

42. Lane SB, Bunch SE: Medical management of recurrent seizures in dogs and cats, *J Vet Intern Med* 4:26-39, 1990.

43. Farnbach GC: Serum concentrations and efficacy of phenytoin, phenobarbital, and primidone in canine epilepsy, *J Am Vet Med Assoc* 184:1117-1120, 1984.

44. Frey HH: Use of anticonvulsants in small animals, *Vet Rec* 118:484-486, 1986.

45. Dayrell Hart B, Steinberg SA, VanWinkle TJ, et al: Hepatotoxicity of phenobarbital in dogs: 18 cases (1985-1989), *J Am Vet Med Assoc* 199:1060-1066, 1991.

46. Levitski RE, Trepanier LA: Effect of timing of blood collection on serum phenobarbital concentrations in dogs with epilepsy, *J Am Vet Med Assoc* 217:200-204, 2000.

47. Pellock JM, Willmore LJ: A rational guide to routine blood monitoring in patients receiving antiepileptic drugs, *Neurology* 41:961-964, 1991.

48. Muller PB, Taboada J, Hosgood G, et al: Effects of long-term phenobarbital on the liver in dogs, *J Vet Intern Med* 14:165-171, 2000.

49. Gieger TL, Hosgood G, Taboada J, et al: Thyroid function and serum hepatic enzyme activity in dogs after phenobarbital administration, *J Vet Intern Med* 14:277-281, 2000.

50. Jacobs G, Calvert C, Kaufman A: Neutropenia and thrombocytopenia in three dogs treated with anticonvulsants, *J Am Vet Med Assoc* 212:681-684, 1998.

51. Kantrowitz LB, Peterson ME, Trepanier LA, et al: Serum total thyroxine, total triiodothyronine, free thyroxine, and thyrotropin concentrations in epileptic dogs treated with anticonvulsants, *J Am Vet Med Assoc* 214:1804-1808, 1999.

52. Gaskill CL, Burton SA, Hans CJ, et al: Effects of phenobarbital treatment on serum thyroxine and thyroid-stimulating hormone concentrations in epileptic dogs, *J Am Vet Med Assoc* 215:489-496, 1999.

53. Schwartz Porsche D, Boenigk HE, Lorenz JH: Bromid Therapie bei den Epilepsien des Hundes: Erste Erfahrungen. Kurzreferate, regionale Arbeitstagung Nord DVG Fachgruppe. Kleintierkrankheiten. Timmendorfer Strand, 1987.

54. Schwartz Porsche D: Epidemiological, clinical, and pharmacokinetic studies in spontaneously epileptic dogs and cats. In Proceedings of the 11th American College of Veterinary Internal Medicine Forum, Washington, DC, 1986, American College of Veterinary Internal Medicine, pp 61-63.

55. Sisson A, LeCouteur RA: Potassium bromide as an adjunct to phenobarbital for the management of uncontrolled seizures in the dog, *Prog Vet Neurol* 1:114-115, 1990.

56. Podell M, Fenner WR: Bromide therapy in refractory canine idiopathic epilepsy, *J Vet Intern Med* 7:318-327, 1993.

57. Nichols ES, Trepanier LA, Linn K: Bromide toxicosis secondary to renal insufficiency in an epileptic dog, *J Am Vet Med Assoc* 208:231-236, 1996.

58. Boothe DM: Anticonvulsant therapy in small animals, *Waltham Focus* 4:25-31, 1995.

59. Trepanier LA, Van Schoick A, Schwark WS, et al: Therapeutic serum drug concentrations in epileptic dogs treated with potassium bromide alone or in combination with other anticonvulsants: 122 cases (1992-1996), *J Am Vet Med Assoc* 213:1449-1453, 1998.

60. Frey HH, Loscher W: Pharmacokinetics of antiepileptic drugs in the dog: a review, *J Vet Pharmacol Ther* 8:219-233, 1985.

61. Farnbach GC: Efficacy of primidone in dogs with seizures unresponsive to phenobarbital, *J Am Vet Med Assoc* 185:867-868, 1984.

62. Sanders JE, Yeary RA: Serum concentrations of orally administered diphenylhydantoin in dogs, *J Am Vet Med Assoc* 172:153-156, 1978.

63. Pasten LJ: Diphenylhydantoin in the canine: clinical aspects and determination of therapeutic blood levels, *J Am Anim Hosp Assoc* 13:247-254, 1977.

64. Nafe LA, Parker A, Kay WJ: Sodium valproate: a preliminary clinical trial in epileptic dogs, *J Am Anim Hosp Assoc* 17:131-133, 1981.

65. Parker AJ: A preliminary report on a new antiepileptic medication for dogs, *J Am Anim Hosp Assoc* 11:437-438, 1975.

66. O'Brien DP, Simpson ST, Longshore RC, et al: Nimodipine for treatment of idiopathic epilepsy in dogs, *J Am Vet Med Assoc* 210:1298-1301, 1997.

67. Saito M, Munana KR, Sharp NJH, et al: Risk factors for development of status epilepticus in dogs with idiopathic epilepsy and effects of status epilepticus on outcome and survival time: 32 cases (1990-1996), *J Am Vet Med Assoc* 219:618-623, 2001.

68. Bateman SW, Parent JM: Clinical findings, treatment, and outcome of dogs with status epilepticus or cluster seizures: 156 cases (1990-1995), *J Am Vet Med Assoc* 215:1463-1468, 1999.

69. Podell M: The use of diazepam per rectum at home for the acute management of cluster seizures in dogs, *J Vet Intern Med* 8:68-74, 1995.

70. Knecht CD, Oliver JE, Redding R, et al: Narcolepsy in a dog and a cat, *J Am Vet Med Assoc* 162:1052-1053, 1973.

71. Richardson JW, Fredrickson P, Lin S: Narcolepsy update, *Mayo Clin Proc* 65:991-998, 1990.

72. Mitler MM, Soave O, Dement WC: Narcolepsy in seven dogs, *J Am Vet Med Assoc* 168:1036-1038, 1976.

73. Katherman AE: A comparative review of canine and human narcolepsy, *Compend Cont Educ Pract Vet* 2:818-822, 1980.

74. Sweeney CR, Hendricks JC, Beech J, et al: Narcolepsy in a horse, *J Am Vet Med Assoc* 183:126-128, 1983.

75. Strain GM, Olcott BM, Archer RM, et al: Narcolepsy in a Brahman bull, *J Am Vet Med Assoc* 185:538-541, 1984.

76. Wauquier A, Verheyen JL, Van Den Broeck WAE, et al: Visual and computer-based analysis of 24 h sleepwaking patterns in the dog, *Electroencephalogr Clin Neurophysiol* 46:33-48, 1979.

77. Cantile C, Baroni M, Arispici M: A case of narcolepsy-cataplexy associated with distemper encephalitis, *J Vet Med Assoc* 46:301-308, 1999.

78. Mitler MM, Dement WC, Guilleminault C, et al: Canine narcolepsy. In Rose FC, Behan PO, editors: *Animal models of neurological disease.* Kent, Great Britain, 1980, Putman Medical.

79. Delashaw JB Jr, Foutz AS, Guilleminault C, et al: Cholinergic mechanisms and cataplexy in dogs, *Exp Neurol* 66:745-757, 1979.

80. Bowersox S, Kilduff K, Zeller DeAmicis L, et al: Brain dopamine receptor levels elevated in canine narcolepsy, *Brain Res* 402:44-48, 1987.

81. Fruhstorfer B, Mignot E, Bowersox S, et al: Canine narcolepsy is associated with an elevated number of α-receptors in the locus coeruleus, *Brain Res* 500:209-214, 1989.

82. Baker TL, Mitler MM, Foutz AS, et al: Diagnosis and treatment of narcolepsy in animals. In Kirk RW, editor: *Current veterinary therapy VIII*. Philadelphia, 1983, WB Saunders.

83. Shores A, Redding R: Narcoleptic hypersomnia syndrome responsive to protriptyline in a labrador retriever, *J Am Anim Hosp Assoc* 23:455-458, 1987.

Chapter
14

Pain

Animals do feel pain, and yet this point has been argued for many years. For a review of the entire spectrum of animal pain, the *Colloquium on Recognition and Alleviation of Animal Pain and Distress* and the text *Animal Pain* are recommended.[1,2]

This chapter reviews the pathophysiology of pain, some diseases that have pain as the primary clinical sign, and the symptomatic treatment of pain.

Definitions of the terms related to the description of pain are essential to communication. Kitchell[3] has provided an excellent working definition: "*Pain* in animals is an aversive sensory and emotional experience (a perception), which elicits protective motor actions, results in learned avoidance, and may modify species-specific traits of behavior, including social behavior." Pain is a perception, not a quantifiable entity. It is also incorrect to refer to painful stimuli or pain receptors, pathways, or nerve fibers. All these are more accurately called *noxious* (noxious means "injurious"). Thus we use the terms *noxious stimuli, nociceptors, nociceptive pathways,* and so on. Other terms frequently used or misused include the following.

Hyperesthesia (hyperalgesia) denotes an increased sensitivity to stimulation. It has often been used to designate an unpleasant response to a nonnoxious stimulus.[3] We use the term more generically than others because of the difficulty in truly knowing whether the animal perceives pain. Throughout this book, we use the term *hyperesthesia* to mean a behavioral reaction of the animal indicating that the stimulus was unpleasant and when we consider the stimulus to be nonnoxious. The most common usage is in describing an animal's response to palpation that does not evoke a reaction in some locations but causes an aversive reaction in others.

Hyperpathia denotes an unpleasant painful response to a noxious stimulus, especially if repeated, and is characterized by delay, overreaction, and aftersensation.[3] This term has been used frequently in veterinary medicine but is far more specific than just a "painful response." Knowing that an animal actually has the sensations associated with hyperpathia would be difficult if not impossible.

Allodynia is pain resulting from a nonnoxious stimulus to normal skin. Because we are often assessing "painful" responses from structures other than skin, this term is not used often.

NEUROANATOMIC BASIS FOR PAIN

Nociception, the neural response to a noxious stimulus, has a specific set of complex pathways. Activation of these pathways leads to the sensation of pain.[3,4] The nociceptive pathway includes peripheral nociceptors; nerve fibers in peripheral nerves, spinal cord, and brainstem relays; spinal cord and brain pathways; and central processing areas in the brainstem, thalamus, and cerebral cortex.

Nociceptors are specific receptors that respond to a variety of stimuli. They include mechanosensitive, thermosensitive, and polymodal (those responding to more than one kind of stimulus) receptors. Nociceptors are usually silent unless stimulated and require more intense stimuli than do many other receptors. They respond to stimuli in proportion to the intensity of the stimulus. The nociceptors of the skin have been studied in the most detail, but nociception clearly occurs from many structures. Nociceptors are generally "free nerve endings," although the endings are never completely free of surrounding structure.[4,5] The nerve fibers associated with nociception are classified as either A delta (small myelinated axons) or C polymodal (nonmyelinated). Excitation of cutaneous A delta receptors causes a "pricking pain" in humans, whereas excitation of C polymodal receptors causes a "burning pain."[6] Release of certain chemicals (acetylcholine, histamine, bradykinin) excites nociceptors, but these chemicals are probably not necessary for all nociception.

Nociceptive afferent fibers generally enter the spinal cord through the dorsal root. The afferent fibers synapse on relay neurons in the dorsal horn of the spinal cord that send axons cranially.

Segmental connections for reflexes such as the flexion reflex are also present. Many of the dorsal horn neurons have synapses from nociceptors in muscles, joints, and other structures. This convergence of nociceptive pathways in the spinal cord may be one of the mechanisms of referred pain.[6]

The nociceptive spinal cord pathways include the spinothalamic, spinoreticular, spinomesencephalic, and spinocervical tracts and the dorsal column postsynaptic system. The relative significance and location of these tracts differ between species. For example, a major part of the spinothalamic tract is in the dorsal lateral funiculus in cats, compared with the ventrolateral funiculus in primates.[4,7] The spinoreticular and spinomesencephalic tracts probably have less discriminative capacity than the spinothalamic tracts. The domestic animals have multisynaptic, bilateral nociceptive pathways, probably in the propriospinal system, that are resistant to destruction. The spinal tracts relay in the thalamus before reaching the cerebral cortex.

Nociception from the head is carried in branches of the trigeminal (V), facial (VII), glossopharyngeal (IX), and vagus (X) nerves. Fibers synapse in the caudal nucleus of the trigeminal nerve and then follow routes to the cerebrum similar to the spinal pathways.

MECHANISMS OF PAIN

Nociceptive stimulation causes two kinds of reactions. *Superficial pain* is discriminative, allowing precise localization of the stimulus. *Deep pain* is motivational, causing the animal to show a change in behavior. Both superficial and deep pain are used clinically to localize lesions. Deep pain is also used as an important test for prognosis in spinal cord lesions. In general, superficial pain comes from the more superficial structures, whereas deep pain comes from receptors in muscle, joints, and bone (Figure 14-1).[8]

Acute pain, also called *nociceptive* or *physiologic pain*, is the immediate response to noxious stimuli. It results from activation of high threshold receptors. Usually minimal tissue damage is present because the animal uses protective reflexes or responses to withdraw from the stimulus.

Chronic pain, also called *clinical* or *pathologic pain*, is described as intense and unrelenting, resulting in extended discomfort. Chronic pain has no beneficial role. It induces biochemical and phenotypic changes in the central nervous system (CNS) that increase the protraction and intensity of pain, and it induces changes that contribute to illness and death. Clinical pain is caused by tissue inflammation that results in abnormal responses to noxious stimuli (hyperalgesia or lowered threshold to noxious stimuli). It is classified as inflammatory or neuropathic or both. Surgical procedures and many inflammatory and ischemic disease processes create pathologic pain through one or both of these mechanisms.

Peripheral sensitization is an important mechanism in the development of chronic pain. This is one explanation for the exaggerated response animals display to normally innocuous stimuli. It results from several inflammatory mediators released from

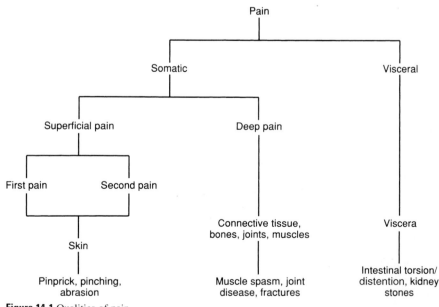

Figure 14-1 Qualities of pain.

damaged tissues that create changes in peripheral sensory receptors.[9] These inflammatory mediators sensitize high-threshold nociceptors to chemical, thermal, and mechanical stimuli.

Central sensitization is a process that develops within dorsal horn neurons secondary to several mechanisms involving inflammatory mediators, neuronal receptors, and neurotransmitter agents. It allows low-threshold sensory fibers to induce pain by increasing the excitability of sensory neurons located in the dorsal horn of the spinal cord.[9] Central sensitization plays a major role in postinjury hypersensitivity.

Peripheral nerve injuries can contribute to acute and chronic pain states through a process termed *disinhibition*.[9] Inhibitory interneurons within the dorsal horns modulate the flow of noxious sensory information within the spinal cord and projections to the brain. The inhibition is modulated by γ aminobutyric acid (GABA) and GABA receptors. Blockage of this GABA-mediated inhibition results in pain. In peripheral nerve injuries, opioid antagonists such as cholecystokinin are also expressed that decrease the analgesic effects of endogenous and exogenous opioids.

Chronic pain may induce phenotypic changes in sensory neurons. Molecular signaling agents produced by sensory neurons and microglial cells modify cell membranes and receptors to increase neuron excitability. Both inflammation and peripheral nerve injuries are capable of inducing neuronal modification, although the specific biochemical mechanisms may vary.

EXAMINATION

The methods for evaluating an animal's ability to perceive pain are discussed in Chapter 1. Recognition of the signs of pain in animals is important for diagnosis and for appropriate, humane care. The perception of pain is apparently similar in most mammalian species, but the relative reaction to pain varies considerably even within the same species. Many animals give little outward indication that they are in pain, although we recognize that the physical abnormality must be painful. For example, a dog with a fractured limb often shows little outward sign of pain and suffering, but we know it must be experiencing considerable pain and suffering.

Animals with severe pain show one or more of the following signs:

Decreased activity
Depressed mentation
Increased respiratory rate
Change in normal attitude (i.e., aggression, withdrawal)
Resistance to handling
Gait abnormality or lameness; stilted, stiff limbs; reluctance to go up or down stairs; reluctance to jump
Unusual posture or restlessness
Chewing, biting, or licking of a painful area
Autonomic signs such as salivation, pupillary dilation, tachycardia, sweating (in the horse), and increased systolic blood pressure
Anorexia

Diffuse or multifocal pain is usually caused by meningitis, polymyositis, polyarthritis, diffuse skeletal disease, or more rarely cancer. Careful palpation of the bones, joints, muscles, and paravertebral region identifies which structures are involved in most animals. Sedation may be necessary if the animal seems hyperesthetic everywhere.

Localization of painful areas is accomplished by a combination of observation, palpation, and manipulation. After observing for the previously listed changes, the clinician systematically palpates the animal. Starting caudally and working cranially to localize pain is usually best. Generally, nervous system disease causes decreased sensation caudal to the lesion, increased sensation at the location of the problem, and normal sensation cranial to the lesion. This finding is especially true of spinal cord lesions. Palpating from caudal to cranial goes from decreased sensation through the painful area to normal sensation, maximizing the ability of the examiner to recognize the abnormal area. If an abnormality is identified, the palpation can be done in the reverse direction to help narrow the location.

Palpation of the vertebral column can be done by pressing one hand on the spinous processes or squeezing the articular or transverse processes, depending on the size of the animal and examiner. Placing the other hand on the abdomen of small animals while palpating detects increased tension in the muscles as painful areas are approached. Pressing on the ribs may also be helpful in recognizing thoracic vertebral pain, such as that in diskospondylitis. Careful palpation can distinguish vertebral from abdominal pain. Some animals are in so much pain that localization is impossible. Sedation often allows a more accurate examination. Diffuse paravertebral pain is a prominent finding in meningitis.

Visceral disorders and peritonitis cause abdominal pain. Vertebral or meningeal pain also causes splinting of the abdomen and a painful response when palpating the abdomen. If a painful response also occurs when palpating the vertebral column, the pain is usually not of abdominal origin.

Manipulation of the limbs and palpation of individual joints are used to identify joint pain. Careful palpation of joints that do not have superimposed muscles differentiates joint from muscle pain. The stifle, hock, elbow, and carpus are good examples. The vertebral column can also be manipulated to elicit pain if palpation is unsuccessful. Flexion, extension, and turning of the head and neck often elicit pain from problems affecting the cervical vertebrae. Extension of the lumbosacral region induces pain in animals with degenerative lumbosacral disease. Extension of the hips usually produces extension of the lumbosacral joint as well as stretching of the lumbosacral nerves. Therefore hip extension is not a good test for differentiating hip pain from lumbosacral pain.

Palpation of individual muscles without pressure on bones or joints identifies muscular pain. The quadriceps, semitendinosus, semimembranosus, and gastrocnemius muscles in the pelvic limb and triceps and carpal flexor muscles in the thoracic limb are good examples.

Palpation of the head, temporal muscles, mandible, and opening the mouth are important in assessing cranial structures.

DISEASES

Table 14-1 lists neurologic diseases that frequently cause pain. Most of these are discussed in other chapters, as indicated in the table. The only neurologic disease that frequently causes pain without other clinical signs is meningitis.

Meningitis

Inflammation of the meninges, or *meningitis,* may be caused by many infectious agents, including bacterial, viral, fungal, protozoal, and rickettsial organisms.[10] A complete list is in the tables in Chapter 15. In addition, autoimmune diseases can cause meningitis, as can some diseases of unknown origin, such as granulomatous meningoencephalomyelitis (GME),[11] a meningitis characterized by an eosinophilic cerebrospinal fluid (CSF),[12] and a suppurative, noninfectious meningitis.[13,14] A vasculitis and meningitis seen in dogs, primarily beagles, has been called the *canine pain syndrome.*[15]

Bacterial meningitis is more common in large animals than in pets. It is most common in neonatal foals, calves, and lambs. *Staphylococcus* organisms may cause bacterial meningitis in dogs, but gram-negative infections are increasing in frequency. Bacterial infections occur by hematogenous spread from infections in other parts of the body; by direct extension from adjacent structures including sinuses, eyes, or ears; and from direct trauma including surgery and CSF collection. The organisms spread through the CSF to both spinal and intracranial meninges. Vasculitis is common, especially in rickettsial infections and immune-mediated disease.[10,15]

Regardless of the cause of meningitis, the potential for the inflammatory process to extend to the nervous tissue is always present. The resulting

Table 14-1   **Neurologic Causes of Pain***

Localization/Class	Acute Nonprogressive	Acute Progressive	Chronic Progressive
Multifocal or Diffuse			
Inflammatory	Meningitis Myositis Neuritis		
Localized			
Degenerative		Disk (type I)	Disk (type II) Spondylosis Lumbosacral stenosis Cervical vertebral spondylopathy
Anomalous		Atlantoaxial instability Hydrocephalus	
Neoplastic			Vertebral Extradural Intradural-extramedullary
Inflammation		Diskospondylitis Osteomyelitis Abscess	
Trauma	Fractures Luxations		
Vascular	Ischemic myopathy		Immune vasculitis

encephalitis, myelitis, or encephalomyelitis causes other clinical signs such as seizures, paresis, ataxia, or altered mental status. Cranial and spinal nerves may be affected. Communicating hydrocephalus may develop because of reduced absorption of CSF in the subarachnoid space and through the venous sinuses. Occlusion of the CSF pathways may also cause obstructive hydrocephalus.

Animals with meningitis are systemically ill. The onset is usually acute, and signs are progressive. The animals may be lethargic and reluctant to eat. Many animals, especially dogs, have rigidity with generalized pain that seems worse in the cervical region. Palpation of the vertebral column and head usually causes the animal to splint the muscles and appear uncomfortable, in contrast to palpation of limb musculature; however, small animals may appear to be in pain everywhere. They frequently walk as if they do not want to jar their body, as if "walking on egg shells." A fever may be present.

The diagnosis is supported by finding increased white blood cells (WBCs) in the CSF. Bacterial infections are generally associated with a WBC count of 500 to 1000 cells per microliter, with a predominance of neutrophils. Rickettsial infections have variable numbers and mixed populations of cells. Ehrlichiosis is more likely to be associated with a predominance of mononuclear cells, whereas Rocky Mountain spotted fever may produce more neutrophils.[10,16] Viral infections generally have a slight increase in WBCs, predominately mononuclear cells. Fungal infections show very high WBC counts with a mixed population of cells, sometimes including many eosinophils.

Antibiotic or corticosteroid therapy may reduce the number of WBCs, especially neutrophils. Organisms may be seen on appropriately stained sediment or on electron microscopy. Cryptococcal organisms are best observed with an India ink preparation. Culture and sensitivity testing in all suspected cases is an important diagnostic aid. Results are most likely to be rewarding when neutrophilic pleocytosis is present. Protein content of the CSF is elevated in meningitis and is highest in bacterial and fungal infections (usually >100 mg/dl). Treatment of infectious diseases is discussed in Chapter 15.

METHODS OF MEASURING PAIN

It is extremely difficult to determine the degree of pain an animal is experiencing, although it is well accepted that animals experience pain in much the same way as humans. Animal caregivers currently use scales adapted for humans. Whereas human patients have the capacity to record the intensity of their pain, in animals pain is measured by using physiologic data and subjective behavioral observation. Clinical variables that can be studied and quantified include heart and respiratory rates; rectal temperature; packed cell volume; and serum concentrations of glucose, cortisol, norepinephrine, and epinephrine. The stress associated with pain may cause increases in heart and respiratory rates and systolic blood pressure.[17] In cats recovering from ovariohysterectomy, increased cortisol concentrations and increased systolic blood pressure were the best indicators of postoperative pain.[17]

The three scales used in animals and humans are the simple descriptive scale (SDS), numeric rating scale (NRS), and visual analog scale (VAS). The SDS allows the observer to rate subjectively the degree of pain from no pain to very severe pain. The NRS is similar to the SDS, except numeric values are assigned to behavioral observations such as vocalization, movement, and agitation.[18] The NRS is commonly modified to include numeric values assigned to physiologic data. A modified NRS has been described that includes physiologic data, response to palpation, activity, mental status, posture, and vocalization.[19] The VAS is a simple scale comprising a straight line (usually 100 mm long) with the limits of the scale written at each end. The observer, or in medicine the patient, marks the line at the point that reflects the degree of pain observed or perceived. Although the VAS is subject to a great deal of variation, it is believed to be more sensitive than either the NRS or SDS in human patients. In veterinary medicine, some variations of SDS or NRS are commonly used. The accuracy of pain-rating scales is usually established by comparing scores with indicators of stress such as increased heart rate and increased concentrations of plasma cortisol. Regardless of the scale used, significant variability exists among trained observers in describing the degree of pain animals experience in the postoperative period.[20]

TREATMENT

Relief of pain in animals was often ignored in the past. Greater awareness of the signs associated with pain has resulted in more aggressive management.[21,22] Pain management in humans includes three categories of therapy: pharmacologic, physical, and psychologic.[23] Pharmacologic and physical methods are used commonly in animals, but psychologic methods are rarely used.

Pharmacologic Management

Analgesic agents include narcotics, antiinflammatory drugs, anesthetics, and psychotropic drugs (Tables 14-2 through 14-7). Anesthetic agents are

Table 14-2   **Analgesic Agents for Dogs**

Analgesic	Dosage (mg/kg) and Route	Duration of Action (hr)	Comments and Side Effects
Opioids			
Morphine	0.1-2.0 IM, SC	3-6	Vomiting, defecation, poor temperature control, increased intracranial pressure
Oxymorphone	0.05-0.22 IV, IM, SC	2-6	Auditory hypersensitivity, increased intracranial pressure
Meperidine	2-6 IM, SC	1-2	Increased intracranial pressure
Codeine	1-2 PO	6	Oral therapy combined with acetaminophen or aspirin
Pentazocine	0.1-0.4 IM	2-4	Poor analgesic
Butorphanol	0.2-0.4 IV, IM, SC	2-6	Minimal side effects
Buprenorphine	0.01-0.02 IV, IM, SC	6-12	
Fentanyl	25, 50, 75, 100 (µg/hr) dermal patches	5 days	Smallest patches are appropriate for small dogs and cats
Nonsteroidal Antiinflammatory Drugs			
Aspirin	10-20 PO	2-4	Combine with codeine, give every 8-12 hr
Acetaminophen	10-20 PO	2-4	Combine with codeine, give every 8-12 hr
Flunixin	0.5-2.2 IM, IV	6-8	Caution with repeated doses
Phenylbutazone	10 PO 22 IV	6-8	Maximum of 800 mg/day
Other Analgesic Agents			
Xylazine	0.05-0.2 IV, IM	1-3	Best when combined with opioid

IM, Intramuscularly; *SC,* subcutaneously; *IV,* intravenously; *PO,* orally.

not discussed. Species variability is important in selecting agents to control pain.[24] For example, the cat, horse, and ruminant may become hyperexcitable with doses of morphine that produce sedation in the dog. These effects may be prevented by combining the narcotic with other agents such as phenothiazine tranquilizers or xylazine.

Narcotics are effective analgesics, providing relief in most cases regardless of the cause of the pain. They are less effective for neurotrophic pain. Their effect occurs primarily in the CNS, and they cause depression of behavior and respiration. Opioid narcotics are controlled drugs. They are frequently given for postoperative and trauma-induced pain. Synthetic agents with both agonist and antagonist opioid effects include butorphanol and buprenorphine.[22,25-27] These agents are not controlled and provide moderate analgesic effects with less depressive effects.

Table 14-3   **Analgesic Agents for Cats**

Analgesic	Dosage (mg/kg) and Route	Duration of Action (hr)	Comments and Side Effects
Opioids			
Morphine	0.1 IM, SC	3-6	Excitement with higher doses
Oxymorphone	0.05-0.22 IV, IM, SC	2-6	Excitement with higher doses, auditory hypersensitivity
Meperidine	2-10 IM, SC	1-2	
Pentazocine	0.75-3.0 IM, SC, IV	2-4	Higher doses have been used
Butorphanol	0.2-0.4 IV, IM, SC	2-6	Minimal side effects
Buprenorphine	0.005-0.01 IM, SC	6-12	
Nonsteroidal Antiinflammatory Drugs			
Aspirin	10 PO	48	Caution with repeated doses
Other Analgesic Agents			
Ketamine	2-4 IV, IM	0.5	Dissociative anesthetic
Xylazine	0.05-0.2 IV, IM	0.5	Best combined with other agents

IM, Intramuscularly; *SC,* subcutaneously; *IV,* intravenously, *PO,* orally.

Table 14-4 **Analgesic Agents for Horses**

Analgesic	Dosage (mg/kg) and Route	Frequency of Administration (hr)	Comments and Side Effects
Opioids			
Morphine	0.2-0.3 IM, IV, SC	4-7	Best after giving xylazine; excitement with higher doses
Meperidine	2-4 IM, IV	0.5-1.0	Excitement, hypotension (IV)
Pentazocine	0.33-0.66 IM, SC, IV	1	
Butorphanol	0.1-0.2 IM	2-4	Excitement with higher doses
Fentanyl	0.1 IV, IM, SC	2	Pacing
Methadone	0.25 IM, IV	6	
Nonsteroidal Antiinflammatory Drugs			
Aspirin	30-50 PO	12	
Dipyrone	5-10 g (total dose) SC, IM, IV	8-24	
Flunixin	1.1 IM, IV, PO	24	Repeat for colic-induced pain, no more than 5 days
Phenylbutazone	4-8 PO 3-6 IV	24 (PO) 12 (IV)	Maximum dose, 8.8 mg/kg daily
Naproxen	10 PO	12	
Meclofenamic acid	2.2 PO	24	Lower dose if used more than 5-7 days
Other Analgesic Agents			
Xylazine	1.1 IV 2.2 IM	0.5	Best combined with other agents

IM, Intramuscularly; *IV*, intravenously; *SC*, subcutaneously; *PO*, orally.

Table 14-5 **Analgesic Agents for Cattle**

Analgesic	Dosage (mg/kg) and Route	Duration of Action (hr)	Comments and Side Effects
Opioids			
Meperidine	3.3-4.4 IM, SC	1-2	Regulatory concern
Nonsteroidal Antiinflammatory Drugs			
Aspirin	50-100 PO	12	
Phenylbutazone	10-20 PO	24	
Other Analgesic Agents			
Xylazine	0.1-0.2 IM	Once	Brahman sensitive, not approved for use (FDA)

IM, Intramuscularly; *SC*, subcutaneously; *PO*, orally; *FDA*, U.S. Food and Drug Administration.

Table 14-6 **Analgesic Agents for Sheep and Goats**

Analgesic	Dosage (mg/kg) and Route	Frequency of Administration (hr)	Comments and Side Effects
Opioids			
Meperidine	1-3 IM	12	
Pentazocine	3.0 IM	4	
Buprenorphine	0.005-0.2 IM	12	
Other Analgesic Agents			
Sodium salicylate	1-4 g (total dose) IV	24	
Xylazine	0.05-0.2 IM	Once	Combinations used

IM, Intramuscularly; *IV*, intravenously.

Table 14-7 **Analgesic Agents for Swine**

Analgesic	Dosage (mg/kg) and Route	Frequency of Administration (hr)
Opioids		
Meperidine	2.0 IM	4
Pentazocine	3.0 IM	4
Buprenorphine	0.005-0.01 IM	12
Nonsteroidal Antiinflammatory Drugs		
Sodium salicylate	1-4 g (total dose) IV	24
Aspirin	10 PO	6

IM, Intramuscularly; *IV,* intravenously; *PO,* orally.

Fentanyl citrate patches provide analgesia for several days.[28,29] The patches are available in four sizes releasing from 25 to 100 µg per hour. The smallest patch maintains a serum level in the therapeutic range for humans. Fentanyl transdermal patches have been used in cats following onychectomy, and the degree of analgesia provided was compared with butorphanol.[30] The fentanyl patch provided analgesia comparable to butorphanol. The potential benefits include avoidance of injections, home use, and adequate serum levels without peaks and troughs. The drug is released faster if body or environmental temperature is elevated.[28] Potential for human abuse is of concern.

Antiinflammatory drugs are most effective in pain associated with inflammation but may be effective in neurotrophic pain as well. The nonsteroidal antiinflammatory drugs (NSAIDs) are widely used, and their action is potentiated by combination with the opioids.[26] A combination of codeine and acetaminophen or aspirin is frequently given for spinal pain associated with disk disease or surgery. NSAIDs are primarily peripherally acting agents that reduce the interaction of humoral substances (e.g., kinins, substance P, histamine, eicosanoids) with pain receptors. These agents have the potential for causing a variety of side effects, especially gastrointestinal hemorrhage and renal failure. Considerable species variability exists in their effectiveness and in the severity of side effects.[25,26] Several studies have compared the effects of injectable NSAIDs and opioid agents.[31-33] These studies generally indicate that carprofen, ketoprofen, and flunixin provide postoperative analgesia at least equal to or sometimes better than the analgesia provided by butorphanol and oxymorphone without creating the sedative side effects characteristic of these opioid agents; however, NSAIDs such as ketoprofen and flunixin are associated with gastrointestinal ulceration in dogs and cats. Renal lesions may also occur, especially in hypovolemic patients.

NSAIDs block prostaglandins that may be protective to the kidney during hypovolemic states. NSAIDs such as carprofen may accentuate postsurgical analgesia when given before surgical procedures; however, NSAIDs may inhibit platelet function, and this causes problems with primary hemostasis. Conventional treatment suggests that the administration of NSAIDs just before surgery or immediately after surgery is best. If NASIDs are used during surgery, maintaining normovolemia and normal renal blood flow are important to prevent renal lesions and potential renal failure.

Xylazine is the most common α_2-agonist currently in use, but detomidine for horses and medetomidine for dogs and cats are also available.[15,25] Xylazine produces mild analgesia in small animals, moderate visceral (but not limb) analgesia in horses, and nearly anesthetic effects in ruminants.

Other psychotropic drugs include tranquilizers and ketamine. The tranquilizers, including phenothiazine derivatives, benzodiazepines, and butyrophenones, are primarily useful in reducing anxiety associated with pain. They may potentiate the effects of other analgesic agents but should not be given alone in the treatment of pain. Ketamine is a dissociative anesthetic and is not generally used for the management of pain.

The issue of pain management is an important dimension in veterinary practice. The willingness to provide pain intervention should be routine in veterinary medicine. Considerable evidence exists that preemptive pain management can be effective in decreasing the development of chronic pain states and is beneficial to the health, recovery, and quality of life of veterinary patients.

Physical Therapy

A variety of therapeutic techniques are helpful in reducing swelling, pain, and discomfort from injury. Commonly available methods are applications of heat or cold, passive exercise, hydrotherapy, and massage. Electrical stimulation is being used in humans with success, but little information is available about its application to veterinary medicine.

Psychologic Therapy

Biofeedback, operant conditioning, hypnosis, and meditation are components of chronic pain therapy in humans. These techniques are probably not applicable to animals.

Acupuncture

Acupuncture is still controversial, although substantial evidence exists for its benefits in treating pain. If it is used for pain relief, and not as a substitute for correction of the cause of pain, it is appropriate.[34-36]

References

1. Colloquium on Recognition and Alleviation of Animal Pain and Distress, *J Am Vet Med Assoc* 191:1184-1298, 1987.
2. Short CE, Poznak AV: *Animal pain.* New York, 1992, Churchill Livingstone.
3. Kitchell R: Problems in defining pain and peripheral mechanisms of pain, *J Am Vet Med Assoc* 191:1195-1199, 1987.
4. Willis WD, Coggeshall RE: *Sensory mechanisms of the spinal cord.* New York, 1991, Plenum Press.
5. Kruger L, Rodin BE: Peripheral mechanisms involved in pain. In Kitchell RL, et al, editors: *Animal pain perception and alleviation.* Bethesda, Md, 1983, American Physiological Society.
6. Willis WD Jr: *The pain system: the neural basis of nociceptive transmission in the mammalian nervous system.* Basel, 1985, S Karger.
7. Willis W, Chung J: Central mechanisms of pain, *J Am Vet Med Assoc* 191:1200-1202, 1987.
8. Schmidt RF: *Fundamentals of sensory physiology.* Berlin, 1986, Springer Verlag.
9. Muir WW, Woolf CJ: Mechanisms of pain and their therapeutic implications, *J Am Vet Med Assoc* 10:1346-1356, 2001.
10. Meric SM: Canine meningitis: a changing emphasis, *J Vet Intern Med* 2:26-35, 1988.
11. Cook JR Jr: Granulomatous meningoencephalomyelitis, *Vet Med Rep* 1:321-327, 1989.
12. Smith Maxie LL, et al: Cerebrospinal fluid analysis and clinical outcome of eight dogs with eosinophilic meningoencephalomyelitis, *J Vet Intern Med* 3:167-174, 1989.
13. Russo E, Lees G, Hall C: Corticosteroid-responsive aseptic suppurative meningitis in three dogs, *Southwest Vet* 35:197-201, 1983.
14. Meric S, Perman V, Hardy R: Corticosteroid responsive meningitis in ten dogs, *J Am Anim Hosp Assoc* 21:677-684, 1985.
15. Burns JC, Felsburg PJ, Wilson H, et al: Canine pain syndrome is a model for the study of Kawaski disease, *Perspect Biol Med* 35:68-73, 1991.
16. Greene CE: Update on neurologic and serologic findings on RMSF in dogs. In *Proceedings of an American College of Veterinary Internal Medicine Forum,* San Diego, 1987, pp 691-692.
17. Smith JD, Allen SW, et al: Indicators of postoperative pain in cats and correlation with clinical criteria, *Am J Vet Res* 57:1674-1678, 1996.
18. Conzemius MG, Hill CM, et al: Correlation between subjective and objective measures used to determine severity of post operative pain in dogs, *J Am Vet Med Assoc* 210:1619-1622, 1999.
19. Firth AM, Haldane SL: Development of a scale to evaluate postoperative pain in dogs, *J Am Vet Med Assoc* 214:651-659, 1998.
20. Holton LL, Scott EM, et al: Comparison of three methods used for assessment of pain in dogs, *J Am Vet Med Assoc* 212:61-66, 1998.
21. Tranquilli WJ, Raffe MR: Understanding pain and analgesic therapy in pets, *Vet Med* 841:680-686, 1989.
22. Potthoff A, Carithers RW: Pain and analgesia in dogs and cats, *Compend Cont Educ Pract Vet* 11:887-897, 1989.
23. Maciewicz R, Mucke L: Pain. In Johnson RT, editor: *Current therapy in neurologic disease.* Philadelphia, 1987, BC Decker.
24. Benson G, Thurmon J: Species difference as a consideration in alleviation of animal pain and distress, *J Am Vet Med Assoc* 191:1227-1230, 1987.
25. Tranquilli WJ, Fikes L, Raffe MR: Selecting the right analgesics: indications and dosage requirements, *Vet Med* 84:692-697, 1989.
26. Jenkins W: Pharmacologic aspects of analgesic drugs in animals: an overview, *J Am Vet Med Assoc* 191:1231-1240, 1987.
27. Raffe MR, Tranquilli WJ: Classifying commonly used analgesic agents, *Vet Med* 84:687-690, 1989.
28. Scherk-Nixon M: A study of the use of a transdermal fentanyl patch in cats, *J Am Anim Hosp Assoc* 32:19-24, 1996.
29. Brock N: Treating moderate and severe pain in small animals, *Can Vet J* 36:658-660, 1995.
30. Gleeasch KL, Kruse-Elliott KT, et al: Comparison of transdermal administration of Fentanyl versus intramuscular administration of butorphanol for analgesia after onychectomy in cats, *J Am Vet Med Assoc* 220:1020-1024, 2002.
31. Mathews KA, Paley DM, et al: A comparison of ketorolac with flunixin, butorphanol, and oxymorphine in controlling postoperative pain in dogs, *Can Vet J* 37:557-567, 1996.
32. Pibarot P, Dupuis J, et al: Comparison of ketoprofen, oxymorphine hydrochloride, and butorphanol in the treatment of postoperative pain in dogs, *J Am Vet Assoc* 211:438-444, 1997.
33. Slingsby LS, Waterman-Pearson AE: Postoperative analgesia in the cat after ovariohysterectomy by use of carprofen, ketoprofen, meloxicam, or tolfenamic acid, *J Small Anim Pract* 41:447-450, 2000.
34. Latshaw W: Current theories of pain perception related to acupuncture, *J Am Anim Hosp Assoc* 11:449-450, 1975.
35. Vincent C, Richardson P: The evaluation of therapeutic acupuncture: concepts and methods, *Pain* 24:1-13, 1986.
36. Martin B, Klide A: Use of acupuncture for the treatment of chronic back pain in horses: Stimulation of acupuncture points with saline solution injections, *J Am Vet Med Assoc* 190:1177-1180, 1987.

Chapter 15

Systemic or Multifocal Signs

The first step in the management of a neurologic problem is localization of the disease process to a single anatomic site. Localization has been emphasized throughout this book; however, a group of diseases that produce more than one lesion or that affect most of the central nervous system (CNS) simultaneously has not yet been discussed. These disorders are categorized as multifocal, systemic, or diffuse diseases. Initially, some of these diseases may appear as focal diseases, but they progress to affect other areas.

LESION LOCALIZATION

The key to recognition of these diseases is a neurologic examination that indicates the involvement of two or more parts of the nervous system that are not closely related anatomically. The most obvious example is an abnormality in both the brain and the spinal cord. All the possible combinations of signs of diffuse or multifocal diseases are too extensive to list, but Table 15-1 outlines some of the more common ones. Anytime the neurologic examination does not strongly indicate a single lesion, this group of diseases becomes more likely.

DISEASES

The major disease categories that produce systemic or multifocal signs are degenerative, metabolic, neoplastic, nutritional, inflammatory, and toxic disorders. Some of these diseases may be chiefly focal in the individual animal, such as primary CNS neoplasms, but they are capable of affecting any part of the nervous system and therefore are included in this section. Diseases that are primarily skeletal in origin are mentioned but not discussed. All these diseases are progressive. The acute or chronic onset and the rate of progression may be of some help in establishing the diagnosis (Table 15-2).

DEGENERATIVE DISEASES

New primary degenerative diseases of the CNS continue to be recognized. These diseases are usually inherited and are relatively rare, but they are important in specific breeds. They are also important because they often serve as excellent models of similar human diseases. Anyone recognizing one of these diseases should contact a neurologist or one of the authors of the papers listed in the references.

Three groups of diseases are discussed: (1) storage diseases, (2) abiotrophies, and (3) degenerations of unknown cause. Primary vascular disease is discussed in Chapter 6 (spinal cord) and Chapter 12 (brain).

Storage Diseases

A large group of diseases are characterized pathologically by the accumulation of metabolic products in cells (Table 15-3). A genetically based deficiency of an enzyme causes accumulation of the product in neurons, glia, or other cells. The effect of the disease may be caused by the accumulation of the product or may be a direct result of the metabolic disturbance.[1] Because the clinical signs and the progression of the disease depend on the pathologic process, many of the conditions are similar. Two groups are commonly recognized: *neuronal storage diseases,* in which the product accumulates in neurons, and *leukodystrophies,* in which progressive destruction of myelin occurs.[2]

The storage diseases are rare, and several have been reported in domestic animals. Most have been recognized in dogs or cats. Animals are usually normal at birth, but they fail to grow normally. Signs typically occur within the first few months of life but may be delayed until adulthood with some conditions.[3] Most of the diseases that have been studied have a recessive mode of inheritance, and so only a portion of the litter is affected. Inbreeding is common in most of the animals studied. Onset of clinical signs is usually in the first few months of life (see Table 15-3). All the disorders are slowly progressive and lead to the animal's death.[4] Bone marrow transplantation may have value in some

Table 15-1 **Examples of Systemic or Multifocal Signs**

Lower motor neuron (LMN) signs (More than one location, may include cranial nerves)
  Diffuse LMN diseases, polyneuropathy (see Chapter 7)
Brain and spinal cord signs
  Pelvic limb paresis and seizures
Systemic disease and CNS signs
  Fever, anorexia, ataxia or seizures
Generalized pain
  Meningitis
Cerebral cortex and brainstem
  Seizures and cranial nerve deficits, blindness, severe gait deficits, head tilt, circling
Bilateral cerebral cortex
  Blindness with normal pupils (may be seen with brain swelling, hydrocephalus) (see Chapter 11)
Cerebellum and paresis
  Head tremor, ataxia, severe gait deficits, paresis
Ascending paralysis
  Pelvic limb paresis progressing to tetraparesis (focal cervical spinal cord lesion must be ruled out)

conditions and has been used experimentally in affected animals.[5]

The lysosomal storage diseases are important diseases because (1) they are genetic disorders and can be eliminated by selective breeding; (2) they may be confused with conditions of nongenetic origin, such as viral diseases; and (3) they are important models for diseases of human. Colonies of animals with some of these diseases have been established at research institutions.

Abiotrophies and Other Degenerative Diseases

The normal neuron is not capable of dividing and reproducing itself but has the capacity to survive for the life of the animal. An abnormality of the metabolic pathways leads to early death of the neuron. This process is termed *abiotrophy*.[6]

The classification proposed by de Lahunta[6] is used in Table 15-4. The degeneration is characterized as primarily motor neuronal, multisystemic, cerebellar, or peripheral. The multisystem disorders are further characterized as to the primary site of the degenerative process—cell body, cell process, myelin, and so forth.

Most of these diseases are seen in young animals, with the exception of degenerative myelopathy of German shepherd dogs (see Chapter 6 and Table 15-4).

Clinical signs relate to the primary site affected. The motor neuron degenerations produce generalized lower motor neuron (LMN) signs (see Chapter 7); myelin disorders cause ataxia that progresses to paresis; and cerebellar degenerations cause ataxia, dysmetria, and tremor (see Chapter 8). The progression is generally slow (over months) but unrelenting.

Table 15-2 **Etiology of Systemic Diseases***

Classification	Acute Progressive	Chronic Progressive
Degenerative		Storage disease
		Abiotrophy
Metabolic	*Hepatic encephalopathy*	*Hepatic encephalopathy*
	Hypoglycemia	Endocrine disease
	Endocrine disease	
	Renal disease	
Neoplastic	Metastatic	*Primary*
		Metastatic
Nutritional		Hypovitaminosis
		Hypervitaminosis
Inflammatory	Infection	Infection (usually viral)
Toxic	Most toxins	*Heavy metals*
		Other toxins, low dosages

*Italics indicate most common diseases seen clinically.
Modified with permission from Oliver JE, Hoerlein BF, Mayhew IG: *Veterinary neurology,* Philadelphia, 1987, WB Saunders, Table 6-1.

Table 15-3 **Storage Diseases**

Disease	Enzyme Deficit (Storage Product)	Signalment (Age When Signs First Occur)	Clinical Signs/ Diagnosis	Human Disease	References
Gangliosidosis GM$_1$ Type 1	β-Galactosidase (ganglioside)	Beagle crosses (3 mo), Portuguese water dogs (5 mo); domestic cats (2-3 mo); Friesian cattle (CNS-1 mo)	Tremor, incoordination, spastic paraplegia, impaired vision; assay enzyme in white blood cells, skin fibroblast cultures, biopsy of lymph node or cerebellum	Norman-Landing disease	168-171
Type 2	β-Galactosidase (ganglioside)	Siamese, Korat, and domestic cats (2-3 mo); Suffolk sheep (4 mo)	Same as Type 1	Derry's disease	172
Gangliosidosis GM$_2$ Type 1	Hexosaminidase A (ganglioside)	German shorthaired pointers (6-9 mo), Japanese spaniels (18 mo)	Ataxia, incoordination, impaired vision, dementia; assay enzyme in white blood cells, biopsy of cerebrum	Tay-Sachs disease	172-174
Type 2	Hexosaminidase A, B (ganglioside)	Domestic cats (2 mo)	Same as cats with GM$_1$ gangliosidosis	Sandhoff's disease	175, 176
Type 3	Hexosaminidase A (ganglioside)	Mixed-breed dogs (1.5 y); Yorkshire swine (CNS-3 mo)	Ataxia, incoordination, tremor, hypermetria	Bernheimer-Seitelberger disease	177
Glucocerebrosidosis	β-Glucosidase (glucocerebroside)	Sydney silky dog (6-8 mo)	Ataxia, incoordination, hypermetria; assay enzyme in white blood cells, skin fibroblast cultures, biopsy of lymph node, liver, bone marrow, cerebellum	Gaucher's disease	178
Sphingomyelinosis	Sphingomyelinase (sphingomyelin)	Siamese, Balinese, domestic cats (2-4 mo); poodles (2-4 mo)	Ataxia, incoordination, tremor, hypermetria, polyneuropathy; assay enzyme in white blood cells, bone marrow, skin fibroblast cultures, biopsy of bone marrow, cerebellum	Niemann-Pick disease	179-182

Continued

Table 15-3 **Storage Diseases**—continued

Disease	Enzyme Deficit (Storage Product)	Signalment (Age When Signs First Occur)	Clinical Signs/ Diagnosis	Human Disease	References
Globoid cell leukodystrophy	β-Galactosidase (galactocerebrosidase)	Cairn terriers, west highland white terriers (2-5 mo); beagles, bluetick coonhounds (4 mo); miniature poodles (2 y); Basset Hounds (1.5-2 y); Pomeranians (1.5 y); domestic cats (5-6 wk); polled Dorset sheep (4-18 mo)	Ataxia, incoordination, tremor, progressive paraparesis, hypermetria, impaired vision; cerebrospinal fluid macrophages with myelin; assay enzyme in white blood cells	Krabbe's disease	183-190
Metachromatic leukodystrophy	Arylsulfatase (sulfatide)	Domestic cats (2 wk)	Progressive motor dysfunction, seizures, opisthotonos		191, 192
Mucopolysaccharidosis	Arylsulfatase B (mucopolysaccharide)	Siamese, domestic cat (4-7 mo)	Progressive paraparesis	Maroteaux-Lamy disease	193-195
	α_1-Iduronidase (mucopolysaccharide)	Domestic cat (10 mo); Plott hounds (3-6 mo), miniature pinschers (6 mo), mixed-breed dogs (4-6 mo)	Progressive paraparesis	Hurler's syndrome	194,196-198
Glycoproteinosis	(? Glycoprotein)	Beagles, Basset hounds, poodles (5 mo-9 yr)	Depression, progressive seizures; biopsy of lymph nodes, liver, cerebellum	Lafora's disease	3,199,200
Mannosidosis	α-Mannosidase (mannoside)	Domestic cats (7 mo); Persian cats (8 wk); Angus, Murray grey cattle, Galloway calves (birth)	Ataxia, incoordination, tremor, and aggression (calves); assay of urine oligosaccharide	Mannosidosis	201-205
	β-Mannosidase (mannoside)	Nubian goats (birth-1 yr)	Ataxia, recumbency	β-Mannosidosis	206, 207

Glycogenosis	α-Glucosidase	Incoordination, exercise intolerance	Lapland dogs (1.5 yr), English springer Spaniels (1 yr); domestic. Norwegian Forest cats (5 mo); Corriedale sheep (6 mo); Shorthorn, Brahman cattle (3-9 mo)	Pompe's disease	208-216
Fucosidosis	α_1-Fucosidase	Incoordination, behavioral changes, dysphonia, dysphagia, seizures; assay enzyme in white blood cells	Springer spaniels (2 yr)		217-219
Ceroid lipofuscinosis	Unknown abnormality	Personality change, visual impairment, ataxia, incoordination, jaw champing, seizures; biopsy of lymph nodes, cerebellum	English setters (1 yr); dachshunds (3.5-7 yr); Cocker Spaniels (1.5 yr); Chihuahuas, Salukis (2 yr); Tibetan terriers (3 yr); Australian Cattle Dogs (14 mo); Border Collies (18-22 mo); Blue Heelers (12 mo); Yugoslavian Sheep Dogs (1 y); mixed-breed dogs (4 mo); Siamese, domestic cats (2-7 y). South Hampshire sheep (6-18 mo); Ramboui let sheep (9-12 mo); Devon cattle (14 mo); Nubian goats (10 mo)	Batten's disease, ceroid lipofuscinosis	220-234

Modified from Oliver JE, Hoerlein BF, Mayhew IG: *Veterinary neurology*, Philadelphia, 1987, WB Saunders, Table 6-1.

Table 15-4 **Abiotrophies and Degenerative Diseases of Unknown Cause**

Anatomic Location	Signalment (Age When Signs First occur)	Clinical Signs	References
Motor neuron	Swedish Laplands (5-7 wk), St. Bernard × Great Dane × Bloodhound crosses (8-14 wk), Brittany Spaniels (6 wk, 6 mo, 1 y), Rottweilers (1-4 wk), English Pointers (5 mo), German Shepherd Dogs (2 wk)	Lower motor neuron (LMN) paralysis and atrophy of muscles of the trunk and limbs	235-240
Multisystem Cell body	Cocker Spaniels (1 y), Cairn Terriers (2.5-5 mo); Angora goats (1 wk-4 mo)	Cerebellar ataxia, spastic paresis	241-244
Cell processes	Smooth Fox Terriers (2.5-4 mo), Jack Russell Terriers (2.5-4 mo)	Cerebellar ataxia, dysmetria, spasticity; rapid early progression, then slow progression	4, 245
	Bullmastiffs (6-9 wk)	Visual abnormality, cerebellar ataxia, primarily in pelvic limbs; head tremor, abnormal nystagmus, behavioral change	246
	German Shepherd Dogs (4-5 y), Siberian Huskies (10-11 y), sporadically in other dog breeds	Progressive pelvic limb ataxia and paresis	247-250
	Simmental (5-8 mo), Limousin crossbred cattle (4 mo)	Progressive ataxia, behavioral change; progresses to recumbency and death by 12 mo	4, 78
	Brown Swiss cattle (5-8 mo)	Progressive pelvic limb paresis and ataxia, thoracic limbs affected late	251, 252
	Appaloosa, Morgan, Przewalski, and other horses; Grant zebras (before 7-14 mo)	Slowly progressive ataxia and paresis of all four limbs; some cases related to vitamin E deficiency	72, 73, 78
Myelin	Rottweilers (1.5-3.5 y)	Ataxia, dysmetria, tetraparesis	253
	Labrador Retrievers (4-6 mo)	Extensor rigidity and opisthotonos, progressive cerebellar ataxia	254
	Dalmatians (3-6 mo)	Progressive visual deficiency and locomotor abnormality	4
	Salukis (3 mo)	Seizures, behavioral change	255
	Afghan hounds (3-13 mo)	Pelvic limb ataxia and paresis, progressing to paraplegia in 7-10 d; varying degrees of thoracic limb involvement later	256
	Egyptian Mau cats (7 wk)	Ataxia, seizures	257
	Charolais cattle (6-36 mo)	Slowly progressive pelvic limb paresis and ataxia	4, 78
	Murray Grey cattle (birth-12 mo)	Spastic pelvic limb paresis and ataxia	4, 78
	Polled Hereford cattle (1-3 d)	Dull, recumbent, opisthotonos	258
Neuroaxonal dystrophy	Collies (2-4 mo), Rottweilers (1-2 yr), Chihuahuas (7 wk)	Progressive cerebellar ataxia, tremor	259-262
	German shepherd dogs (15 mo)	Progressive pelvic limb paresis and ataxia	263, 264
	Boxers (1-7 mo)	Spastic pelvic limb paresis, late tetraparesis	265, 266
	Siamese and domestic cats (5 wk)	Progressive cerebellar ataxia	267
	Suffolk (1.5-5 mo), Merino (1-4 y), Coopworth (1-6 mo) sheep	Progressive paresis and ataxia	268
	Morgan horses (6-12 mo)	Spastic pelvic limb paresis and ataxia	269, 270

Table 15-4 **Abiotrophies and Degenerative Diseases of Unknown Cause**—continued

Anatomic Location	Signalment (Age When Signs First occur)	Clinical Signs	References
Neurofilaments	Collies (3 wk)	Paresis of limbs	271
	Domestic cats (3 wk)	Progressive paresis of all four limbs	272
	Yorkshire pigs (5 wk)	Progressive paresis	273
	Grant zebras (2 wk)	Progressive tetraparesis	4
	Hereford cattle (birth)	Progressive spastic paraplegia	274
Cerebellum			
Autosomal recessive	Kerry Blue terriers (8-16 wk), Gordon setters (6-30 mo), rough-coated Collies (4-12 wk), Australian Kelpies (6-12 wk), Bullmastiffs (4-9 wk)	Progressive cerebellar ataxia, dysmetria, tremor	275-281
Multiple litters	Airedale terriers, Bernese Mountain dogs, Finnish Harriers, Brittany spaniels, Border collies, beagles, Samoyeds, Clumber Spaniels, Akitas, Bern Running Dogs	Progressive cerebellar ataxia, dysmetria, tremor	3, 4, 281-283
Single dog or litter	Miniature poodles, Fox Terriers, Cairn terriers, Cocker spaniels, Labrador retrievers, Golden retrievers, great Danes, Schnauzer/beagle crosses, mixed-breed dogs	Progressive cerebellar ataxia, dysmetria, tremor	3, 4, 284
Cats	Domestic cats	Progressive cerebellar ataxia	285
Cattle	Aberdeen Anguses, Ayrshires, Charolais, Herefords, Holsteins, Shorthorns	Progressive cerebellar ataxia	3, 286-288
Horses	Arabians, Gotland ponies, Oldbergs	Progressive cerebellar ataxia	78
Sheep	Corriedales, Merinos, Welsh Mountain sheep, Border Leicesters	Progressive cerebellar ataxia	3, 4, 78, 289, 290
Swine	Yorkshires, Saddlebacks	Progressive cerebellar ataxia	3, 78, 291
Astrocytes	Labrador retrievers, Scottish terriers, Alpine sheep	Progressive spasticity and ataxia	4, 292
Schwann cells	Tibetan mastiffs (7-12 wk)	Pelvic limb paresis	293, 294
Nociceptive neurons	English pointers, European Shorthaired Pointers (11-12 wk)	Mutilation of digits, analgesia of distal extremity	295, 296
Sensory neuropathy	Longhaired Dachshunds, boxers, Pyrenean mountain dogs, Jack Russell terriers, Collies	Ataxia, urinary incontinence, proprioceptive deficits, decreased nociception	297
Distal neuropathy	Doberman pinschers (3 yr)	Pelvic limb gait and stance abnormality	298

Like the storage diseases, the abiotrophies are rare, usually inherited, and eventually fatal. The course of disease is usually longer than that with the storage diseases.

Differential Diagnosis of Degenerative Diseases

Many of these diseases have a similar clinical history and course. The findings on a neurologic examination may indicate a predominance of cerebral, cerebellar, or spinal cord signs. These findings and the age and breed of the animal should suggest a small number of possibilities (see Tables 15-3 and 15-4). In the early stages, neuronal diseases often can be differentiated from demyelinating diseases. Neuronal diseases (storage disease, abiotrophy) are more likely to have cerebral or LMN signs. Demyelinating diseases are more likely to have ascending ataxia and paresis of an upper motor neuron (UMN) type, often with tremors of the limbs. Proprioceptive positioning is commonly affected in demyelinating diseases but is rarely involved in the early stages of neuronal disease.

The degenerative diseases also must be differentiated from inflammatory, neoplastic, and toxic disorders. Specific diagnostic tests are available for most of these conditions and are discussed later in this chapter.

Metabolic Disorders

Normal nervous system function depends on a closely regulated environment. Conversely, the homeostasis of the body is coordinated by the nervous system through the neuroendocrine, autonomic, and somatic systems. Disorders altering homeostasis often have profound effects on the nervous system.

Liver Diseases

Hepatic encephalopathy is a complex metabolic disorder resulting from abnormal liver function.

Pathogenesis. Hepatic encephalopathy has been reported in three types of liver disease: (1) severe parenchymal liver damage, either acute or chronic (cirrhosis, neoplasia, toxicosis); (2) anomalous portal venous circulation (rare in large animals); and (3) congenital urea-cycle enzyme deficiencies (rare).[7] Parenchymal liver diseases other than cirrhosis (fatty infiltration, chronic active hepatitis, and so forth) usually do not cause hepatic encephalopathy except in the terminal stages of the disease. Pyrrolizidine alkaloids in certain plants such as *Senecio* spp. and *Crotalaria* spp. cause parenchymal liver damage and hepatic encephalopathy in herbivores. Parenchymal disease severely reduces the capacity of the liver to perform its normal metabolic functions. Portosystemic venous shunts divert a significant portion of the portal blood past the liver into the vena cava. Potentially toxic substances that normally are absorbed from the gastrointestinal (GI) tract and detoxified in the liver enter the systemic circulation. Urea-cycle enzyme deficiencies prevent the metabolism of ammonia to urea.

The metabolic changes that cause the clinical syndrome of hepatic encephalopathy result from failure of the liver to (1) remove toxic products of gut metabolism and (2) synthesize factors necessary for normal brain function.[7] The exact cause of hepatic encephalopathy is unknown, but current theories of the pathogenesis include (1) ammonia as the primary putative neurotoxin, although other synergistic toxins may be involved; (2) disorders of aromatic amino acid metabolism resulting from alterations in monoamine neurotransmitters; (3) disorders of γ-aminobutyric acid (GABA) or glutamate; and (4) increased cerebral concentrations of an endogenous benzodiazepine-like substance.[8] Ammonia is probably the most important

toxic substance, although the level of ammonia in the blood does not necessarily correlate with the severity of the CNS disturbance.[9]

Clinical Signs. Most animals with liver disease severe enough to produce hepatic encephalopathy have other clinical signs such as GI disturbances, anorexia, weight loss, stunted growth, ascites, and polyuria-polydipsia.

The neurologic signs are frequently worse after feeding, especially if high-protein food is given. The release of nitrogenous materials into the portal circulation exacerbates the signs. Depression that may progress to stupor and coma is the most common neurologic sign. Other signs of cerebral involvement such as behavior change, continuous pacing and head pressing, blindness, and seizures also are common. Frequently, the clinical picture is that of a waxing and waning diffuse cerebral abnormality. The postural reactions and reflexes are only minimally involved except when the animal is nearly comatose. The cranial nerves are not markedly affected except that vision may be impaired. Ptyalism is common, especially in cats.

A variety of factors can precipitate the neurologic signs of hepatic encephalopathy in an animal with marginal liver function (Table 15-5). Any source of protein in the digestive tract is a common cause. Hemorrhage in the GI tract, constipation, or increased fatty acids also may precipitate a crisis. Alterations in fluids, electrolytes, or pH may increase the blood and tissue ammonia levels. Decreased renal function reduces elimination of ammonia and other metabolites. Fever and infection cause increased tissue catabolism and increased nitrogen release. Stored blood for transfusions may have an excess of ammonia. Depressant drugs directly affect the brain and frequently are metabolized in the liver. The first evidence of hepatic dysfunction often is slow recovery from anesthesia. Diuretics used to treat ascites may cause hepatic encephalopathy through their effect on potassium, renal output of ammonia, and alkalosis.

Diagnosis. A variety of clinicopathologic abnormalities may be present, depending on the cause. Microcytosis with normochromic erythrocytes, ammonium biurate crystals in the urine, lowered cholesterol, and lowered blood glucose levels may occur in portacaval shunts. Frequently, serum albumin and serum urea nitrogen levels are low. Parenchymal disease often causes elevations in liver enzymes such as serum alanine aminotransferase (ALT), aspartate aminotransferase (AST), and alkaline phosphatase (AP). These enzymes usually are not elevated significantly in portacaval shunts.[10] Hepatic dysfunction may be confirmed with tests such as the ammonia tolerance test or serum bile acids measured after a 12-hour fast and 2 hours

Table 15-5 **Management of Hepatic Encephalopathy (HE)**

Factors that Exacerbate HE	Management of HE
Increased dietary protein and fatty acids	Low-protein, low-fat diet
Bacterial production of ammonia in large bowel	Diet, antibiotics
Constipation leading to bacterial production of ammonia in large bowel	Diet, laxatives, enemas in acute problems, lactulose
Gastrointestinal hemorrhage	Monitoring and treatment of ulcers, bleeding disorders, hookworms, whipworms
Hypokalemia, hypovolemia, alkalosis—aggravated by diuretics	Monitoring and correction of fluid and electrolyte imbalance, use of potassium-sparing diuretics with caution or not at all
Transfusion of stored blood	Use of fresh blood (only if essential)
Sedatives, narcotics, anesthetics	Use of depressant drugs with extreme caution (in lowest possible dosages), monitoring carefully
Infections, fever	Monitoring and vigorous treatment

after a meal.[11,12] Hepatic ultrasonography (US) is a sensitive indicator of liver size, and the definitive diagnosis of a shunt requires US or contrast-enhanced radiography. Depending on the experience of the operator, abdominal US has a sensitivity of about 80% and a specificity of about 65% for the detection of extrahepatic portosystemic shunts. The sensitivity for detection of intrahepatic shunts is nearly 100%.[13] Radiocolloid scintigraphy using technetium[99m] sulfur colloid (TcSC) is used to evaluate liver size and shape. Transcolonic TcSC procedures have been described for the diagnosis of macrovascular shunts in dogs, cats, and potbellied pigs.[14,15] Biopsy is required for confirmation of parenchymal disease.

Management. The successful medical management of hepatic encephalopathy depends on the cause of the liver disorder and the degree of liver malfunction. Animals with marginal liver function may be managed by reducing the sources of nitrogenous products in the GI tract (see Table 15-5). A high-carbohydrate, low-fat, low-protein diet with high biologic value is indicated. If dietary management alone is inadequate, then oral, nonabsorbable antibiotics (such as neomycin) may be given to reduce the bacterial flora that split urea. Mild laxatives or lactulose (a nonabsorbable disaccharide) may be helpful.[16,17] In addition to its laxative effects, lactulose creates an acid environment in the colon that allows NH_3 to be trapped as NH_4^+ in the gut lumen.

Acute crises of hepatic encephalopathy require more vigorous treatment. Protein sources must be removed completely. Enemas and laxatives are used to remove all nitrogenous material from the GI tract. Sedative drugs, methionine, and diuretics are discontinued. Sources of GI hemorrhage are corrected if they are present. Dehydration, hypokalemia, and alkalosis are managed with intravenous (IV) fluid therapy. Renal output must be maintained to

eliminate nitrogenous products. Oxygen therapy may be necessary, especially in cases of coma. The prognosis for herbivores with hepatic encephalopathy from pyrrolizidine toxicity is poor.

Specific treatment of the cause is instituted, if possible. Unfortunately, most chronic liver diseases and the urea-cycle enzyme deficiencies cannot be treated specifically. Portosystemic shunts may be corrected surgically if portal circulation to the liver is adequate. Partial occlusion of the shunt may be effective. Seizures may occur in dogs after shunt ligation[18,19]; pretreatment with phenobarbital may be indicated.[19] For details of the management of hepatic encephalopathy, the reader should consult the references.[8,9,17,20-23]

Renal Diseases

The terminal stages of renal failure may cause tetany or seizures. Chronic renal disease may be associated with muscle wasting and weakness. Encephalopathy, polyneuropathy, and polymyopathy have been seen in humans with chronic renal disease, especially those receiving hemodialysis. Renal encephalopathy has been reported in cows and dogs.[24,25] Alterations in electrolyte metabolism, especially calcium and potassium, may cause signs that are related to the nervous system (discussed later in this chapter).

L-2-Hydroxyglutaric Aciduria

This disease is an inborn error of metabolism that affects humans and Staffordshire bull terriers.[26] In Staffordshire bull terriers, neurologic signs developed between 4 months and 7 years of age. Four of six dogs had chronic progressive disease, and two dogs were presented with an acute onset of seizures between 4 and 6 months of age.[26] Neurologic signs include seizures, ataxia, dementia, and head tremor. Levels of L-2-hydroxyglutaric acid and lysine were elevated in urine, cerebrospinal fluid (CSF), and plasma. Magnetic resonance imaging (MRI) showed symmetrical and extensive polioencephalopathy suggestive of a metabolic or toxic disorder. CSF analysis for cells and protein concentrations were normal. No definitive treatment is available.

Endocrine Disorders

Endocrine disorders that affect electrolyte and glucose homeostasis may produce neurologic signs in affected animals. Hormonal excess or deficiency may affect the function of nerves or muscles directly. Pituitary lesions may cause signs of hormonal and brain dysfunction if the disease extends into the hypothalamus. In this section, specific endocrine and metabolic diseases that produce prominent neurologic signs of weakness are discussed. Those that cause involuntary movements, tremor, tetany, and spasticity are discussed in Chapter 10. Readers should seek other textbooks for in-depth descriptions of each disorder.

Generalized Weakness. Many endocrine and metabolic diseases result in generalized weakness because they affect neuromuscular functions. With certain conditions, clinical signs improve with rest and are exacerbated by exercise. The term *episodic weakness* has been applied to this condition (see Chapter 7).

This section addresses endocrine and metabolic diseases that produce episodic or generalized weakness.

Hypocalcemia. Parturient paresis, or milk fever, is a hypocalcemic metabolic disorder that occurs in mature dairy cows, sows, sheep, and, rarely, horses, usually within 48 hours of parturition. The affected cows are usually more than 5 years old, and incidence is increased in heavy milk producers and in the Jersey breed. Many dairy cows are marginally hypocalcemic at parturition, and any factor that decreases the metabolic adjustment to this hypocalcemia may cause paresis. Such factors include milk yield versus calcium mobilization from bone and gut, the ratios of calcium to phosphorus in the diet, anorexia and decreased intestinal motility, and dietary pH.

The onset of parturient paresis (stage 1) is often missed and is characterized by apprehension, anorexia, ataxia, and limb stiffness. Stage 2 is marked by progressive muscular weakness, recumbency, and depression. The head is usually turned to the flank, and an S-shaped curvature of the neck may be present. Other signs include dilated pupils, decreased pupillary light reflexes, reduced anal reflex, decreased defecation and urination, no ruminal motility, protrusion of the tongue, and frequent straining.

Stage 3 occurs in about 20% of cases and is characterized by lateral recumbency; severe depression or coma; subnormal temperature; a weak, irregular heart rate; and slow, irregular, shallow respirations. The pupils are dilated and unresponsive to light. Bloating may occur. Changes in serum ions include hypocalcemia, hypophosphatemia, and hypomagnesemia. With prolonged anorexia, serum sodium and potassium levels may decrease.

Intravenous calcium salts (Ca, 1 g per 45 kg of body weight) are usually effective. Calcium borogluconate is commonly used; a 25% solution contains 10.4 g of calcium per 500 ml. Milk fever can be prevented in susceptible cows or herds by the administration of vitamin D or its analogs or by the manipulation of the prepartum dietary calcium and phosphorus levels.

Hypocalcemic syndromes are well documented in dogs and cats.[27] In both species, primary hypoparathyroidism is a documented cause of chronic hypocalcemia. In cats hypoparathyroidism is sometimes caused by inadvertent surgical resection of the parathyroid glands during thyroidectomy for the treatment of hyperthyroidism. Hypocalcemia may be associated with chronic renal disease in dogs and cats. It is the major biochemical abnormality in dogs with eclampsia and may be observed in animals receiving blood transfusions containing calcium-chelating anticoagulants. Enema solutions that contain phosphate may cause hypocalcemia in cats.

When the total serum calcium concentration falls below 6 to 7 mg/dl (ionized <2.5 mg/dl), the clinical signs of hypocalcemia are likely to occur.[28] Tetanic muscle contractions are the most common clinical signs, but some dogs develop muscle weakness early in the disease. Hypocalcemia is suspected when the total serum calcium concentration is less than 9.0 mg/dl and the serum albumin concentration is normal. Serum ionized calcium concentrations help to confirm the diagnosis. Once the diagnosis of hypocalcemia is confirmed, the underlying cause should be identified. The diagnosis of both eclampsia and iatrogenic hypoparathyroidism is usually obvious from the history and physical findings. Primary hypoparathyroidism may be confirmed through parathormone (PTH) assays conducted at specialized laboratories.[27]

Animals experiencing seizures should be given 10% calcium gluconate solution IV at a dose of 0.5 to 1.5 ml/kg. The dosage should be slowly infused over a 10- to 20-minute period, and the heart rate and QT interval should be closely monitored. The calcium dose can be repeated every 6 to 8 hours as a bolus injection.

Oral maintenance therapy is instituted when the total serum calcium concentration is consistently less than 6.5 mg/dl. Calcium gluconate or calcium lactate is administered orally in doses of 1 to 4 g for dogs and 0.5 to 1.0 g for cats. In parathyroid deficiency, vitamin D therapy is required. Dihydrotachysterol is a synthetic vitamin D that is active in the absence of PTH. The loading dose is 0.03 mg/kg daily administered orally for 3 to 4 days. The maintenance dose is 0.01 to 0.02 mg/kg per day. Each patient should be closely monitored because hypercalcemia may be a complication of vitamin D therapy, especially when supplemental calcium salts are administered.[29]

Ketonemic Syndromes. These diseases occur primarily in ruminants and are characterized by hypoglycemia and the accumulation of ketones in body fluids. Conditions that have been recognized include bovine ketosis (acetonemia) and pregnancy toxemia of cattle, sheep, and goats. Unlike most monogastric animals, ruminants produce most of their glucose supplies from the gluconcogenesis of volatile fatty acids (acetic, propionic, and butyric acids). Nearly 50% of the glucose in a cow is normally derived from dietary propionic acid that is converted to glucose in the gluconeogenic pathway. Reduction of propionic acid production in the rumen can result in hypoglycemia and the subsequent mobilization of free fatty acids and glycerol from fat stores. The liver has a limited ability to utilize these fatty acids because the levels of oxaloacetate are low. Acetyl coenzyme A, therefore, is not incorporated into the tricarboxylic acid cycle and is converted into the ketone bodies acetoacetate and β-hydroxybutyrate. When the production of ketones by the liver exceeds peripheral utilization, pathologic ketosis results.

Both ketosis and primary hypoglycemia are involved in the development of the clinical signs. The most common signs include depression, partial to complete anorexia, weight loss, and decreased milk production. The neurologic signs present in some cows include ataxia, apparent blindness, salivation, tooth grinding, excessive licking, muscle twitching, head pressing, and hyperesthesia. Cows may charge blindly if they are disturbed.

The diagnosis of bovine ketosis is based on the presence of elevated ketone levels in blood and milk with concomitant hypoglycemia. The odor of ketones may be perceived on the breath and in the urine. The immediate therapy is an IV injection of glucose, followed by oral administration of 125 to 250 g of propylene glycol twice a day. Glucocorticoids are also beneficial in cows that are not septic. Cows with severe neurologic signs can be treated with 2 to 8 g of chloral hydrate orally twice a day for 3 to 5 days.

Pregnancy toxemia is a condition that is closely related pathophysiologically to bovine ketosis. It occurs in ewes during the last 6 weeks of pregnancy, when the demand for glucose by developing fetuses is large. Pregnancy toxemia occurs in pastured or housed beef cows during the last 2 months of pregnancy. Overweight cows or those bearing twin calves are especially susceptible. In ewes and cows, the basic cause is nutrition insufficient to maintain normal blood glucose concentrations when fetal glucose demands are high. Hypoglycemia precipitates the ketosis, as has been described earlier in this section.

In sheep, clinical signs may develop in a flock and may extend for several weeks. Ewes become depressed and develop weakness, ataxia, and loss of muscle tone. Terminally, recumbency and coma develop. Neuromuscular disturbances include fine muscle tremors of the ears and the lips. In some cases, seizures develop. "Stargazing" postures and grinding of the teeth are common. The neurologic signs in cattle include depression, excitability, and ataxia. The diagnosis of pregnancy toxemia is based on the history, clinical signs, and presence of ketosis and hypoglycemia.

In sheep, flock treatment consists of increasing the availability of glucose precursors in the diet or drenching affected ewes twice daily with 200 ml of a warm 50% glycerol solution. The anabolic steroid trienbolone acetate also is beneficial in 30-mg doses administered intramuscularly (IM). Induction of parturition or fetal removal by cesarean section also may be needed to reduce the metabolic drain on the ewe. Cattle are treated by the method described for bovine ketosis. Pregnancy toxemia can be prevented by ensuring adequate nutrition during pregnancy.

Diabetes Mellitus. Diabetes mellitus may result in neurologic signs from at least four mechanisms. Insulin deficiency results in failure of glucose transport into muscle and adipose tissue. An early sign of diabetes may be exercise intolerance and weakness. If severe insulin deficiency occurs, ketonemia develops from a marked increase in lipolysis and serum fatty acids. The ensuing metabolic acidosis results in depressed cerebral function that culminates in coma and death. In the untreated ketoacidotic dog or cat, hyperkalemia may be a serious complication that depresses neuromuscular and cardiovascular function. With therapy and correction of the acidosis, potassium ions reenter cells, and hypokalemia may be a complication that fosters muscle weakness and depression. In some animals, the hyperglycemia may be severe, even though acidosis is absent. This syndrome is called *hyperosmolar nonketotic coma.* Clinical signs result from the hyperosmolar effects of glucose on the cerebral cortex. Diabetic animals may also develop neuropathies with associated LMN signs in affected muscles (see Chapter 7).

The comatose diabetic animal is a difficult therapeutic challenge. The clinician must exercise great care in performing insulin, acid-base, electrolyte, and fluid therapy. Interested readers should consult other texts for an in-depth discussion of the diagnosis and management of the diabetic patient.

Hypothyroidism. Deficiencies of thyroxine result in a marked decrease in cerebral function and basal metabolic rate. Severely hypothyroid dogs may become very depressed or may appear dull and unresponsive. Coma may occur in severe cases.[30-32] A very-low-voltage electroencephalogram (EEG) usually is seen. The cerebral signs improve dramatically after replacement thyroid medication. Polyneuropathies have been recognized in dogs without the usual signs of hypothyroidism. Syndromes include laryngeal paralysis, vestibular and auditory dysfunction, and various peripheral and cranial nerve palsies (see Chapter 7). The fact that the animal has a polyneuropathy rather than a single problem may be defined by electromyography (EMG) or other electrodiagnostic tests. Measurement of free thyroxine and thyroid stimulating hormone (TSH) concentrations or TSH response testing are necessary to confirm a diagnosis.[33,34] Many of these animals respond well to thyroid hormone supplementation, but weeks to months may be required for nerve function to recover.[35]

Hyperadrenocorticism. Hyperadrenocorticism (Cushing's disease/syndrome) occurs in dogs, horses, and cats. In dogs and horses, pituitary adenomas that hypersecrete adrenocorticotropic hormone (ACTH) are the most common cause, but functional cortisol-secreting adrenal tumors also produce this syndrome in dogs and cats. The clinical signs are caused by the metabolic effects of hypercortisolemia. Generalized muscle weakness resulting from the catabolic effects of glucocorticoids is a common finding. Some dogs develop muscle degeneration, known as *steroid-induced* myopathy (see Chapter 7).

This condition produces spontaneous muscle contractions *(myotonia)* and a stiff gait. Pituitary adenomas *(macroadenomas)* may create neurologic signs by growth and expansion into the hypothalamus.[36] Signs of pituitary macroadenomas include depression, confusion, circling, ataxia, and seizure. Macroadenomas are more common in older, large-breed dogs.

In dogs and cats, hyperadrenocorticism is confirmed with screening tests such as the low-dose dexamethasone suppression test, the ACTH stimulation test, or the urine cortisol:creatinine ratio. Pituitary-dependent hyperadrenocorticism is differentiated from functional adrenocortical tumors with the high-dose dexamethasone suppression test or ACTH assay or both. Similar tests, as well as measurement of increased plasma ACTH concentrations, are useful in the diagnosis of equine Cushing's disease.[37] Abdominal US may also be helpful in the diagnosis of adrenal gland disease. Macroadenomas can be accurately diagnosed with MRI.[38] In dogs pituitary-dependent hyperadrenocorticism responds well to the adrenocorticolytic drug mitotane. Side effects of this drug include neurologic signs that may be similar to those produced by macroadenomas. The direct toxic effects of mitotane peak within 24 hours and subside within 48 hours after administration.

Episodic Weakness. Chapter 7 introduces the problem of episodic weakness and discusses the primary neuromuscular causes of this problem. This section briefly addresses the endocrinologic and metabolic causes of episodic weakness.

Hypercalcemia. An increased concentration of serum calcium may result in neuromuscular, cardiovascular, and renal dysfunction. When the level of calcium in body fluids rises above normal, excitable cell membranes are depressed. Reflex activities of the CNS become sluggish, and muscles also become sluggish and weak. Hypercalcemia decreases the QT interval of the electrocardiogram (ECG) and decreases myocardial function. Hypercalcemia impairs renal concentrating ability. In prolonged hypercalcemia, mineralization of soft tissue may occur. The syndrome of hypercalcemic nephropathy is well documented in animals and culminates in chronic renal failure. In dogs calcium levels above 12.5 mg/dl result in hypercalcemic signs. In some cases, muscle weakness is markedly worse during exercise and improves with rest.

Several causes of hypercalcemia exist, including primary hyperparathyroidism, paraneoplastic syndromes, vitamin D rodenticide intoxication, and iatrogenic calcium therapy.[39] Primary hyperparathyroidism results from autonomously functioning parathyroid adenomas. These tumors secrete PTH in the presence of increasing serum calcium concentrations. Certain nonendocrine tumors such as lymphosarcoma, anal sac adenocarcinoma, squamous cell carcinoma, and thymoma secrete substances with PTH-like activity that results in hypercalcemia.[39-41] This syndrome is called the *hypercalcemia of malignancy* and is the most common cause for hypercalcemia in dogs and cats. Rodenticides that contain analogues of vitamin D promote increased absorption of calcium and may produce hypercalcemia.[42]

The symptomatic therapy of hypercalcemia includes diuresis with fluids and furosemide. Corticosteroids also are beneficial because they promote the renal excretion of calcium. Salmon calcitonin may also be given to decrease serum calcium concentrations.[43]

Hyperkalemia. Increased serum concentrations of potassium reduce the activity of excitable membranes, especially cardiac muscle. Excessive extracellular potassium causes cardiac flaccidity and decreases the conduction of impulses through the atrioventricular (AV) node. Thus, heart rate and cardiac output may be severely depressed. In addition, the contraction of skeletal muscle may be somewhat depressed. Hyperkalemia therefore manifests as generalized weakness that becomes worse with exercise.

Hyperkalemia may occur secondary to severe acidosis; however, the usual cause is adrenal insufficiency. Adrenal insufficiency, a chronic immune-mediated adrenalitis, may result in aldosterone deficiency secondary to atophy of the zona glomerulosis. Hyperkalemia and hyponatremia contribute to the typical signs of depression, anorexia, vomiting, diarrhea, weakness, bradycardia, and decreased cardiac output. The disease responds well to fluid therapy and replacement adrenocortical hormone therapy.

Hyperkalemic periodic paralysis, an episodic syndrome of muscular weakness and fasciculations, occurs in quarter horses (see Chapter 7).[44]

This disease is caused by a genetic mutation in the muscle sodium-channel protein gene.[45] It is associated with marked hyperkalemia without major acid-base imbalance or high serum activity of enzymes derived from muscle. The episodes occur spontaneously or can be induced by administration of potassium chloride orally. EMG changes include fibrillation potentials, positive sharp waves, and complex repetitive discharges. Histologic changes in muscle are minimal but may include vacuolation of type-2b fibers or mild degenerative changes. Marked hyperkalemia is present during episodes. IV administration of calcium, glucose, or bicarbonate results in recovery. Administration of acetazolamide, 2.2 mg/kg orally every 8 to 12 hours, prevents the episodes. Decreasing the potassium content of the feed may also be effective. This can be done by feeding oat hay, feeding grain two to three times daily, and providing free access to salt.[44]

Hypokalemia. Decreased serum concentrations of potassium decrease the activity of skeletal muscle because the membranes are hyperpolarized. Muscle weakness and even paralysis may occur. The primary causes of hypokalemia include diuretic therapy, vomiting, diarrhea, alkalosis, excessive mineralocorticoid therapy for adrenal insufficiency, renal failure, and diabetic ketoacidosis. Hypokalemic myopathy is well documented in cats with renal failure, in cats with chronic anorexia, and in cats receiving low potassium diets. Most patients respond well to potassium supplementation (see Chapter 7).

Hypoglycemia. Hypoglycemia causes altered CNS function similar to that associated with hypoxia. The blood glucose concentration is of prime importance for normal neuronal metabolism because glucose oxidation is the primary energy source. No glycogen stores are present in the CNS. Glucose enters nervous tissue by diffusion rather than by insulin facilitation. The severity of the CNS signs is related more to the rate of decrease than to the actual concentration of glucose. Sudden drops in glucose levels are more likely to cause seizures, whereas slowly developing hypoglycemia may cause weakness, paraparesis, behavioral changes, or severe depression.

Hypoglycemia in young animals may be secondary to malnutrition, parasitism, stress, or some GI abnormality. Puppies are frequently extremely depressed or comatose when brought for consultation. The blood glucose level is usually very low (<30 mg/100 ml). Serum glucose should be determined, and IV glucose is administered immediately (2 to 4 ml of 20% glucose per kilogram of body weight). If seizures are present, diazepam should be administered if no immediate response occurs to the glucose (see the section on the treatment of status epilepticus in Chapter 13). Continued signs of stupor or coma indicate brain swelling and are treated with corticosteroids and mannitol (see Chapter 12). Dietary regulation, including tube feeding if necessary, must be established to maintain normoglycemia.

Glycogen-storage diseases also have been reported in puppies (see Chapter 7). Persistent recurrent hypoglycemia, hepatomegaly, acidosis, and ketosis suggest a glycogen-storage disease. Liver and muscle biopsies are required to make a definitive diagnosis. The management of these cases is frequently unsuccessful.

Adult-onset hypoglycemia usually is caused by a functional tumor of the pancreatic beta cells (insulinoma).[46-48] Excessive insulin produces an increased transfer of blood glucose into the nonneuronal cellular compartments, resulting in hypoglycemia and abnormal CNS metabolism. Although insulinomas are relatively rare, increasing awareness has resulted in more frequent diagnosis. Most of the tumors in dogs are carcinomas and have metastasized to the liver and other sites by the time a definitive diagnosis is made. In addition to hypoglycemia, beta-cell tumors may also induce peripheral neuropathies. Other neoplasms also may induce hypoglycemia.[49]

Seizures are more frequently related to exercise, fasting (or, conversely, eating), and excitement.

Other signs such as weakness, muscle tremor, disorientation, and behavioral changes are also common. The signs are episodic until irreversible neuronal damage occurs. LMN paresis can be detected in dogs with peripheral neuropathies induced by beta-cell tumors (see Chapter 7).

Hypoglycemia can mimic the other causes of seizures. Blood glucose concentrations after a 12-hour fast are usually below normal (<60 mg/100 ml). Longer fasts (24 to 48 hours) may be necessary in some cases, but animals should be monitored closely during this time. Plasma insulin levels are more specific for making a diagnosis.[46] Serum insulin concentrations are near zero when plasma glucose concentrations are less than or equal to 30 mg/dl. Plasma insulin levels should be measured when the blood glucose concentrations are below 60 mg/100 ml. Normal or increased plasma insulin concentrations in hypoglycemic dogs are strongly suggestive of insulinoma. The glucagon tolerance test may be used as an alternative procedure, but it carries a greater risk of profound hypoglycemia during the test. Abdominal US may detect pancreatic masses in some cases and help localize the lesion for surgical resection.

The management of patients in coma and status epilepticus is discussed in Chapters 12 and 13, respectively.

Surgical removal of the tumor is indicated when the patient's condition has stabilized. The reported incidence of malignancy ranges from 56% to 82%; therefore, the prognosis is poor even with successful removal of the pancreatic focus.[46,47] Animals with insulinoma should be fed several small meals each day. Diets high in simple sugars should be avoided. Glucocorticoids such as prednisolone, given at a dosage of 0.25 to 0.50 mg/kg per day, help to normalize the blood glucose concentration because of their anti-insulin effects. Diazoxide may be useful in the management of insulinoma because it increases blood glucose concentrations through several mechanisms. The initial dose is 10 mg/kg divided twice a day orally. The dose may be gradually increased but should not exceed 60 mg/kg daily.[29,49] Streptozotocin is effective in dogs with metastatic disease, but the dose must be monitored carefully to prevent renal toxicity. Seizures may persist because of prior neuronal injury even though serum glucose levels have been normalized.[50]

Neoplasms

Neoplasia that affects the nervous system is classified into three groups (Table 15-6). *Primary tumors* arise from cells that normally are found in the cranial vault, vertebral canal, or peripheral nerves. *Secondary tumors* metastasize from a primary tumor to the nervous system. *Tumors of surrounding structures* such as the skull or vertebrae may be

Table 15-6   **Classification of Neoplasia of the Nervous System**

Tumor Type	Predilection Site	Species (Breed)	Incidence
Primary tumors			
Tumors of nerve cells			
Ganglioneuroma	Variable (cerebellum, cranial nerve roots, eye, cervical region)	Dogs, pigs, horses, cattle	Rare
Tumors of neuroepithelium			
Ependymoma	Ependymal surfaces	Dogs, cats, horses, cattle	Uncommon
Blastoma (neuroepithelioma)	Thoracolumbar spinal cord	Dogs	Uncommon
Plexus papilloma	Fourth ventricle	Dogs, horses, cattle	Common (dogs)
Tumors of glia			
Astrocytoma	Piriform area, convexity of cerebral hemispheres, thalamus, hypothalamus	Dogs (brachycephalic), cats, cattle	Common (dogs)
Oligodendroglioma	Cerebral hemispheres	Dogs (brachycephalic)	Common (dogs)
Glioblastoma	As for astrocytoma	Dogs (brachycephalic), cattle, pigs	Uncommon
Medulloblastoma	Cerebellum	Dogs, cats, pigs, calves,	Common (dogs)
Gliomas, unclassified	Periventricular areas, especially subependymal plate	Dogs (brachycephalic), cattle, horses, sheep, pigs	Common (dogs)
Tumors of peripheral nerves and nerve sheaths			
Neurinoma (schwannoma)	Peripheral nerves	Dogs, cattle	Uncommon
Neurofibroma	Peripheral nerves	Dogs, cattle, horses, pigs, sheep	Common (dogs, cattle)
Neurofibrosarcoma	Peripheral nerves	Dogs, cats, horses	Common (dogs, cattle)

Table 15-6   Classification of Neoplasia of the Nervous System—continued

Tumor Type	Predilection Site	Species (Breed)	Incidence
Tumors of the meninges, vessels, and other mesodermal structures			
Meningioma	Falx cerebri, cerebral hemispheres, brainstem, cervical spinal cord	Dogs (dolichocephalic), cats, horses, cattle, sheep	Common (dogs, cats)
Angioblastoma	Variable (cerebral hemispheres, choroid plexus, medulla, spinal cord)	Dogs, horses, pigs	Rare
Sarcoma	Variable (meninges, brain, spinal cord)	Dogs, cats, horses, cattle, sheep	Common (dogs, cats)
Focal granulomatous meningoencephalomyelitis (reticulosis)	Cerebral hemispheres, brainstem	Dogs, cats, horses, cattle	Common (dogs)
Tumors of the pineal and pituitary glands and of the craniopharyngeal duct			
Pinealoma	Pineal body	Dogs, horses, cattle	Rare
Pituitary adenoma	Pituitary gland	Dogs (brachycephalic), cats, horses, cattle, sheep	Common (dogs, horses)
Craniopharyngioma (germ cell tumors)	Hypophyseal-infundibular areas	Dogs	Rare
Tumors of heterotopic tissues (malformation tumors)			
Epidermoid, dermoid, teratoma	Variable (fourth ventricle and cerebellopontine angle for epidermoid)	Dogs, horses, cattle, sheep	Rare
Secondary tumors			
Metastatic tumors Mammary gland adenocarcinoma, pulmonary carcinoma, chemodectoma, prostatic carcinoma, hemangiosarcoma, fibrosarcoma, malignant melanoma, salivary gland adenocarcinoma	Variable	Dogs, cats, cattle, horses, sheep	Common
Lymphosarcoma	Spinal cord	Cats, cattle, dogs	Common (cattle, cats)
Primary tumors from surrounding tissues			
Osteoma, osteosarcoma, chondroma, chondrosarcoma, hemangioma, hemangiosarcoma, fibrosarcoma, calcifying aponeurotic fibromatosis, epidermoid cyst, lipoma	Variable (brain, spinal cord)	Dogs, cats, horses, cattle, pigs	Common (dogs, cats)

Modified from Oliver JE, Hoerlein BF, Mayhew IG: *Veterinary neurology*, Philadelphia, 1987, WB Saunders, p 279.

considered a form of secondary tumor. Peripheral nerve and spinal cord tumors were also discussed in Chapters 5 and 6, respectively.

Pathogenesis

Tumors affect the function of the nervous system by (1) the destruction of nervous tissue, (2) compression of surrounding structures (Figure 15-1), (3) interference with circulation and subsequent development of vasogenic cerebral edema, and (4) disturbance of CSF circulation. Increased intracranial pressure resulting from the combined effects of mass effect, edema, and CSF accumulation may cause herniation of the cerebrum ventral to the tentorium cerebelli or herniation of the cerebellum into the foramen magnum (Figure 15-2;

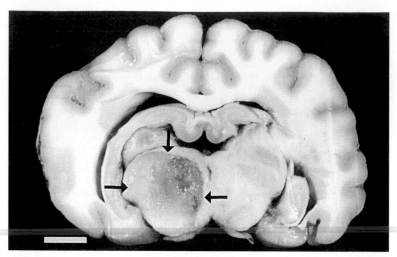

Figure 15-1 Transverse section of the brain at the level of the thalamus from an 8-year-old male German shepherd dog with a 4-week history of progressive signs of left forebrain dysfunction. Using computed tomography, a homogeneously enhancing mass was identified in the thalamus. Irradiation was recommended but declined by the owner. The dog was euthanized, and a necropsy was done. A somewhat gelatinous mass is seen in the left thalamus *(arrows)*. On histologic examination, the tumor had features of an oligodendroglioma. Bar = 0.7 cm. (From Bagley RS, et al: Central nervous system neoplasia. In Slatter DH, editor: *Textbook of small animal surgery*, Philadelphia, 1993, WB Saunders.)

see Chapter 12). Primary tumors usually grow slowly, producing chronic, progressive clinical signs. Vascular involvement may lead to infarction or hemorrhage and acute neurologic deficits (see Figure 15-2; also see Figure 12-7). Metastatic tumors tend to be aggressive biologically and are more likely to cause acute dysfunction.[51]

Incidence

Because the nervous system typically is not completely evaluated at necropsy, estimating the true incidence of neoplasia in the general population of any species is difficult. Brain tumors are estimated to occur at a rate of 14.5 and 3.5 per 100,000 dogs and cats at risk, respectively.[52]

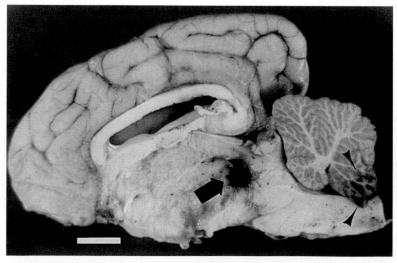

Figure 15-2 Midsagittal section of brain from a 2-year-old male German shepherd dog with acutely progressive depression, circling, blindness, apnea, and death over an 11-hour period. Much of the thalamus is occupied by a poorly defined mass with histologic features of a pituitary carcinoma. A focus of black discoloration *(arrow)* shown to be hemorrhage microscopically is noted dorsocaudally in the thalamus. The caudal cerebellar vermis *(arrowheads)* is discolored subsequent to foramen magnum brain herniation. Caudal transtentorial brain herniation was also present. Tumor necrosis and hemorrhage were presumed to contribute to the herniation and the dog's acute clinical deterioration. Bar = 0.8 cm. (From Bagley RS, et al: Central nervous system neoplasia. In Slatter DH, editor: *Textbook of small animal surgery*, Philadelphia, 1993, WB Saunders.)

Table 15-7 **Common Sites and Signs of Brain Tumors**

Site	Signs
Cerebrum	
Frontal lobe	Seizures, abnormal behavior, contralateral postural reaction deficits
Occipital lobe	Seizures, contralateral visual field deficit
Temporal lobe	Seizures, abnormal behavior
Pituitary-hypothalamus	Behavioral, autonomic and endocrine signs: polyuria, polydipsia, changes in eating, sleeping, and behavior patterns, and so forth; later visual deficits
Brainstem	Gait and postural reaction deficits, cranial nerve (CN) signs
Cerebellopontine angle	CN V, CN VII, and CN VIII signs, hemiparesis

Brain tumors are infrequently reported in food animals and horses.

Astrocytoma and meningioma are the most common brain tumors in dogs; meningioma has been reported more frequently in later studies.[51] Astrocytoma occurs more commonly in brachycephalic breeds such as boxers, Boston terriers, and English bulldogs. The incidence of meningioma may be higher in dolichocephalic breeds such as German shepherd dogs and collies.[53-55] Neoplastic reticulosis is seen in all breeds.

In general, the risk of neoplasia increases with age.[56] In one study, the risk of glial tumors in dogs peaked at 10 to 14 years of age, the risk of meningeal tumors peaked at 7 to 9 years of age, and the risk of peripheral nerve tumors peaked at 2 to 3 and 7 to 9 years of age. Younger dogs may have epidermoid-dermoid cysts, medulloblastomas, and teratomas. Astrocytomas have been reported in dogs as young as 1.4 years that presented with signs of forebrain disease.[57]

Clinical Signs

The signs of CNS tumors depend on the location of the mass (Table 15-7). In contrast to the other diseases discussed in this chapter, signs of focal disease are expected with CNS neoplasia. Metastatic disease and the diffuse neoplastic disorders (reticulosis, lymphosarcoma) may cause multifocal involvement. Sites of predilection for tumors are given in Table 15-6.

Cerebral tumors can become relatively large (i.e., greater than 1 cm in diameter) before clinical signs are recognized (see Figures 15-1 and 15-2). Many animals with brain tumors, however, may have vague signs such as behavioral changes for up to a year before showing overt neurologic signs.[55] Seizures may be the first sign of a cerebral tumor. As the tumor expands, other signs are noted. Seizures usually become more frequent despite the use of anticonvulsants.

Pituitary tumors in animals tend to expand dorsally into the hypothalamus, producing seizures and changes in metabolic and endocrine function in the early stages. These tumors can become quite large before cranial nerve or motor signs are observed (Figure 15-3). Blindness from compression of the optic nerves does not occur frequently, but it can occur.[58]

Brainstem tumors are characterized by gait deficits and cranial nerve signs (Figure 15-4). Behavioral changes and seizures are usually absent with tumors of the brainstem and cerebellum until the mass affects the reticular activating system or alters intracranial pressure by obstructing CSF circulation. In addition to signs related to the location of the lesion (see Table 15-7), signs due to increased intracranial pressure (depression, papilledema) are frequently present.[59]

Peripheral nerve and spinal cord tumors are discussed in Chapters 5 and 6, respectively.

Diagnosis

Brain Tumors. The primary groups of diseases that must be considered in the differential diagnosis of brain tumors are outlined in Table 15-8. The more common degenerative diseases can be excluded on the basis of age at onset; however,

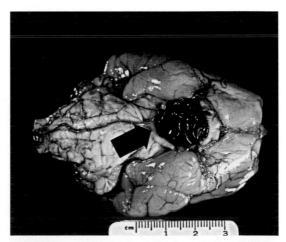

Figure 15-3 A pituitary tumor *(arrow)* in a Labrador retriever with visual and postural reaction deficits and Horner's syndrome.

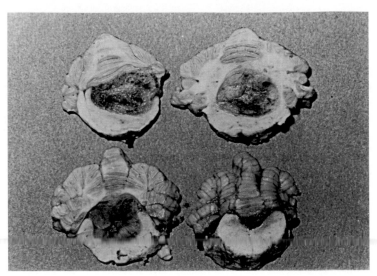

Figure 15-4 Oligodendroglioma in the medulla oblongata. The dog had left facial paralysis, right hemiparesis, and a forced gaze deviation to the right. This is an exception to the usual rule of paresis ipsilateral to cranial nerve involvement with brainstem lesions, possibly related to the central location of the mass.

tumors occasionally are seen in young animals.[57] The other diseases, except for inflammation and vascular lesions, may be excluded when focal signs develop. Most inflammatory diseases, with the exception of brain abscesses and granulomatous meningoencephalomyelitis, are multifocal or diffuse; but focal signs may occur early in the course of the disease. Hemorrhages and infarcts are usually acute in onset and nonprogressive.

Computed tomography (CT) (Figures 15-5 and 15-6) or MRI (Figure 15-7) is used most commonly to diagnose brain neoplasia.[60] The features of most brain tumors have been relatively well characterized in dogs and cats.[61,62] Images are obtained before and after administration of contrast media (CT, meglumine iothalamate, 600 to 900 mg iodine/kg, IV; MRI, gadolinium-diethylenetriaminepentaacetic acid [DTPA], 0.1 to 0.2 mmol/kg, IV). Contrast agents are excluded by the normal blood-brain barrier but leak through an abnormal or damaged barrier associated with a tumor. Secondary effects of brain tumors, such as vasogenic edema and hydrocephalus, also can be defined (see discussion of CT and MR imaging, in Chapter 4).

Cerebrospinal fluid analysis may provide limited information in the diagnosis of neoplasia but also increases the risk of brain herniation. Tumors generally cause an increase in CSF pressure and protein content with no increase in cells. Inflammation may be seen, however, particularly with meningiomas.[63] Pleocytosis may portend a poorer prognosis.[64] Generally, CSF evaluation should be done only if CT is normal or inflammatory disease is suspected because of clinical features or results of other diagnostic tests.

Electroencephalography may aid in the diagnosis of cortical tumors by showing a focal abnormality.

Increased intracranial pressure may cause generalized high-voltage slow waves. Lateralization may be demonstrated in a small portion of cases.

Radiographic procedures other than CT or MRI are rarely used today (see Chapter 4). These include arteriography and radioisotope brain scans for cerebral lesions and sinus venography and positive contrast thecography for lesions on the floor of the skull. If neoplasia is suspected early, thoracic and abdominal radiographs may help to identify primary malignancy that may have metastasized to the brain.

The diagnosis of peripheral nerve and spinal cord tumors is discussed in Chapters 5 through 7.

Management

The objectives of therapy for a brain tumor are eradication of the tumor and control of secondary tumor effects such as edema.[55] Corticosteroids are often effective in reducing peritumoral edema and also can reduce the growth of some types of tumors. Improvement may be significant and last for weeks to months. Acute episodes may be treated with IV methylprednisolone (30 mg/kg) or dexamethasone (2 mg/kg), whereas long-term treatment is usually with oral prednisolone (0.5 mg/kg every 48 hours; increased gradually until improvement occurs and then reduced to the smallest effective dosage). Anticonvulsant therapy may also be needed. Eventually growth of the tumor causes severe clinical signs, often acutely after a period of relative normalcy.[56]

Four principal methods of treatment are available for eradication or reduction of the tumor mass: surgery, chemotherapy, radiation therapy, and immunotherapy. Surgery and radiation therapy are used in most cases, although the use of chemotherapy is increasing.

Table 15-8 **Differential Diagnosis of Brain Tumors**

Characteristic	Brain Tumor	Degenerative Disease	Metabolic Disease	Inflammatory Disease	Toxic Disease	Vascular Disease
Age	Adult to old	Young	Any	Any	Any	Any
Progression	Slow	Slow	Variable, often waxing and waning	Usually fast	Slow (heavy metal)	Acute onset, not progressive
Focal signs	Yes	No	No	Maybe, especially abscess	No	Yes
CSF	Increased protein, variable cells	Increased protein (variable), normal cells	Normal	Increased protein, increased cells	Increased protein, normal cells (heavy metal)	Increased protein, normal cells, may be xanthochromic
EEG	May be focal (cortical) or diffuse HVSW	Diffuse abnormality	Diffuse abnormality	Diffuse abnormality	Diffuse abnormality	May be focal abnormality
CT, MRI	Positive	Variable	Negative	Variable	Negative	Positive, infarct or hemorrhage

HVSW, High-voltage slow waves; *CT,* computed tomography; *MRI,* magnetic resonance imaging.

373

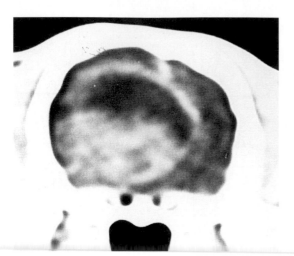

Figure 15-5 Contrast-enhanced computed tomography scan of a 10-month-old domestic cat with a 5-month history of seizures. The cat became acutely worse 5 days before the scan, with severe depression, proprioceptive deficits of the right limbs, and a decreased menace reaction on the right. A massive lesion (3 cm in diameter) occupies most of the forebrain on the left side. The ventral portion and dorsal rim enhance with contrast material. The falx cerebri is displaced to the right. The histologic diagnosis was malignant ependymoma.

The criteria for successful surgery include (1) a solitary, noninvasive tumor, (2) a tumor that is on or near the surface of the cerebral hemisphere, (3) a neurologic status that is compatible with life, (4) an accurate localization, (5) a careful and complete surgical resection, and (6) an intensive postoperative care regimen. Meningiomas are most likely to meet the first two requirements (Figure 15-8). Newer techniques such as laser

surgery, microsurgery, and intraoperative US are likely to enhance the chance of success.[56]

Radiation therapy has been used with moderate success. It may be the primary mode of treatment or may be used after surgical resection of both gliomas and meningiomas.[64-66] Lymphoma and granulomatous meningoencephalomyelitis may also be sensitive to radiation.[55,65] Doses of 45.6 to 48 Gy have generally been administered to the whole brain using 12 fractions of 3.8 to 4.0 Gy three times weekly. Clinical improvement may occur within 2 weeks of initiating irradiation, although actual reduction in tumor mass may not be noted on CT for several months. Significant improvement may be seen in some dogs despite persistence of considerable tumor volume on CT. Complications of radiation include brain necrosis, damage to extracranial structures such as the eyes and skin, and tumor necrosis and hemorrhage. Brain necrosis in humans is typically seen with total doses of 50 to 60 Gy. Effects of irradiation can be augmented by various methods, including sensitizers such as misonidazole, hyperthermia, boron neuron-capture therapy, and interstitial implants (brachytherapy).[51]

Few data are available regarding the medical treatment of brain tumors in animals, aside from information about the use of corticosteroids (see preceding). Specific chemotherapeutic agents that achieve adequate penetration of the brain include the nitrosoureas, carmustine, lomustine, and semustine. Several dogs with histologically confirmed gliomas have improved after the administration of the nitrosourea lomustine (CCNU) (50 to 80 mg/m² of body surface area at intervals of 6 to 8 weeks)

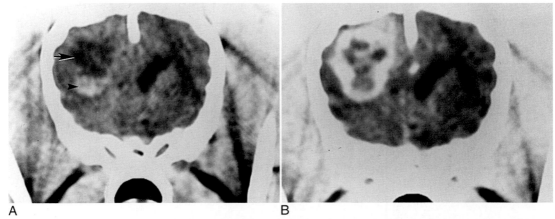

A   B

Figure 15-6 Computed tomography scans before (**A**) and after (**B**) iodine enhancement at the level of the basal nuclei from an 8-year-old female boxer with altered attitude and circling. A poorly defined lucent area *(arrow)*, potentially corresponding to necrosis that may be contiguous with the lateral ventricle, and a focus of increased density *(arrowhead)*, presumed to be hemorrhage, are present in **A** before contrast enhancement. After contrast administration, a ring pattern of enhancement is noted in **B**. The mass was partially resected and had features of an anaplastic mixed glioma. (From Kornegay JN: Central nervous system neoplasia. In Kornegay JN, editor: *Neurologic disorders* [Contemporary Issues in Small Animal Practice, vol 5.], Philadelphia, 1986, WB Saunders.)

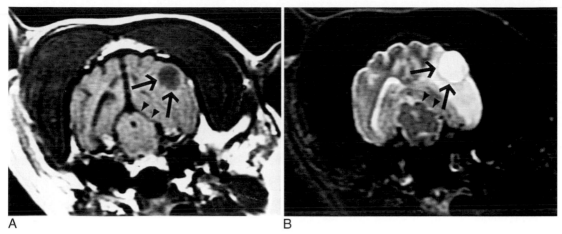

Figure 15-7 Transverse magnetic resonance images at the level of the midbrain and occipital cortex from a 12-year-old female mixed-breed dog with seizures, left hemiparesis, and decreased vision in the left eye of 3 weeks' duration. A tumor *(arrows)* and secondary effects are seen in both images. **A,** T1-weighted; as a result, the cerebrospinal fluid (CSF) and the tumor appear dark. **B,** T2 weighted; the tumor and the CSF appear bright. Collapse of the right lateral ventricle and flattening of the ipsilateral rostral colliculus *(arrowheads)* subsequent to caudal transtentorial brain herniation are seen in **A** and **B.** Collapse of the ventricle has occurred because of the effects of both the tumor mass and the surrounding edema. The edema is poorly appreciated because of its low signal intensity in **A** but appears bright in **B.** The tumor was surgically resected and identified histopathologically as a meningioma. Spin echo: TR, 0.5 seconds in **A** and 2.5 seconds in **B;** TE, 25 milliseconds in **A** and 80 milliseconds in **B.** (From Kornegay JN: Imaging brain neoplasms: computed tomography and magnetic resonance imaging, *Vet Med Rep* 2:372-390, 1990.)

alone or in combination with other forms of treatment.[51]

Immunotherapy consisting of stimulating and culturing the patient's lymphocytes and returning them to the tumor bed during surgery is another

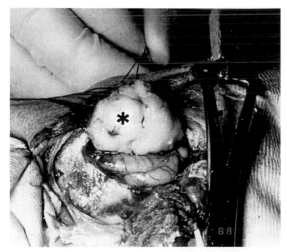

Figure 15-8 Photograph at the time of a craniotomy in a 13-year-old female domestic cat with episodes of depression, torticollis, and circling of approximately 8 months' duration. A mass *(asterisk)* that markedly displaces the cerebral hemisphere is being elevated from the brain by sutures passing from the tumor to between the surgeon's fingers at the top. The mass was diagnosed histologically as a meningioma. The cat was clinically normal 18 months after surgery. (From Kornegay JN: *Feline neurology* [Problems in Veterinary Medicine Series], Philadelphia, 1991, JB Lippincott.)

therapeutic approach.[67] Limited trials suggest that this may be an effective treatment modality.

Although some improvement in outcome of treatment is being reported as protocols are refined, published studies are not encouraging. One review of 86 brain tumors in dogs is illustrative.[64] Median survival time was 1 month (range, 1 day to 42.4 months). The median survival time of seven untreated dogs was 0.2 months. In dogs that underwent surgery alone, median survival time was 0.9 months, and in dogs treated with cobalt 60 radiation (some with hyperthermia or surgery in addition), it was 4.9 months. Dogs with a solitary tumor had a better prognosis than those with multiple tumors. As protocols improve with experience, these results should also improve. Owners should be made aware of the limitations of therapy.

Treatment of peripheral nerve and spinal cord tumors is discussed in Chapters 5 and 6, respectively.

Nutritional Disorders

Nervous system disorders caused by nutritional deficiencies or excesses are uncommon in companion animals, but they are more common in food animals. Severe malnutrition can cause a variety of abnormalities that are related to multiple deficiencies. Vitamin deficiencies and excesses and mineral imbalances are the most common nutritional abnormalities seen in practice.

Hypovitaminosis

Vitamin A. Deficiencies in vitamin A can produce night blindness. Hypovitaminosis A in young animals may cause excessive thickening of the skull and the vertebrae with secondary compression of nervous tissue (especially of the cranial nerves as they pass through the foramina). Poor absorption of CSF may result in communicating hydrocephalus.[68] Hypovitaminosis A is rare or rarely recognized in companion animals but has been reported in food animals.[68-70] Blindness in cattle with vitamin A deficiency is caused by several pathologic mechanisms.[71]

Papilledema occurs in adult animals secondary to increased CSF pressure, which is secondary to poor absorption. Photoreceptor abnormalities, especially affecting the rods, lead to night blindness. Similar changes occur in growing calves, but, in addition, the optic nerves are compressed by narrowing of the optic canals, resulting in ischemia and direct interference with the nerve.

Vitamin E. A noninflammatory myopathy may be produced by vitamin E deficiency. Although myopathies are seen fairly often, vitamin E deficiency is rare in companion animals. Calves and sheep have a myopathy associated with a deficiency in vitamin E and selenium. Swine may die suddenly because of degeneration of cardiac muscle. An association of vitamin E deficiency with degenerative myelopathy in horses has been proposed (see Chapter 7).[72,73]

Vitamin B Complex. Deficiencies in all the B vitamins can cause pathologic changes in both the central and peripheral nervous systems. Thiamine deficiency has been reported in dogs, cats, and ruminants.[69,74-77] The syndrome in dogs progresses from anorexia to pelvic limb paresis, tetraparesis, seizures, and coma in approximately 1 week.[77] Malacia and hemorrhage were found in multiple sites in the brain and the spinal cord, with the most severe lesions in the brainstem. Animals treated with thiamine recovered. A peripheral neuropathy with LMN paralysis also has been seen.[74]

Cats with thiamine deficiency often have characteristic ventral flexion of the head and the neck, sometimes causing the chin to touch the sternum. Ataxia and seizures may be present. The lesions are similar to those that occur in dogs.[69] The deficiency in dogs was produced by a diet consisting entirely of cooked meat or a specific thiamine-deficient diet.[77] Cat foods with fish as the primary ingredient contain thiaminase, which destroys thiamine in the diet.[69]

Treatment should be instituted immediately for any animal suspected of having thiamine deficiency. In dogs and cats, 50 to 100 mg of thiamine should be given IV and then repeated IM daily until a response is obtained or another diagnosis is established. Larger doses are required in cattle and horses.

Polioencephalomalacia (symmetric necrosis of the cerebral cortex) is caused by thiamine deficiency in ruminants. The deficiency results from increased breakdown of thiamine in the rumen by thiaminase-secreting bacteria. Animals have usually been moved from a marginal pasture to a lush pasture, are in a feed lot, or have had some similar change in feeding patterns. Animals younger than 2 years of age are most commonly affected.[76]

Clinical signs are primarily cerebral in origin and include depression, pacing, head pressing, blindness, ataxia, teeth grinding, opisthotonos, and seizures. Dorsomedial strabismus has been attributed to trochlear nerve (cranial nerve [CN] IV) paralysis. Increased intracranial pressure is common and may lead to transtentorial herniation. Symmetric laminar cortical necrosis is the most prominent pathologic finding. Edema of the brain with flattening of the gyri may be present. Autofluorescence of the cut surface of the cerebral cortex under ultraviolet light is usually present.

Measurement of transketolase, the thiamine-dependent coenzyme, is helpful for making a diagnosis. The condition should be treated with thiamine, 250 to 1,000 mg administered IV or IM for 3 to 5 days. Steroids should be given if CNS signs are severe. Severely affected animals may have permanent cortical damage.[78]

Niacin and riboflavin deficiencies are less common, but because animals with thiamine deficiency also may have deficiencies in these vitamins, multiple B–complex preparations are indicated. The diet should be corrected to prevent recurrences.

Hypervitaminosis

Vitamin A. Increased levels of vitamin A have been reported in cats with predominantly liver diets. Hypertrophic vertebral bone formation causes ankylosing spondylosis, usually of the cervical vertebrae but in some cases extending to the lumbar region. The clinical signs relate primarily to the rigidity of the vertebral column. Nerve compression occurs in severely affected cats. Dietary correction stops the progression of the spondylosis but does not significantly reduce the spondylosis that is present. Anti-inflammatory and analgesic drugs have been recommended but must be used with caution, especially in cats.[69]

Toxic Disorders

Toxicities causing CNS dysfunction are common in both small and large animals. Many cause biochemical changes and are potentially reversible, whereas others produce structural damage. The more common toxicants are listed in Table 15-9. Toxicologic disorders, including those caused by poisonous plants, are discussed in detail in several texts.[69,79,80]

Diagnosis

A history of exposure to a toxin is the most important factor in establishing the diagnosis in cases of poisoning. CNS signs of intoxication include (1) seizures; (2) depression or coma; (3) tremors, ataxia, and paresis; and (4) LMN signs. Animals that show any of these four signs must be considered as possible poisoning victims until proved otherwise. Metabolic and inflammatory disorders are most commonly confused with toxicosis.

When an animal shows signs suggestive of poisoning, the owner must be questioned carefully to find a possible source. Animals in status epilepticus must be treated immediately, and the history must be obtained later (see Chapter 13). Direct questions regarding agents that are capable of

Table 15-9 **Common Toxicants**

Use	Toxicant	Primary Effect
Pesticides	Chlorinated hydrocarbons	CNS stimulation
	Organophosphates	Binding of acetylcholinesterase
	Carbamates	Binding of acetylcholinesterase
	Pyrethrins	Blocking of nerve conduction and GABA inhibition
	Metaldehyde	CNS stimulation
	Arsenic	GI irritation
Rodenticides	Strychnine	Blocking of inhibitory interneurons
	Thallium	GI irritation, CNS stimulation, peripheral neuropathy, skin lesions
	α-Naphthyl thiourea (ANTU)	GI irritation, pulmonary edema, depression, coma
	Sodium fluoroacetate (1080)	CNS stimulation
	Warfarin	Anticoagulation
	Zinc phosphide	GI irritation, depression
	Phosphorus	GI irritation, CNS stimulation, coma
	Cholecalciferol	CNS depression, cardiac depression
	Bromethalin	Acute—CNS stimulation; chronic—CNS depression
Herbicides and fungicides	Numerous	GI irritation, CNS depression, some are stimulants
Heavy metals	Lead (see arsenic and thallium, above)	GI irritation, CNS stimulation or depression
Drugs	Narcotics	CNS depression
	Amphetamines	CNS stimulation
	Barbiturates	CNS depression
	Tranquilizers	CNS depression
	Aspirin	GI irritation, coma
	Marijuana	Abnormal behavior, depression
	Anthelmintics	GI irritation, CNS stimulation
	Ivermectin	Depression, tremors, ataxia, coma
Garbage	Staphylococcal toxin	GI irritation, CNS stimulation
	Botulinus toxin	LMN paralysis
Poisonous plants	Various	Various
Antifreeze	Ethylene glycol	GI irritation, CNS stimulation, renal failure
Detergents and disinfectants	Hexachlorophene	CNS stimulation or depression, tremors
	Phenols	GI irritation, CNS degeneration
Animal origin	Snake bite	Necrotizing wound, shock, CNS depression
	Toad (*Bufo* spp.)	Digitoxin-like action, CNS stimulation
	Lizards	GI irritation, CNS stimulation or depression
	Tick paralysis (*Dermacentor* spp., *Ixodes* in Australia)	LMN paralysis

producing the signs must be asked. Owners usually are aware of common agents such as insecticides and rodenticides, but they may have difficulty identifying a source of lead poisoning and may be reluctant to admit a source of drug intoxication.

The clinical signs may be sufficient for the clinician to establish a presumptive diagnosis (e.g., intoxication from strychnine and organophosphates). Other agents, such as lead and drugs, may require laboratory confirmation (Tables 15-10 through 15-13).

Toxicants Causing Seizures. The most common sign of poisoning in small animals is seizures (see Table 15-10). The animal may show continuous or

Table 15-10 **Common Toxicants Causing Seizures**

Toxicants	Diagnosis	Management	Prognosis
Organochlorines	Exposure; muscle fasciculations common; laboratory confirmation difficult	Removal of toxicant—washing, gastric lavage; sedation or anesthesia with barbiturates	Poor with seizures
Organophosphates and carbamates	Exposure; salivation, diarrhea, constricted pupils, muscle weakness; blood cholinesterase level decreased; tissue analysis poor	Removal of toxicant; atropine; pralidoxime chloride (2-PAM) (not for carbamates)	Good if treated early
Pyrethrins	Exposure; tremor, salivation, ataxia, seizures; analysis of tissues	Removal of toxicant; sedation	Good if treated early
Strychnine	Exposure; tetany without loss of consciousness, increased by stimulation or noise; laboratory analysis of stomach contents, urine, tissues	Removal of toxicant—gastric lavage or emesis; sedation—barbiturates; respiratory support if needed	Good if treated early
Bromethalin	Exposure; high dose—excitement, tremor, seizures; low dose—tremor, depression, ataxia	Removal of toxicant—activated charcoal; corticosteroids, mannitol	Fair if treated vigorously for several days
Sodium fluoroacetate (1080)	Exposure; seizures are clonic and severe; laboratory confirmation difficult	Removal of toxicant; sedation—barbiturates	Poor with seizures
Thallium	Exposure; GI signs, seizures only in severe poisonings; laboratory analysis of urine and tissues	Removal of toxicant; diphenylthiocarbazone (Dithion) early, ferric ferrocyanide (Prussian blue) late	Poor with seizures, fair with other signs, good with treatment
Lead	Exposure (may be difficult to document); chronic intoxication may cause intermittent seizures, behavioral change, tremor, GI signs; blood lead level >0.4 ppm; basophilic stippling, nucleated red blood cells (RBCs) with no anemia	Removal of toxicant; calcium ethylenediaminetetraacetic acid	Good with treatment
Staphylococcal toxin	Exposure to garbage; severe GI signs; isolation of toxins and testing in laboratory animals	Removal of toxicant; sedation	Poor with seizures; animals usually die rapidly
Toad (*Bufo* spp.—reported only in southern Florida)	Exposure; severe buccal irritation	Wash mouth; sedation—anesthesia	Fair if treated within 15-30 min, otherwise poor
Amphetamines	Exposure to prescription or "street" drugs; hyperactivity, dilated pupils; analysis of urine	Removal of toxicant; sedation or anesthesia—barbiturates	Good if treated early
Metaldehyde	Exposure to snail bait; tremor, ataxia, salivation; seizures are tonic, similar to strychnine, but not changing with stimuli; laboratory analysis of stomach contents	Removal of toxicant; sedation or anesthesia; support respiration	Fair if treated early
Caffeine and other methylxanthines	Ataxia, tachycardia, seizures, coma; laboratory analysis of stomach contents and tissues	Removal of toxicant; sedation, fluids	Fair with treatment
Zinc phosphide	Exposure to rodenticide; behavioral changes, hysteria followed by seizures; GI irritation; analysis of stomach contents and tissues	Removal of toxicant; oral and intravenous bicarbonate; sedation—barbiturates	Poor

Table 15-11   Common Toxicants Causing Behavioral Changes, CNS Depression, or Coma

Toxicants	Diagnosis	Management	Prognosis
Drugs—narcotics, barbiturates, tranquilizers, marijuana	Degree of depression depends on dose; source of pharmaceuticals or "street" drugs; laboratory analysis of blood or urine	Removal of toxicant, narcotic antagonists, diuresis, support respiration	Good with treatment
α-Naphthyl thiourea (ANTU)	Exposure; pulmonary edema; depression and coma terminal; laboratory analysis of stomach contents and tissues	Removal of toxicant, treatment of pulmonary edema	Poor
Ethylene glycol	Exposure; GI irritation, renal failure; oxalate crystals in urine	IV ethanol (30%) with sodium bicarbonate; alternative for dogs—4-methylpyrazole	Poor if coma, fair to good if treated early
Cholecalciferol	Exposure; depression, weakness, cardiac depression, renal failure	Removal of intoxicant; IV saline diuresis, furosemide, corticosteroids	Fair with treatment
Many poisons produce coma terminally			

closely spaced convulsions (e.g., from organophosphates, strychnine) or may have a history of intermittent seizures (e.g., from lead). Animals in status epilepticus must be treated immediately (see Chapter 13).

The tetany produced by strychnine is differentiated from the seizures produced by other agents in this group. Despite the severe muscle spasms, the animal is conscious. Tetany caused by strychnine may be confused with hypocalcemic tetany seen in lactating animals of all species or in tetanus. Intravenous calcium provides immediate

relief in cases of hypocalcemia. Tetanus is much slower in onset than is strychnine poisoning and generally causes more continuous contraction of the muscles. Seizures from other agents produce clonus (alternating flexion and extension).

Organophosphates may be distinguished from organochlorines by their profound effect on the autonomic nervous system, producing profuse salivation, constricted pupils, and diarrhea. Organochlorines frequently produce fine-muscle fasciculations, even between seizures. Pyrethrins and pyrethroids are being used more frequently and

Table 15-12   Common Toxicants Causing Tremor, Ataxia, or Paresis

Toxicants	Diagnosis	Management	Prognosis
Hexachlorophene	Exposure; usually young, nursing animal; large dose causes GI irritation, severe depression; chronic exposure causes cerebellar signs and CNS edema	Removal of toxicant, supportive care; treatment for cerebral edema	Fair; may be residual effects
Lead	Chronic lead poisoning may produce cerebellar signs and dementia (see Table 15-10)	See Table 15-10	Good
Organophosphates	Chronic low doses (flea collars, dips) may produce tremor and weakness (see Table 15-10)	See Table 15-10	Good
Organochlorines	Low-dose exposure may produce weakness and muscle fasciculation (see Table 15-10)	See Table 15-10	Fair to good
Tranquilizers	Ataxia common with tranquilizers (see Table 15-10)	None needed	Good
Marijuana	Behavioral changes and ataxia common	Removal of toxicant	Good
Ergot alkaloids	Cattle and other herbivores grazing on Dallis grass or ryegrass; ataxia, uncoordinated gait	Removal from pasture	Good
Nitro-bearing plants (e.g., *Astragalus* spp., locoweed)	Cattle, sheep, and horses; ataxia, weakness or hyperexcitability, death	Removal from pasture	Fair in ruminants; may be permanent CNS damage
Yellow star thistle	Horses have an acute onset of rigidity of muscles of mastication and involuntary movement of the lips; ataxia, circling, and pacing may occur; lesions are necrosis of the globus pallidus and substantia nigra	No treatment known	Poor

Table 15-13   **Common Toxicants Causing LMN Signs**

Toxicants	Diagnosis	Management	Prognosis
Botulinus toxin	Exposure to contaminated food, carrion, and so forth; ascending LMN paralysis (see Chapter 7)	See Chapter 7	Good
Tick paralysis (*Dermacentor* spp., *Ixodes* species in Australia)	Presence of ticks; ascending LMN paralysis (see Chapter 7)	Removal of ticks (see Chapter 7)	
Drug reaction (nitrofurantoins, doxorubicin, vincristine)	Exposure; rare in animals	Removal of source	Fair
Cyanide (from *Sorghum* species grass)	Cauda equina syndrome with dysuria, flaccid anus and tail, prolapsed penis; may progress to paraplegia; usually occurs in horses	Removal from pasture; no treatment available	May improve after removal from source; residual deficits common
Organophosphates	Chronic exposure may cause LMN signs; axonopathy affecting pelvic limbs first	Removal of source; atropine and pralidoxime if acute signs present; no treatment for peripheral neuropathy	Fair to poor
Heavy metals (lead, arsenic, mercury, thallium)	Chronic exposure, rare in animals (see Table 15-10)	See Table 15-10	See Table 15-10
Industrial chemicals (acrylamide, carbon disulfide, polychlorinated biphenyls)	Not reported in animals; presumably could cause distal axonopathy	Removal from source	Unknown

may cause seizures. The seizure may be preceded by tremors, ataxia, salivation, and other signs. Ingestion of products containing caffeine and other methylxanthines, including chocolate, may also cause seizures. Metaldehyde, a common snail bait, can cause continuous seizures.[81]

Central nervous system signs of lead intoxication are seen most often in cases of chronic exposure.[82-86] The seizures are intermittent. The differential diagnosis of recurrent seizure disorders is discussed in Chapter 13. Laboratory analysis of the blood for evidence of lead is diagnostic. If the blood lead values are in the high normal range and lead poisoning is suspected, treatment followed by measurement of urine lead levels is diagnostic. Other toxicants causing seizures are seen infrequently.

Metronidazole is an antimicrobial, antiprotozoal agent that causes neurotoxicity in dogs and cats.[87-89] The drug is also used in the chronic treatment of inflammatory bowel disease. Neurologic signs include seizures, tremors, ataxia, and peripheral neuropathies. Doses of metronidazole reported to be toxic in cats ranged from 111 mg/kg of body weight per day for 9 weeks to 58 mg/kg of body weight per day for 6 months.[88] The neurologic signs resolved within days of drug withdrawal and supportive treatment. In dogs, doses as low as 67.3 mg/kg of body weight per day for 3 to 14 days caused neurotoxicity.[87] In this report of five dogs, two were euthanized because of severe CNS disease, and three recovered after several months.

Most dogs recover within 7 to 14 days. Diazepam may be effective in treatment of the neurologic signs because it facilitates the effects of GABA, a potent inhibitory neurotransmitter.[89] Diazepam, 0.43 mg/kg PO every 8 hours for 3 days, decreased response time from 4.25 days for untreated dogs to 13.4 hours for treated dogs. In addition, the time to recovery was reduced from 11 days to 38.8 hours.[89]

Ivermectin is widely used as an antihelminthic and preventative of dirofilariasis. It is also used in higher doses for the treatment of sarcoptic and demodectic mange in dogs. In most breeds of dogs, ivermectin has a wide margin of safety. Collies, Australian shepherds, shelties, and old English sheepdogs have an increased sensitivity to ivermectin and related compounds. Some collies have a genetic mutation that results in a nonfunctional P-glycoprotein.[90,91] P-glycoprotein plays an important neuroprotective role in the blood-brain barrier in that it enhances the transport of drugs from the CSF back into circulation. Ivermectin is a GABA agonist that inhibits activity at presynaptic and postsynaptic neurons in the CNS. Clinical signs of ivermectin neurotoxicity include depression, disorientation, tremors, ataxia, blindness, mydriasis, seizures, and coma.[91,92] Clinical signs are dose dependent in that susceptible breeds rarely develop clinical signs at 6 μg/kg once a month, which is the standard dose for heartworm prevention. Doses exceeding 200 μg/kg may cause clinical signs in susceptible breeds and doses above 400 µg/kg may cause death.[92] The recovery period may take more than 3 weeks. There is no specific treatment for ivermectin toxicity.

Toxicants Causing Behavioral Change, Depression, or Coma. Depression or coma may be seen with almost any poison in the terminal stages. Drugs such as narcotics, barbiturates, and tranquilizers most frequently cause depression or coma and also may cause behavioral changes in smaller doses (see Table 15-11). Some other agents such as chlorpyrifos and lead also can produce behavioral changes with chronic intoxication.[86,93] The diagnosis may be obvious if the source is known (e.g., with accidental overdosing with an anticonvulsant or ingestion by an animal of its owner's tranquilizers). Reports of animals that have ingested "street" drugs are increasing, and the owner is usually reluctant to admit the source of the intoxication in these cases. Laboratory analysis of blood or urine may be necessary to confirm the diagnosis.

Toxicants Causing Tremors, Ataxia, and Paresis. Chronic organophosphate poisoning from flea collars and topical or systemic insecticides frequently causes signs that are suggestive of cerebellar disease or muscle weakness (see Table 15-12). The finding of weakness is not consistent with pure cerebellar disease; so when both are present, poisoning must be considered.[94] Chronic lead poisoning also may cause tremor and ataxia (see Chapter 10).

Hexachlorophene toxicity has been seen in puppies with signs of tremor and ataxia.[95-97] Severe depression may follow. The usual source has been repeated washing of the bitch's mammary glands with a soap containing hexachlorophene. Bathing young dogs or cats of any age in hexachlorophene soap also has produced the syndrome. Hexachlorophene is rarely available now.

Metaldehyde poisoning, which produces tremor and ataxia progressing to depression and coma, is seen frequently in areas where the substance is used for snail bait. Numerous plant toxicities cause tremor and ataxia (Table 15-14).

Toxicants Causing LMN Signs. Botulism and tick paralysis cause generalized LMN paralysis by blockade of the neuromuscular junction (see Table 15-13). These conditions are discussed in Chapter 7.

Some drugs (e.g., nitrofurans and anticonvulsants) and some chronic toxicities (such as lead, organophosphate, and arsenic poisoning) can produce peripheral neuropathies. Other signs usually predominate, however.

Treatment

Removal of the toxic substance is the most important part of the treatment for many toxicities. Agents that have entered the animal through the skin, such as insecticides, should be removed by thorough washing and rinsing. Ingested agents may be removed by inducing emesis, performing gastric lavage, or administering laxatives or enemas. Diuresis may promote excretion when absorption has occurred. Activated charcoal is an effective adsorbing agent.[98] Status epilepticus is a life-threatening emergency and must be treated accordingly (see Chapter 13).

Specific treatments for the various toxicities are outlined in Tables 15-10 through 15-14. The reader should consult the references for details.[69,79,80,99]

Inflammatory Diseases

The inflammatory diseases of the nervous system are caused by infectious or parasitic organisms or immune reactions. Canine distemper, granulomatous meningoencephalomyelitis, feline infectious peritonitis (Figure 15-9), equine protozoal myeloencephalitis, and bacterial infections, including thromboembolic meningoencephalitis and listeriosis, are common causes of disease. Some of the fungal diseases are common in endemic areas. Most of the other diseases are relatively uncommon. Inflammatory diseases are discussed in many textbooks.[100-105] The differential diagnosis is outlined in Figure 15-10 and is discussed in the next section. The more common inflammatory diseases are outlined in Tables 15-15 to 15-22.

Text continued on p. 395

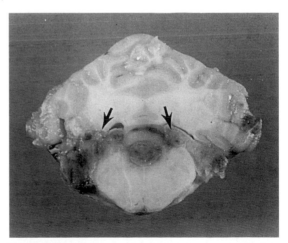

Figure 15-9 Transverse section of the brain at the level of the medulla oblongata and cerebellum from a 3-year-old male domestic cat with chronic wasting and vague neurologic dysfunction. Fibrinopurulent material is within the fourth ventricle and extends to the lateral apertures *(arrows)* bilaterally. Microscopic examination revealed acute necrotizing ventriculitis and choroiditis. Feline infectious peritonitis was suspected. (From Kornegay JN: Pathogenesis of central nervous system disease. In Slatter DH, editor: *Textbook of small animal surgery,* Philadelphia, 1985, WB Saunders.)

Table 15-14 Examples of Several Plant (and Fungal) Toxicoses of Domestic Herbivores that Can Result in Syndromes Characterized by Neurologic Signs

Plant	Species Affected	Neurologic Signs	Pathophysiology	Neural Legions	Treatment	Prognosis
Ryegrass	Sheep, cattle, horses	Ataxia, tremor, tetany	Pentrem and fumi tremorgen mycotoxins from *Penicillium* spp.	Secondary Purkinje cell degeneration	Diazepam	Good
Phalaris spp.	Sheep, cattle	Ataxia, tremor, weakness, seizures	Dimethyltryptamine alkaloids act as monoamine oxidase inhibitors	Neuronal pigmentation (indole melanins)	?Diazepam	Bad
Paspallum, Dallas grass	Cattle, sheep	Ataxia, tremor	*Claviceps paspalli* ergot alkaloids probably neurotoxic	None	—	Good
Swainsona spp. and locoweeds	Sheep, cattle, horses	Weight loss, ataxia, aggressiveness	Indolizidine alkaloid (swainsonine) induces α-mannosidosis	Neuroaxonal dystrophy, neurovisceral storage products	Reserpine (locoweed)	Fair to very good
Sorghum spp.	Horses, cattle, sheep	Ataxia, bladder paralysis	Possibly HCN or lathyrogenic toxins	Spinal cord fiber degeneration	—	Poor to fair
Solanum esuriale	Sheep	Exercise intolerance, weakness, arched back (humpyback)	Unknown (suspected toxin in *S. esuriale*)	Spinal cord fiber degeneration; myopathy	—	Bad
Solanum fastigiatum, S. dimidiatum, S. kwebense	Cattle	Cerebellar ataxia, "cerebellar seizures"	Suspected induction of gangliosidosis	Purkinje cell vacuolation and degeneration	—	Poor
Cycad palms	Cattle, goats, horses	Ataxia, recumbency	Possibly toxic glycosides, cycasin and macrozamin	Spinal cord fiber degeneration	—	Bad

Plant	Species	Clinical signs	Mechanism/toxin	Lesions	Treatment	Prognosis
Melochia pyramidata	Cattle	Ataxia, recumbency	Unknown	Spinal and nerve fiber degeneration	—	Bad
Tribulus terrestris	Sheep	Asymmetric pelvic limb weakness	Possibly neuromuscular process	None	—	Bad
Karwinskia humboldana	Goats	Hypermetria, weakness	Unknown	Peripheral neuropathy, central neuroaxonal dystrophy, myopathy	—	Bad
Nardoo fern, *Marsilea drummondi*	Sheep	Depression, blindness, convulsions	Probably a thiaminase	Polioencephalomalacia	Thiamine	Good if early
Birdsville indigo, *Indigofera linnaei*	Horses	Weight loss, ataxia, weakness	Arginine antagonist alkaloids; indospicine, canavine	None	Arginine-rich feeds (gelatine, Lucerne)	Good
Mexican fireweed, *Kochia scoparia*	Cattle	Blindness (nephrosis, hepatitis)	Saponins, alkaloids, oxalates; possibly thiaminase	Polioencephalomalacia	—	Poor
Buckeye, *Aesculus* spp.	Cattle	Staggering, convulsions	Glycosides and alkaloids described	Unknown	—	Fair
Helichrysum argyrosphaerum	Sheep, cattle	Peripheral blindness, nystagmus, weakness	Unknown	Patchy status spongiosus, white matter	—	Fair for life, bad for vision
Yellow star thistle, *Centaurea solstitialis*	Horses	Depression, pacing, dystonia of muscles of prehension, mastication, and deglutition	Unknown	Nigropallidal encephalomalacia	Tube feed	Poor, starve

Modified from Kornegay JN, Mayhew IG: Metabolic, toxic, and nutritional diseases of the nervous system. In Oliver JE, Hoerlein BF, Mayhew IG, editors: *Veterinary neurology*, Philadelphia, 1987, WB Saunders.

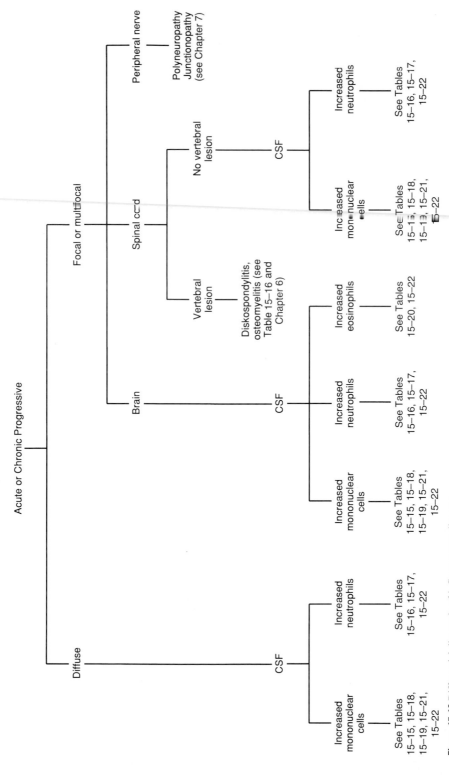

Figure 15-10 Differential diagnosis of inflammatory diseases.

Table 15-15 Viral Diseases of the CNS

Disease	Cause	Incidence	Clinical Signs and Pathology	Course and Prognosis	Diagnostic Tests	Treatment	Prevention
Dogs and Cats							
Canine distemper	Morbilli virus	Common; dogs	Young dogs: systemic illness; respiratory, gastrointestinal, and CNS signs; cerebellum, cerebellar peduncles, optic nerves and tracts, and spinal cord commonly affected; CNS signs may occur early or weeks to months after systemic illness	Acute to subacute, progressive; poor prognosis if CNS signs	History, EEG, CSF (increased lymphocytes, increased protein, especially IgG), CSF antibody, tissue fluorescent antibody (FA), ophthalmoscopy	Supportive; antibacterial agents, anticonvulsants	Vaccine
	Morbilli virus	Common; dogs	Mature dogs: similar to above or may have CNS disease without systemic illness; may start with focal signs (spinal cord, cerebellum) and progress to involve other areas	Subacute to chronic, progressive; poor prognosis if CNS signs	See above	See above	Vaccine
"Old dog" encephalitis	Morbilli virus	Uncommon but not rare; dogs	Mature to older dogs: chronic distemper encephalitis; cerebral signs at onset	Chronic; poor prognosis	History, EEG, ophthalmoscopy, CSF antibody	Supportive	Vaccine
Rabies	Rhabdovirus	Variable; all mammals	Initially behavioral changes; rapid progression to either furious or dumb form; atypical variants may be seen, especially in large animals *Furious:* restlessness, wandering, biting anything encountered, convulsions *Dumb:* progressive paralysis, pharyngeal and hypoglossal paralysis, respiratory paralysis	Acute, progresses to death in 3-8 d from onset	Necroscopy—FA of brain, mouse inoculation; dermal tissue FA is possible	None	Vaccine

Continued

Table 15-15 **Viral Diseases of the CNS**—continued

Disease	Cause	Incidence	Clinical Signs and Pathology	Course and Prognosis	Diagnostic Tests	Treatment	Prevention
Pseudorabies (Aujeszky's disease)	Herpesvirus	Rare except in swine; May affect all animals	May be subclinical in swine; Other animals: early excitement progresses rapidly to coma and death; intense pruritus and self-mutilation, especially at portal of entry, contact with swine in history	Peracute, progression to death in 1-2 d usually	History, signs, necropsy (FA)	None	None available except vaccine for swine
Infectious canine hepatitis	Canine adenovirus type I	Rare CNS; dogs	Affects vascular endothelium, potentially causing signs of CNS disease; primarily liver, kidney, and respiratory signs; hepatic encephalopathy terminally	Acute to chronic	Signs, clinical laboratory profile (liver)	Supportive	Vaccine
Feline infectious peritonitis	Coronavirus	Relatively common; cats	Two forms: *wet* (diffuse, fibrinous peritonitis) and *dry* (disseminated pyogranulomatous lesions in viscera, CNS, and eye); dry form may have only CNS signs, which may be focal in onset; meningeal involvement is common	Slowly progressive; eventually fatal	Signs, clinical laboratory profile (increased white blood cell [WBC] count, neutrophils, plasma protein >8 g/dl), increased globulin, ocular lesions, CSF (increased protein, increased cells, neutrophils or mixed), antibody titer	Supportive	Vaccine marginally effective; isolate infected cats

Disease	Cause	Occurrence	Clinical Signs	Course/Prognosis	Diagnosis	Treatment	Prevention
Postvaccinal rabies	Inadequately attenuated virus in vaccines	Rare; most common in cats	Progressive ascending paralysis to diffuse meningoencephalomyelitis	Acute onset; rapid progression; poor prognosis	History, necropsy	None	Use proper vaccine
Postvaccinal canine distemper	Inadequately attenuated virus in vaccine	Rare; usually young dogs	Usually occurs 1-2 wk after vaccination; behavioral changes common; ataxia, depression, seizures; brainstem lesions predominate	Acute, poor prognosis	History, necropsy	None	None
Canine herpesvirus	Canine herpesvirus	Sporadic; neonates and young puppies	In utero or early exposure; multisystemic signs, depression, diarrhea, rhinitis, loss of consciousness, opisthotonus, seizures; may have residual neurologic deficits if they survive	Acute, progressive; frequently fatal	History, signs, virus isolation, histopathology	Supportive	Administer colostrums and hyperimmune serum in high-incidence kennels
Feline panleukopenia	Parvovirus	Sporadic; neonatal cats	CNS affected primarily in prenatal or neonatal; cerebellar hypoplasia common in prenatal (see Chapter 8)	Present at birth, non-progressive	History, age, signs, necropsy	None	Vaccine
Feline leukemia virus	Retrovirus	Common; cats	CNS affected in some cases; epidural lymphoma causes spinal cord signs; diffuse brain disease may be present; systemic involvement usually apparent; immunosuppression may allow other infections	Chronic, progressive; usually fatal	History, signs, complete blood cell count, cytology of aspirates of CSF; extradural spinal masses should be considered likely for lymphoma	Combination chemotherapy	Vaccine
Feline immunodeficiency virus	Lentivirus	Rare to see neurologic signs	Behavioral abnormalities	Chronic, poorly characterized	History, signs	None	None
Feline paramyxovirus	Paramyxovirus	Unusual; cats	Signs similar to canine distemper encephalitis; demyelination, myoclonus reported	Chronic progressive	Virus isolation	None	None

Continued

Table 15-15 **Viral Diseases of the CNS**—continued

Disease	Cause	Incidence	Clinical Signs and Pathology	Course and Prognosis	Diagnostic Tests	Treatment	Prevention
Horses and Food Animals							
Encephalomyelitis	Togavirus	Variable; horses, dogs	Depression, fever, anorexia, lack of coordination, pacing, circling; primarily	Acute, progressive; recovery variable; may be permanent brain damage	History, CSF, serology, virus isolation	Supportive	Vaccine, horses
Enteroviral encephalomyelitis	Enterovirus	Variable; swine	Pelvic limb ataxia and paresis, paralysis, seizures	Acute, progressive; recovery or progression to death in 1-3 wk	History, virus isolation, serology	Supportive	Vaccine, swine
Equine herpesvirus (rhinopneumonitis)	Herpesvirus Type 1	Variable; horses	Upper respiratory infection; ataxia, cauda equina signs, tetraplegia or paraplegia	Acute, progressive; fair to good prognosis	History, signs, CSF (xanthochromia, increased protein, few cells), serology, virus isolation	Supportive, corticosteroids	Vaccine
Scrapie	"Slow" virus	Sporadic; sheep >2 yr old	Pruritus, cerebellar ataxia, death; neuronal and spongiform degeneration of brain	Chronic, progressive; always fatal	History and signs, histopathology	None	None
Visna, maedi	Lentivirus	Variable; sheep >2 yr old	Ataxia, pelvic limb paresis, progressive to tetraparesis	Chronic, progressive; usually fatal	History, signs, CSF (increased cells, lymphocytes), histopathology, virus isolation, circulating antibody	None	None
Malignant catarrhal fever	Herpesvirus	Sporadic; adult cattle	Depression, blindness, pacing, seizures, death; nasal and ocular discharge	Acute, progressive; usually fatal	History and signs, histopathology	None	None
Hemagglutinating encephalomyelitis virus	Coronavirus	Young swine	Depression, ataxia, tremors, seizures, and hyperesthesia	Acute, CNS form, others more chronic	Serology and virus isolation	None	None

Disease	Cause	Occurrence	Signs	Course	Diagnosis	Treatment	Prevention
Pseudorabies (Aujeszky's disease)	Herpesvirus	Rare except in swine; May affect all mammals	May be subclinical in swine; Other animals: early excitement, progresses rapidly to coma and death; intense pruritus and self-mutilation, especially at portal of entry; contact with swine in history	Peracute, progression to death in 1-2 d	History, signs, necropsy (FA)	None	None available except vaccine for swine
Porcine (paramyxovirus)	Paramyxovirus	Rare; nursing pigs	Depression, ataxia, seizures, weakness, tremor, blindness, panophthalmitis	Acute, progressive; usually fatal	History and signs	None	None
Bovine spongiform encephalopathy	Possibly scrapie virus (prion)	Primarily Holstein-Friesian cattle in United Kingdom	Behavioral disorders, gait and postural abnormalities, hyperreactive to stimuli, aggressive	Chronic, progressive; usually fatal	Signs, histopathology, mouse inoculation	None	None
Equine infectious anemia	Retrovirus	Rare CNS; horses	Behavioral changes, blindness, ataxia, weakness	Chronic, progressive	Serology	Supportive	None
Caprine arthritis-encephalomyelitis	Retrovirus	Sporadic; young goats	Arthritis, ataxia and paresis, affects pelvic limbs first and progresses to all four limbs; some have cerebellar brainstem or cranial nerve signs	Acute to chronic, progressive; frequently fatal	History, signs, CSF, serology	Supportive	None
Infectious bovine rhinotracheitis	Bovine herpesvirus type 1	Rare; young calves	Depression, ataxia, blindness, tremor, seizures	Acute, progressive; fatal	Other animals with upper respiratory disease, serology, virus isolation	Supportive	Vaccine
Louping ill	Flavivirus	Primarily sheep in Great Britain	Ataxia of head and trunk, leaping gait	Acute, progressive; about 50% fatal	Presence of ticks; serology, virus isolation	Supportive	Vaccine

Table 15-16 **Bacterial Diseases of the CNS**

Disease	Cause	Incidence	Clinical Signs and Pathology	Course and Prognosis	Diagnostic Tests	Treatment
Meningitis	*Staphylococcus, Pasteurella,* others	Variable, but generally uncommon	Generalized or localized (especially cervical) hyperesthesia; degree of illness variable; temperature and white blood cell (WBC) count may be normal	Usually acute onset, but may be chronic; prognosis good with early treatment	CSF (protein often >200 mg/dl, increased cells, primarily neutrophils), culture and sensitivity testing	Antibiotics according to sensitivity: ampicillin, trimethoprim, chloramphenicol
Meningoencephalo-myelitis	As in meningitis	Uncommon	As in meningitis, plus signs of brain or spinal cord disease; often includes blindness, seizures, ataxia, cranial nerve deficits	Usually acute: prognosis good with early treatment, but neurologic deficits are common	Same as meningitis; EEG may indicate encephalitis	Same as for meningitis; seizures—diazepam, phenobarbital; acute cerebral edema—mannitol
Abscess	As in meningitis	Rare	May have focal signs or focal signs plus signs of meningitis or meningoencephalitis	May be chronic; progression may be rapid once signs are obvious	Same as in meningo-encephalitis	Same as for meningo-encephalitis
Vertebral osteomyelitis, diskospondylitis (see Chapter 6)	*Staphylococcus, Brucella canis,* others	Moderately frequent in dogs	Pain, usually focal; may have spinal cord compression; usually clinically ill, often over weeks to months	Chronic, may become acute when spinal cord is compressed	Radiography, myelography, *Brucella* serology; blood and urine culture and sensitivity	Antibiotics, preferably bactericidal; curettage, decompression if spinal cord is compressed

390

Tetanus (see Chapter 10)	*Clostridium tetani*	Rare except in horses	Extensor rigidity of all limbs, often with opisthotonos; contraction of facial muscles, prolapsed nictitating membrane; usually infected wound	Acute onset, often lasts 1-2 wk, animals may die; prognosis fair if treated	Signs, history, isolation of organism from wound	Penicillin, tetanus antitoxin, tranquilizers or muscle relaxants; quiet environment; treat wound, nursing
Botulism	*Clostridium botulinum*	Sporadic	LMN-type paralysis, often beginning with pelvic limbs, progressing to tetraparesis in less than 24 hr; caused by toxin blocking neuromuscular junction	Acute onset, lasts about 2 wk; good prognosis unless respiratory paralysis is present early	Serum, fecal analysis, history, EMG, and nerve conduction velocity	Enemas and laxatives early, supportive care, antitoxin usually not effective
Thromboembolic meningoencephalitis	*Haemophilus somnus*	Cattle, primarily young in feedlot	Fever, depression, blindness, lack of coordination, cranial nerve signs, seizures	Acute progressive; fair prognosis with early treatment	History, CSF (increased protein, increased neutrophils), culture	Antibiotics, vaccine available
Listeriosis	*Listeria monocytogenes*	Sporadic in ruminants	Depression, asymmetric ataxia and paresis, cranial nerve signs, central vestibular signs	Acute progressive in sheep and goats, more chronic in cattle; poor prognosis if CNS signs are present	History, signs, CSF (increased protein, increased mononuclear cells), histopathology, fluorescent antibody, isolation of organism	Antibiotics (penicillin, sulfonamides, tetracyclines) for 2-4 wk

Table 15-17 **Mycotic Diseases of the CNS**

Disease	Cause	Incidence	Clinical Signs and Pathology	Course and Prognosis	Diagnostic Tests	Treatment
Cryptococcosis	*Cryptococcus neoformans*	Low; primarily in eastern and Midwestern U.S. but not reported throughout U.S.	Nose and sinuses usually are infected, with extension to brain; ocular lesions and blindness common; CNS involvement common	Chronic; guarded prognosis	Smears and culture of exudates, serum titers, CSF (increased protein, increased cells, neutrophils and mononuclear cells, possibly organisms)	Itraconazole, fluconazole[*]
Blastomycosis	*Blastomyces dermatitidis*	Low; primarily in eastern and midwestern U.S.	Rarely involves CNS; pyogranulomatous encephalitis or single or multifocal granulomas; frequently involves lungs, skin, and eyes	Chronic; poor prognosis	See Cryptococcosis	Amphotericin B,[*] 5-fluorocytosine, ketoconazole, itraconazole, fluconazole
Histoplasmosis	*Histoplasma capsulatum*	Low; primarily in central U.S.	CNS involvement uncommon; involves reticuloendothelial cells of most viscera	Chronic; poor prognosis	See Cryptococcosis	Amphotericin B,[*] 5-fluorocytosine, ketoconazole, itraconazole, fluconazole
Coccidioidomycosis	*Coccidioides immitis*	Can be relatively common in endemic areas of southwestern U.S.	CNS involvement uncommon; pulmonary infection common	Chronic; poor prognosis	See Cryptococcosis	Amphotericin B,[*] 5-fluorocytosine, ketoconazole, itraconazole, fluconazole
Nocardiosis	*Nocardia* species	Low throughout U.S.	Systemic disease, signs similar to canine distemper; respiratory or cutaneous forms; CNS abscesses and vertebral osteomyelitis reported	Chronic; poor prognosis	Smears, cultures, CSF (increased protein, increased cells, neutrophils)	Penicillin, sulfonamides, trimethoprim
Actinomycosis	*Actinomyces* species	Low throughout U.S.	Similar to nocardiosis	Chronic; poor prognosis	Similar to nocardiosis	Penicillin, clindamycin, erythromycin, lincomycin
Paecilomycosis	*Paecilomyces* species	Rare	Disseminated form of diskospondylitis	Chronic; poor prognosis	Culture, biopsy	None
Aspergillosis	*Aspergillus* species	Primarily in large animals	Encephalitis can develop after immunosuppression or guttural pouch infection	Chronic; poor prognosis	Culture, CSF	Amphotericin B,[*] 5-fluorocytosine, ketoconazole, itraconazole, fluconazole
Phaeohyphomycosis	*Cladosporium* species	Rare	Encephalitis with granulomas has been reported in dogs and cats	Chronic; poor prognosis	Culture, biopsy	Amphotericin B,[*] 5-fluorocytosine, ketoconazole, itraconazole, fluconazole Unknown efficacy

[*]Itraconazole and fluconazole have been used effectively in some cats with cryptococcal encephalitis and are the preferred treatment. Data for other fungal CNS infections are largely lacking.

Table 15-18 **Protozoal Diseases of the CNS**

Disease	Cause	Incidence	Clinical Signs and Pathology	Course and Prognosis	Diagnostic Tests	Treatment
Toxoplasmosis	*Toxoplasma gondii*	Common infection but infrequent clinical problem	Clinical manifestations usually associated with another disease or immunosuppression; CNS, eyes, lungs, gastrointestinal tract and skeletal muscles often affected	Chronic; fair to poor prognosis	Serum titer, oocysts in stool, biopsy, CSF (increased protein, increased cells, mononuclear cells and neutrophils)	Sulfonamides, pyrimethamine, clindamycin
Neosporosis	*Neospora caninum*	Uknown frequency, cases of toxoplasmosis reported in past were sometimes *Neospora*; reported in dogs and rarely in cats, cattle, and horses	Similar to toxoplasmosis; ascending paralysis of limbs with extension of the pelvic limbs is frequent in young pups	Chronic progressive; fair to poor prognosis	CSF, biopsy, isolation of organism	Sulfonamides, pyrimethamine, clindamycin are probably effective if given early
Babesiosis	*Babesia* spp.	Rare in U.S.	Parasite of red blood cells; rarely causes CNS disease, hemorrhage; more severe with other infections, such as *Ehrlichia*	Acute to chronic; poor prognosis	Peripheral blood smears	Diminazene, phenamidine, or imidocarb
Encephalitozoonosis	*Encephalitozoon cuniculi*	Rare; primarily affects dogs < 2 mo old	Acute encephalitis, ataxia, tremors, behavioral changes	Acute; poor prognosis	Serum titers, culture, histopathology	None
Trypanosomiasis	*Trypanosoma cruzi*	Rare in U.S.	Parasite of red blood cells; rarely causes CNS disease	Chronic, fair prognosis with treatment	Peripheral blood smears	Nifurtimox
Equine protozoal myeloencephalitis	*Sarcocystis neurona* (*Sarcocystis falcatula*)	Fairly common in horses	Systemic, multifocal, involving almost any part of the nervous system: commonly spinal cord, cauda equina, and cranial nerve signs	Chronic, progressive; usually poor prognosis; treatment may be effective	Rule out other causes, CSF (sometimes increased protein, increased cells, mononuclear; titer, PCR)	Pyrimethamine, trimethoprim-sulfonamide
Coccidiosis	Several species	Common enteric, rare CNS, several species of animals affected	Enteric coccidiosis is reported to cause CNS signs in some cases; *Sarcocystis* spp. may cause myopathy	Variable	Fecal identification, organism in muscle biopsy or necropsy	Sulfonamides, amprolium
Hepatozoonosis	*Hepatozoon canis*	Rare; dogs	Muscle pain and gait abnormalities may be seen	Chronic; poor prognosis	Biopsy	Possibly sulfonamides, pyrimethamine (efficacy not known)

Table 15-19 **Rickettsial and Chlamydial Diseases of the CNS**

Disease	Cause	Incidence	Clinical Signs and Pathology	Course and Prognosis	Diagnostic Tests	Treatment
Rocky Mountain spotted fever	*Rickettsia rickettsii*	Fairly common in endemic areas of U.S.; dogs	Meningitis, ataxia, other CNS signs; can look like canine distemper	Acute; good prognosis with treatment	History of ticks, signs, thrombocytopenia, serum titer	Doxycycline, chloramphenicol
Ehrlichiosis	*Ehrlichia canis*	Rarely CNS signs in dogs	Meningitis, encephalitis	Acute to chronic; good prognosis if treated early	Pancytopenia, thrombocytopenia, serum titer	Doxycycline, chloramphenicol
Salmon poisoning	*Neorickettsia helminthoeca*	Rare, Pacific Northwest U.S.	Depression and convulsions terminally; paresis of pelvic limbs less common; nonsuppurative meningoencephalitis	Acute; fair to good prognosis if treated early	History of eating salmon, fluke eggs in feces	Doxycycline, chloramphenicol
Sporadic bovine encephalomyelitis (Buss disease)	*Chlamydia psittaci*	Sporadic, young cattle	Respiratory disease, polyarthritis, diffuse cerebral signs	Acute progressive; mortality approximately 50%	History, signs, CSF (increased protein, increased mononuclear cells), serology	Tetracycline, tylosin
Neuroborreliosis (Lyme disease)	*Borrelia burgdorferi*	Rare, except in endemic areas	Depression, meningitis	Acute to chronic (poorly characterized)	Antibodies to *B. burgdorferi* (especially in CSF)	Third generation cephalosporins, tetracyclines

Table 15-20 **Parasitic Diseases of the CNS**

Disease	Cause	Incidence	Clinical Signs and Pathology	Course and Prognosis	Diagnostic Tests	Treatment
Dirofilariasis	*Dirofilaria immitis,* microfilaria or aberrant adult	Rare, areas with heartworm disease	CNS signs rare; microfilaria or migrating adult heartworms may cause infarction; seizures and other cerebral signs	Acute onset; prognosis poor	Blood smear or serology to confirm heartworm disease, CSF (increased eosinophils suggestive), difficult to prove antemortem	None proved
Larva migrans	*Toxocara canis* and other species	Rare	Granulomas in brain or spinal cord from migrating larvae; signs related to location of lesion	Acute or chronic; prognosis depends on severity of signs	None, necropsy	None
Cuterebra	*Cuterebra* spp.	Rare	CNS signs depend on location of lesion	Acute to chronic; poor prognosis	None, necropsy	None
Coenurosis	*Coenurus* spp.	Rare; most often reported in sheep	CNS signs depend on location of lesion	Acute to chronic; poor prognosis	None, sheep have softening of skull that can be palpated or seen on radiographs	Surgical removal in sheep

Diagnosis

Most of the inflammatory diseases are characterized by an acute onset. All are progressive, and some are chronic-progressive. Diffuse or multifocal involvement is characteristic of most of the diseases in this group, but localized signs also occur. The minimum database (see Chapter 1) may provide evidence of systemic infection (e.g., alterations in white blood cell [WBC] count), although many primary CNS inflammatory diseases do not produce a systemic response. Therefore, positive findings in laboratory data are useful, but negative findings do not rule out infectious disease. Focal deficits should be investigated according to the location of the lesion (see Chapters 5 through 15).

Analysis of CSF is a useful test for establishing the diagnosis of inflammatory disease (see Chapter 4). Increases in CSF protein concentrations range from low (50 to 100 mg/dl) in chronic viral diseases to very high (300+ mg/dl) in bacterial and fungal infections. Characteristic cell changes are increased mononuclear cells in viral diseases; increased neutrophils in bacterial diseases; increased numbers of both mononuclear cells and neutrophils in mycotic and protozoal diseases and feline infectious peritonitis; and increased numbers of mononuclear cells, neutrophils, and some eosinophils in parasitic and immune-mediated diseases. Exceptions do exist. For example, chronic bacterial infections may cause a mononuclear cell response, especially increases in macrophages, whereas some viral diseases cause increased neutrophils in the CSF. The presence of neutrophils in the CSF is not necessarily abnormal. The only cell

Table 15-21 **Immune-mediated Diseases of the CNS**

Disease	Cause	Incidence	Clinical Signs and Pathology	Course and Prognosis	Diagnostic Tests	Treatment
Coonhound paralysis	Probable immune reaction to transmissible agent in raccoon saliva or environment	Fairly high in some areas, dogs	Ascending LMN paralysis; may last approximately 6 wk; ventral roots and peripheral nerves have segmental demyelination and some axon loss	Acute onset, lasts approximately 6 wk; good prognosis with good nursing	History, EMG, nerve conduction velocity	Supportive
Postvaccinal rabies	CNS tissues in vaccine	Rare—these vaccines are no longer used	Ascending paralysis; demyelination from immune reaction to myelin in brain-origin vaccines	Acute onset, progressive; poor prognosis	None	None

Table 15-22 Unclassified Inflammatory Diseases of the CNS

Disease	Cause	Incidence	Clinical Signs and Pathology	Course and Prognosis	Diagnostic Tests	Treatment
Granulomatous meningoencephalo-myelitis (inflammatory reticulosis)	Unknown, probably immune-mediated	Relatively common; dogs	Nonsuppurative inflammation of brain or spinal cord and meninges; may be disseminated, focal, or multifocal; neoplastic forms are usually called reticulosis; signs depend on location of the predominant lesions	Chronic progressive, poor prognosis	CSF (increased cells of a mixed population), histopathology	Cytosine arabinoside and prednisone
Feline polioencephalo-myelitis	Unknown	Rare; cats	Paresis, especially of the pelvic limbs, tremor, hyperesthesia; spinal cord neurons and white matter predominantly affected; brain lesions are scattered	Chronic progressive, poor prognosis	Some cats have leukopenia and nonregenerative anemia, histopathology	None
Pug and Maltese terrier encephalitis	Unknown, possibly immune-mediated	Rare; pugs, usually less than 2 y old	Seizures, cerebral signs; mononuclear inflammatory changes in cerebrum and meninges	Chronic progressive, poor prognosis	Breed, CSF (increased mononuclear cells), histopathology	Corticosteroids may give transient improvement
Corticosteroid-responsive meningitis	Unknown, probably immune-mediated	Uncommon; usually large-breed dogs	Hyperesthesia, especially cervical; anorexia, muscular rigidity, and fever common	Acute; fair to good prognosis with therapy	CSF (increased protein and cells, especially neutrophils), neutrophilia in blood also	Corticosteroids may be needed for several months
Pyogranulomatous meningoencephalo-myelitis	Unknown, probably immune-mediated	Uncommon; reported in pointers only	Hyperesthesia, especially cervical, atrophy of cervical muscles, rigidity, some incoordination; both brain and spinal cord affected, worse in cervical spinal cord; mixed mononuclear and neutrophil infiltrations in meninges and parenchyma	Acute progressive; poor prognosis	Breed, CSF (increased neutrophils), histopathology	None; some remission with antibiotics
Yorkshire terrier encephalitis	Unknown, possibly immune-mediated	Rare, Yorkshire terriers	Acute progressive with variable presentation; seizures, abnormal gait, vestibular signs, postural reaction deficits; multifocal perivascular cuffing of mononuclear cells; gliosis and malacia	Progressive, over weeks to months	Breed, CSF (mononuclear pleocytosis, mild increase in protein), histopathology	None effective
Necrotizing vasculitis of beagles and Bernese Mountain dogs	Unknown, probably immune-mediated	Rare, beagles and Bernese Mountain dogs 3-12 mo old	Acute progressive, pyrexia, cervical pain, paresis; suppurative meningitis, vasculitis; infarction may occur in Bernese Mountain dogs	Progressive	Breed, CSF (neutrophilic pleocytosis, increased protein)	Immunosuppressive levels of corticosteroids may control signs

whose presence in the CSF seems consistently abnormal is the macrophage. The CSF can be normal in CNS inflammation.

Clinical suspicion of an infection is an adequate indication for bacterial and fungal cultures and bacterial sensitivity tests. The presence of antibodies in the CSF to specific viruses or to other infectious agents provides evidence of infection because they are not present in normal vaccinated animals or those with systemic infection but without CNS disease (also see Chapter 4).[101] In CSF samples contaminated by blood (hemorrhage), serum albumin and antibody concentrations should be compared with concentrations in the CSF. When the level of CSF antibodies exceeds that of serum, CNS infection is more likely. Inflammation may increase the permeability of the blood-brain barrier, allowing serum antibodies to leak into the CSF.

PRINCIPLES OF MEDICAL TREATMENT

Medical treatment is most commonly indicated for infections involving the nervous system. Physical therapy also is necessary for rehabilitation. Seizures (see Chapter 13) and other diseases requiring specific treatment are covered in the descriptions of the diseases. The management of CNS edema is discussed in Chapter 12 in the section on brain trauma. Management of pain is reviewed in Chapter 14.

Management of Central Nervous System Infections

Effective therapy for CNS infections depends on the identification of the cause and selection of the appropriate antimicrobial agent. Identification is based on CSF analysis and culture. Selection of the appropriate antimicrobial agent depends on two principles: (1) the agent must be effective against the microbial target without severely injuring the patient; and (2) it must be delivered to, and must penetrate, the CNS. Unfortunately, anatomic and physiologic barriers to successful therapy for CNS infections exist, especially when certain drugs are used. The combined effects of these obstacles create a functional blood-brain barrier.

The Blood-Brain Barrier

The combined functions of the CNS capillaries and the choroid plexus create a barrier to the movement of drugs from the capillary or pericapillary fluid into nervous tissue or CSF. Discrepancies between serum and CNS drug concentrations occur because of two factors: the special anatomy of CNS capillaries and the secretory selectivity of the choroid

plexus. In capillaries outside the CNS, drugs and other agents pass from the blood through clefts between endothelial cells and through fenestrations in the capillary basement membrane. In the CNS, capillary endothelial cells are joined by tight junctions that seal the intercellular clefts. The capillary basement membrane has no fenestrations and glial cell foot processes surround the capillaries.

In the CNS, a drug must penetrate an inner bimolecular lipid membrane, the endothelial cell cytoplasm, an outer lipid membrane, and a basement membrane and then traverse the glial foot processes.[106] Penetration of a drug is largely a function of its endothelial membrane solubility. Membrane solubility is favored by (1) a low degree of ionization at physiologic pH, (2) a low degree of plasma protein binding, and (3) a high degree of lipid solubility of the unionized drug.[107,108] Certain highly lipid-soluble drugs bind strongly to tissue sites in the brain, permitting high concentrations to be achieved within nervous tissue.

Regulation of CSF solutes occurs at the choroid plexus. Plasma dialysate that filters through fenestrated capillaries is selectively secreted by choroid epithelial cells. Certain CSF constituents also are actively reabsorbed by the choroidal epithelial cell, which tends to clear these substances from the CSF and from nervous tissue. This active transport system for weak organic acids removes drugs such as penicillin and gentamicin. Inflammation may block this system, allowing drug concentrations to increase. In addition, inflammation may increase the permeability of endothelial membranes to certain antibiotics, allowing these drugs to penetrate nervous tissue in cases of disease. In the normal animal, these antibiotics penetrate poorly. As the inflammation decreases, penetration of the antibiotic also decreases.

ANTIMICROBIAL AGENTS IN TREATING INFECTIONS

Antimicrobial agents are grouped by their capacity to achieve concentrations in CSF sufficient to inhibit microorganisms throughout the period of therapy.[108] Table 15-23 lists these drugs relative to achievable concentrations in CSF. Microbicidal drugs are preferred to microbistatic drugs whenever possible. Antibiotics such as the aminoglycosides diffuse poorly, even in the presence of inflammation. Intrathecal administration may be required for adequate CSF concentrations to be achieved, but this route is rarely used in animals because of the necessity for anesthesia with each injection. Placement of intraventricular catheters can facilitate the injection of drugs into the CSF.

Table 15-23 **Antimicrobial Drugs: Ability to Penetrate the Blood-Brain Barrier**

	Good	Intermediate	Poor
Microbicidal	Trimethoprim	Penicillin G*	Penicillin G
	Moxalactam	Ampicillin*	benzathine
	Cefotaxime	Methicillin*	Cephalosporins[‡]
	Ceftazidime	Nafcillin*	Aminoglycosides
	Metronidazole	Carbenicillin*	
	Enrofloxacin	Oxacillin	
	Vancomycin		
Microbistatic	Chloramphenicol	Tetracycline	Amphotericin B
	Sulfonamides	Flucytosine	Erythromycin[§]
	Isoniazid	Clindamycin	
	Minocycline[†]		
	Doxycycline[†]		
	Rifampin		

*High intravenous doses are needed to achieve the maximal effect.
[†]Lipid-soluble tetracyclines that achieve higher concentrations in CSF than do other tetracyclines.
[‡]First and second generation, may be effective early in bacterial meningitis; concentrations dramatically decrease with repair of the blood-brain barrier.
[§]Penetration in the face of inflammation is unpredictable.

Bacterial Infections

Bacterial Meningoencephalomyelitis

The pathogenesis, pathophysiology, and implications of treatment of bacterial meningitis in humans and experimental animals have been reviewed.[109] Bacteria must be able to survive in the intravascular space, penetrate the blood-brain barrier, and colonize in the meninges or CSF. Breakdown of the blood-brain barrier causes exudation of albumin into the CSF and facilitates the development of brain or spinal cord edema. Experiments in rats suggest that bacteria in the CSF elicit the release of endogenous inflammatory mediators that are important in the development and progression of clinical signs.[109] Experimental studies in rabbits reveal that the inflammatory process causes brain edema, probably secondary to loss of cerebrovascular autoregulation, direct cytotoxicity, and increased CSF outflow resistance.[110]

These findings may have important therapeutic implications. Rapidly acting bactericidal therapy delivered into the CSF is mandatory because only bactericidal therapy is associated with a cure in humans and experimental animal models. Rapid destruction of bacteria could release high concentrations of inflammatory bacterial fragments or toxins (lipopolysaccharides), which might exacerbate the inflammatory process.[110-112]

These studies also suggest that adjunctive therapy with antiinflammatory agents may be beneficial in bacterial meningitis.[110] In animals with experimental *Streptococcus pneumoniae* meningitis, methylprednisolone reduced CSF outflow resistance and both methylprednisolone and dexamethasone reduced brain edema.[110] Pretreatment with dexamethasone followed in 15 to 20 minutes with third-generation cephalosporins resulted in decreased inflammatory mediator release in laboratory animals with *Haemophilus influenzae* CNS infections.[111] Several controlled studies in children with bacterial meningitis demonstrated the benefits of adjunctive corticosteroid therapy, especially when corticosteroids are administered 15 to 20 minutes before bactericidal antibiotic therapy.[112] In these studies dexamethasone was given 15 to 20 minutes before cefotaxime therapy and was continued every 6 hours for 4 days.

Other antiinflammatory agents that might be useful include indomethacin, pentoxifylline, and superoxide dismutase. Specific monoclonal antibodies have shown promise in experimental models of bacterial meningitis, especially when dexamethasone is also administered.[113]

Although these studies may have therapeutic implications for bacterial meningitis in domestic animals, controlled studies regarding these species have not been published. Furthermore, these studies involve specific neurotrophic bacteria that may behave differently than the agents producing meningitis in animals.

Bacterial Meningoencephalomyelitis in Dogs and Cats. Bacterial meningoencephalomyelitis (Figure 15-11) is not common in dogs and cats. It usually occurs in association with bacteremia secondary to endocarditis, urinary tract infections, and pulmonary infections. Critically ill patients may have added risk of CNS infection. Meningitis

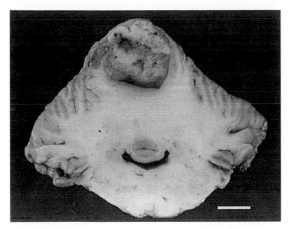

Figure 15-11 Transverse section of brain at the medulla oblongata and cerebellum from a 9-year-old female Vizsla with acute, progressive neurologic dysfunction. The dorsal cerebellar vermis contains a roughly circular area of caseous necrosis. On microscopic examination, a marked infiltrate of neutrophils was noted. *Enterobacter* spp. were cultured from the lesion. A diagnosis of focal cerebellar abscess was made. Bar = 2 cm. (From Kornegay JN: Pathogenesis of central nervous system disease. In Slatter DH, editor: *Textbook of small animal surgery,* Philadelphia, 1985, WB Saunders.)

may also occur from extension of infection in structures adjacent to the nervous system, such as the nasal passages, sinuses, and internal ears. Aerobic bacteria associated with bacterial meningitis in dogs and cats include *Pasteurella multocida, Staphylococcus intermedius, Streptococcus* spp., and *Escherichia coli.*[108,114,115] Uncommonly, *Proteus, Pseudomonas, Salmonella,* and *Klebsiella* organisms may be the causative agents. These gram-negative organisms are more common in nosocomial infections of critically ill patients. Anaerobic bacteria isolated from dogs and cats with CNS infection include *Bacteroides, Fusobacterium, Peptostreptococcus,* and *Eubacterium.*[116]

Definitive treatment of bacterial meningitis is based on isolation of the organism from the CSF and determination of its antibiotic sensitivity. The source of infection should be identified and managed therapeutically. Blood and urine cultures may be useful to identify the causative agent. Pending the outcome of CSF cultures, the initial antibiotic therapy in small animals is based on clinical findings of concomitant infection and the most likely causative agent present. Broad-spectrum bactericidal antibiotics that penetrate the CSF are chosen.

Trimethoprim-sulfonamide combinations and enrofloxacin are good initial choices. Both are available to veterinarians, penetrate the CSF in good concentrations, and are not expensive compared with third-generation cephalosporins. Enrofloxacin has greater activity against gram-negative bacteria and very little activity against anaerobes.[117] The dosage for enrofloxacin is 5 mg/kg twice a day for 7 to 10 days, then 5 mg/kg once a day for 10 to 14 days. The initial dose for trimethoprim-sulfonamides is 30 mg/kg every 12 hours for 5 to 7 days and then 15 mg/kg every 12 hours for 10 to 14 days.

Third-generation cephalosporins such as cefotaxime and ceftazidime penetrate the CSF in good concentrations and are effective against many resistant gram-negative bacteria.[118] They are usually effective against anaerobes but have reduced activity against gram-positive cocci. Ceftiofur, approved for use in animals, does not cross the blood-brain barrier unless inflammation is present, and, in this regard, is similar to the aminopenicillins. When gram-negative sepsis is suspected as the cause of the meningitis, the third-generation cephalosporins are the drugs of choice.

Meningitis caused by gram-positive bacteria may respond to high doses of aminopenicillins.[115] Many isolates of *S. intermedius* and *Staphylococcus aureus* secrete beta lactamase, which inactivates most aminopenicillins. Aminopenicillins combined with clavulanic acid and lactamase-resistant penicillins such as methicillin or oxacillin are better choices for staphylococcal infections.

Rifampin is bactericidal, readily penetrates the CSF, and has very good activity against staphylococci.[119] It is also effective against many gram-negative bacteria. Bacterial resistance to rifampin develops readily, especially when it is given as a single agent. For staphylococcal infections, rifampin is best combined with beta-lactam antibiotics. The human dose of 10 mg/kg daily produces a concentration in canine serum four times that required in people to inhibit bacteria but also causes adverse side effects in dogs. A dose less than 10 mg/kg daily is recommended, but definitive pharmacologic studies have not been published.[119] Rifampin also may be useful in treating chronic abscesses and pyogranulomatous infections.

Imipenem is a beta-lactam compound that belongs to the carbapenem family of antibiotics. It has broad-spectrum activity against most gram-positive and gram-negative aerobes and anaerobes. Imipenem is useful in the treatment of nosocomial gram-negative infections that do not respond to other antibiotic regimens.[118,120] After intravenous administration, imipenem penetrates the CSF in good concentrations.

Occasionally, systemic infection with *Brucella canis* extends to the nervous system. The best therapy for brucellosis includes a combination of streptomycin and minocycline. Streptomycin should be administered for 2 weeks by parenteral injection. Minocycline should be given orally for 4 weeks in combination with the 2-week course for strepto-mycin.[121,122]

Bacterial Meningitis in Horses. Bacterial meningitis occurs most commonly in septicemic foals that do not acquire passive transfer of immunity.[123-125] Common primary sites of infection include the GI tract, lung, and umbilicus. Pneumonia, peritonitis, hypopyon, septic arthritis, and omphalophlebitis are common. Extension to the brain and spinal cord frequently occurs if treatment is not aggressive.

The diagnosis of meningitis in foals is confirmed by cytologic evaluation and bacterial culture of the CSF. A neutrophilic pleocytosis is typical, and cell counts may exceed 1,000 cells/mm^3 (normal <5 cells/mm^3).[123,124] The total CSF protein level is usually more than 100 mg/dl. *E. coli* and *Klebsiella* spp. are the most frequently isolated organisms.[125,126]

Although definitive antibiotic therapy is based on bacterial culture and sensitivity testing, initial empiric therapy is based on the assumption that gram-negative enteric bacteria are the most likely cause. Third-generation cephalosporins are the antimicrobials recommended in foals. These include cefotaxime sodium (40 mg/kg IV every 8 hours) and ceftazidime (50 mg/kg IV every 12 hours). Ceftiofur (2 to 4 mg/kg IV every 12 hours) is available to veterinarians but does not penetrate the CSF in normal horses. Although very expensive, these antibiotics can rapidly sterilize the CSF and may shorten the total treatment time and thus reduce overall costs of therapy.[123] Trimethoprim-sulfonamide combinations may be effective but are less so than the third-generation cephalosporins previously described.

Adjunctive antiinflammatory therapy in foals with progressive neurologic dysfunction includes the use of glucocorticoids (dexamethasone, 0.15 mg/kg every 6 hours IV). Because glucocorticoid therapy can cause rapid bacterial dissemination in septicemic foals, great caution is advised in their use.[123] Dimethyl sulfoxide (1 g/kg IV every 24 hours) may help to reduce CNS inflammation and edema and protect against reperfusion injury when cerebral ischemia is present. Mannitol (0.25 to 1.0 g/kg IV every 24 hours) helps to reduce CNS edema. Plasma transfusions (1 to 2 L IV) and enteral hyperalimentation may be indicated. Diazepam (0.2 to 0.5 mg/kg every 15 minutes) or phenobarbital (10 to 20 mg/kg IV every 8 hours) or both can be given to control seizures.[123]

Bacterial Meningoencephalomyelitis in Cattle. Bacterial meningitis is the most common CNS disease in neonatal calves.[127] It develops secondary to septicemia and bacteremia associated with failure of passive transfer of colostral antibodies. *E. coli* is the organism most frequently responsible in clinical cases.[127] Isolates may be resistant to trimethoprim-

sulfonamides, and many, if not most, are now resistant to triple sulfonamide drugs. Most affected calves die or are euthanized, usually within 2 to 3 days after diagnosis and initiation of therapy. Neutrophilic pleocytosis and increased protein are present in the CSF of 60% to 70% of affected calves. Mononuclear pleocytosis may be present in chronic disease. Free bacteria are present in the CSF in less than 50% of cases examined.

Although trimethoprim-sulfonamides and triple sulfonamide drugs are frequently chosen to treat bacterial meningitis in calves, studies indicate an emerging resistance of gram-negative bacteria to these drugs. Although expensive, the third-generation cephalosporins are the rational empiric drugs of choice for treatment. Because of their cost, these drugs may not be economically feasible in many cases.

Haemophilus somnus is the major cause of thromboembolic meningoencephalitis (TEME) in cattle.[128] Exposure to this organism is widespread, and up to 25% of cattle may harbor serum antibodies to the organism. *H. somnus* persists in the urinary and reproductive tracts of cattle and is shed in urine and reproductive secretions. The disease is most common in weaned calves, and outbreaks of hemophilosis occur 1 to 2 weeks after cattle arrive at the feedyard.[129] Bronchopneumonia is the most common form of hemophilosis; but arthritis, myelitis, retinitis, myocarditis, laryngitis, otitis media interna, and conjunctivitis also occur. The TEME usually follows the occurrence of pneumonia by 1 to 2 weeks. Morbidity is low, and mortality is high.

As with the neurotrophic bacteria that infect people, *H. somnus* possesses several virulent factors (mucopolysaccharide capsule, outer membrane proteins, and endotoxin concentrated in the cell wall) that enhance its penetration into, and subsequent injury to, the CNS.

H. somnus colonizes the small vessels of the meninges, brain, and spinal cord. Fibrin thrombi and brain infarction cause the neurologic signs. The most effective antibiotics for TEME include the aminopenicillins and ceftiofur. Both are approved for use in food animals and penetrate the CSF when active inflammation is present. Trimethoprim-sulfonamides may be effective but must be given parenterally to ruminants because trimethoprim is sequestered in the rumen when given orally. Oxytetracycline is used for non-CNS infections.

Listeria monocytogenes is a resistant and ubiquitous bacterium capable of causing CNS disease in people and domestic animals.[130] Ruminants appear more susceptible to infection than do other domestic animals. The organism can be transmitted in silage and other feed. Food-borne infection is common in humans. Although meningitis and encephalitis are the classic manifestations of listeriosis in ruminants, spinal cord disease, abortion, and mastitis also occur. Diagnosis is confirmed by isolation of the organism from body fluids or tissues. Cold enrichment methods are used to isolate the organism. The aminopenicillins are frequently given to treat listeriosis. In ruminants, the tetracyclines may also be effective even though they poorly penetrate the CSF. Doxycycline may be a reasonable choice because it does penetrate the CSF.

Bacterial Brain Abscess

Brain abscesses are more common in large animals than in dogs and cats (see Figure 15-11). Neurologic signs relate to the specific location of the abscess and compression or necrosis of surrounding neurologic structures. Large abscesses may create signs similar to any other intracranial mass. Increased intracranial pressure, cerebral edema, and brain herniation may occur.

The pituitary abscess syndrome has been described in cattle, goats, sheep, and swine.[131] The anatomy of the *rete mirabilis* and its close association to the pituitary gland may explain the predilection for pituitary abscesses in cattle. The primary clinical signs include depression, ataxia, blindness, dysphagia, head pressing, bradycardia, nystagmus, and strabismus. The CSF may contain increased total protein concentrations and pleocytosis. Bacterial cultures of CSF are usually negative. *Corynebacterium pyogenes* and *Streptococcus* spp. are most commonly isolated from abscesses at necropsy.[131] Infection at other sites with the same organisms occurs in about 50% of cases. The mortality rate is nearly 100%, and successful therapy is rare.

In horses brain abscesses are usually caused by *Streptococcus equi,* but other streptococci are occasionally isolated.[132] The prognosis is generally poor. If diagnosed by CT, successful surgical drainage is possible.[133] Brain abscesses are rare in dogs and cats but may result from extension of purulent otitis media interna, rhinitis, sinusitis, open skull fractures, and foreign-body penetration of the brain. The causative agents are usually *Staphylococcus* spp., *Streptococcus* spp., and *Pasteurella* spp. Anaerobes may also be isolated in some cases. Localization of the abscess with CT or MRI may allow surgical drainage or excision. Methicillin, oxacillin, and rifampin may be useful for gram-positive infections. Clindamycin and metronidazole may be given in anaerobic infections. A guarded prognosis should be made.

Cats may have meningitis secondary to abscesses that are frequently caused by anaerobic bacteria. Penicillin or amoxicillin is effective and reasonable in cost. Clindamycin or metronidazole is a good alternative for resistant infections.[134]

Diskospondylitis

The most common cause of diskospondylitis in dogs is *Staphylococcus intermedius*; occasionally *Brucella canis* organisms are the source.[135] The disease may be associated with urinary tract infection and bacteremia. In staphylococcal diskospondylitis, penicillinase-resistant antibiotics should be chosen. Cephalosporins or methicillin or oxacillin is usually effective. Medical treatment should be tried before surgical treatment is considered. Severe paresis may require decompression. Vertebral curettage, in addition to antibiotic therapy for 4 to 6 weeks, may achieve resolution if medical treatment is unsuccessful. In *Brucella canis* diskospondylitis, therapy is expensive and may not eradicate the infection effectively. Streptomycin-minocycline combinations are used as described for meningitis.[122] The dog should be neutered and isolated from other dogs.

Mycotic Infections

The more common mycotic infections of the CNS are caused by *Cryptococcus neoformans*, *Blastomyces dermatitidis*, and *Coccidioides immitis*. A definitive diagnosis is made by isolation or identification of the organism in the CSF or other body secretions. Treatment regimens are similar for the various deep mycotic agents.

Cryptococcal Meningitis

For many years the mainstay of therapy for the deep mycotic pathogens has been amphotericin B. This drug is poorly absorbed from the GI tract and must be given IV for a full therapeutic effect. Amphotericin B diffuses poorly into the CSF. For this reason, although amphotericin B has value in fulminating systemic infections, agents such as itraconazole and fluconazole are preferred for cryptococcal meningitis. Several therapeutic regimens of amphotericin B have been described.

Flucytosine, when combined with amphotericin B, acts synergistically in vitro against *Cryptococcus neoformans*. It achieves satisfactory concentrations in the CSF. The oral dose of flucytosine is 50 to 75 mg/kg every 8 hours.[136,137] The rate of relapse is considerably lower with the combined therapy. Side effects include leukopenia, thrombocytopenia, vomiting, and diarrhea.

Successful management of cryptococcal meningitis has been reported with the azole and trizole antifungal compounds.[138,139] At usual concentrations in the plasma these compounds are considered fungistatic, but at higher concentrations they may be fungicidal.[138] The azoles and trizoles inhibit synthesis of ergosterol in the fungal cell membrane. Ketoconazole, itraconazole, and fluconazole have been studied in dogs and cats. All are well absorbed from the GI tract. Absorption of itraconazole is enhanced by food in the intestinal tract.

Ketoconazole does not penetrate the CSF in adequate concentrations to be effective, and yet reports exist of success with this agent in the treatment of cryptococcal meningitis, especially when combined with flucytosine.[140] Ketoconazole therapy is associated with hepatic dysfunction, elevated liver enzymes, and suppression of endogenous steroid synthesis. It has a slow onset of action, and in life-threatening conditions ketoconazole is often combined with amphotericin B to provide immediate fungicidal activity in all tissues except the eye and the CNS. The dose of ketoconazole for dogs and cats is 10 to 15 mg/kg daily.

Itraconazole has a broad spectrum of activity against many fungal organisms and has been effective in the treatment of cryptococcal meningitis in cats.[141] In systemic blastomycosis, itraconazole produces a cure rate equal to or greater than that of combined therapy with ketoconazole and amphotericin B. Itraconazole is less toxic than ketoconazole but is more expensive. Fluconazole is a bistriazole compound with broad-spectrum antifungal activity. It is well absorbed from the GI tract and has a bioavailability greater than 90%.[139] It penetrates into the meninges and CSF with or without inflammation. Fluconazole is the drug of choice in the treatment of cryptococcal meningitis in humans and is recommended in dogs and cats with mycotic infections of the CNS. Serious side effects are uncommon. The recommended dose in dogs and cats for both itraconazole and fluconazole is 10 mg/kg daily divided twice daily for 2 to 3 months beyond the resolution of all signs.[142]

Coccidioidal Meningitis

Coccidioides immitis is not susceptible to the synergistic activity of combined amphotericin B and flucytosine therapy but may respond to ketoconazole administered at 10 mg/kg every 24 hours for 9 to 12 months.[143] Although in some cases treatment resolved the clinical signs, recurrences were common when treatment was discontinued. Similar results were found in a few cases treated with itraconazole and fluconazole.[143]

Other Systemic Fungal Infections of the Meninges

Histoplasma capsulatum, *Blastomyces dermatitidis*, *Aspergillus* spp., *Candida* spp., and *Sporothrix schenckii* occasionally are involved in meningitis. Treatment is the same as for cryptococcosis and coccidioidomycosis.[144-147]

Actinomycetes Infections

Tuberculous Meningitis

Although it is nearly nonexistent in dogs and cats, tuberculous meningitis occurs occasionally in primates. Most of the antituberculous drugs readily penetrate the CNS. A combination of isoniazid and ethambutol is suggested. Other effective drugs include rifampin, ethionamide, pyrazinamide, and cycloserine.

Nocardiosis

The drugs of choice have been triple sulfonamides or trimethoprim-sulfa combinations. Their in vitro effect, however, has not been duplicated in vivo. The drugs should be given in high doses, and precautions should be taken to prevent nephrotoxicity. Alternative drugs include minocycline, amikacin, and erythromycin combined with ampicillin.[148]

Actinomycosis

The drug of choice is ampicillin given IV at 10 to 20 mg/kg every 6 hours.[148] Therapy is continued with clindamycin, chloramphenicol, or minocycline.

Protozoan Infections

Toxoplasma gondii is an intracellular coccidian parasite that produces systemic infection in dogs and cats and occasionally in other domestic animals. Cats are the definitive host and pass oocysts in the feces. In cats infection may occur through ingestion of any of the three life stages of the organism or transplacentally.[149] The organism may infect the muscle, CNS, liver, lung, and eye. A variety of clinical signs may occur, including uveitis, retinitis, myositis, pneumonia, and encephalitis. The diagnosis of clinically active toxoplasma infection is based on suggestive clinical signs, demonstration of *T. gondii* tachyzoites or bradyzoites in tissue biopsy sections, or immune testing for antibodies or antigen in serum, ocular fluid, or CSF. Although several immunologic tests are commercially available, the *T. gondii*–specific immunoglobulin M (IgM) and IgG enzyme-linked immunosorbent assays (ELISA) are most often used in dogs and cats. IgM levels tend to increase within 2 to 4 weeks of infection but are negative by 16 weeks.[150] IgM titers more than 1:256 indicate recent or active infection. A fourfold increase in IgG titers also indicates recent or active disease. Both IgG and IgM titers can be assessed in samples of CSF and compared with serum concentrations of albumin, IgG, and IgM. When the levels in CSF exceed those in serum, active or recent CNS infection should be suspected.

Clindamycin hydrochloride is the primary antimicrobial selected to treat clinical toxoplasmosis in dogs and cats. The dose in cats is 12.5 to 25 mg/kg orally or IM every 12 hours. The dose in dogs is 10 to 20 mg/kg orally or IM every 12 hours. Although clindamycin does not adequately penetrate the CSF of humans, the drug may penetrate the CSF of cats in sufficient levels to be effective for neurologic disease.[151] Transient vomiting is a common side effect in some cats. Cats should be treated for at least 4 to 5 weeks.

Neosporosis is caused by the protozoan *Neospora caninum.* Natural infections have been reported in dogs and calves. The muscles and the CNS are the most common sites of infection. Affected animals typically develop nonsuppurative encephalomyelitis, polyradiculoneuritis, and myositis. A positive diagnosis is based on demonstration of the organism in blood, CSF, or tissues. A fluorescent antibody test can detect *N. caninum*–specific antibodies. Clinical experience with treatment is limited, but treatment with clindamycin should be tried early in the course of illness. Sulfadiazine may also be effective (see also Chapter 7).[149]

Equine protozoal myeloencephalitis is described in Chapter 6. It is the most common neurologic disease in horses with multifocal or asymmetric neurologic deficits. Infection of the CNS may occur anywhere, but the spinal cord is most commonly affected.[152] The causative organism has been termed *Sarcocystis neurona*; however, based on DNA studies, this organism seems identical to *Sarcocystis falcatula*, a protozoal organism found in the opossum and small birds. Horses are aberrant dead-end hosts. The opossum is the primary host, and small birds are secondary hosts. Horses are most likely infected by fecal-oral transmission or by contamination of feed with dead birds that have the organism encysted in their muscles. Diagnosis is made by analysis of CSF using Western blot techniques to identify antibodies specific to the organism. Polymerase chain reaction may be used to identify antigen in the CSF. The prognosis is poor. Pyrimethamine, 1 mg/kg every 24 hours, combined with sulfamethoxazole, 12.5 to 25 mg/kg every 24 hours, is recommended. Treatment should be continued for 60 to 90 days and at least 2 weeks beyond complete clinical remission.[153]

Viral Infections

The viral diseases causing encephalomyelitis are summarized in Table 15-15. Viral infection of the CNS may fit into one of four categories: (1) viral invasions resulting in inflammation (viral meningitis, encephalitis, encephalomyelitis, or poliomyelitis); (2) postinfectious, noninflammatory encephalopathic states; (3) postinfectious and postvaccinal inflammatory states ("old dog" encephalitis, perhaps polyradiculoneuritis, brachial plexus neuropathy); and (4) slow virus infections (scrapie, bovine spongiform encephalopathy, Aleutian mink disease).

West Nile virus is a Flavivirus that causes acute polioencephalomyelitis in birds, horses, and humans and rarely in other animal species.[154-156] The disease is transmitted by multiple mosquito species, and birds are the major reservoir. Horses and humans are considered dead-end hosts. In horses the most common clinical signs are fever, paresis, ataxia, and muscle fasciculations.[154] The lesions are most severe in the spinal cord and are usually asymmetrical and multifocal. Abnormal mentation and cranial nerve abnormalities occur in 44% to 67% of affected horses.[154] Confirmation is based on positive viral isolation from blood, tissue or CSF, an associated fourfold or greater increase in plaque reduction neutralization tests (PRNTs), or concomitant single positive results with IgM capture ELISA test and PRNT test.[154] CSF abnormalities are found in about 70% of affected horses.[156] As in other acute viral infections, increased concentrations of protein, lymphocytes, and large mononuclear cells are the most common findings.[156] CSF collected from the lumbosacral region may be abnormal more often than CSF collected from other regions.[156] No definitive treatment is available and an approved vaccine is available. There are reports of horses developing disease despite vaccination.[154]

Few reports address the use of antiviral agents in animals. Acyclovir is an antiherpes viral agent that inhibits the enzyme thymidine kinase and thus inhibits DNA synthesis. This effect is 200 times greater for the viral enzyme than for the enzyme in mammalian cells.[157] Acyclovir can be given orally and intravenously. It penetrates into the CSF and aqueous humor at 30% to 50% of the plasma concentration. In human herpes encephalitis, the IV dose is 10 mg/kg every 8 hours. The dose should be reduced with renal failure because the drug is excreted in the urine. Encephalopathy is a rare side effect with high doses.

Foscarnet is effective against herpesvirus, cytomegalovirus, and the human immunodeficiency virus. It penetrates the CNS in good concentrations.[157]

Rickettsial Infections

The agents that cause Rocky Mountain spotted fever (RMSF) and canine ehrlichiosis may cause meningitis and encephalitis in addition to vasculitis and hematologic disorders.[158,159] Both diseases are transmitted by ticks and are limited to areas harboring the appropriate vector. Dogs with RMSF may have acute cervical pain and minimal signs related to brain or spinal cord disease. Dogs with neurologic ehrlichiosis usually have signs related to brainstem or spinal cord lesions. CSF may be normal or reveal increased protein and a mixed pleocytosis.[158] Confirmation of ehrlichiosis may be difficult in some dogs and is based on serologic tests and isolation of the organism.[160] Treatment is with tetracycline, minocycline, or doxycycline. Chloramphenicol is usually effective, but our experience suggests that better results are achieved with the tetracyclines, especially doxycycline, because it penetrates the CSF in good concentrations. The dose is 5 to 10 mg/kg every 12 hours IV or orally. In the treatment of CNS ehrlichiosis, concomitant administration of antiinflammatory doses of corticosteroids seems to improve clinical response.

NONSEPTIC INFLAMMATORY DISEASES

Several nonseptic inflammatory diseases may respond to medical therapy.[161,162] The causes of these diseases are not currently known, but immune-mediated mechanisms are suspected. Accordingly, corticosteroids and other immunosuppressive drugs may be beneficial with certain diseases. Differentiating these diseases from bacterial or viral infections is difficult because the clinical signs and CSF findings may be similar with both types of inflammation (see Chapter 4).

Steroid-responsive meningitis-arteritis (SRMA) occurs in large-breed dogs, usually less than 2 years of age. Spinal hyperesthesia occurs in more than 90% of affected dogs. Neutrophilic leukocytosis with left shift and fever occurs in two thirds of affected dogs. Boxers and Bernese mountain dogs may be predisposed to this disease.[161] Dogs with noninfectious, nonerosive, idiopathic immune-mediated polyarthritis (IMPA) commonly have spinal pain, and about 50% of these dogs have concurrent SRMA.[163] Analysis of CSF usually reveals marked increases in protein and neutrophils. Bacterial cultures from the CSF are negative. IgA concentrations are increased in both the plasma and the CSF. Most dogs respond dramatically to prednisone, 2 to 4 mg/kg every 24 hours. Once the signs are controlled, the dose is decreased to alternate-day therapy, and then the total dose is gradually reduced. Relapses are common when the steroid dose is too low or is discontinued.

Necrotizing meningeal vasculitis is a severe form of steroid-responsive meningitis-arteritis.[161,162] Necrotizing vasculitis also occurs in young dogs, especially beagles, Bernese mountain dogs, and German shorthaired pointers. Although the prognosis in affected beagles is guarded, other breeds may respond well to prednisone at 2 to 4 mg/kg every 24 hours using the aforementioned reducing-dosage regimen.

Granulomatous meningoencephalomyelitis (GME) is a common inflammatory disease that affects young to middle-aged toy and terrier breed dogs.[161,162,164,165] The exact cause is unknown, but studies of inflammatory cells in dogs with GME suggest a T cell–mediated delayed-type hypersensitivity.[166] Neurologic signs may be acute or chronic and focal, disseminated, or ocular. Cervical pain is a common finding. About 50% of affected dogs have focal signs referable to the forebrain, and about 50% have forebrain and brainstem disease.[164] Central vestibular signs are common manifestations of acute disease.[165] Mononuclear pleocytosis, activated macrophages, occasionally mast cells and increases in protein are common CSF abnormalities.

A definitive diagnosis is based on histopathologic examination of the CNS. Response to prednisone therapy is highly variable. Some dogs respond to prednisone (2 to 4 mg/kg every 24 hours, using the aforementioned reducing-dosage regimen), but relapses and progression of neurologic signs are common in many dogs. Cytosine arabinoside, given as a single agent or in combination with prednisone, is an effective treatment.[166a] A dose of 50 mg/m² is given subcutaneously twice a day for 2 consecutive days. The regimen is repeated initially every 3 weeks. To monitor for myelosuppression, a CBC should be performed 10 to 14 days following the first course of treatment and every 2 to 3 months throughout the course of therapy. Radiation treatment is effective for dogs with focal GME.[164] The prognosis for survival is better for dogs with focal disease.[164]

PHYSICAL THERAPY

Physical rehabilitation is often as important as specific medical or surgical treatment in the outcome of a patient with neurologic disease. Physical therapy is often neglected, however, in veterinary practice. It is time consuming, labor intensive, and often boring. Pet owners can be taught to help, and many do a better job than veterinarians.

Hydrotherapy

Exercises performed in water or whirlpools are very effective for relaxing contracted muscles, maintaining joint mobility, and stimulating circulation in atrophied muscles. Most important, they also help to keep the patient clean. Paralyzed dogs should undergo hydrotherapy sessions twice a day.

Muscles and limbs should be exercised passively. Sodium hypochlorite is used as a disinfectant in bathtubs and whirlpools to help suppress wound infections.

Exercise

Exercise can be passive or active, depending on the degree of neurologic dysfunction. If possible, dogs should be exercised outdoors, with a towel used as a sling. Walkers, dog carts, or slings may be useful for long-term rehabilitation. Limbs should be massaged vigorously to stimulate muscle tone and delay muscle contracture. Muscle massage with warm mineral oil is also helpful. Proper exercise encourages dogs to walk and improves their mental status.

Bladder Care

Many neurologic lesions disrupt voluntary micturition, resulting in urinary incontinence, retention cystitis, and bladder atony. Urinary bladders should be expressed or emptied by intermittent catheterization at least three times a day. Urinary tract infections should be treated with appropriate antibiotics. See Chapter 3 for details and for pharmacologic agents to assist micturition.

Cage Care

Paralyzed dogs must be turned frequently and must be kept on soft beds to prevent decubital ulcers and wound infections. Waterbeds, sealed foam mattresses, and air mattresses are helpful. The primary concern is to keep the cage clean and free of bacterial contamination. Paralyzed dogs, especially large breeds, are predisposed to wound infections, respiratory infections, and urine soilings. They must be cleaned frequently and nursed compassionately to be rehabilitated.

SUPPORTIVE CARE OF RECUMBENT LARGE ANIMALS

Horses and cattle are especially prone to develop secondary complications caused by recumbency. Self-trauma, decubital ulceration, myopathy, neuropathy, pneumonia, malnutrition, colic, and urinary tract infections are common complications in recumbent horses.[167] Cattle are also prone to bloat.

Horses and cattle should be protected from self-trauma. Limbs should be wrapped with thick layers of sheet cotton or quilted limb wraps. The head should be protected with a padded and properly fitted helmet. Tranquilizing agents such as chloral hydrate, detomidine, and xylazine may be required early in the course of treatment. These agents may hamper neurologic evaluation and may produce hypotension. To the greatest extent possible, large animals should be maintained in sternal recumbency because this position improves ventilation and peripheral circulation. Hay bales make good props for this purpose. Slings and overhead hoists may be helpful, but horses must be monitored continually to avoid injury and asphyxiation.

Decubital ulceration over bony prominences can be minimized by distributing pressure; applying pads over pressure points; using liberal amounts of clean, dry bedding; and turning the patient every 2 hours. Because eye injuries are common, the eyes should be examined two to three times a day. Padded helmets are useful in preventing eye injuries. Artificial tears and triple-antibiotic ointment should be applied when patients cannot lubricate their corneas.

Impaction of the large or small colon and rectum are common complications. Water should be offered every 4 hours, and a highly digestible diet of quality hay and pelleted feeds is recommended. Pelleted feed should contain ground alfalfa, bran, and psyllium. Water should be given by nasogastric intubation if a horse has trouble drinking and swallowing. Laxative agents such as mineral oil, dioctyl sodium sulfosuccinate, and magnesium sulfate can be provided on a regular basis.

Urine retention should be evaluated by observation and rectal palpation. Chronic catheterization is best accomplished using an aseptic closed system. The use of prophylactic urinary antibiotics is controversial and may contribute to resistant infections. Pneumonia and pleuritis are fatal complications in recumbent horses. Frequent turning is the best way to prevent pulmonary complications.

Case Histories

The cases involve the same disorders as those covered in this chapter; however, because this is the last chapter, other entities might be included to test the reader's aptitude in making a neurologic diagnosis.

CASE HISTORY 15A

Signalment
Canine, German shepherd dog, male, 10 months old.

History
Vaccinations were given on schedule. The dog had a "cold" 6 weeks ago that lasted for 1 week. One week ago the owner noticed a lack of coordination and falling to the left side. Yesterday the dog developed a head tilt to the left side.

Physical Examination
No abnormalities are found.

Neurologic Examination*

A. Observation
  1. Mental status: Depressed
  2. Posture: Head tilt to left
  3. Gait: Ataxia; the dog stumbles on the left thoracic limb at times
B. Palpation: Normal
C. Postural reactions

Left	Reactions	Right
	Proprioceptive positioning	
+1	PL	+2
+1	TL	+2
	Hopping	
+1	PL	+2
+1	TL	+2
+1	Extensor postural thrust	+2
+0 to +1	Hemistand-hemiwalk	+2
	Placing, tactile	
+1	PL	+2
+1	TL	+2
	Placing, visual	
+1	TL	+2

D. Spinal reflexes

Left	Reflex (Spinal Segment)	Right
+3	Quadriceps (L4-6)	+2
+2	Extensor carpi radialis (C7-T1)	+2
+2	Flexion, PL (L5-S1)	+2
+2	Flexion, TL (C6-T1)	+2
+0	Crossed extensor	+0
+2	Perineal (S1-2)	+2

E. Cranial nerves

Left	Nerve—Function (Response/Test)	Right
+2	CN II—vision (menace)	+2
+2 +2 +2	CN II, III—pupil size (Stimulus left eye) (Stimulus right eye)	+2 +2 +2
NE	CN II—fundus	NE
+2	CN III, IV, VI (Strabismus)	+2
Changes direction	(Nystagmus)	Changes direction
+2	CN V—sensation	+2
+2	CN V—mastication	+2
+2 +2	CN VII—facial muscles (Palpebral)	+2 +2
+2	CN IX, X—swallowing	+2
+2	CN XII—tongue	+2

F. Sensation: Location
  Hyperesthesia: The dog resents palpation of the neck
  Superficial pain: +2
  Deep pain: +2
Complete sections G and H before reviewing the case summary.
G. Assessment (anatomic diagnosis and estimation of prognosis)
H. Plan (diagnostic)

Rule-outs	Procedure
1.	
2.	
3.	
4.	

CASE HISTORY 15B

Signalment
Yorkshire terrier litter: two female puppies, one male puppy; 4 weeks old.

History
Second litter of a 3-year-old bitch. The sire is different from that of the first litter. The bitch was the only dog in the household. One week ago the puppies were observed shaking. The condition progressed to coarse muscular twitching. The puppies are still nursing. The bitch is in good health and has had all immunizations. No vaccinations were given during pregnancy.

Physical Examination
Normal.

Neurologic Examination*
A. Observation
  1. Mental status: Alert
  2. Posture: Generalized tremor is worse when the puppies are active; usually stops when they are at rest
  3. Gait: Dysmetria

---

*0, Absent; +1, decreased; +2, normal; +3, exaggerated; +4, very exaggerated or clonus; PL, pelvic limb; TL, thoracic limb; NE, not evaluated.

*0, Absent; +1, decreased; +2, normal; +3, exaggerated; +4, very exaggerated or clonus; PL, pelvic limb; TL, thoracic limb; NE, not evaluated.

B. Palpation: Normal
C. Postural reactions: All present, but dysmetric
D. Spinal reflexes: All normal
E. Cranial nerves: All normal
F. Sensation: Location
    Hyperesthesia: No
    Superficial pain: +2
    Deep pain: +2
Complete sections G and H before reviewing the case summary.
G. Assessment (anatomic diagnosis and estimation of prognosis)
H. Plan (diagnostic)

Rule-outs	Procedure
1.	
2.	
3.	
4.	

CASE HISTORY 15C

Signalment
Canine, Doberman pinscher, male, 3 years old.

History
Intermittent lameness for several weeks.

Physical Examination
Normal except for findings described below.

Neurologic Examination
A. Observation
    1. Mental status: Alert
    2. Posture: Normal
    3. Gait: The dog walks gingerly, as if he does not want to bear weight; slight sway of pelvis
B. Palpation: Pain is elicited from deep palpation of limbs. No muscle atrophy is present.
C. Postural reactions: All normal, although he resents manipulation.
D. Spinal reflexes: All normal
E. Cranial nerves: All normal
F. Sensation: Location
    Hyperesthesia: Pain is elicited from deep palpation of limbs
    Superficial pain: +2
    Deep pain: +2
Complete sections G and H before reviewing the case summary.
G. Assessment (anatomic diagnosis and estimation of prognosis)
H. Plan (diagnostic)

Rule-outs	Procedure
1.	
2.	
3.	
4.	

CASE HISTORY 15D

Signalment
English pointer, male, 6 years old.

History
The dog has been depressed and ataxic for 1 week. His appetite is poor. Vaccinations are current.

Physical Examination
The dog is depressed and thin.

Neurologic Examination[*]
A. Observation
    1. Mental status: Alert
    2. Posture: Normal
    3. Gait: Slight truncal ataxia
B. Palpation: Normal
C. Postural reactions

Left	Reactions	Right
	Proprioceptive positioning	
+2	PL	+2
+2	TL	+2
+2	Wheelbarrowing	+2
	Hopping	
+1	PL	+1
+1	TL	+1
+2	Extensor postural thrust	+2
+2	Hemistand-hemiwalk	+2
	Placing, tactile	
+2	PL	+2
+2	TL	+2
	Placing, visual	
+2	TL	+2

D. Spinal reflexes: All normal
E. Cranial nerves: All normal
F. Sensation: Location
    Hyperesthesia: Resists turning of neck
    Superficial pain: +2
    Deep pain: +2
Complete sections G and H before reviewing the case summary.
G. Assessment (anatomic diagnosis and estimation of prognosis)
H. Plan (diagnostic)

Rule-outs	Procedure
1.	
2.	
3.	
4.	

CASE HISTORY 15E

Signalment
Canine, cairn terrier, male, 4 months old.

History
The dog is one of a litter of four; the others are normal. At 9 weeks he had a wide-based gait that gradually progressed to a swaying of the pelvis and a stumbling of the pelvic limbs.

---

[*]*0, Absent; +1, decreased; +2, normal; +3, exaggerated; +4, very exaggerated or clonus; PL, pelvic limb; TL, thoracic limb; NE, not evaluated.*

Examination by another veterinarian was otherwise negative. Now pelvic limb paresis is present.

Physical Examination
Normal.

Neurologic Examination*
A. Observation
   1. Mental status: Alert
   2. Posture: The dog cannot stand; tremors of the head, trunk, and limbs occur when the dog is active
   3. Gait: The dog pulls around with the thoracic limbs; some voluntary movements of the pelvic limbs (primarily hip flexion) are present
B. Palpation: Normal
C. Postural reactions

Left	Reactions	Right
	Proprioceptive positioning	
+0	PL	+0
+1	TL	+1
+1	Wheelbarrowing	+1
	Hopping	
+0	PL	+0
+1	TL	+1
+0	Extensor postural thrust	+0
NE	Hemistand-hemiwalk	NE
	Placing, tactile	
+0	PL	+0
	Placing, visual	
+1	TL	+2

D. Spinal reflexes: All normal
E. Cranial nerves: All normal
F. Sensation: Location
   Hyperesthesia: No
   Superficial pain: +2
   Deep pain: +2
Complete sections G and H before reviewing the case summary.
G. Assessment (anatomic diagnosis and estimation of prognosis)
H. Plan (diagnostic)

Rule-outs	Procedure
1.	
2.	
3.	
4.	

ASSESSMENT 15A

The dog has ataxia and hemiparesis from central vestibular disease on the left side (see Chapter 7 for a review of localization). The only finding not explained by a single lesion is the

---

*0, Absent; +1, decreased; +2, normal; +3, exaggerated; +4, very exaggerated or clonus; *PL*, pelvic limb; *TL*, thoracic limb; *NE*, not evaluated.

suggestion of hyperesthesia along the cervical vertebral column. The disease has a moderately acute onset and is progressive. In a young dog, the most common cause of an acute progressive disease is inflammation. The hyperesthesia suggests meningitis. The history of a respiratory problem several weeks ago should not be ignored. An alternative cause might be neoplasia, but this condition is much less likely. The primary question is the kind of infection: viral, bacterial, fungal, rickettsial, or protozoal. Canine distemper must be considered despite the apparent focal neurologic deficit. Focal brainstem disease and meningitis could also be bacterial (abscess plus subarachnoid involvement). Rickettsial diseases are possible if the dog was from an endemic area.

Localization
Left brainstem, vestibular nuclei, meninges.

Rule-outs
Inflammation: viral (distemper), bacterial, or other. How does a clinician differentiate these types of infection? If the examiner starts with simple, noninvasive methods, fundic and otoscopic examinations might reveal chorioretinitis from distemper or a middle-ear infection that has progressed to the brainstem. The results of both examinations are normal, however. Laboratory data might be of value but are frequently normal when either of our choices are present, as they are in this case. Rickettsial diseases frequently cause thrombocytopenia, which was not found. EEG might be useful if cerebral disease is also present, but it would not really differentiate viral from bacterial inflammation. The best test is an examination of the CSF. In this case, a cerebellomedullary sample produced the following results:

Protein	65 mg/dl
Red blood cells (RBCs)	2/µl
WBCs	12/µl
Differential	All lymphocytes

These findings are suggestive of a viral infection. A bacterial infection usually would cause more protein and more cells to be present, and the cells would be predominantly neutrophils. A fluorescent antibody examination of blood, conjunctival scrapings, or cells in the CSF might be used to confirm the diagnosis of distemper.

Chloramphenicol was administered. The day after hospitalization, head tremors were observed, indicating involvement of the cerebellum. On the third day the dog had generalized seizures. The owners requested euthanasia. Necropsy confirmed the diagnosis of distemper encephalomyelitis.

ASSESSMENT 15B

The signs are compatible with cerebellar disease. Cerebellar hypoplasia or in utero damage to the cerebellum must be considered; however, toxic products also can produce cerebellar signs. The progressive nature of the syndrome suggests something other than a congenital defect, which is usually static with some improvement as compensation occurs. Other progressive diseases such as storage diseases are degenerative. None has been reported in the Yorkshire terrier.

Localization
Cerebellum.

Rule-outs
   1. Toxic disorders
   2. Degenerative diseases
   3. Cerebellar hypoplasia

Further questioning of the owners revealed that they did not believe any toxic products were available because they had small children and were very careful. They were specifically asked to describe their management routine of the bitch and the puppies. They said that they were extremely careful and in fact washed the bitch's mammary glands every day because she went outside and got dirty. They were using a hexachlorophene soap to wash the bitch. They were instructed to wash her with a mild soap, rinse thoroughly, and discontinue cleaning the mammary glands. The pups gradually improved until they were normal, about 4 weeks later.

Diagnosis
Hexachlorophene toxicity.

ASSESSMENT 15C

A normal neurologic examination in the presence of a gait abnormality is suggestive of a musculoskeletal disease. Although the history and the breed predilection suggest cervical spondylopathy or cervical disk disease, the neurologic examination does not. Palpation of the head and spine was normal, but the dog experienced pain on palpation of the long bones of the limbs. A radiographic examination confirmed the diagnosis of panosteitis.

Differentiating musculoskeletal problems from neurologic diseases is very important. Dogs with musculoskeletal problems and no neurologic disease have a normal neurologic examination. Severe hip dysplasia does not cause a proprioceptive deficit. Conversely, if a deficit is found on the neurologic examination, it is rarely due to musculoskeletal disease.

ASSESSMENT 15D

The neurologic findings are not localizing. Depression and slowing of the hopping reactions could be indicative of generalized disease not affecting the CNS or of a mild CNS disease. Resistance to manipulation of the neck and the strong panniculus reaction may be indicative of pain. Deep palpation along the vertebral column elicits strong guarding reactions of the paraspinal muscles. Absolute evidence of pain cannot be demonstrated, but the breed must be considered. Hunting dogs are often stoic. Systemic disease must be considered, with meningitis included as a strong possibility. Laboratory data are needed to rule out the former and CSF analysis to rule out the latter.

Rule-outs
1. Systemic disease
2. Meningitis, possibly with mild encephalomyelitis
3. Polymyositis

Laboratory Examination
The results of a blood chemistry profile and a urinalysis are normal.

Blood	
WBCs	31,000/µl
Neutrophils	24,500/µl
Bands	240/µl
Lymphocytes	6,260/µl
CSF	
Protein	235 mg/dl
RBCs	5/µl
WBCs	2,435/µl
Neutrophils	94%
Mononuclear cells	6%

Blood and CSF cultures were submitted.

The findings are indicative of bacterial meningitis. IV ampicillin therapy was started pending the results of the cultures. The dog improved in 48 hours. Blood cultures were negative, but CSF cultures revealed *Staphylococcus intermedius* sensitive to ampicillin. IV therapy was continued for 4 days, followed by oral ampicillin for 3 weeks. The dog recovered completely. The source of the infection was not found.

ASSESSMENT 15E

The head tremor suggests cerebellar disease. The paresis is caused by either brainstem or spinal cord dysfunction. No other signs of brainstem disease are present. The progression from pelvic limb paresis to tetraparesis can be seen with cervical spinal cord lesions or with progressive generalized myelopathy. The progression from spinal cord signs to cerebellar signs should suggest multifocal or systemic disease. The disorder is chronic and progressive in a young dog. These characteristics should prompt consideration of the inherited degenerative diseases. The next step is to review which diseases might be present in Cairn terriers. Globoid cell leukodystrophy, a demyelinating disease, has been reported in this breed. The rule-outs might also include viral diseases such as distemper. Lead toxicity should be considered, although paresis is unusual with this condition.

Localization
Cerebellum, spinal cord.

Rule-outs
1. Degenerative disease (globoid cell leukodystrophy)
2. Inflammation (viral)
3. Toxicity (lead)

Laboratory Examination
The complete blood count, serum chemistry profile, and urinalysis are normal.

CSF	
Protein	95 mg/dl
Cells	
RBCs	4/µl
WBCs	2/µl
Blood	
Lead concentration	0.02 ppm

The blood lead level is normal. The CSF results are indicative of a degenerative process without active inflammation (increased protein level, normal cell counts). This finding does not rule out viral diseases of the CNS, especially canine distemper, because the active inflammatory process may have been present several weeks earlier. Globoid cells may be seen in the CSF in some cases of globoid cell leukodystrophy, but their absence does not exclude the diagnosis. A biopsy of a peripheral nerve might reveal the pathologic changes characteristic of this disease. The owners elected euthanasia because all the possible diseases had a very poor prognosis. No significant lesions were found on gross necropsy. Histopathologic examination confirmed the diagnosis of globoid cell leukodystrophy.

References

1. Baker HJ, et al: The gangliosidoses: Comparative features and research applications, *Vet Pathol* 16:635-649, 1979.

2. Kornegay JN: Congenital and degenerative diseases of the central nervous system. In Kornegay JN, editor: *Neurologic disorders.* New York, 1986, Churchill Livingstone.

3. Evans RJ: Lysosomal storage diseases in dogs and cats, *J Small Anim Pract* 30:144-150, 1989.

4. Braund KG: Degenerative and developmental diseases. In Oliver JE, Hoerlein BF, Mayhew IG, editors: *Veterinary neurology.* Philadelphia, 1987, WB Saunders.

5. Taylor RM, Farrow BRH, Stewart GJ: Correction of enzyme deficiency by allogenic bone marrow transplantation following total lymphoid irradiation in dogs with lysosomal storage disease (fucosidosis). *Transplant Proc* 18:326-329, 1986.

6. de Lahunta A: Abiotrophy in domestic animals: A review, *Can J Vet Res* 54:65-76, 1990.

7. Hardy RM: Pathophysiology of hepatic encephalopathy, *Semin Vet Med Surg* 5:100-106, 1990.

8. Maddison JE: Hepatic encephalopathy: Current concepts of the pathogenesis, *J Vet Intern Med* 6:341-353, 1992.

9. Bunch SE: Hepatic encephalopathy, *Prog Vet Neurol* 2:287-296, 1992.

10. Center SA, Magne ML: Historical, physical examination, and clinicopathologic features of portosystemic vascular anomalies in the dog and cat, *Semin Vet Med Surg* 5:83-93, 1990.

11. Center SA, et al: Evaluation of twelve-hour preprandial and two-hour post prandial serum bile acids concentrations for diagnosis of hepatobiliary diseases in dogs, *J Am Vet Med Assoc* 199:217-226, 1991.

12. Center SA, Erb HN, Joseph SA: Measurement of serum bile acids concentrations of hepatobiliary disease in cats, *J Am Vet Med Assoc* 207:1048-1054, 1995.

13. Holt DE, Schelling CG, Saunders HM, et al: Correlation of ultrasonographic findings with surgical, portographic, and necropsy findings in dogs and cats with portosystemic shunts: 63 cases (1987-1993), *J Am Vet Med Assoc* 207:1190-1193, 1995.

14. Koblik PD, et al: Use of 99m technetium-pertechnetate as a screening test for portosystemic shunts in dogs, *J Am Vet Med Assoc* 196:925-930, 1990.

15. Koblik PD, Hornof WJ: Transcolonic sodium pertechnetate Tc 99m scintigraphy for diagnosis of macrovascular portosystemic shunts in dogs, cats, and potbellied pigs: 176 cases (1988-1992), *J Am Vet Med Assoc* 207:729-733, 1995.

16. Tyler JW: Hepatoencephalopathy, Part II: Pathophysiology and treatment, *Compend Cont Educ Pract Vet* 12:1260-1270, 1990.

17. Taboada J: Medical management of animals with portosystemic shunts, *Semin Vet Med Surg* 5:107-119, 1990.

18. Matushek KJ, Bjorling D, Mathews K: Generalized motor seizures after portosystemic shunt ligation in dogs: Five cases (1981-1988), *J Am Vet Med Assoc* 196:2014-2017, 1990.

19. Hardie EM, Kornegay JN, Cullen JM: Status epilepticus after ligation of portosystemic shunts, *Vet Surg* 19:412-417, 1990.

20. Johnson C, Armstrong P, Hauptman J: Congenital portosystemic shunts in dogs: 46 cases (1979-1986), *J Am Vet Med Assoc* 191:1478-1483, 1987.

21. Matushek KJ, Bjorling D, Mathews K: Generalized motor seizures after portosystemic shunt ligation in dogs: Five cases (1981-1988), *J Am Vet Med Assoc* 196:2014-2017, 1990.

22. Van Gundy TE, Boothe HW, Wolf A: Results of surgical management of feline portosystemic shunts, *J Am Anim Hosp Assoc* 25:55-62, 1990.

23. Lawrence D, Bellah JR, Diaz R: Results of surgical management of portosystemic shunts dogs: 20 cases (1985-1990), *J Am Vet Med Assoc* 201:1750-1753, 1992.

24. Dunigan C, Tyler J, Valdez R, et al: Apparent renal encephalopathy in a cow, *J Vet Intern Med* 10:39-41, 1996.

25. Wolf AM: Canine uremic encephalopathy, *J Am Anim Hosp Assoc* 16:735-738, 1980.

26. Abramson CJ, et al: L-2-hydroxyglutaric aciduria in Staffordshire bull terriers, *J Vet Intern Med* 17:551-556, 2003.

27. Lorenz MD, Cornelius LM: *Small animal medical diagnosis.* Philadelphia, 1987, JB Lippincott.

28. Kornegay JN: Hypocalcemia in dogs, *Compend Cont Educ Pract Vet* 4:103-110, 1982.

29. Lorenz MD, Cornelius LM, Ferguson DC: *Small animal medical therapeutics.* Philadelphia, 1992, JB Lippincott.

30. Kelly M, Hill J: Canine myxedema stupor and coma, *Compend Cont Educ Pract Vet* 6:1049-1057, 1984.

31. Kelly MJ: Canine myxedema stupor and coma. In Kirk RW, editor: *Current veterinary therapy, X: Small animal practice.* Philadelphia, 1989, WB Saunders.

32. Panciera DL: Hypothyroidism in dogs: 66 cases (1987-1992), *J Am Vet Med Assoc* 204:761-767, 1994.

33. Nelson RW, et al: Serum free thyroxine concentrations in healthy dogs, dogs with hypothyroidism, and euthyroid dogs with concurrent illness, *J Am Vet Med Assoc* 198:1401-1407, 1991.

34. Peterson ME, Gamble DA: Effect of nonthyroid illness on serum thyroxine concentrations in cats: 494 cases (1988), *J Am Vet Med Assoc* 197:1203-1208, 1990.

35. Jaggy A, et al: Neurologic manifestations of hypothyroidism: A retrospective study of 29 dogs. *J Vet Intern Med* 8:328-336, 1994.

36. Sarfaty DS, Carillo JM, Peterson ME: Neurologic, endocrinologic, and pathologic findings associated with large pituitary tumors in dogs: Eight cases (1976-1984), *J Am Vet Med Assoc* 193:854-856, 1988.

37. Love S: Equine Cushing's disease, *Br Vet J* 149:139-153, 1993.

38. Duesberg CA, et al: Magnetic resonance imaging for diagnosis of pituitary macroadenomas in dogs, *J Am Vet Med Assoc* 206:657-662, 1995.

39. Feldman EC, Nelson RW: Hypercalcemia and primary hyperparathyroidism. In *Canine and feline endocrinology and reproduction.* Philadelphia, 1996, WB Saunders.

40. Harris CL, et al: Hypercalcemia in a dog with thymoma, *J Am Anim Hosp Assoc* 27:281-284, 1991.

41. Klausner JS, et al: Hypercalcemia in two cats with squamous cell carcinoma, *J Am Vet Med Assoc* 196:103-105, 1990.

42. Foosbee SK, Forrester SD: Hypercalcemia secondary to cholecalciferol rodenticide toxicosis in two dogs, *J Am Vet Med Assoc* 196:1265-1268, 1990.

43. Dougherty SA, Center SA, Dzanis DA: Salmon calcitonin as adjunct treatment for vitamin D toxicosis in a dog, *J Am Vet Med Assoc* 196:1269-1272, 1990.

44. Spier SJ, et al: Hyperkalemic periodic paralysis in horses, *J Am Vet Med Assoc* 197:1009-1017, 1990.

45. Rudolph JA, et al: Periodic paralysis in Quarter Horses: A sodium channel mutation disseminated by selective breeding, *Nat Genet* 2:144-147, 1992.

46. Elie MS, Zerbe CA: Insulinoma in dogs, cats, and ferrets, *Compend Cont Educ Pract Vet* 17:51-59, 1995.

47. Caywood DD, et al: Pancreatic insulin-secreting neoplasms: Clinical, diagnostic, and prognostic features in 73 dogs, *J Am Anim Hosp Assoc* 24:577-584, 1988.

48. Hawks D, Peterson ME, Hawkins KL: Insulin-secreting pancreatic (islet cell) carcinoma in a cat, *J Vet Intern Med* 6:193-196, 1992.

49. Dyer DR: Hypoglycemia: A common metabolic manifestation of cancer, *Vet Med* 87:40-47, 1992.

50. Chrisman CL: Postoperative results and complications of insulinomas in dogs, *J Am Anim Hosp Assoc* 16:677-684, 1980.

51. Bagley RS, et al: Central nervous system. In Slatter D, editor: *Textbook of small animal surgery*. Philadelphia, 1993, WB Saunders.

52. Vandevelde M: Brain tumors in domestic animals: An overview. In *Proceedings of a Conference on Brain Tumors in Man and Animals*, Research Triangle Park, NC, 1984.

53. Hayes HM, Priester WA, Pendergrass TW: Occurrence of nervous-tissue tumors in cattle, horses, cats and dogs, *Int J Cancer* 15:39-47, 1975.

54. Luginbuhl H, Fankhauser R, McGrath JT: Spontaneous neoplasms of the nervous system in animals, *Prog Neurol Surg* 2:85-164, 1968.

55. LeCouteur RA: Brain tumors of dogs and cats: Diagnosis and management, *Vet Med Report* 2:332-342, 1990.

56. LeCouteur RA: Tumors of the nervous system. In Withrow SJ, MacEwen EG, editors: *Clinical veterinary oncology*. Philadelphia, 1989, JB Lippincott.

57. Kube SA, Brutette DS, Hanson, SM: Astrocytomas in young dogs, *J Am Anim Hosp Assoc* 39:288-293, 2003.

58. Davidson MG, et al: Acute blindness associated with intracranial tumors in dogs and cats: Eight cases (1984-1989), *J Am Vet Med Assoc* 199:755-758, 1991.

59. Palmer AC, Malinowski W, Barnett KC: Clinical signs including papilloedema associated with brain tumors in twenty-one dogs, *J Small Anim Pract* 15:359-386, 1974.

60. Kornegay JN: Imaging brain neoplasms: Computed tomography and magnetic resonance imaging, *Vet Med Report* 2:372-390, 1990.

61. Turrel J, Fike J, LeCouteur R, et al: Computed tomographic characteristics of primary brain tumors in 50 dogs, *J Am Vet Med Assoc* 188:851-856, 1986.

62. Thomas WB, et al: Magnetic resonance imaging features of primary brain tumors in dogs. *Vet Radiol Ultrasound* 37:20-27, 1996.

63. Bailey C, Higgins R: Characteristics of cisternal cerebrospinal fluid associated with primary brain tumors in the dog: A retrospective study, *J Am Vet Med Assoc* 188:414-417, 1986.

64. Heidner GL, Kornegay JN, Page RL, et al: Analysis of survival in a retrospective study of 86 dogs with brain tumors, *J Vet Intern Med* 5:219-226, 1991.

65. Turrel J, Fike J, LeCouteur R, et al: Radiotherapy of brain tumors in dogs, *J Am Vet Med Assoc* 184:82-86, 1984.

66. Lester NV, et al: Radiosurgery using a stereotactic headframe system for irradiation of brain tumors in dogs, *J Am Vet Med Assoc* 219:1562-1567, 2001.

67. Ingram M, et al: Adoptive immunotherapy of brain tumors in dogs, *Vet Med Report* 2:398-402, 1990.

68. Frier H, et al: Formation and absorption of cerebrospinal fluid in adult goats with hypo and hypervitaminosis A, *Am J Vet Res* 35:45-55, 1974.

69. Kornegay JN, Mayhew IG: Metabolic, toxic, and nutritional diseases of the nervous system. In Oliver JE, Hoerlein BF, Mayhew IG, editors: *Veterinary neurology*. Philadelphia, 1987, WB Saunders.

70. van Donkersgoed J, Clark EG: Blindness caused by hypovitaminosis A in feedlot cattle, *Can Vet J* 29:925-927, 1988.

71. Anderson WI, et al: The ophthalmic and neuro-ophthalmic effects of a vitamin A deficiency in young steers, *Vet Med* 86:1143-1148, 1991.

72. Mayhew I, et al: Equine degenerative myeloencephalopathy: A vitamin E deficiency that may be familial, *J Vet Intern Med* 1:45-50, 1987.

73. Dill SG, et al: Serum vitamin E and blood glutathione peroxidase values of horses with degenerative myeloencephalopathy, *Am J Vet Res* 50:166-168, 1989.

74. Anderson WI, Morrow LA: Thiamine deficiency encephalopathy with concurrent myocardial degeneration and polyradiculoneuropathy in a cat, *Cornell Vet* 77:251-257, 1987.

75. Houston DM, Hulland TJ: Thiamine deficiency in a team of sled dogs, *Can Vet J* 29:383-385, 1988.

76. Rammell C, Hill J: A review of thiamine deficiency and its diagnosis, especially in ruminants, *N Z Vet J* 34:202-204, 1987.

77. Read DH, Harrington DD: Experimentally induced thiamine deficiency in beagle dogs: Pathologic changes of the central nervous system, *Am J Vet Res* 47:2281-2289, 1986.

78. Mayhew IG: *Large animal neurology: A handbook for veterinary clinicians*. Philadelphia, 1989, Lea & Febiger.

79. Osweiler GD, Carson TL, Buck WB, et al: *Clinical and diagnostic veterinary toxicology*, 3rd ed. Dubuque, IA, 1985, Kendall/Hunt Publishing.

80. Grauer GF, Hjelle JJ. Section 16: Toxicology. In Morgan RV, editor: *Handbook of small animal practice*. New York, 1988, Churchill Livingstone.

81. Dorman DC: Toxins that induce seizures in small animals. In *Proceedings of the Eighth Annual Veterinary Medical Forum*, Washington, DC, 1990, pp 361-364.

82. Bratton GR, Kowalczyk DF: Lead poisoning. In Kirk RW, editor: *Current veterinary therapy, X: Small animal practice*. Philadelphia, 1989, WB Saunders.

83. Dollahite JW, et al: Chronic lead poisoning in horses, *Am J Vet Res* 39:961-964, 1978.

84. Zook BC, Carpenter JL, Leeds EB: Lead poisoning in dogs, *J Am Vet Med Assoc* 155:1329-1342, 1969.

85. Knecht CD, Crabtree J, Katherman A: Clinical, clinicopathologic, and electroencephalographic features of lead poisoning in dogs, *J Am Vet Med Assoc* 175:196-201, 1979.

86. Nicholls TJ, Handson PD: Behavioural change associated with chronic lead poisoning in working dogs, *Vet Rec* 112:607, 1983.

87. Dow SW, et al: Central nervous system toxicosis associated with metronidazole treatment of dogs: Five cases (1984-1987), *J Am Vet Med Assoc* 195:365-368, 1989.

88. Caylor KB, Cassimatis MK: Metronidazole neurotoxicosis in two cats, *J Am Anim Hosp Assoc* 37:258-262, 2001.

89. Evans, J, et al: Diazepam as a treatment for metronidazole toxicosis in dogs: A retrospective study of 21 cases, *J Vet Intern Med* 17:302-310, 2003.

90. Mealey KL: Role or P-glycoprotein in the blood-brain barrier. In *Proceedings of the 19th Veterinary Medical Forum*, Denver, CO, 2001, pp 396-398.

91. Nelson OL, et al: Ivermectin toxicity in an Australian shepherd dog with MDR1 mutation associated with ivermectin sensitivity in collies, *J Vet Intern Med* 17:354-356, 2003.

92. Hopper K, Aldrich J, Haskins SC: Ivermectin toxicity in 17 collies, *J Vet Intern Med* 16:89-94, 2002.

93. Jaggy A, Oliver JE: Chlorpyrifos toxicosis in two cats, *J Vet Intern Med* 4:135-139, 1990.

94. Farrow BRH: Tremor syndromes in dogs. In *Proceedings of the Sixth Annual Veterinary Medical Forum*, Washington, DC, 1988, pp 57-60.

95. Bath ML: Hexachlorophene toxicity in dogs, *J Small Anim Pract* 19:241-244, 1978.

96. Scott DW, Bolton GR, Lorenz MD: Hexachlorophene toxicosis in dogs, *J Am Vet Med Assoc* 162:947-949, 1973.

97. Thompson J, Senior D, Pinson D, et al: Neurotoxicosis associated with the use of hexachlorophene in a cat, *J Am Vet Med Assoc* 190:1311-1312, 1987.

98. Dorman DC: Initial management of toxicoses. In *Proceedings of the Eighth Annual Veterinary Medical Forum*, Washington, DC, 1990, pp 419-422.

99. Hamir A, Sullivan N, Handson P, et al: A comparison of calcium disodium ethylene diamine tetraacetate (Ca EDTA) by oral and subcutaneous routes as a treatment of lead poisoning in dogs, *J Small Anim Pract* 27:39-43, 1990.

100. Munana KR: Encephalitis and meningitis, *Vet Clin North Am (Sm Anim Pract)* 26:857-874, 1996.

101. Greene CE: Infectious diseases affecting the nervous system. In Kornegay JN, editor: *Neurologic disorders.* New York, 1986, Churchill Livingstone.

102. Braund KG: Granulomatous meningoencephalomyelitis. In Kirk RW, editor: *Current veterinary therapy, X: Small animal practice.* Philadelphia, 1989, WB Saunders.

103. Braund KG, Brewer BD, Mayhew IG: Inflammatory, infectious, immune, parasitic, and vascular diseases. In Oliver JE, Hoerlein BF, Mayhew IG, editors: *Veterinary neurology.* Philadelphia, 1987, WB Saunders.

104. Fenner W: Meningitis. In Kirk RW, editor: *Current veterinary therapy, IX: Small animal practice.* Philadelphia, 1986, WB Saunders.

105. Timoney JF, et al: *Hagan and Bruner's microbiology and infectious diseases of domestic animals.* Ithaca, NY, 1988, Comstock Publishing Associates, 1988.

106. Milhorat TH: *Cerebrospinal fluid and the brain edemas.* New York, 1987, Neuroscience Society of New York, 1987.

107. Webb AA, Muir GD: The blood-brain barrier and its role in inflammation, *J Vet Intern Med* 14:399-411, 2000.

108. Fenner WR: Bacterial infections of the central nervous system. In Greene CE, editor: *Infectious diseases of the dog and cat.* Philadelphia, 1990, WB Saunders.

109. Quagliarello V, Scheld WM: Bacterial meningitis: Pathogenesis, pathophysiology, and progress, *N Engl J Med* 327:864-872, 1992.

110. Scheld WM, et al: Cerebrospinal fluid outflow resistance in rabbits with experimental meningitis: Alterations with penicillin and methylprednisolone, *J Clin Invest* 66:243-253, 1980.

111. Mustafa MM, et al: Modulation of inflammation and cachectin activity in relation to treatment of experimental *Hemophilus influenza* type B meningitis, *J Infect Dis* 160:818-825, 1989.

112. Odio CM, et al: The beneficial effects of early dexamethasone administration in infants and children with bacterial meningitis, *N Engl J Med* 324:1535-1531, 1991.

113. Saez-Llorens X, Jafari HS, Severien C, et al: Enhanced attenuation of meningeal inflammation and brain edema by concomitant administration of anti-CD 18 monoclonal antibodies and dexamethasone in experimental *Hemophilus* meningitis, *J Clin Invest* 88:2003-2011, 1991.

114. Radaelli ST, Platt SR: Bacterial meningoencephalomyelitis in dogs: A retrospective study of 23 cases (1990-1999), *J Vet Intern Med* 16:159-163, 2002.

115. Kornegay JN, Lorenz MD, Zenoble RD: Bacterial meningoencephalitis in two dogs, *J Am Vet Med Assoc* 173:1334-1336, 1978.

116. Dow SW, et al: Central nervous system infection associated with anaerobic bacteria in two dogs and two cats, *J Vet Intern Med* 2:171-176, 1988.

117. Bahri LE, Blouin A: Fluoroquinolones: A new family of antimicrobials, *Compend Cont Educ Pract Vet* 13:1429-1434, 1991.

118. Orsini JA, Perkons S: New beta-lactam antibiotics in critical care medicine, *Compend Cont Educ Pract Vet* 16:183-186, 1994.

119. Frank LA: Clinical pharmacology of rifampin, *J Am Vet Med Assoc* 197:114-117, 1990.

120. Haskins SC: Management of septic shock, *J Am Vet Med Assoc* 200:1915-1924, 1992.

121. Greene CE: Infectious diseases affecting the nervous system. In Kornegay JN, editor: *Neurologic disorders.* New York, 1986, Churchill Livingstone.

122. Carmichael LE, Greene CE: Canine brucellosis. In Greene CE, editor: *Infectious diseases of the dog and cat.* Philadelphia, 1990, WB Saunders.

123. Moore BR: Update on equine therapeutics: Bacterial meningitis in foals, *Compend Cont Educ Pract Vet* 17:1417-1420, 1995.

124. Morris DD, Rutkowski J, Lloyd KC: Therapy in two cases of neonatal foal septicemia and meningitis with cefotaxim96 sodium, *Equine Vet J* 19:151-154, 1987.

125. Santschi EM, Foreman JH: Equine bacterial meningitis, Part I, *Compend Cont Educ Pract Vet* 11:479-483, 1989.

126. Foreman JH, Santschi EM: Equine bacterial meningitis, Part II, *Compend Cont Educ Pract Vet* 11:640-644, 1989.

127. Green SL, Smith LL: Meningitis in neonatal calves: 32 cases (1983-1990), *J Am Vet Med Assoc* 201:125-128, 1992.

128. Harris FW, Janzen ED: The *Haemophilus somnus* disease complex (Haemophilosis): A review, *Can Vet J* 30:816-822, 1989.

129. Donkersgoed JV, Janzen ED, Harland RJ: Epidemiological features of calf mortality due to hemophilosis in a large feedlot, *Can Vet J* 31:821-825, 1990.

130. Blenden DC, Kampelmacher EH, Torres-anjel MJ: Listeriosis [zoonosis update], *J Am Vet Med Assoc* 1:79-84, 1990.

131. Perdizet JA, Dinsmore P: Pituitary abscess syndrome, *Compend Cont Educ Pract Vet* 8:311-318, 1986.

132. Raphel CF: Brain abscess in three horses, *J Am Vet Med Assoc* 180:874-877, 1982.

133. Allen JR, Barbee DD, Boulton MD: Brain abscess in a horse: Diagnosis by computed tomography and successful surgical treatment, *Equine Vet J* 19:552-555, 1987.

134. Greene CE, editor: *Infectious diseases of the dog and cat.* Philadelphia, 1990, WB Saunders.

135. Kornegay JN: Diskospondylitis. In Slatter DH, editor: *Textbook of small animal surgery.* Philadelphia, 1993, WB Saunders.

136. Medleau L, Barsanti JA: Cryptococcosis. In Greene CE, editor: *Infectious diseases of the dog and cat.* Philadelphia, 1990, WB Saunders.

137. Cook JR, Evinger JV, Wagner LA: Successful combination chemotherapy for cryptococcal meningoencephalitis, *J Am Anim Hosp Assoc* 27:61-64, 1991.

138. Hill PB, Moriello KA, Shaw SE: A review of systemic antifungal agents, *Vet Dermatol* 6:59-66, 1995.

139. Heit MC, Riviere JE: Antifungal therapy: Ketoconazole and other azole derivatives, *Compend Cont Educ Pract Vet* 1:21-31, 1995.
140. Mikiciuk MG, Fales WH, Schmidt DA: Successful treatment of feline cryptococcosis with ketoconazole and flucytosine, *J Am Anim Hosp Assoc* 26:199-201, 1990.
141. Medleau L, Jacobs GJ, Marks MA: Itraconazole for the treatment of cryptococcosis in cats, *J Vet Intern Med* 9:39-42, 1995.
142. Legendre A, Berthelin C: How do I treat central nervous system cryptococcosis in dogs and cats? *Prog Vet Neurol* 6:32-34, 1995.
143. Greene RT, Troy GC: Coccidioidomycosis in 48 cats: A retrospective study (1984-1993), *J Vet Intern Med* 2:86-91, 1995.
144. Clinkenbeard KD, Cowell RL, Tyler RD: Disseminated histoplasmosis in dogs: 12 cases (1981-1986), *J Am Vet Med Assoc* 193:1443-1447, 1988.
145. Sharp NJH, Sullivan M: Use of ketoconazole in the treatment of canine nasal aspergillosis, *J Am Vet Med Assoc* 194:782-786, 1989.
146. Miller PE, Miller LM, Schoster JV: Feline blastomycosis: A report of three cases and literature review (1961 to 1988), *J Am Anim Hosp Assoc* 26:417-424, 1990.
147. Hodges RD, et al: Itraconazole for the treatment of histoplasmosis in cats, *J Vet Intern Med* 8:409-413, 1994.
148. Hardie EM: Actinomycosis and nocardiosis. In Greene CE, editor: *Infectious diseases of the dog and cat*. Philadelphia, 1990, WB Saunders.
149. Dubey JP, Greene CE, Lappin MR: Toxoplasmosis and neosporosis. In Greene CE, editor: *Infectious diseases of the dog and cat*. Philadelphia, 1990, WB Saunders.
150. Lappin MR, Greene CE, Winston S, et al: Clinical feline toxoplasmosis: Serologic diagnosis and therapeutic management of 15 cases, *J Vet Intern Med* 3:139-143, 1989.
151. Lappin MR: Feline toxoplasmosis, *Waltham Focus* 4:2-8, 1992.
152. Fenger CK: PCR-based detection of *Sarcocystis neurona*: Implications for diagnosis and research. In *Proceedings of the 12th American College of Veterinary Internal Medicine Forum*, 1994, pp 550-552.
153. Fenger CK: Update on the diagnosis and treatment of equine protozoal myeloencephalitis (EPM). In *Proceedings of the 13th American College of Veterinary Internal Medicine Forum*, 1995, pp 597-599.
154. Porter MB, et al: West Nile virus encephalomyelitis in horses: 46 cases (2001), *J Am Vet Med Assoc* 222:1241-1247, 2003.
155. Tyler JW, et al: West Nile virus encephalomyelitis in a sheep, *J Vet Intern Med* 17:242-244, 2003.
156. Wamsley HL, et al: Findings in cerebrospinal fluids of horses infected with West Nile virus: 30 cases (2001), *J Am Vet Med Assoc* 221:1303-1305, 2002.
157. Gilman AG, et al: Antiviral agents. In Goodman and Gilman, editors: *The pharmacological basis of therapeutics*. New York, 1990, Pergamon Press.
158. Meinkoth JH, et al: Morphologic and molecular evidence of a dual species ehrlichial infection in a dog presenting with inflammatory central nervous system disease, *J Vet Intern Med* 12:389-393, 1989.
159. Maretzki CH, Fisher DJ, Greene CE: Granulocytic ehrlichiosis and meningitis in a dog, *J Am Vet Med Assoc* 205:1554-1556, 1994.
160. Neer TM, et al: Consensus statement on ehrlichial disease of small animals from the infectious disease study group of the ACVIM, *J Vet Intern Med* 16:309-315, 2002.
161. Meric SM: Canine meningitis: A changing emphasis, *J Vet Intern Med* 2:26-35, 1988.
162. Tipold A: Diagnosis of inflammatory and infectious diseases of the central nervous system in dogs: A retrospective study, *J Vet Intern Med* 9:304-314, 1995.
163. Webb AA, Taylor SM, Muir GD: Steroid-responsive meningitis-arteritis in dogs with noninfectious, nonerosive, idiopathic, immune-mediated polyarthritis, *J Vet Intern Med* 16:269-273, 2002.
164. Munana K, Luttgen PJ: Prognostic factors for dogs with granulomatous meningoencephalomyelitis: 42 cases (1982-1996), *J Am Vet Med Assoc* 212:1902-1906, 1998.
165. Demierre S, et al: Correlation between the clinical course of granulomatous meningoencephalomyelitis in dogs and the extent of mast cell infiltration, *Vet Rec* 148:467-472, 2001.
166. Kipar A, Baumgartner W, Vogil C: Immunohistochemical characterization of inflammatory cells in brains of dogs with granulomatous meningoencephalitis, *Vet Pathol* 35:43-52, 1998.
166a. Cuddon PA, et al: New treatments for granulomatous meningoencephalomyelitis. In *Proceedings of the 20th Annual Veterinary Medical Forum*, Dallas, TX, 2002.
167. McConnico RS, Clem MF, DeBowes RM: Supportive medical care of recumbent horses, *Compend Cont Educ Pract Vet* 8:1287-1295, 1991.
168. Shell LG, et al: Neuronal-visceral GM$_1$ gangliosidosis in Portuguese water dogs, *J Vet Intern Med* 3:1-7, 1989.
169. Baker HJ, et al: Animal models of human ganglioside storage diseases, *FASEB J* 35:1193-1201, 1976.
170. Read DH, et al: Neuronal-visceral GM$_1$ gangliosidosis in a dog with β-galactosidase deficiency, *Science* 194:442-445, 1976.
171. Donnelly WJC, Sheahan BJ, Rogers TA: GM$_1$ gangliosidosis in Friesian calves, *J Pathol* 111:173-179, 1973.
172. Baker HJ, et al: Neuronal GM$_1$ gangliosidosis in a Siamese cat with β-galactosidase deficiency, *Science* 174:838-839, 1971.
173. Cummings JF, Wood PA, Walkley SU, et al: GM$_2$ gangliosidosis in a Japanese spaniel, *Acta Neuropathol* 67:247-253, 1985.
174. Singer HS, Cork LC: Canine GM$_2$ gangliosidosis: Morphological and biochemical analysis. *Vet Pathol* 26:114-120, 1989.
175. Cork LC, Munnell JF, Lorenz MD: The pathology of feline GM$_2$ gangliosidosis, *Am J Pathol* 90:723-734, 1978.
176. Cork LC, et al: GM$_2$ ganglioside lysosomal storage in cats with β-hexosaminidase deficiency, *Science* 196:1014-1017, 1977.
177. Read WK, Bridges CH: Neuronal lipodystrophy: Occurrence in an inbred strain of cattle, *Pathol Vet* 6:235-243, 1969.
178. Hartley WJ, Blakemore WF: Neurovisceral glucocerebroside storage (Gaucher's disease) in a dog, *Vet Pathol* 10:191-201, 1973.
179. Cuddon PA, Higgins RJ, Duncan ID: Feline Niemann-Pick disease associated polyneuropathy. In *Proceedings of the Sixth Annual Veterinary Medical Forum*, Washington, DC, 1988, p 726.
180. Baker H, et al: Sphingomyelin lipidosis in a cat, *Vet Pathol* 24:386-391, 1987.
181. Bundza A, Lowden JA, Charlton KM: Niemann-Pick disease in a poodle dog, *Vet Pathol* 16:530-538, 1979.
182. Chrisp CE, et al: Lipid storage disease in a Siamese cat, *J Am Vet Med Assoc* 156:616-622, 1970.
183. Johnson KH: Globoid leukodystrophy in the cat, *J Am Vet Med Assoc* 157:2057-2067, 1970.

184. Selcer ES, Selcer RR: Globoid cell leukodystrophy in two West Highland white terriers and one Pomeranian, *Compend Cont Educ Pract Vet* 6:621-624, 1984.

185. Luttgen PJ, Braund KG, Storts RW: Globoid cell leukodystrophy in a basset hound, *J Small Anim Pract* 24:153-160, 1983.

186. Zaki F, Kay WJ: Globoid cell leukodystrophy in a miniature poodle, *J Am Vet Med Assoc* 163:248-250, 1973.

187. Pritchard DH, Napthine DV, Sinclair AJ: Globoid cell leukodystrophy in polled Dorset sheep, *Vet Pathol* 17:399-405, 1980.

188. Johnson GR, Oliver JE, Selcer R: Globoid cell leukodystrophy in a beagle, *J Am Vet Med Assoc* 167:380-384, 1975.

189. Fletcher TF: Electroencephalographic features of leukodystrophic disease in the dog, *J Am Vet Med Assoc* 157:190-198, 1970.

190. Fletcher TF, Kurtz HJ, Low DG: Globoid cell leukodystrophy (Krabbe type) in the dog, *J Am Vet Med Assoc* 149:165-172, 1966.

191. Fatzer R: Leukodystrophische Ershrankungen im Gehirn junger Katzen, *Schweiz Arch Tierheilkd* 117:641-648, 1975.

192. Hegreberg GA, Thuline HC, Francis BH: Morphologic changes in feline leukodystrophy, *FASEB J* 30:341, 1971.

193. Cowell KR, et al: Mucopolysaccharidosis in a cat, *J Am Vet Med Assoc* 169:334-339, 1976.

194. Haskins ME, Jezyk PF, Desnick RJ, et al: Animal models of mucopolysaccharidosis. In Desnick RJ, Patterson DF, Scarpelli DG, editors: *Animal models of inherited metabolic diseases.* New York, 1982, Alan R Liss.

195. Haskins ME, et al: The pathology of the feline model of mucopolysaccharidosis VI, *Am J Pathol* 101:657-674, 1980.

196. Shull RM, et al: Morphologic and biochemical studies of canine mucopolysaccharidosis I, *Am J Pathol* 114:487-495, 1984.

197. Haskins ME, et al: The pathology of the feline model of mucopolysaccharidosis I, *Am J Pathol* 112:27-36, 1983.

198. Shull RM, et al: Animal model of human disease: Canine a-L-iduronidase deficiency—A model of mucopolysaccharidosis I, *Am J Pathol* 109:244-248, 1982.

199. Hegreberg GA, Padget GA: Inherited progressive epilepsy of the dog with comparisons to Lafora's disease of man, *FASEB J* 35:1202-1205, 1976.

200. Cusick PK, Cameron AM, Parker AJ: Canine neuronal glycoproteinosis: Lafora's disease in the dog, *J Am Anim Hosp Assoc* 12:518-521, 1976.

201. Cummings JF, Wood PA, de Lahunta A, et al: The clinical and pathologic heterogeneity of feline a-mannosidosis, *J Vet Intern Med* 2:163-170, 1988.

202. Maenhout T, et al: Mannosidosis in a litter of Persian cats, *Vet Rec* 122:351-354, 1988.

203. Blakemore W: A case of mannosidosis in the cat: Clinical and histopathological findings, *J Small Anim Pract* 27:447-455, 1986.

204. Embury DH, Jerrett IV: Mannosidosis in Galloway calves, *Vet Pathol* 22:548-551, 1985.

205. Vandevelde M, Fankhauser R, Bichsel P, et al: Hereditary neurovisceral mannosidosis with associated mannosidase deficiency in a family of Persian cats, *Acta Neuropathol* 58:64-68, 1982.

206. Shapiro JL, et al: Caprine β-mannosidosis in kids from an Ontario herd, *Can Vet J* 26:155-158, 1985.

207. Healy PJ, et al: β-Mannosidase deficiency in Anglo Nubian goats, *Aust Vet J* 57:504-507, 1981.

208. Fyfe JC, et al: Familial glycogen storage disease type IV (GSD IV) in Norwegian forest cats (NWFC), *J Vet Intern Med* 4:127, 1990.

209. Harvey JW, et al: Polysaccharide storage myopathy in canine phosphofructokinase deficiency (type VII glycogen storage disease), *Vet Pathol* 27:1-8, 1990.

210. Walvoort HC, et al: Canine glycogen storage disease type II: A clinical study of four affected Lapland dogs, *J Am Anim Hosp Assoc* 20:279-286, 1984.

211. O'Sullivan BM, et al: Generalised glycogenosis in Brahman cattle, *Aust Vet J* 57:227-229, 1981.

212. Manktelow CD, Hartley WJ: Generalized glycogen storage disease in sheep, *J Comp Pathol* 85:139-145, 1975.

213. McHowell J, Dorling PR, Cook RD, et al: Infantile and late onset form of generalised glycogenosis type II in cattle, *J Pathol* 134:266-277, 1981.

214. Mostafa IE: A case of glycogenic cardiomegaly in a dog, *Acta Vet Scand* 11:197-208, 1970.

215. Sandstrom B, Westman J, Ockerman PA: Glycogenosis of the central nervous system in the cat, *Acta Neuropathol (Berl)* 14:194-200, 1969.

216. Jolly RD, Hartley WJ: Storage diseases of domestic animals, *Aust Vet J* 43:1-8, 1977.

217. Herrtage ME: Canine fucosidosis, *Vet Annu* 28:223-227, 1988.

218. Taylor R, Farrow B, Healy P: Canine fucosidosis: Clinical findings, *J Small Anim Pract* 28:291-300, 1987.

219. Kelly WR, et al: Canine L fucosidosis: A storage disease of Springer spaniels, *Acta Neuropathol (Berl)* 60:9-13, 1983.

220. Taylor RM, Farrow BRH: Ceroid lipofuscinosis in border collie dogs, *Acta Neuropathol (Berl)* 75:627-631, 1988.

221. Harper PAW, et al: Neurovisceral ceroid lipofuscinosis in blind Devon cattle, *Acta Neuropathol (Berl)* 75:632-636, 1988.

222. Cho D, Leipold H, Rudolph R: Neuronal ceroidosis (ceroid lipofuscinosis) in a blue heeler dog, *Acta Neuropathol (Berl)* 69:161-164, 1986.

223. Nimmo Wilkie JS, Hudson EB: Neuronal and generalized ceroid lipofuscinosis in a cocker spaniel, *Vet Pathol* 19:623-628, 1982.

224. Vandevelde M, Fatzer R: Neuronal ceroid-lipofuscinosis in older dachshunds, *Vet Pathol* 17:686-692, 1980.

225. Koppang N: Canine ceroid lipofuscinosis in English setters, *J Small Anim Pract* 10:639-644, 1970.

226. Armstrong D, Koppang N, Jolly R: Ceroid lipofuscinosis, *Comp Pathol Bull* 12:2-4, 1980.

227. Appleby EC, Longstaffe JA, Bell FR: Ceroid lipofuscinosis in two Saluki dogs, *J Comp Pathol* 92:375-380, 1982.

228. Hoover D, Little P, Cole W: Neuronal ceroid-lipofuscinosis in a mature dog, *Vet Pathol* 21:359-361, 1984.

229. Fiske RA, Storts RW: Neuronal ceroid-lipofuscinosis in Nubian goats, *Vet Pathol* 25:171-173, 1988.

230. Green P, Little P: Neuronal ceroid-lipofuscin storage in Siamese cats, *Can J Comp Med* 38:207-212, 1974.

231. Mayhew I, Jolly R: Ovine ceroid lipofuscinosis. In *Proceedings of the 11th Annual Veterinary Medical Forum,* 1986, pp 57-59.

232. Reece RL, MacWhirter P: Neuronal ceroid lipofuscinosis in a lovebird, *Vet Rec* 122:187, 1988.

233. Sisk DB, et al: Clinical and pathologic features of ceroid lipofuscinosis in two Australian cattle dogs, *J Am Vet Med Assoc* 197:361-364, 1990.

234. Cummings JF, de Lahunta A, Riis RC, et al: Neuropathologic changes in a young adult Tibetan terrier with subclinical neuronal ceroid-lipofuscinosis, *Prog Vet Neurol* 1:301-309, 1990.

235. Shell L, Jortner B, Leib M: Familial motor neuron disease in Rottweiler dogs: Neuropathologic studies, *Vet Pathol* 24:135-139, 1987.

236. Shell L, Jortner B, Leib M: Spinal muscular atrophy in two Rottweiler littermates, *J Am Vet Med Assoc* 190:878-880, 1987.

237. Cummings JF, George C, de Lahunta A, et al: Focal spinal muscular atrophy in two German shepherd pups, *Acta Neuropathol (Berl)* 79:113-116, 1989.

238. Cork LC, Griffin JW, Munnell JF, et al: Hereditary canine spinal muscular atrophy, *J Neuropathol Exp Neurol* 38:209-221, 1979.

239. Inada S, Sakamoto H, Haruta K, et al: A clinical study on hereditary progressive neurogenic muscular atrophy in pointer dogs, *Jpn J Vet Sci* 40:539-547, 1978.

240. Sandefeldt E, Cummings JF, de Lahunta A, et al: Hereditary neuronal abiotrophy in the Swedish Lapland dog, *Cornell Vet* 63:1-71, 1973.

241. Lancaster M, Gill I, Hooper P: Progressive paresis in Angora goats, *Aust Vet J* 64:123, 1987.

242. Palmer AC, Blakemore WF: A progressive neuronopathy in the young cairn terrier, *J Small Anim Pract* 30:101-106, 1989.

243. Jaggy A, Vandevelde M: Multisystem neuronal degeneration in cocker spaniels, *J Vet Intern Med* 2:117-120, 1988.

244. Cummings JF, de Lahunta A, Moore JJ: Multisystemic chromatolytic neuronal degeneration in a cairn terrier pup, *Cornell Vet* 78:301-314, 1988.

245. Hartley WJ, Palmer AC: Ataxia in Jack Russell terriers, *Acta Neuropathol (Berl)* 26:71-74, 1973.

246. Carmichael S, Griffiths IR, Harvey MJA: Familial cerebellar ataxia with hydrocephalus in bull mastiffs, *Vet Rec* 112:354-358, 1983.

247. Matthews NS, de Lahunta A: Degenerative myelopathy in an adult miniature poodle, *J Am Vet Med Assoc* 186:1213-1214, 1985.

248. Waxman FJ, Clemmons RM, Johnson G, et al: Progressive myelopathy in older German shepherd dogs, I: Depressed response to thymus-dependent mitogens, *J Immunol* 124:1209-1215, 1980.

249. Averill DR: Degenerative myelopathy in the aging German shepherd dog, *J Am Vet Med Assoc* 162:1045-1051, 1973.

250. Griffiths IR, Duncan ID: Chronic degenerative radiculomyelopathy in the dog, *J Small Anim Pract* 16:461-471, 1975.

251. Aitchison S, Westfall J, Leipold H, et al: Ultrastructural alterations of motor cortex synaptic junctions in Brown Swiss cattle with weaver syndrome, *Am J Vet Res* 46:1733-1736, 1985.

252. Baird JD, Sarmiento UM, Basrur PK: Bovine progressive degenerative myeloencephalopathy (weaver syndrome) in brown Swiss cattle in Canada: A literature review and case report, *Can Vet J* 29:370-377, 1988.

253. Gamble DA, Chrisman CL: A leukoencephalomyelopathy of Rottweiler dogs, *Vet Pathol* 21:274-280, 1984.

254. Zachary JF, O'Brien DP: Spongy degeneration of the central nervous system in two canine littermates, *Vet Pathol* 22:561-571, 1985.

255. Luttgen PJ, Storts RW: Central nervous system status spongiosus, In *Proceedings of the 5th Veterinary Medical Forum,* San Diego, 1987, p 841.

256. Cockrell BY, et al: Myelomalacia in Afghan hounds, *J Am Vet Med Assoc* 162:362-365, 1973.

257. Kelly DF, Gaskell CJ: Spongy degeneration of the central nervous system in kittens, *Acta Neuropathol (Berl)* 35:151-158, 1976.

258. Harper P, et al: Maple syrup urine disease in calves: A clinical, pathological and biochemical study, *Aust Vet J* 66:46-49, 1989.

259. Clark RG, et al: Suspected neuroaxonal dystrophy in collie sheep dogs, *N Z Vet J* 30:102-103, 1982.

260. Cork LC, et al: Canine neuroaxonal dystrophy, *J Neuropathol Exp Neurol* 42:286-296, 1983.

261. Chrisman CL, Cork LC, Gamble DA: Neuroaxonal dystrophy of Rottweiler dogs, *J Am Vet Med Assoc* 184:464-467, 1984.

262. Blakemore W, Palmer A: Nervous disease in the chihuahua characterised by axonal swellings, *Vet Rec* 117:498-499, 1985.

263. Duncan ID, Griffiths IR: Canine giant axonal neuropathy: Some aspects of its clinical, pathological and comparative features, *J Small Anim Pract* 22:491-501, 1981.

264. Duncan ID, Griffiths IR: Canine giant axonal neuropathy, *Vet Rec* 101:438-441, 1977.

265. Griffiths IR: Progressive axonopathy: An inherited neuropathy of boxer dogs, 1: Further studies of the clinical and electrophysiological features, *J Small Anim Pract* 26:381-392, 1985.

266. Griffiths IR, Duncan ID, Barker J: A progressive axonopathy of boxer dogs affecting the central and peripheral nervous system, *J Small Anim Pract* 21:29-43, 1980.

267. Woodard JC, Collins GH, Hessler JR: Feline hereditary neuroaxonal dystrophy, *Am J Pathol* 74:551-560, 1974.

268. Nuttall WO: Ovine neuroaxonal dystrophy in New Zealand, *N Z Vet J* 36:5-7, 1988.

269. Beech J, Haskins M: Genetic studies of neuroaxonal dystrophy in the Morgan, *Am J Vet Res* 48:109-113, 1987.

270. Beech J: Neuroaxonal dystrophy of the accessory cuneate nucleus in horses, *Vet Pathol* 21:384-393, 1984.

271. de Lahunta A, Shively GN: Neurofibrillary accumulation in a puppy, *Cornell Vet* 65:240-247, 1975.

272. Vandevelde M, Greene C, Hoff E: Lower motor neuron disease with accumulation of neurofilaments in a cat, *Vet Pathol* 13:428-435, 1976.

273. Higgins RJ, et al: Spontaneous lower motor neuron disease with neurofibrillary accumulation in young pigs, *Acta Neuropathol (Berl)* 59:288-294, 1983.

274. Rousseaux CG, et al: Shaker calf syndrome: A newly recognized inherited neurodegenerative disorder of horned Hereford calves, *Vet Pathol* 22:104-111, 1985.

275. Cork LC, Troncoso JC, Price DL: Canine inherited ataxia, *Ann Neurol* 9:492-499, 1981.

276. de Lahunta A, et al: Hereditary cerebellar cortical abiotrophy in the Gordon setter, *J Am Vet Med Assoc* 177:538-541, 1980.

277. Montgomery D, Storts R: Hereditary striatonigral and cerebel-olivary degeneration of the Kerry blue terrier, II: Ultrastructural lesions in the caudate nucleus and cerebellar cortex, *J Neuropathol Exp Neurol* 43:263-275, 1984.

278. Montgomery D, Storts R: Hereditary striatonigral and cerebello-olivary degeneration of the Kerry blue terrier, *Vet Pathol* 20:143-159, 1983.

279. de Lahunta A, Averill DR: Hereditary cerebellar cortical and extrapyramidal nuclear abiotrophy in Kerry blue terriers, *J Am Vet Med Assoc* 168:1119-1124, 1976.

280. Steinberg S, et al: Clinical features of inherited cerebellar degeneration in Gordon setters, *J Am Vet Med Assoc* 179:886-890, 1981.

281. de Lahunta A: Comparative cerebellar disease in domestic animals, *Compend Cont Educ Pract Vet* 2:8-19, 1980.

282. de Lahunta A: *Veterinary neuroanatomy and clinical neurology,* 2nd ed. Philadelphia, 1983, WB Saunders.

283. LeCouteur RA, Kornegay JN, Higgins RJ: Late onset progressive cerebellar degeneration of Brittany spaniel dogs. In *Proceedings of the Sixth Annual Veterinary Medical Forum,* Washington, DC, 1988, pp 657-658.

284. Chrisman CL, et al: Late-onset cerebellar degeneration in a dog, *J Am Vet Med Assoc* 182:717-720, 1983.

285. Haskins ME, et al: Mucopolysaccharidosis in a domestic short haired cat: A disease distinct from that seen in the Siamese cat, *J Am Vet Med Assoc* 175:384-387, 1979.

286. Barlow R: Genetic cerebellar disorders in cattle. In Rose FC, Behan PO, editors: *Animal models of neurological disease.* Kent, Great Britain, 1980, Pitman Medical.

287. Barlow R: Morphogenesis of cerebellar lesions in bovine familial convulsions and ataxia, *Vet Pathol* 18:151-162, 1981.

288. White ME, Whitlock RH, de Lahunta A: A cerebellar abiotrophy of calves, *Cornell Vet* 65:476-491, 1975.

289. Terlecki S, et al: A congenital disease of lambs clinically similar to "inherited cerebellar cortical atrophy" (daft lamb disease), *Br Vet J* 134:299-308, 1978.

290. Harper P, et al: Cerebellar abiotrophy and segmental axonopathy: Two syndromes of progressive ataxia of Merino sheep, *Aust Vet J* 63:18-21, 1986.

291. Kidd A, et al: A new genetically determined congenital nervous disorder in pigs, *Br Vet J* 142:275-285, 1986.

292. Sorjonen D, Cox N, Kwapien R: Myeloencephalopathy with eosinophilic refractile bodies (Rosenthal fibers) in a Scottish terrier, *J Am Vet Med Assoc* 190:1004-1006, 1987.

293. Cooper BJ, et al: Canine inherited hypertrophic neuropathy: Clinical and electrodiagnostic studies, *Am J Vet Res* 45:1172-1177, 1984.

294. Cooper B, et al: Defective Schwann cell function in canine inherited hypertrophic neuropathy, *Acta Neuropathol (Berl)* 63:51-56, 1984.

295. Cummings JF, et al: Animal model of human disease: Hereditary sensory neuropathy: Nociceptive loss and acral mutilation in pointer dogs: Canine hereditary sensory neuropathy, *Am J Pathol* 112:136-138, 1983.

296. Cummings JF, de Lahunta A, Winn SS: Acral mutilation and nociceptive loss in English pointer dogs, *Acta Neuropathol (Berl)* 53:119-127, 1981.

297. Duncan ID, Griffiths IR, Munz M: The pathology of a sensory neuropathy affecting long haired dachshund dogs, *Acta Neuropathol (Berl)* 58:141-151, 1982.

298. Chrisman CL: Distal polyneuropathy of doberman pinschers. In *Proceedings of the Third Annual Medical Forum,* American College of Veterinary Internal Medicine, San Diego, 1985.

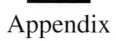

Appendix

BREED SPECIFIC NEUROMUSCULAR DISEASES IN DOMESTIC ANIMALS

Bovine Diseases

Breed	Disease	Chapter	Inherited	References
Aberdeen angus	Cerebellar degeneration	8		1
	Cerebellar hypoplasia	8	S	2
	Epilepsy	13	Y	3
	Mannosidosis	15	Y	4-6
Angus & shorthorn	Hypomyelination	10	Y	7, 8
Ayrshire	Cerebellar degeneration	8	Y	9, 10
	Cerebellar hypoplasia	8		10
Ayrshire cross	Atlanto-occipital malformation	7		11
Beefmaster	Ceroid lipofuscinosis	15		12
	Neuronal lipodystrophy	15	Y	6
Brahman	Glycogenosis	15	Y	13
	Narcolepsy/cataplexy	13		14
Brown Swiss	Cerebellar degeneration	8		15
	Degenerative mycloencephalopathy	7	S	15-17
	Epilepsy	13	Y	18
Charolais	Cerebellar hypoplasia	8		19
	Demyelination	7, 15	Y	6, 20-23
	Cerebellar degeneration and epilepsy	13		6
	Myelodysplasia	6	Y	24, 25
Charolais cross	Atlanto-occipital malformation	7		11
Devon	Atlanto-occipital malformation	7		26
	Ceroid lipofuscinosis	15		12, 27
Galloway	Mannosidosis	15		28
Guernsey	Narcolepsy/cataplexy	13		29
Hereford	Cerebellar degeneration	8	Y	30
	Cerebellar hypoplasia	8	Y	6, 30, 31
	Ceroid lipofuscinosis	15		6
	Epilepsy	13		32
	Hydrocephalus	12	Y	33-35
	Hypomyelination	10		8, 36
	Neuronal degeneration	7	Y	37, 38
	Spinocerebellar degeneration	15		37
Holstein Friesian	Atlanto-occipital malformation	7		39, 40
	Atlantoaxial luxation	7	S	39

Continued

Bovine Diseases *(Continued)*

Breed	Disease	Chapter	Inherited	References
Holstein Friesian	Cerebellar brainstem malformation	8		41
	Cerebellar degeneration	8	Y	6, 30, 42
	Cerebellar hypoplasia	8		43
	Gangliosidosis GM$_1$	15	Y	4, 44-47
	Hypomyelination	10		555
	Myopathy of diaphragmatic muscles		Y	556
	Spinal dysraphism	6		48
	Spongiform degeneration	12		49
Jersey	Cerebellar degeneration	8		6
	Hypomyelination	10	Y	8, 50
Limousin	Epilepsy	13		6
Limousin cross	Neuronal degeneration	15	Y	51, 52
Murray grey	Demyelination	7, 15	Y	53, 54
	Mannosidosis	15	Y	5
Norwegian red poll	Pelvic limb paralysis	6	Y	52
Polled Hereford	Congenital myoclonus (neuraxial edema)	15	Y	55-59
	Neuronal degeneration	15	Y	60
Polled shorthorn	Congenital myoclonus (neuraxial edema)	15	Y	557
Red Danish	Paralysis		Y	61
Salers	ß-Mannosidosis	15	Y	62, 63
Shorthorn	Cerebellar degeneration	8, 15	Y	6
	Cerebellar hypoplasia	8	Y	6, 30, 64, 65
	Glycogenosis	15	Y	6, 66, 67
	Hydrocephalus	12	Y	33, 34, 68
	Hypomyelination	10	Y	8, 36
	Retinal dysplasia	11	Y	69
Simmental	Neuronal degeneration	15	Y	51, 52
	Spongiform myelopathy			558
Swedish red	Epilepsy	13		70
Various	Arthrogryposis	7		71
	Cerebellar brainstem malformation	8		72
	Myelodysplasia	6		73, 74
	Neurofibromatosis	15		75

Y, Yes; *S,* suspected.

Canine Diseases

Breed	Disease	Chapter	Inherited	References
Afghan hound	Myelopathy	6	Y	76-79
	Retinal degeneration	11	Y	69
Airedale terrier	Cerebellar hypoplasia	8		80-82
	Cerebellar degeneration	8	Y	30
	Congenital myasthenia gravis	7	Y	83
Akita	Cerebellar degeneration	8, 15		30
	Congenital vestibular disease	8	S	84
Alaskan malamute	Peripheral neuropathy	7	Y	552
	Retinal degeneration	11	Y	69
Australian cattle dog	Ceroid lipofuscinosis	15	Y	85
	Dermatomyositis	7	Y	551
	Portosystemic shunt	13		559
Australian heeler	Deafness	9	Y	86
Australian kelpie	Cerebellar degeneration	8	Y	551
Australian shepherd dog	Chorioretinal dysplasia	11	Y	69
	Deafness	9	Y	86, 87
Basenji	Coloboma	11	Y	69
Basset hound	Cervical malformation	7	S	88-90
	Globoid cell leukodystrophy	15	S	91
	Glycoproteinosis	13	S	92
Beagle	Agenesis vermis cerebellum	8	S	93
	Cerebellar degeneration	8	Y	30, 84
	Congenital vestibular disease	8		94, 95
	Epilepsy	13	Y	81, 95-105
	Gangliosidosis GM$_1$	15	Y	45, 46, 106
	Globoid cell leukodystrophy	15	S	107
	Glycoproteinosis	13	S	92, 96, 97, 108
	Necrotizing vasculitis	15	Y	553
	Retinal degeneration	11	Y	69
	Retinal dysplasia	11		69
Beagle-schnauzer cross	Cerebellar degeneration	8		551
Bedlington terrier	Retinal dysplasia	11	Y	69, 81, 109
Belgian sheepdog (Groenendaeler shepherd dog)	Muscular dystrophy	7	Y	573
Belgian Tervuren	Epilepsy	13	Y	81, 98, 382
Bern running dog	Cerebellar degeneration	8	Y	30
Bernese mountain dog	Aggression			110
	Cerebellar degeneration	8	Y	84

Continued

Canine Diseases (Continued)

Breed	Disease	Chapter	Inherited	References
Bernese mountain dog	Fibrinous encephalomyelopathy (Alexander's disease)	15		560
	Hypomyelination	10		111
	Malignant histiocytosis	15		112
	Necrotizing vasculitis	14		561
Bichon frise	Steroid responsive tremor syndrome	10		551
Blue heeler	Ceroid lipofuscinosis	15		113, 114
Bluetick coonhound	Globoid leukodystrophy	15	Y	81, 115
Border collie	Cerebellar degeneration	8	Y	116
	Ceroid lipofuscinosis	15	Y	84, 117, 118
	Deafness	9		87
	Retinal degeneration	11	Y	69, 81, 109
	Sensory neuropathy	17		119
Borzoi	Cervical vertebral malformation	7		120
Boston terrier	Deafness	9	Y	86
	Gliomas	15	S	75, 121, 122
	Hemivertebrae	6	Y	81, 123, 124
	Hydrocephalus	12	P	125, 126
	Myelodysplasia	6	Y	123
	Pituitary tumors	15	S	75
Bouvier des Flandres	Laryngeal paralysis	9	Y	127, 128
Boxer	Ependymoma	15		75
	Glioma	15	S	75, 121, 122
	Pituitary tumors	15	S	75
	Progressive axonopathy	7	Y	129, 130
	Sensory neuronopathy	7	Y	551
	Sphingomyelinosis	15		562
Briard	Retinal degeneration	11	Y	69, 109
Brittany	Cerebellar degeneration	8		31
	Muscular dystrophy	7		563
	Neurogenic muscular dystrophy	7	Y	132, 133
	Retinal dysplasia	11		69
	Sensory ganglioradiculitis	14		551
Bullmastiff	Cerebellar and neuronal degeneration	8	Y	134
	Cervical vertebral malformation	7		135
Bull terrier	Cerebellar hypoplasia	8		136
	Deafness	9	Y	81, 87, 137, 138
	Hyperkinesis	10		139
	Laryngeal paralysis	9		551

Breed	Disease	Chapter	Inherited	References
Cairn terrier	Cerebellar degeneration	8		8
	Globoid cell leukodystrophy	15	Y	81, 140-144
	Hydrocephalus	12	P	126
	Neuronal degeneration	7		145, 146
Cardigan Welsh corgi	Retinal degeneration	11	Y	69, 81
Catahoula	Deafness	9		551
Cavalier King Charles spaniel	Muscular hypertonicity, Scotty cramp	7	Y	147-149
Chesapeake Bay retriever	Degenerative myelopathy	6		551
	Retinal degeneration	11		69
Chihuahua	Ceroid lipofuscinosis	15	Y	12
	Hydrocephalus	12	P	81, 126, 150
	Neuroaxonal dystrophy	7		151
Chondrodystrophic breeds	Intervertebral disk disease	6	S	152-158
Chow chow	Cerebellar hypoplasia	8	S	30, 159, 160
	Hypomyelination	10	Y	161-164
	Myotonia	10	Y	165-171
Clumber spaniel	Cerebellar degeneration	15		30
	Mitochondrial myopathy	7		551
Cocker spaniel	Aggression			110, 172
	Cerebellar degeneration	8, 15		8
	Ceroid lipofuscinosis	15	Y	173
	Congenital vestibular disease	8	S	84, 94
	Deafness	9	S	86
	Esophageal hypomotility		Y	174, 175
	Facial paralysis	9	S	176, 177
	Phosphofructokinase deficiency myopathy	7	Y	564
	Hydrocephalus	12		81
	Portosystemic shunt	12	Y	565
	Retinal degeneration	11	Y	69, 81, 109
	Retinal dysplasia	11	Y	69, 109
	Neuronal degeneration	7		178
Collie	Cerebellar degeneration	8	Y	30, 179, 180
	Chorioretinal dysplasia	11	Y	69
	Collie eye syndrome	11	Y	
	Deafness	9	Y	181
	Dermatomyositis	7	Y	167, 182-187
	Myelodysplasia	6		188

Continued

Canine Diseases *(Continued)*

Breed	Disease	Chapter	Inherited	References
Collie	Neuroaxonal dystrophy	7	Y	180
	Neuronal degeneration	7		189
	Retinal degeneration	11	Y	109
	Sensory ganglioradiculitis	10		551
Corgi	Ceroid lipofuscinosis	15		566
Corgi, Welsh	Sensory ganglioradiculitis	7		551
Dachshund	Cerebellar hypoplasia	8		136
	Ceroid lipofuscinosis	15	Y	190
	Epilepsy	13	Y	191
	Esophageal hypomotility	13		174, 175
Dachshund, longhaired	Ceroid lipofuscinosis	15	Y	192
	Sensory neuropathy	7	Y	193, 194
Dachshund, miniature, longhaired	Retinal degeneration	11	Y	69, 109
Dalmatian	Ceroid lipofuscinosis	15		566
	Deafness	9	Y	81, 86, 87, 137, 138, 181, 195-200
	Globoid cell leukodystrophy	15		81
	Hyperkinesis	10	S	201
	Hypomyelination	10	Y	202
	Leukodystrophy	15	Y	203
	Myelodysplasia	6	S	204
	Polyneuropathy, laryngeal paralysis	7, 9		567
Doberman pinscher	Aggression			205
	Cervical vertebral malformation	7	S	88-90, 206-212
	Congenital vestibular disease	8	S	84, 94, 95
	Deafness	9		213
	Distal polyneuropathy	7		214
	Hemivertebrae	6		215
	Narcolepsy-cataplexy	13	Y	216-220
	Sensory neuropathy	7		221
Dolichocephalic breeds	Meningioma	15		75, 222
English bulldog	Deafness	9	S	86
	Hemivertebrae	6	Y	81, 123, 124
	Hydrocephalus	12	P	81, 125, 126
	Myelodysplasia	6	Y	81, 188, 223-225
	Vertebral canal stenosis	6		226
English pointer	Hyperkinesis	10	Y	227-229

Canine Diseases *(Continued)*

Breed	Disease	Chapter	Inherited	References
English pointer	Sensory neuropathy	7	Y	81, 194, 230-232
English setter	Ceroid lipofuscinosis	15	Y	233-237
	Deafness	9	Y	86, 238
English springer spaniel	Cerebellar degeneration	8		551
	Gangliosidosis GM$_1$	15	Y	239
	Phosphofructokinase deficiency myopathy	7	Y	240, 241
	Polymyopathy, dyserythropoiesis	7		242
Finnish harrier	Cerebellar degeneration	8	Y	30, 243
Foxhound	Deafness	9	Y	81, 137, 244
Fox terrier	Congenital myasthenia gravis	7	Y	167, 245, 246
	Deafness	9		81
	Spinocerebellar degeneration	15	S	81
French bulldog	Hemivertebrae	6		81, 123
Gamel Dansk honsehund	Myasthenia gravis	7	Y	569
German shepherd dog	Aggression		S	205
	Cerebellar degeneration	8		551
	Congenital vestibular disease	8	S	84, 94, 95, 247
	Degenerative myelopathy	6	S	248-257
	Epilepsy	13	Y	81, 98, 270
	Esophageal hypomotility		S	174, 175, 258-260
	Giant axonal neuropathy	7	Y	261-265
	Glycogenosis	15	Y	551
	Lumbosacral malformation	6	S	266-268
	Myelodysplasia	6		269
	Peripheral neuropathy	7		570
German shorthaired pointer	Gangliosidosis GM$_2$	15	Y	4, 44-46, 271
	Hemivertebrae	6		272
	Necrotizing vasculitis	14		551
Golden retriever	Ceroid lipofuscinosis	15		566
	Horner's syndrome	11		571
	Hydrocephalus and hypertrichosis	12	S	554
	Muscular dystrophy	7	Y	167, 273-276
	Myotonia	10	S	166
	Retinal degeneration	11	Y	69, 81
	Sensory neuropathy	15		277

Continued

Canine Diseases *(Continued)*

Breed	Disease	Chapter	Inherited	References
Gordon setter	Cerebellar degeneration	8	Y	30, 278-281
	Retinal degeneration	11	Y	69, 81, 109
Great Dane	Central core myopathy	7		572
	Cerebellar degeneration	8, 15		8
	Cervical vertebral malformation	7	S	27, 88-90, 206- 212, 282-284
	Esophageal hypomotility		S	175, 258, 285, 286
	Myotonia	10		551
	Retinal dysplasia	11		69
Great Dane cross	Neuronal degeneration	7	Y	287
Greyhound	Esophageal hypomotility			260
	Retinal degeneration	11	Y	69
Horak's	Epilepsy	13	Y	98, 288
Irish setter	Cerebellar degeneration	8	Y	30, 84
	Cerebellar hypoplasia	8	S	30
	Esophageal hypomotility		S	286
	Lissencephaly	13	S	30
	Quadriplegia and amblyopia	7	Y	30, 81
	Retinal degeneration	11	Y	69, 81, 109
Irish terrier	Muscular dystrophy	7	Y	167, 289
Irish wolfhound	Portosystemic shunt	12		575
Jack Russell terrier	Congenital myasthenia gravis	7	Y	167, 290, 291
	Neuroaxonal dystrophy	7		576
	Sensory neuronopathy	14		551
	Spinocerebellar degeneration	15	Y	81, 292
Japanese chin	Gangliosidosis GM_2	15		294
Japanese retriever	Ceroid lipofuscinosis	15		293
Keeshond	Epilepsy	13	Y	81, 98, 295
Kerry blue terrier	Cerebellar degeneration	8	Y	30
	Degenerative myelopathy	6		551
	Striatonigral olivocerebellar degeneration	8		296-298
Kooiker	Leukodystrophy	7		577, 578
Labrador retriever	Axonopathy	7	Y	579
	Cerebellar hypoplasia	8		136
	Cerebellar degeneration	8	P	299
	Fibrinoid encephalopathy (Alexander's disease)	12		551
	Leucoencephalomalacia	12		580
	Muscular dystrophy	7	Y	166, 300-306

Canine Diseases *(Continued)*

Breed	Disease	Chapter	Inherited	References
Labrador retriever	Narcolepsy/cataplexy	13	Y	216, 218-220, 307, 308
	Reflex myoclonus	10	S	309
	Retinal degeneration	11	Y	69, 81, 109
	Retinal dysplasia	11	Y	69, 81, 109
	Spongiform (myelin) degeneration	12		310, 311
Lapland dog	Glycogenosis	15	Y	312, 313
	Neuronal degeneration	7	Y	81, 314, 315
Lhaso apso	Hydrocephalus	12	P	126, 316, 317
	Lissencephaly	13	S	318, 319
Lurcher	Hypomyelination	10	S	162, 164, 320
Maltese	Steroid responsive tremor syndrome	10		551
	Hydrocephalus	12	Y	126, 321, 322
	Portosystemic shunt	12		559
Miniature pinscher	Mucopolysaccharidosis	15		551
	Retinal degeneration	11	Y	69
Miniature schnauzer	Esophageal hypomotility		Y	174, 175, 323, 324
	Ceroid lipofuscinosis	15		566
	Muscular dystrophy	7		581
Mixed breed dogs	Cerebellar brainstem malformation	13		72
	Gangliosidosis GM$_2$	15		325
	Mucopolysaccharidosis	15	Y	326
Newfoundland	Esophageal hypomotility		Y	175, 327
Norwegian dunkerhound	Deafness	9	Y	137
Norwegian elkhound	Retinal degeneration	11	Y	69, 81
Old English sheepdog	Deafness	9	Y	86, 328
	Mitochondrial myopathy	7		551
Papillon	Neuroaxonal dystrophy	7		582
Pekingese	Hydrocephalus	12	P	126
Plott hound	Mucopolysaccharidosis	15	Y	326, 329
Pointer	Neurogenic muscular atrophy	7	Y	330-332
	Retinal degeneration	11		69
Pomeranian	Globoid cell leukodystrophy	15		333
	Hydrocephalus	12	P	126
Poodle	Agenesis vermis cerebellum	8	S	334
	Cerebellar hypoplasia	8	S	334, 335
	Demyelination	7	S	336
	Globoid cell leukodystrophy	15	Y	81, 337

Continued

Canine Diseases *(Continued)*

Breed	Disease	Chapter	Inherited	References
Poodle	Glycoproteinosis	13	S	92
	Sphingomyelinlipidosis	15	Y	338
Poodle, miniature or toy	Retinal degeneration	11	Y	69, 81, 109
Poodle, miniature	Cerebellar degeneration	7		551
	Fibrinoid encephalomyelopathy (Alexander's disease)	15		551
Poodle, standard	Polymicrogyria and hydrocephalus	12		583
Poodle, toy	Hydrocephalus	12	P	322
Portuguese water dog	Gangliosidosis GM$_1$	15		339
Pug	Encephalitis	15	Y	584-586
	Esophageal hypomotility			259
	Hemivertebrae	6		123
	Hydrocephalus	12	P	126, 317
Pyrenean mountain dog	Demyelination	7		340
	Sensory neuronopathy	7		551
Redbone coonhound	Retinal degeneration	11	Y	69
Rhodesian ridgeback	Myotonic myopathy	10		551
Rottweiler	Distal sensory neuropathy	7		587
	Leukoencephalomyelopathy	15	Y	341, 342
	Muscular dystrophy	7		551
	Neuroaxonal dystrophy	7	Y	342-345
	Neuronal degeneration	7		346-348
	Retinal dysplasia	11		69, 109
	Spinal dysraphism	6		349
Saluki	Ceroid lipofuscinosis	15	Y	350
	Retinal degeneration	11	Y	69
	Spongiform degeneration	12		351
Samoyed	Cerebellar degeneration	8	Y	30, 84
	Steroid responsive tremor syndrome	10		551
	Hypomyelination	10		162, 164, 352
	Muscular dystrophy	7		588
	Myasthenia gravis	7		551
	Retinal degeneration	11	Y	69
	Spongiform degeneration	12	S	353
Schipperke	Galactosialidosis	15		590
Scottish terrier	Deafness	9		81
	Fibrinoid myeloencephalopathy (Alexander's disease)	7		354
	Neuroaxonal dystrophy	7		589
	Sensory ganglioradiculitis	7		551

Canine Diseases *(Continued)*

Breed	Disease	Chapter	Inherited	References
Scottish terrier	Scotty cramp	10	Y	81, 355-362
Sealyham terrier	Retinal dysplasia	11	Y	69, 81, 109
Shetland sheepdog	Dermatomyositis	7		167, 363
	Retinal degeneration	11	Y	69
	Chorioretinal dysplasia	11	Y	69
Shropshire terrier	Deafness	9		87
Siberian husky	Cerebellar hypoplasia	8		364
	Degenerative myelopathy	6		365
	Laryngeal paralysis	9	Y	366
	Sensory neuropathy	7		221
Silky terrier	Agenesis vermis cerebellum	8		93
	Glucocerebrosidosis	15	Y	367, 368
	Spongiform degeneration	12	S	369
Spitz	Steroid responsive tremor syndrome	10		551
Springer spaniel	Aggression		S	110, 205
	Congenital myasthenia gravis	7	Y	167, 370
	Fucosidosis	15	Y	371-377
	Glycogenosis	15	Y	551
	Hypomyelination	10	Y	162, 164, 378
	Retinal degeneration	11	Y	69, 379, 380
	Retinal dysplasia	11	Y	69, 109
Staffordshire terrier	Myotonic myopathy	10		551
Sussex spaniel	Mitochondrial myopathy	7	S	551
Terrier cross	Ceroid lipofuscinosis	15		381
Tibetan mastiff	Hypertrophic neuropathy	7	Y	383-386
Tibetan spaniel	Retinal degeneration	11	Y	109
Tibetan terrier	Ceroid lipofuscinosis	15		591
	Retinal degeneration	11	Y	69, 109, 387
Toy breeds	Atlantoaxial luxation	7	S	81, 388-392
	Hydrocephalus	12	P	126
	Occipital dysplasia	8	S	393, 394
Various	Cartilaginous exostoses	6		395-398
West Highland white terrier	Steroid responsive tremor syndrome	10		551
	Globoid cell leukodystrophy	15	Y	81, 142-144, 333, 399
	Myotonic myopathy	10		551

Continued

Canine Diseases *(Continued)*

Breed	Disease	Chapter	Inherited	References
Weimaraner	Cerebellar hypoplasia	8		136
	Hypomyelination	10		162, 164, 400-402
	Spinal dysraphism	6	Y	81, 403-408
Whippet	Sensory neuropathy	14		221
Wire fox terrier	Lissencephaly	13	S	30
	Cerebellar hypoplasia	8	S	30
	Esophageal hypomotility		Y	174, 175, 258, 260, 286, 409
Yorkshire terrier	Steroid responsive tremor syndrome	10		551
	Hydrocephalus	12	Y	126
	Necrotizing encephalitis	15		592
	Portosystemic shunt	12		575
	Retinal dysplasia	11		69
Yugoslavian sheepdog	Ceroid lipofuscinosis	15		551

Y, Yes; *P,* probable; *S,* suspected.

Caprine Diseases

Breed	Disease	Chapter	Inherited	References
Goats	Myotonia	10	Y	300, 410, 411
Nubian	Ceroid lipofuscinosis	15	Y	416, 417
	Mannosidosis	15	Y	412-414
Angora	Atlantoaxial luxation	7		415

Y, Yes.

Equine Diseases

Breed	Disease	Chapter	Inherited	References
Appaloosa	Myeloencephalopathy	7, 15		418
	Night blindness	11	S	69
	Retinal degeneration, nyctalopia	11	Y	69
Arabian	Atlanto-occipital malformation	7	Y	419-421
	Cerebellar degeneration	8	Y	30, 422-424
	Cerebellar dysplasia	8		422, 423
Arabian foals	Epilepsy	13	S	425
Donkey	Myeloencephalopathy	7		426
Gotland pony	Cerebellar degeneration	8	Y	30, 427
Horses	Atlanto-occipital malformation	7		419, 428, 429

Equine Diseases *(Continued)*

Breed	Disease	Chapter	Inherited	References
Horses	Cartilaginous exostoses	6		430, 431
	Cervical vertebral malformation	7	S	419, 421, 432-436
	Degenerative myeloencephalopathy	7	S	418, 426, 437, 438
	Myotonia	10	S	439
Miniature horses	Narcolepsy	13	Y	593
Morgan	Myeloencephalopathy	7		418
	Neuroaxonal dystrophy	7		440, 441
Oldberg	Cerebellar degeneration	8, 15		51
Przewalski's horse	Myeloencephalopathy	7		418
Shetland ponies	Narcolepsy-cataplexy	13	S	421
Standardbred	Muscular dystrophy	7	Y	442
	Myeloencephalopathy	7		418
Suffolk draft horses	Narcolepsy/cataplexy	13	S	421
Thoroughbred	Cerebellar dysplasia	8		443
	Cervical vertebral malformation	7	S	419, 421, 435, 444-447
Thoroughbred (and others)	Laryngeal paralysis	9	S	448- 460
Various	Peripartum asphyxia syndrome	12		461
Welsh pony	Myeloencephalopathy	7		426
Zebra	Cervical vertebral malformation	7		462
	Degenerative myeloencephalopathy	7	S	418

Y, Yes; *S,* suspected.

Feline Diseases

Breed	Disease	Chapter	Inherited	References
Abyssinian	Glucocerebrosidosis	15	Y	463, 464
	Retinal degeneration	11	Y	109
	Retinal dysplasia	11	Y	109
Balinese	Sphingomyelin lipidosis	15		465
Birman	Distal central peripheral axonopathy	7	Y	551
	Spongiform encephalopathy	12		594
Burmese	Congenital vestibular disease	8	S	84, 94, 95
	Encephalocele	12	Y	466, 467
Cats (white, blue eyes)	Deafness	9	Y	196, 468-475
Devon rex	Muscular dystrophy	7	Y	574

Continued

Feline Diseases *(Continued)*

Breed	Disease	Chapter	Inherited	References
Domestic	Atlanto-occipital-axial malformation	7		476
	Cartilaginous exostoses	6		475
	Cerebellar degeneration	8, 15		30
	Cerebellar hypoplasia	8		475, 477-479
	Degenerative myelopathy	6		480
	Hyperoxaluria-associated polyneuropathy	7	Y	551
	Gangliosidosis GM_1	15	Y	4, 44-46
	Gangliosidosis GM_2	15	Y	45, 46, 481, 482
	Globoid cell leukodystrophy	15	Y	4, 483
	Glycogenosis	15	Y	4, 484
	Laryngeal paralysis	9		485-487
	Leukodystrophy	15	Y	488, 489
	Lissencephaly	13		490
	Mannosidosis	15	Y	491, 492
	Meningioma	15	S	75, 121, 493-495
	Mucopolysaccharidosis	15	Y	496, 497
	Muscular dystrophy	7		595-597
	Myasthenia gravis	7		551
	Neuronal ceroid lipofuscinosis	15		598
	Neuroaxonal dystrophy	7	Y	498
	Neuronal degeneration	7	Y	499
	Olivopontocerebellar degeneration	8		30
	Retinal degeneration	11		69
	Sphingomyelin lipidosis	15	Y	500, 501
Egyptian Mau	Spongiform (myelin) degeneration	12	Y	502
Himalayan	Esophageal hypomotility			503
Korat	Gangliosidosis GM_1	15	Y	44-46
	Laryngeal paralysis	9		486
Manx	Myelodysplasia	6	Y	123, 504-507
Norwegian forest cat	Glycogenosis	15	Y	508
Persian	Laryngeal paralysis	9		486
	Mannosidosis	15	Y	509-511
Siamese	Ceroid lipofuscinosis	15	Y	512
	Congenital vestibular disease	8	S	84, 94, 95
	Esophageal hypomotility		S	175
	Gangliosidosis GM_1	15	Y	44-46, 77
	Hydrocephalus	12	Y	475

Feline Diseases *(Continued)*

Breed	Disease	Chapter	Inherited	References
Siamese	Hypomyelination	10		599
	Myasthenia gravis	7		551
	Mucopolysaccharidosis	15	Y	513-519
	Neuroaxonal dystrophy	15		498
	Optic pathway anomaly	11	Y	69
	Sphingomyelin lipidosis	15	Y	520, 521
	Strabismus	11		475

Y, Yes; *S,* suspected.

Ovine Diseases

Breed	Disease	Chapter	Inherited	References
Border Leicester	Cerebellar degeneration	8		522
Coopworth	Neuroaxonal dystrophy	7	Y	523
Corriedale	Cerebellar degeneration	8	Y	30
	Glycogenosis	15	Y	524
Merino	Agenesis vermis cerebellum	8		93
	Anencephaly	12		525
	Cerebellar degeneration	8		526
	Muscular dystrophy	7	Y	527-529
	Neuroaxonal dystrophy	7		526
	Thalamic cerebellar neuropathy	8		600
Polled Dorset	Globoid cell leukodystrophy	15	Y	530
Rambouillet	Ceroid lipofuscinosis	15	Y	531
Sheep	Arthrogryposis	7		532, 533
	Atlantoaxial luxation	7		534
	Cerebellar hypoplasia	8		532
	Glucocerebrosidosis	15	Y	24
	Hydrocephalus	12		532
	Hypomyelination	10		532
	Myelodysplasia	6		532
South Hampshire	Ceroid lipofuscinosis	15	Y	12
Suffolk	Congenital myopathy	7	Y	527, 535
	Gangliosidosis GM$_1$	15	Y	536
	Neuroaxonal dystrophy	7	Y	523, 537
Welsh mountain	Cerebellar degeneration	8	Y	30
Various	Agenesis vermis cerebellum	8		532
	Cerebellar brainstem malformation	13		72, 532

Y, Yes.

Porcine Diseases

Breed	Disease	Chapter	Inherited	References
British saddleback	Hypomyelination	10	Y	538
Landrace	Hypomyelination	10	Y	538-540
	Malignant hyperthermia	15	Y	541-545
Pietrain	Malignant hyperthermia	15	Y	541
	Myopathy, hypertrophy	7	Y	546
Poland China	Malignant hyperthermia	15	Y	541, 545
Saddleback—large white	Cerebellar degeneration	8		547
Swine	Encephalocele	12		548
	Glucocerebrosidosis	15	S	24
	Hydrocephalus	12		540
	Lissencephaly	13		518
Yorkshire	Cerebellar degeneration	8	Y	30
	Gangliosidosis GM$_2$	15	Y	44-46, 549
	Neuronal degeneration	7	S	550

Y, Yes; *S,* suspected.

References

1. Barlow R: Morphogenesis of cerebellar lesions in bovine familial convulsions and ataxia, *Vet Pathol* 18:151-162, 1981.
2. Edmonds L, Crenshaw D, Selby LA: Micrognathia and cerebellar hypoplasia in an Aberdeen Angus herd, *J Hered* 64:62-64, 1973.
3. Barlow RM, Linklater KA, Young GB: Familial convulsions and ataxia in Angus calves, *Vet Rec* 83:60-65, 1968.
4. Jolly RD, Hartley WJ: Storage diseases of domestic animals, *Aust Vet J* 43:1-8, 1977.
5. Healy PJ, Cole AE: Heterozygotes for mannosidosis in Angus and Murray grey cattle, *Aust Vet J* 52:385-386, 1976.
6. Barlow R: Genetic cerebellar disorders in cattle. In Rose FC, Behan PO, editors: *Animal models of neurological disease.* Kent, Great Britain, 1980, Pitman Medical.
7. Young S: Hypomyelinogenesis congenital (cerebellar ataxia) in Angus shorthorn calves, *Cornell Vet* 52:84-93, 1962.
8. Braund KG: Degenerative and developmental diseases. In Oliver JE, Hoerlein BF, Mayhew IG, editors: *Veterinary neurology.* Philadelphia, 1987, WB Saunders.
9. Jennings A, Summer G: Cortical cerebellar disease in an Ayrshire, *Vet Rec* 63:60, 1951.
10. Howell J, Ritchie H: Cerebellar malformations in two Ayrshire calves, *Pathol Vet* 3:159-168, 1966.
11. Boyd J, McNeil P: Atlanto-occipital fusion and ataxia in the calf, *Vet Rec* 120:34-37, 1987.
12. Mayhew I, Jolly R: Ovine ceroid lipofuscinosis. In Proceedings of the Fourth Annual Veterinary Medical Forum, American College of Veterinary Internal Medicine. Washington, DC, 1986.
13. O'Sullivan BM, et al: Generalised glycogenosis in Brahman cattle, *Aust Vet J* 57:227-229, 1981.
14. Strain GM, et al: Narcolepsy in a Brahman bull, *J Am Vet Med Assoc* 185:538-541, 1984.
15. Aitchison S, et al: Ultrastructural alterations of motor cortex synaptic junctions in Brown Swiss cattle with weaver syndrome, *Am J Vet Res* 46:1733-1736, 1985.
16. Baird JD, Sarmiento UM, Basrur PK: Bovine progressive degenerative myeloencephalopathy ("weaver syndrome") in Brown Swiss cattle in Canada: A literature review and case report, *Can Vet J* 29:370-377, 1988.
17. Stuart LD, Leipold HW: Lesions in bovine progressive degenerative myeloencephalopathy ("weaver") of Brown Swiss cattle, *Vet Pathol* 22:13-23, 1985.
18. Atkeson FW, Ibsen HL, Eldridge E: Inheritance of an epileptic type character in Brown Swiss cattle, *J Hered* 34:45, 1944.
19. Cho DY, Leipold HW: Cerebellar cortical atrophy in a Charolais calf, *Vet Pathol* 15:264-266, 1978.
20. Palmer AC, et al: Progressive ataxia of Charolais cattle associated with a myelin disorder, *Vet Rec* 91:592-594, 1972.
21. Montgomery D, Mayer J: Progressive ataxia of Charolais cattle, *Southwest Vet* 37:247-250, 1986.
22. Cordy D: Progressive ataxia of Charolais cattle: An oligodendroglial dysplasia, *Vet Pathol* 23:78-80, 1986.
23. Zickeer SC, et al: Progressive ataxia in a Charolais bull, *J Am Vet Med Assoc* 192:1590-1592, 1988.
24. Done JT: Developmental disorders on the nervous system in animals, *Adv Vet Sci Comp Med* 21:69-114, 1977.
25. Leipold HW, et al: Spinal dysraphism, arthrogryposis and cleft palate in newborn Charolais calves, *Can Vet J* 10:268-273, 1969.
26. McCoy D, et al: Stabilization of atlantoaxial subluxation secondary to atlantooccipital malformation in a Devon calf, *Cornell Vet* 76:277-286, 1986.
27. Harper PAW, et al: Neurovisceral ceroid-lipofuscinosis in blind Devon cattle, *Acta Neuropathol* 75:632-636, 1988.
28. Embury DH, Jerrett IV: Mannosidosis in Galloway calves, *Vet Pathol* 22:548-551, 1985.
29. Palmer AC, Smith GF, Turner S: Cataplexy in a Guernsey bull, *Vet Rec* 106:421, 1980.

30. de Lahunta A: Comparative cerebellar disease in domestic animals, *Compend Cont Educ Pract Vet* 8:8-19, 1980.

31. O'Sullivan BM, McPhee CP: Cerebellar hypoplasia of genetic origin in calves, *Aust Vet J* 51:469-471, 1975.

32. Strain GM, Olcott BM, Turk MA: Diagnosis of primary generalized epilepsy in a cow, *J Am Vet Med Assoc* 191:833-836, 1987.

33. Greene HJ, Leipold HW, Hibbs CM: Bovine congenital defects: Variations of internal hydrocephalus, *Cornell Vet* 64:596-616, 1974.

34. Leech RW, Haugse CN, Christoferson LA: Congenital hydrocephalus, *Am J Pathol* 92:567-570, 1978.

35. Axthelm MK, Leipold HW, Phillips RM: Congenital internal hydrocephalus in polled Hereford cattle, *Vet Med Small Anim Clin* 76:567-570, 1981.

36. Hulland TJ: Cerebellar ataxia in calves, *Can J Comp Med* 21:72-76, 1957.

37. Rousseaux CG, et al: "Shaker" calf syndrome: A newly recognized inherited neurodegenerative disorder of horned Hereford calves, *Vet Pathol* 22:104-111, 1985.

38. Rousseaux CG, Klavano GG, Johnson ES, et al: A newly recognized neurodegenerative disorder of horned Hereford calves, *Can Vet J* 24:296-297, 1983.

39. Watson AG, et al: Occipito-atlanto-axial malformation with atlanto-axial subluxation in an ataxic calf, *J Am Vet Med Assoc* 187:740-742, 1985.

40. Leipold HW, et al: Congenital defect of the atlantooccipital joint in a Holstein Friesian calf, *Cornell Vet* 62:646-671, 1972.

41. Hiraga T, Abe M: Two calves of Arnold-Chiari malformation and their craniums, *Jpn J Vet Sci* 49:651-656, 1987.

42. White ME, Whitlock RH, de Lahunta A: A cerebellar abiotrophy of calves, *Cornell Vet* 65:476-491, 1975.

43. Umemura T, et al: Histopathology of congenital and perinatal cerebellar anomalies in twelve calves, *Jpn J Vet Sci* 49:95-104, 1987.

44. Baker HJ, et al: Animal models of human ganglioside storage diseases, *FASEB J* 35:1193-1201, 1976.

45. Baker HJ, et al: Feline gangliosidoses as models of human lysosomal storage diseases. In Desnick RJ, Patterson DF, Scarpelli DG, editors: *Animal models of inherited metabolic diseases.* New York, 1982, Alan R. Liss.

46. Baker HJ, et al: The gangliosidoses: Comparative features and research applications, *Vet Pathol* 16:635-649, 1979.

47. Donnelly WJC, Sheahan BJ, Rogers TA: GM1 gangliosidosis in Friesian calves, *J Pathol* 111:173-179, 1973.

48. Henninger RW, Sigler RE: Spinal dysraphism in a calf, *Compend Cont Educ Pract Vet* 5:5488-5491, 1983.

49. Wells G, et al: A novel progressive spongiform encephalopathy in cattle, *Vet Rec* 121:419-420, 1987.

50. Saunders LZ, et al: Hereditary congenital ataxia in Jersey calves, *Cornell Vet* 42:559-591, 1952.

51. Mayhew IG: *Large animal neurology: A handbook for veterinary clinicians.* Philadelphia, 1989, Lea & Febiger.

52. de Lahunta A: Abiotrophy in domestic animals: A review, *Can J Vet Res* 54:65-76, 1990.

53. Richards R, Edwards J: A progressive spinal myelinopathy in beef cattle, *Vet Pathol* 23:35-41, 1986.

54. Edwards JR, Richards RB, Carrick MJ: Inherited progressive spinal myelinopathy in Murray Grey cattle, *Aust Vet J* 65:108-109, 1988.

55. Healy P, Harper P, Dennis J: Diagnosis of neuraxial oedema in calves, *Aust Vet J* 63:95-96, 1986.

56. Duffell S: Neuraxial oedema of Hereford calves with and without hypomyelinogenesis, *Vet Rec* 117:95-98, 1986.

57. Donaldson C, Mason R: Hereditary neuraxial oedema in a Poll Hereford herd, *Aust Vet J* 61:188-189, 1984.

58. Healy PJ, Harper PAW, Bowler JK: Prenatal occurrence and mode of inheritance of neuraxial oedema in Poll Hereford calves, *Res Vet Sci* 38:96-98, 1985.

59. Gundlach AL, et al: Deficit of spinal cord glycine/strychnine receptors in inherited myoclonus of poll Hereford calves, *Science* 241:1807-1810, 1988.

60. Harper P, et al: Maple syrup urine disease in calves: A clinical, pathological and biochemical study, *Aust Vet J* 66:46-49, 1989.

61. Innes JRM, Saunders LA: *Comparative neuropathology.* New York, 1962, Academic Press.

62. Abbitt B, et al: ß-Mannosidosis in twelve Salers calves, *J Am Vet Med Assoc* 198:109-113, 1991.

63. Jolly RD, et al: ß-Mannosidosis in a Salers calf: A new storage disease of cattle, *N Z Vet J* 38:102-105, 1990.

64. Swan R, Taylor E: Cerebellar hypoplasia in beef shorthorn calves, *Aust Vet J* 59:95-96, 1982.

65. O'Sullivan B, McPhee C: Cerebellar hypoplasia of genetic origin in calves, *Aust Vet J* 51:469-471, 1975.

66. Richards RB, et al: Bovine generalized glycogenosis, *Neuropathol Appl Neurobiol* 3:45-56, 1977.

67. McHowell J, et al: Infantile and late onset form of generalized glycogenosis type II in cattle, *J Pathol* 134:266-277, 1981.

68. Greene HJ, et al: Internal hydrocephalus and retinal dysplasia in shorthorn cattle, *Ir Vet* 32:65-69, 1978.

69. Slatter D. *Fundamentals of veterinary ophthalmology.* Philadelphia, 1981, WB Saunders.

70. Chrisman CL: Epilepsy and seizures. In Howard JL, editor: *Current veterinary therapy: Food animal practice.* Philadelphia, 1981, WB Saunders.

71. Russell RG, Oteruelo FT: Ultrastructural abnormalities of muscle and neuromuscular junction differentiation in a bovine congenital neuromuscular disease, *Acta Neuropathol* 62:112-120, 1983.

72. Van den Akker S: Arnold-Chiari malformation in animals, *Acta Neuropathol (Berl)* (suppl. 1):39-44, 1962.

73. Boyd JS: Unusual case of spina bifida in a Friesian cross calf, *Vet Rec* 116:203-205, 1985.

74. Wasserman C: Myelodysplasia in a calf, *Mod Vet Pract* 67:879-883, 1986.

75. Luginbuhl H, Fankhauser R, McGrath JT: Spontaneous neoplasms of the nervous system in animals, *Prog Neurol Surg* 2:85-164, 1968.

76. Averill DR, Bronson RT: Inherited necrotizing myelopathy of Afghan hounds, *J Neuropathol Exp Neurol* 36:734-747, 1977.

77. Baker HJ, et al: Neuronal GM1 gangliosidosis in a Siamese cat with ß-galactosidase deficiency, *Science* 174:838-839, 1971.

78. Cockrell BY, et al: Myelomalacia in Afghan hounds, *J Am Vet Med Assoc* 162:362-365, 1973.

79. Cummings JF, de Lahunta A: Hereditary myelopathy of Afghan hounds: A myelinolytic disease, *Acta Neuropathol* 42:173-181, 1978.

80. Cordy DR, Snelbaker HA: Cerebellar hypoplasia and degeneration in a family of Airedale dogs, *J Neuropathol Exp Neurol* 11:324-328, 1952.

81. Erickson F, Leipold HW, McKinley J: Congenital defects in dogs, Part 2. *Canine Pract* 14:51-61, 1977.

82. Dow RW: Partial agenesis of the cerebellum in dogs, *J Comp Neurol* 72:569-586, 1940.

83. Duncan ID, Griffiths I: Neuromuscular diseases. In Kornegay JN, editor: *Neurologic disorders.* New York, 1986, Churchill Livingstone.

84. de Lahunta A: *Veterinary neuroanatomy and clinical neurology,* 2nd ed. Philadelphia, 1983, WB Saunders.

85. Sisk DB, et al: Clinical and pathologic features of ceroid lipofuscinosis in two Australian cattle dogs, *J Am Vet Med Assoc* 197:361-364, 1990.

86. Hayes HM, et al: Canine congenital deafness: Epidemiologic study of 272 cases, *J Am Anim Hosp Assoc* 17:473, 1981.

87. Igarashi M, et al: Inner ear anomalies in dogs, *Ann Otol Rhinol Laryngol* 81:249-255, 1972.

88. Shores A: Canine cervical vertebral malformation/malarticulation syndrome, *Compend Cont Educ Pract Vet* 6:326-333, 1984.

89. Wright F, Rest JR, Palmer AC: Ataxia of the Great Dane caused by stenosis of the cervical vertebral canal: Comparison with similar conditions in the basset hound, Doberman pinscher, ridgeback and the thoroughbred horse, *Vet Rec* 92:1-6, 1973.

90. Denny H, Gibbs C, Gaskell C: Cervical spondylopathy in the dog: A review of thirty-five cases, *J Small Anim Pract* 10:117-132, 1977.

91. Luttgen PJ, Braund KG, Storts RW: Globoid cell leukodystrophy in a basset hound, *J Small Anim Pract* 24:153-160, 1983.

92. Cusick PK, Cameron AM, Parker AJ: Canine neuronal glycoproteinosis: Lafora's disease in the dog, *J Am Anim Hosp Assoc* 12:518-521, 1976.

93. Pass DA, Howell JM, Thompson RR: Cerebellar malformation in two dogs and a sheep, *Vet Pathol* 18:405-407, 1981.

94. Lane SB: Vestibular disease in companion animals, *Pedigree Forum* 6:11-16, 1987.

95. Chrisman CL: Disorders of the vestibular system, *Compend Cont Educ Pract Vet* 1:744-757, 1979.

96. Hegreberg GA, Padget GA: Inherited progressive epilepsy of the dog with comparisons to Lafora's disease of man, *FASEB J* 35:1202-1205, 1976.

97. Edmonds HL, et al: Spontaneous convulsions in beagle dogs, *FASEB J* 39:2424-2428, 1979.

98. Holliday TA: Epilepsy in animals. In Frey HH, Janz D, editors: *Handbook of experimental pharmacology, vol 74.* Berlin, 1985, Springer-Verlag.

99. Biefelt SW, Redman HC, Broadhurst JJ: Sire and sex-related differences in rates of epileptiform seizures in a purebred beagle dog colony, *Am J Vet Res* 32:2039-2048, 1971.

100. Montgomery DL, Lee AC: Brain damage in the epileptic beagle dog, *Vet Pathol* 20:160-169, 1983.

101. Edmonds HL Jr, et al: Spontaneous convulsions in beagle dogs, *FASEB J* 38:2424-2428, 1979.

102. Redman HC, Wilson GL, Hogan JE: Effect of chlorpromazine combined with intermittent light stimulation on the electroencephalogram and clinical response of the beagle dog, *Am J Vet Res* 34:929-936, 1973.

103. Redman HC, Weir JE: Detection of naturally occurring neurologic disorders of beagle dogs by electroencephalography, *Am J Vet Res* 30:2075-2082, 1969.

104. Redman HC, Hogan JE, Wilson GL: Effect of intermittent light stimulation singly and combined with pentylenetetrazol on the electroencephalogram and clinical response of the beagle dog, *Am J Vet Res* 33:677-685, 1972.

105. Wiederholt WC: Electrophysiologic analysis of epileptic beagles, *Neurology* 24:149-155, 1974.

106. Read DH, et al: Neuronal-visceral GM_1 gangliosidosis in a dog with ß-galactosidase deficiency, *Science* 194:442-445, 1976.

107. Johnson GR, Oliver JE, Selcer R: Globoid cell leukodystrophy in a beagle, *J Am Vet Med Assoc* 167:380-384, 1975.

108. Tomchick T: Familial Lafora's disease in the beagle dog, *FASEB J* 32:8-21, 1973.

109. Barnett KC: Inherited eye disease in the dog and cat, *J Small Anim Pract* 29:462-475, 1988.

110. Voith VL: Diagnosis and treatment of aggressive behavior problems in dogs. In Proceedings of the 47th Annual Meeting of the American Animal Hospital Association, 1980.

111. Palmer A, et al: Recognition of 'trembler,' a hypomyelination condition in the Bernese mountain dog, *Vet Rec* 120:609-612, 1987.

112. Rosin A, Moore P, Dubielzig R: Malignant histiocytosis in Bernese mountain dogs, *J Am Vet Med Assoc* 188:1041-1046, 1986.

113. Cho D, Leipold H, Rudolph R: Neuronal ceroidosis (ceroid-lipofuscinosis) in a blue heeler dog, *Acta Neuropathol* 69:161-164, 1986.

114. Wood PA, et al: Animal model: Ceroidosis (ceroid-lipofuscinosis) in Australian cattle dogs, *Am J Med Genet* 26:891-898, 1987.

115. Boysen BG, Tryphonas L, Harries NW: Globoid cell leukodystrophy in the bluetick hounds dog, 1: Clinical manifestations, *Can Vet J* 15:303-308, 1974.

116. Gill JM, Hewland ML: Cerebellar degeneration in the border collie, *N Z Vet J* 8:170, 1980.

117. Taylor RM, Farrow BRH: Ceroid lipofuscinosis in border collie dogs, *Acta Neuropathol* 75:627-631, 1988.

118. Studdert VP, Mitten RW: Clinical features of ceroid lipofuscinosis in border collies, *Aust Vet J* 68:137-140, 1991.

119. Wheeler SJ: Sensory neuropathy in a border collie puppy, *J Small Anim Pract* 28:281-289, 1987.

120. Jaggy A, et al: Hereditary cervical spondylopathy (wobbler syndrome) in the Borzoi dog, *J Am Anim Hosp Assoc* 24:453-460, 1988.

121. Hayes KC, Schiefer B: Primary tumors in the CNS of carnivores, *Pathol Vet* 6:94-116, 1969.

122. Hayes HM, Priester WA, Pendergrass TW: Occurrence of nervous-tissue tumors in cattle, horses, cats and dogs, *Int J Cancer* 15:39-47, 1975.

123. Bailey CS: An embryological approach to the clinical significance of congenital vertebral and spinal cord abnormalities, *J Am Anim Hosp Assoc* 11:426-434, 1975.

124. Morgan JP: Congenital anomalies of the vertebral column of the dog: A study of the incidence and significance based on a radiographic and morphometric study, *J Am Vet Radiol Soc* 9:21-29, 1968.

125. de Lahunta A, Cummings JF: The clinical and electroencephalographic features of hydrocephalus in three dogs, *J Am Vet Med Assoc* 146:954-964, 1965.

126. Selby L, Hayes H, Becker S: Epizootiologic features of canine hydrocephalus, *Am J Vet Res* 40:411-413, 1979.

127. Venker-van Haagen AJ, Bouw J, Hartman W: Hereditary transmission of laryngeal paralysis in young Bouviers, *J Am Anim Hosp Assoc* 17:75-76, 1981.

128. Venker-van Haagen AJ, Hartman W, Goedegebuure SA: Spontaneous laryngeal paralysis in young Bouviers, *J Am Anim Hosp Assoc* 14:714-720, 1978.

129. Griffiths I: Progressive axonopathy of boxer dogs. In Proceedings of the Fifth Annual Veterinary Medical Forum, American College of Veterinary Internal Medicine. San Diego, 1987.

130. Griffiths IR, Duncan ID, Barker J: A progressive axonopathy of boxer dogs affecting the central and peripheral nervous system, *J Small Anim Pract* 21:29-43, 1980.

131. LeCouteur RA, Kornegay JN, Higgins RJ: Late onset progressive cerebellar degeneration of Brittany spaniel dogs. In Proceedings of the Sixth Annual Veterinary

Medical Forum, American College of Veterinary Internal Medicine. Washington, DC, 1988.

132. Cork LC, et al: Hereditary canine spinal muscular atrophy, *J Neuropathol Exp Neurol* 38:209-221, 1979.

133. Lorenz MD, et al: Hereditary muscular atrophy in Brittany spaniels: Clinical manifestations, *J Am Vet Med Assoc* 175:833-839, 1986.

134. Carmichael S, Griffiths IR, Harvey MJA: Familial cerebellar ataxia with hydrocephalus in bull mastiffs, *Vet Rec* 112:354-358, 1983.

135. Raffe M, Knecht C: Cervical vertebral malformation in bull mastiffs, *J Am Anim Hosp Assoc* 14:593-594, 1978.

136. Kornegay J: Cerebellar vermian hypoplasia in dogs, *Vet Pathol* 23:374-379, 1986.

137. Hudson W, Ruben R: Hereditary deafness in the Dalmatian dog, *Arch Otolaryngol Head Neck Surg* 75:213-219, 1962.

138. Anderson H, Henricson B, Lundquist P, et al: Genetic hearing impairment in the Dalmatian dog, *Acta Otolaryngol Suppl (Stockh)* 232:1-34, 1968.

139. Brown S, et al: Naloxone-responsive compulsive tail chasing in a dog, *J Am Vet Med Assoc* 190:884-886, 1987.

140. Kurtz HJ, Fletcher TF: The peripheral neuropathy of canine globoid-cell leukodystrophy (Krabbe type), *Acta Neuropathol* 16:226-232, 1970.

141. Howell JM: Globoid cell leucodystrophy in two dogs, *J Small Anim Pract* 12:633-642, 1971.

142. Fletcher TF, Kurtz HJ, Low DG: Globoid cell leukodystrophy (Krabbe type) in the dog, *J Am Vet Med Assoc* 149:165-172, 1966.

143. McGrath JT, et al: A morphologic and biochemical study of canine globoid cell leukodystrophy, *J Neuropathol Exp Neurol* 28:171, 1969.

144. Suzuki Y, et al: Studies in globoid leukodystrophy: Enzymatic and lipid findings in the canine form, *Exp Neurol* 29:65-75, 1970.

145. Palmer AC, Blakemore WF: Progressive neuronopathy in the cairn terrier, *Vet Rec* 123:39, 1988.

146. Cummings JF, de Lahunta A, Moore JJ: Multisystemic chromatolytic neuronal degeneration in a cairn terrier pup, *Cornell Vet* 78:301-314, 1988.

147. Wright J, et al: Muscle hypertonicity in the Cavalier King Charles spaniel: Myopathic features, *Vet Rec* 118:511-512, 1986.

148. Jones BR, Johnstone AC: An unusual myopathy in a dog, *N Z Vet J* 30:119-121, 1982.

149. Herrtage ME, Palmer AC: Episodic falling in the Cavalier King Charles spaniel, *Vet Rec* 112:458-459, 1983.

150. Few AB: The diagnosis and surgical treatment of canine hydrocephalus, *J Am Vet Med Assoc* 149:286-293, 1966.

151. Blakemore W, Palmer A: Nervous disease in the chihuahua characterised by axonal swellings, *Vet Rec* 117:498-499, 1985.

152. Hansen HJ: A pathologic-anatomical study on disk degeneration in the dog, *Acta Orthop Scand Suppl* 11, 1952.

153. Ghosh P, et al: A comparative chemical and histochemical study of the chondrodystrophoid and nonchondrodystrophoid canine intervertebral disc, *Vet Pathol* 13:414-427, 1976.

154. Priester W: Canine intervertebral disc disease: Occurrence by age, breed, and sex among 8,117 cases, *Theriogenology* 6:293-303, 1976.

155. Brown N, Helphrey M, Prata R: Thoracolumbar disk disease in the dog: A retrospective analysis of 187 cases, *J Am Anim Hosp Assoc* 13:665-672, 1977.

156. Hoerlein B: Comparative disk disease: Man and dog, *J Am Anim Hosp Assoc* 15:535-545, 1979.

157. Hoerlein B: Intervertebral disc protrusions in the dog, I: Incidence and pathological lesions, *Am J Vet Res* 51:260-283, 1953.

158. Braund KG: Intervertebral disk disease. In Kornegay JN, editor: *Neurologic disorders.* New York, 1986, Churchill Livingstone.

159. Knecht CD, et al: Cerebellar hypoplasia in chow chows, *J Am Anim Hosp Assoc* 15:51, 1979.

160. Knecht C, et al: Cerebellar hypoplasia in chow chows, *J Am Anim Hosp Assoc* 15:51-53, 1979.

161. Vandevelde M, et al: Dysmyelination of the central nervous system in the chow chow dog, *Acta Neuropathol* 42:211-215, 1978.

162. Duncan I: Congenital tremor and abnormalities of myelination. In Proceedings of the Fifth Annual Veterinary Medical Forum, American College of Veterinary Internal Medicine. San Diego, 1987.

163. Vandevelde M, et al: Dysmyelination in chow chow dogs: Further studies in older dogs, *Acta Neuropathol (Berl)* 55:81-87, 1981.

164. Duncan I: Abnormalities of myelination of the central nervous system associated with congenital tremor, *J Vet Intern Med* 1:10-23, 1987.

165. Shores A, et al: Myotonia congenita in a chow chow pup, *J Am Vet Med Assoc* 188:532-533, 1986.

166. Braund KG: Identifying degenerative and developmental myopathies, *Vet Med* 81:713-718, 1986.

167. Shelton G, Cardinet H: Pathophysiologic basis of canine muscle disorders, *J Vet Intern Med* 1:36-44, 1987.

168. Farrow BRH: Canine myotonia. In Proceedings of the Sixth Annual Veterinary Medical Forum, American College of Veterinary Internal Medicine. Washington, DC, 1988.

169. Nafe LA, Shires P: Myotonia in the dog. In Proceedings of the Second Annual Veterinary Medical Forum, American College of Veterinary Internal Medicine, 1984.

170. Jones BR, et al: Myotonia in related chow chow dogs, *N Z Vet J* 25:217-220, 1977.

171. Farrow BRH, Malik R: Hereditary myotonia in the chow chow, *J Small Anim Pract* 22:451-465, 1981.

172. Mugford RA: Aggressive behavior in the English cocker spaniel, *Vet Ann* 24:310-314, 1984.

173. Nimmo Wilkie JS, Hudson EB: Neuronal and generalized ceroid-lipofuscinosis in a cocker spaniel, *Vet Pathol* 19:623-628, 1982.

174. Clifford DH, Malek R: Diseases of the canine esophagus due to prenatal influence, *Am J Dig Dis* 14:578-602, 1969.

175. Clifford DH: Esophageal achalasia, *Comp Pathol Bull* 10:2-3, 1978.

176. Kern TJ, Erb HN: Facial neuropathy in dogs and cats: 95 cases (1975-1985), *J Am Vet Med Assoc* 191:1604-1609, 1987.

177. Braund KG, et al: Idiopathic facial paralysis in the dog, *Vet Rec* 105:297-299, 1979.

178. Jaggy A, Vandevelde M: Multisystem neuronal degeneration in cocker spaniels, *J Vet Intern Med* 2:117-120, 1988.

179. Hartley WJ, et al: Inherited cerebellar degeneration in the rough coated collie, *Aust Vet Pract* 8:79-85, 1978.

180. Clark RG, et al: Suspected neuroaxonal dystrophy in collie sheep dogs, *N Z Vet J* 30:102-103, 1982.

181. Lurie M: The membranous labyrinth in the congenitally deaf collie and dalmatian dog, *Laryngoscope* 58:279-287, 1948.

182. Hargis AM, Haupt KH, Hegreberg GA, et al: Familial canine dermatomyositis, *Am J Pathol* 116:234-244, 1984.

183. Haupt KH, et al: Familial canine dermatomyositis: Clinical, electrodiagnostic, and genetic studies, *Am J Vet Res* 46:1861-1869, 1985.

184. Hargis A, et al: Postmortem findings in four litters of dogs with familial canine dermatomyositis, *Am J Pathol* 123:480-496, 1986.

185. Hargis A, et al: Prospective study of familial canine dermatomyositis, *Am J Pathol* 123:465-479, 1986.

186. Hargis AM, et al: Dermatomyositis: Familial canine dermatomyositis, *Am J Pathol* 120:323-325, 1985.

187. Kunkle GA, et al: Dermatomyositis in collie dogs, *Compend Cont Educ Pract Vet* 7:185-192, 1985.

188. Wilson JW, et al: Spina bifida in the dog, *Vet Pathol* 16:165-179, 1979.

189. de Lahunta A, Shively GN: Neurofibrillary accumulation in a puppy, *Cornell Vet* 65:240-247, 1975.

190. Cummings JF, de Lahunta A: An adult case of canine neuronal ceroid-lipofuscinosis, *Acta Neuropathol* 39:43-51, 1977.

191. Holliday TA, Cunningham JG, Gutnick MJ: Comparative clinical and electroencephalographic studies of canine epilepsy, *Epilepsia* 11:281-292, 1971.

192. Vandevelde M, Fatzer R: Neuronal ceroid-lipofuscinosis in older dachshunds, *Vet Pathol* 17:686-692, 1980.

193. Duncan ID, Griffiths IR, Munz M: The pathology of a sensory neuropathy affecting long haired dachshund dogs, *Acta Neruopathol* 58:141-151, 1982.

194. Braund KG: Identifying degenerative peripheral neuropathies in pets, *Vet Med* 88:352-380, 1987.

195. Johnsson L, et al: Vascular anatomy and pathology of the cochlea in Dalmatian dogs. In Darin de Lorenzo AJ, editor: *Vascular disorders and hearing defects.* University Park, MD, 1973, University Park Press.

196. Suga F, Hattler K: Physiological and histopathological correlates of hereditary deafness in animals, *Laryngoscope* 80:80-104, 1970.

197. Marshall A: Use of brain stem auditory-evoked response to evaluate deafness in a group of Dalmatian dogs, *J Am Vet Med Assoc* 188:718-722, 1986.

198. Ferrara ML, Halnan CRE: Congenital brain defects in the deaf Dalmatian, *Vet Rec* 112:344-346, 1983.

199. Mair IWS: Hereditary deafness in the Dalmatian dog, *Arch Otol* 212:1-14, 1976.

200. Branis M, Burda H: Inner ear structure in the deaf and normally hearing Dalmatian dog, *J Comp Pathol* 95:295-299, 1985.

201. Woods CB: Hyperkinetic episodes in two Dalmatians, *J Am Anim Hosp Assoc* 13:255-257, 1977.

202. Greene CE, Vandevelde M, Hoff EJ: Congenital cerebrospinal hypomyelinogenesis in a pup, *J Am Vet Med Assoc* 171:534-536, 1977.

203. Bjerkas I: Hereditary "cavitating" leukodystrophy in Dalmatian dogs, *Acta Neuropathol* 40:163-169, 1977.

204. Neufeld JL, Little PB: Spinal dysraphism in a Dalmatian dog, *Can Vet J* 15:335-336, 1974.

205. Houpt KA: Aggression in dogs, *Compend Cont Educ Pract Vet* 1:123-128, 1979.

206. Seim H: Ventral decompression and stabilization for the treatment of caudal cervical spondylomyelopathy in the dog. In Proceedings of the Fifth Annual Veterinary Medical Forum, American College of Veterinary Internal Medicine. San Diego, 1987.

207. Lyman R: Continuous dorsal laminectomy for treatment of Doberman pinschers with caudal cervical vertebral instability and malformation. In Proceedings of the Fifth Annual Veterinary Medical Forum, American College of Veterinary Internal Medicine. San Diego, 1987.

208. Seim H, Withrow S: Pathophysiology and diagnosis of caudal cervical spondylo-myelopathy with emphasis on the Doberman pinscher, *J Am Anim Hosp Assoc* 18:241-251, 1982.

209. Read R, Robins G, Carlisle C: Caudal cervical spondylo-myelopathy (wobbler syndrome) in the dog: A review of thirty cases, *J Small Anim Pract* 24:605-621, 1983.

210. Trotter E, et al: Caudal cervical vertebral malformation-malarticulation in Great Danes and Doberman pinschers, *J Am Vet Med Assoc* 168:917-930, 1976.

211. Mason T: Cervical vertebral instability (wobbler syndrome) in the dog, *Vet Rec* 104:142-145, 1979.

212. Raffe M, Knecht C: Cervical vertebral malformation: A review of 36 cases, *J Am Anim Hosp Assoc* 16:881-883, 1980.

213. Wilkes M, Palmer A: Congenital deafness in Dobermans, *Vet Rec* 118:218, 1986.

214. Chrisman CL: Distal polyneuropathy of Doberman pinschers. In Proceedings of the Third Annual Veterinary Medical Forum, American College of Veterinary Internal Medicine. San Diego, 1985.

215. Leyland A: Ataxia in a Doberman pinscher, *Vet Rec* 116:414-415, 1985.

216. Baker TL, et al: Diagnosis and treatment of narcolepsy in animals. In Kirk RW, editor: *Current veterinary therapy VIII. Small animal practice.* Philadelphia, 1983, WB Saunders.

217. Bowersox S, et al: Brain dopamine receptor levels elevated in canine narcolepsy, *Brain Res* 402:44-48, 1987.

218. Kaitin KI, Kilduff TS, Dement WC: Evidence for excessive sleepiness in canine narcoleptics, *Electroencephalogr Clin Neurophysiol* 65:447-454, 1986.

219. Foutz AS, Mitler MM, Dement WC: Narcolepsy, *Vet Clin North Am* 10:65-80, 1980.

220. Bakr TL, et al: Canine model of narcolepsy: Genetic and developmental determinants, *Exp Neurol* 75:729-742, 1982.

221. Wouda W, et al: Sensory neuronopathy in dogs: A study of four cases, *J Comp Pathol* 93:437-450, 1983.

222. Patnaik A, Kay W, Hurvitz A: Intracranial meningioma: A comparative pathologic study of 28 dogs, *Vet Pathol* 23:369-373, 1986.

223. Parker AJ, et al: Spina bifida with protrusion of spinal cord tissue in a dog, *J Am Vet Med Assoc* 163:158-160, 1973.

224. Parker AJ, Byerly CS: Meningomyelocoele in a dog, *Vet Pathol* 10:266-273, 1973.

225. Kornegay JN: Congenital and degenerative diseases of the central nervous system. In Kornegay JN, editor: *Neurologic disorders.* New York, 1986, Churchill Livingstone.

226. Knecht C, Blevins W, Raffe M: Stenosis of the thoracic spinal canal in English bulldogs, *J Am Anim Hosp Assoc* 15:182-183, 1979.

227. Klein E, et al: Adenosine receptor alterations in nervous pointer dogs: A preliminary report. *Clin Neuropharmacol* 10:462-469, 1987.

228. Murphree OD, Dykman RA: Litter patterns in the offspring of nervous and stable dogs. I: Behavioral tests, *J Nerv Ment Dis* 141:321-332, 1965.

229. Dykman RA, Murphree OD, Ackerman PT: Litter patterns in the offspring of nervous and stable dogs. II: Autonomic and motor conditioning, *J Nerv Ment Dis* 141:419-431, 1966.

230. Cummings JF, et al: Reduced substance P-like immunoreactivity in hereditary sensory neuropathy of pointer dogs, *Acta Neuropathol (Berl)* 63:33-40, 1984.

231. Cummings JF, et al: Animal model of human disease: Hereditary sensory neuropathy: Nociceptive loss and acral mutilation in pointer dogs: Canine hereditary sensory neuropathy, *Am J Pathol* 112:136-138, 1983.

232. Cummings JF, de Lahunta A, Winn SS: Acral mutilation and nociceptive loss in English pointer dogs, *Acta Neuropathol* 53:119-127, 1981.

233. Koppang N: Canine ceroid-lipofuscinosis in English setters, *J Small Anim Pract* 10:639-644, 1970.

234. Watson B, Watson G: Electroretinograms in English setters with neuronal ceroid lipofuscinosis, *Invest Ophthalmol Vis Sci* 19:87-90, 1980.

235. Armstrong D, Koppang N, Jolly R: Ceroid-lipofuscinosis. *Comp Pathol Bull* 12:2-4, 1980.

236. Armstrong D, Koppang N, Nilsson S: Canine hereditary ceroid lipofuscinosis, *Eur Neurol* 21:147-156, 1982.

237. Jasty V, et al: An unusual case of generalized ceroid-lipotuscinosis in a cynomolgus monkey, *Vet Pathol* 21:46-50, 1984.

238. Sims MH, Shull-Selcer E: Electrodiagnostic evaluation of deafness in two English setter littermates, *J Am Vet Med Assoc* 187:398-404, 1985.

239. Alroy J, et al: Neurovisceral and skeletal Gm$_1$ gangliosidosis in dogs with ß-galactosidase deficiency, *Science* 229:470-472, 1985.

240. Giger U, Argov Z: Metabolic myopathy in phosphofructokinase deficient English springer spaniels. In Proceedings of the Fifth Annual Veterinary Medical Forum, American College of Veterinary Internal Medicine. San Diego, 1987.

241. Giger U, Roudebush P: Inherited phosphofructokinase deficiency in English springer spaniels causes hemolytic disorder with hemolytic crises. In Proceedings of the Fifth Annual Veterinary Medical Forum, American College of Veterinary Internal Medicine. San Diego, 1987.

242. Holland CT, et al: Dyserythropoiesis, polymyopathy, and cardiac disease in three related English springer spaniels, *J Vet Intern Med* 5:151-159, 1991.

243. Tontitila P, Lindberg LA: ETT Fall av cerebellar ataxi hos finsk stovare, *Svoman Elainlaakarilehti* 77:135, 1971.

244. Adams EW: Hereditary deafness in a family of foxhounds, *J Am Vet Med Assoc* 128:302-303, 1956.

245. Jenkins WL, Van Dyk E, McDonald CB: Myasthenia gravis in a fox terrier litter, *J S Afr Vet Assoc* 47:59-62, 1976.

246. Miller LM, et al: Congenital myasthenia gravis in 13 smooth fox terriers, *J Am Vet Med Assoc* 182:694-697, 1983.

247. Lee M: Congenital vestibular disease in a German shepherd dog, *Vet Rec* 113:571, 1983.

248. Braund KG, Vandevelde M: German shepherd dog myelopathy: A morphologic and morphometric study, *Am J Vet Res* 39:1309-1315, 1978.

249. Williams DA, Sharp NJH, Batt RM: Enteropathy associated with degenerative myelopathy in German shepherd dogs. In Scientific Proceedings of the American College of Veterinary Internal Medicine, 1983.

250. Waxman FJ, et al: Progressive myelopathy in older German shepherd dogs, I: Depressed response to thymus-dependent mitogens, *J Immunol* 124:1209-1215, 1980.

251. Waxman FJ, Clemmons RM, Hinrichs DJ: Progressive myelopathy in older German shepherd dogs, II: Presence of circulating suppressor cells, *J Immunol* 124:1216-1222, 1980.

252. Averill DR: Degenerative myelopathy in the aging German shepherd dog, *J Am Vet Med Assoc* 162:1045-1051, 1973.

253. Griffiths IR, Duncan ID: Chronic degenerative radiculomyelopathy in the dog, *J Small Anim Pract* 16:461-471, 1975.

254. Braund KG: Hip dysplasia and degenerative myelopathy: Making the distinction in dogs, *Vet Med* 82:82-89, 1987.

255. Clemmons RM: Degenerative myelopathy. In Kirk RW, editor: *Current veterinary therapy X. Small animal practice.* Philadelphia, 1989, WB Saunders.

256. Williams DA, Prymak C, Baughan J: Tocopherol (vitamin E) status in canine degenerative myelopathy. In Proceedings of the Third Annual Veterinary Medical Forum, American College of Veterinary Internal Medicine. San Diego, 1985.

257. Amanai H: Leukomyelodegeneration in two aged German shepherd littermates: Patho-morphological observations, *Jpn J Vet Res* 35:121, 1987.

258. Clifford DH, Pirsch JG: Myenteric ganglial cells in dogs with and without hereditary achalasia of the esophagus, *Am J Vet Res* 32:615-619, 1971.

259. Boudrieau RJ, Rogers WA: Megaesophagus in the dog: A review of 50 cases, *J Am Anim Hosp Assoc* 21:33-40, 1985.

260. Clifford DH, Gyorkey F: Myenteric ganglial cells in dogs with and without achalasia of the esophagus, *J Am Vet Med Assoc* 150:205-211, 1967.

261. Duncan ID, Griffiths IR: Canine giant axonal neuropathy, *Vet Rec* 101:438-441, 1977.

262. Duncan ID, Griffiths IR: Peripheral nervous system in a case of canine giant axonal neuropathy, *Neuropathol Appl Neurobiol* 5:25-39, 1979.

263. Duncan ID, Griffiths IR: Canine giant axonal neuropathy: Some aspects of its clinical, pathological and comparative features, *J Small Anim Pract* 22:491-501, 1981.

264. Griffiths IR, et al: Further studies of the central nervous system in canine giant axonal neuropathy, *Neuropathol Appl Neurobiol* 6:421-432, 1980.

265. Julien JP, et al: Giant axonal neuropathy: Neurofilaments isolated from diseased dogs have a normal polypeptide composition, *Exp Neurol* 72:619-627, 1981.

266. Jaggy A, Lang J, Schawalder P: Cauda equina syndrom beim Hund, *Schweiz Arch Tierheilkd* 129:171-192, 1987.

267. Oliver J, Selcer R, Simpson S: Cauda equina compression from lumbosacral malarticulation and malformation in the dog, *J Am Vet Med Assoc* 173:207-214, 1978.

268. Lenehan T: Canine cauda equina syndrome, *Compend Cont Educ Pract Vet* 5:941-951, 1983.

269. Clayton HM, Boyd JS: Spina bifida in a German shepherd puppy, *Vet Rec* 112:13-15, 1983.

270. Falco MJ, Barker J, Wallace ME: The genetics of epilepsy in the British Alsatian, *J Small Anim Pract* 15:685-692, 1974.

271. Karbe E: Animal model of human disease: GM$_2$ gangliosidosis (amaurotic idiocies) types I, II, and III. Animal model: Canine GM$_2$ gangliosidosis, *Am J Pathol* 71:151-154, 1973.

272. Kramer JW, et al: Characterization of heritable thoracic hemivertebra of the German shorthaired pointer, *J Am Vet Med Assoc* 181:814-815, 1982.

273. Kornegay JN: Golden retriever myopathy. In Proceedings of the Second Annual Veterinary Medical Forum, American College of Veterinary Internal Medicine. Washington, DC, 1984.

274. Kornegay JN: Golden retriever myopathy. In Kirk RW, editor: *Current veterinary therapy IX: Small animal practice.* Philadelphia, 1986, WB Saunders.

275. Kornegay JN: Golden retriever muscular dystrophy. In Proceedings of the Sixth Annual Veterinary Medical Forum, American College of Veterinary Medicine. Washington, DC, 1988.

276. Valentine B, et al: Progressive muscular dystrophy in a golden retriever dog: Light microscope and ultrastructural features at 4 and 8 months, *Acta Neuropathol* 71:301-310, 1986.

277. Steiss JE, et al: Sensory neuropathy in a dog. *J Am Vet Med Assoc* 190:205-208, 1987.

278. Cork LC, Troncoso JC, Price DL: Canine inherited ataxia, *Ann Neurol* 9:492-499, 1981.

279. de Lahunta A, et al: Hereditary cerebellar cortical abiotrophy in the Gordon setter, *J Am Vet Med Assoc* 177:538-541, 1980.

280. Steinberg S, et al: Clinical features of inherited cerebellar degeneration in Gordon setters, *J Am Vet Med Assoc* 179:886-890, 1981.

281. Troncoso JC, Cork LC, Price DL: Canine inherited ataxia: Ultrastructural observations, *J Neuropathol Exp Neurol* 44:165-175, 1985.

282. Hedhammer A, et al: Overnutrition and skeletal disease: An experimental study in growing great Dane dogs, *Cornell Vet* (Suppl 5) 64:1-60, 1974.

283. Olsson S, Stavenhorn M, Hoppe F: Dynamic compression of the cervical spinal cord: A myelographic and pathologic investigation in Great Dane dogs, *Acta Vet Scand* 23:65-78, 1982.

284. Wright F, Rest J, Palmer A: Ataxia of the Great Dane caused by stenosis of the cervical vertebral canal: Comparison with similar conditions in the basset hound, Doberman pinscher, ridgeback and the thoroughbred horse, *Vet Rec* 92:1-6, 1973.

285. Strombeck DR, Troya L: Evaluation of lower motor neuron function in two dogs with megaesophagus, *J Am Vet Med Assoc* 169:411-414, 1976.

286. Strombeck DR: Pathophysiology of esophageal motility disorders in the dog and cat, *Vet Clin North Am* 8:229-244, 1978.

287. Stockard C: An hereditary lethal factor for localized motor and preganglionic neurons, *Am J Anat* 59:1-53, 1936.

288. Cunningham JG, Farnbach GC: Inheritance and idiopathic canine epilepsy, *J Am Anim Hosp Assoc* 24:421-424, 1988.

289. Wentink GH, et al: Myopathy with a possible recessive X-linked inheritance in a litter of Irish terriers, *Vet Pathol* 9:328-349, 1972.

290. Palmer AC, Goodyear JV: Congenital myasthenia in the Jack Russell terrier, *Vet Rec* 103:433-434, 1978.

291. Wilkes MK, et al: Ultrastructure of motor endplates in canine congenital myasthenia gravis, *J Comp Pathol* 97:247-256, 1987.

292. Hartley WJ, Palmer AC: Ataxia in Jack Russell terriers, *Acta Neuropathol (Berl)* 26:71-74, 1973.

293. Umemura T, et al: Generalized lipofuscinosis in a dog, *Jpn J Vet Sci* 47:673-677, 1985.

294. Cummings JF, et al: GM$_2$ gangliosidosis in a Japanese spaniel, *Acta Neuropathol (Berl)* 67:247-253, 1985.

295. Wallace ME: Keeshonds: A genetic study of epilepsy and EEG readings, *J Small Anim Pract* 16:1-10, 1975.

296. de Lahunta A, Averill DR: Hereditary cerebellar cortical and extrapyramidal nuclear abiotrophy in Kerry blue terriers, *J Am Vet Med Assoc* 168:1119-1124, 1976.

297. Montgomery D, Storts R: Hereditary striatonigral and cerebello-olivary degeneration of the Kerry blue terrier, *Vet Pathol* 20:143-159, 1983.

298. Montgomery D, Storts R: Hereditary striatonigral and cerebello-olivary degeneration of the Kerry blue terrier II: Ultrastructural lesions in the caudate nucleus and cerebellar cortex, *J Neuropathol Exp Neurol* 43:263-275, 1984.

299. Perille AL, et al: Postnatal cerebellar cortical degeneration in Labrador retriever puppies, *Can Vet J* 32:619-621, 1991.

300. Atkinson JB, LeQuire VS: Myotonia congenita, *Comp Pathol Bull* 17:3-4, 1985.

301. McKerrell RE, Braund KG: In Kirk RW, editor: *Current veterinary therapy X. Small animal practice.* Philadelphia, 1989, WB Saunders.

302. Moore M, et al: Electromyographic evaluation of adult Labrador retrievers with type II muscle fiber deficiency, *Am J Vet Res* 48:1332-1336, 1987.

303. Braund KG: Labrador retriever myopathy. In Proceedings of the Sixth Annual Veterinary Medical Forum, American College of Veterinary Internal Medicine. Washington, DC, 1988.

304. McKerrell R, Braund K: Hereditary myopathy in Labrador retrievers: Clinical variations, *J Small Anim Pract* 28:479-489, 1987.

305. McKerrell R, Braund K: Hereditary myopathy in Labrador retrievers: A morphologic study, *Vet Pathol* 23:411-417, 1986.

306. Amann JF, Laughlin MH, Korthuis RJ: Muscle hemodynamics in hereditary myopathy of Labrador retrievers, *Am J Vet Res* 49:1127-1130, 1988.

307. Shores A, Redding R: Narcoleptic hypersomnia syndrome responsive to protriptyline in a Labrador retriever, *J Am Anim Hosp Assoc* 23:455-458, 1987.

308. Katherman AE: A comparative review of canine and human narcolepsy, *Compend Cont Educ Pract Vet* 2:818-822, 1980.

309. Fox JG, et al: Familial reflex myoclonus in Labrador retrievers, *Am J Vet Res* 45:2367-2370, 1984.

310. O'Brien DP, Zachary JF: Clinical features of spongy degeneration of the central nervous system in two Labrador retriever littermates, *J Am Vet Med Assoc* 186:1207-1210, 1985.

311. Zachary JF, O'Brien DP: Spongy degeneration of the central nervous system in two canine littermates, *Vet Pathol* 22:561-571, 1985.

312. Walvoort HC, et al: Canine glycogen storage disease type II: A clinical study of four affected Lapland dogs, *J Am Anim Hosp Assoc* 20:279-286, 1984.

313. Mostafa IE: A case of glycogenic cardiomegaly in a dog, *Acta Vet Scand* 11:197-208, 1970.

314. Sandefeldt E, et al: Hereditary neuronal abiotrophy in the Swedish Lapland dog, *Cornell Vet* 63:1-71, 1973.

315. Sandefeldt E, et al: Hereditary neuronal abiotrophy in Swedish Lapland dogs, *Am J Pathol* 82:649-652, 1976.

316. Schmahl W, Kaiser E: Hydrocephalus, syringomyelia, and spinal cord angiodysgenesis in a Lhasa Apso dog, *Vet Pathol* 21:252-254, 1984.

317. Sahar A, et al: Spontaneous canine hydrocephalus: Cerebrospinal fluid dynamics, *J Neurol Neurosurg Psychiatry* 34:308-315, 1971.

318. Greene CE, Vandevelde M, Braund K: Lissencephaly in two Lhasa Apso dogs, *J Am Vet Med Assoc* 169:405-410, 1976.

319. Zaki FA: Lissencephaly in Lhasa Apso dogs, *J Am Vet Med Assoc* 169:1165-1168, 1976.

320. Mayhew IG, et al: Tremor syndromes and hypomyelination in Lurcher pups, *J Small Anim Pract* 25:551-559, 1984.

321. Simpson ST: Hydrocephalus in the Maltese dog: Electroencephalographic and C.T. correlations. In Proceedings of the Fourth Annual Veterinary Medical Forum, American College of Veterinary Internal Medicine. Washington, DC, 1986.

322. Simpson ST, et al: Hydrocephalus. In Proceedings of the Fifth Annual Veterinary Medical Forum, American

College of Veterinary Internal Medicine. San Diego, 1987.

323. Cox VS, et al: Hereditary esophageal dysfunction in the miniature schnauzer dog, *Am J Vet Res* 41:326-330, 1980.

324. Clifford DH, et al: Management of esophageal achalasia in miniature schnauzers, *J Am Vet Med Assoc* 161:1012-1020, 1972.

325. Rotmistrovsky RA, et al: GM_2 gangliosidosis in a mixed-breed dog, *Prog Vet Neurol* 2:203-208, 1991.

326. Shull RM, et al: Morphologic and biochemical studies of canine mucopolysaccharidosis I, *Am J Pathol* 114:487-495, 1984.

327. Schwartz A, et al: Congenital neuromuscular esophageal disease in a litter of Newfoundland puppies, *J Am Vet Radiol Soc* 17:101-105, 1976.

328. Coulter DB: A dog with a partial merle coat, white iris, and bilaterally impaired hearing, *Calif Vet* 12:9-11, 1982.

329. Shull RM, et al: Animal model of human disease: Canine alpha-iduronidase deficiencyA model of mucopolysaccharidosis I, *Am J Pathol* 109:244-248, 1982.

330. Inada S, et al: Canine storage disease characterized by hereditary progressive neurogenic muscular atrophy: Breeding experiments and clinical manifestation, *Am J Vet Res* 47:2294-2299, 1986.

331. Inada S, et al: A clinical study on hereditary progressive neurogenic muscular atrophy in pointer dogs, *Jpn J Vet Sci* 40:539-547, 1978.

332. Izumo S, et al: Morphological study on the hereditary neurogenic amyotrophic dogs: Accumulation of lipid compound-like structures in the lower motor neuron, *Acta Neuropathol* 61:270-276, 1983.

333. Selcer ES, Selcer RR: Globoid cell leukodystrophy in two West Highland white terriers and one pomeranian, *Compend Cont Educ Pract Vet* 6:621-624, 1984.

334. Oliver JE, Geary JC: Cerebellar anomalies: Two cases, *Vet Med Small Anim Clin* 60:697, 1965.

335. Kay WJ, Budzilovich GN: Cerebellar hypoplasia and agenesis in the dog, *J Neuropathol Exp Neurol* 29:156, 1970.

336. Matthews NS, de Lahunta A: Degenerative myelopathy in an adult miniature poodle, *J Am Vet Med Assoc* 186:1213-1214, 1985.

337. Zaki F, Kay WJ: Globoid cell leukodystrophy in a miniature poodle, *J Am Vet Med Assoc* 163:248-250, 1973.

338. Bundza A, Lowden JA, Charlton KM: Niemann-Pick disease in a poodle dog, *Vet Pathol* 16:530-538, 1979.

339. Shell LG, et al: Neuronal visceral GM_1 gangliosidosis in Portuguese water dogs. In Proceedings of the Sixth Annual Veterinary Medical Forum, American College of Veterinary Internal Medicine. Washington, DC, 1988.

340. Wright JA, Brownlie S: Progressive ataxia in a Pyrenean mountain dog, *Vet Rec* 116:410-411, 1985.

341. Gamble DA, Chrisman CL: A leukoencephalomyelopathy of Rottweiler dogs, *Vet Pathol* 21:274-280, 1984.

342. Chrisman C: Neuroaxonal dystrophy and leukoencephalomyelopathy of Rottweiler dogs. In Kirk RW, editor: *Current veterinary therapy IX. Small animal practice.* Philadelphia, 1986, WB Saunders.

343. Chrisman CL, Cork LC, Gamble DA: Neuroaxonal dystrophy of Rottweiler dogs, *J Am Vet Med Assoc* 184:464-467, 1984.

344. Cork LC, et al: Canine neuronaxonal dystrophy, *J Neuropathol Exp Neurol* 42:286-296, 1983.

345. Evans MG, Mullaney TP, Lowrie CT: Neuroaxonal dystrophy in a Rottweiler pup, *J Am Vet Med Assoc* 192:1560-1562, 1988.

346. Shell L, Jortner B, Leib M: Familial motor neuron disease in Rottweiler dogs: Neuropathologic studies, *Vet Pathol* 24:135-139, 1987.

347. Shell L, Jortner B, Leib M: Spinal muscular atrophy in two Rottweiler littermates, *J Am Vet Med Assoc* 190:878-880, 1987.

348. Shell LG: Spinal muscular atrophy in Rottweiler pups. In Proceedings of the Sixth Annual Veterinary Medical Forum, American College of Veterinary Internal Medicine. Washington, DC, 1988.

349. Shell LG, et al: Spinal dysraphism, hemivertebra, and stenosis of the spinal canal in a Rottweiler puppy, *J Am Anim Hosp Assoc* 24:341-344, 1988.

350. Appleby EC, Longstaffe JA, Bell FR: Ceroid lipofuscinosis in two Saluki dogs, *J Comp Pathol* 92:375-380, 1982.

351. Luttgen PJ, Storts RW: Central nervous system status spongiosus. In Proceedings of the Fifth Annual Veterinary Medical Forum, American College of Veterinary Internal Medicine. San Diego, 1987.

352. Cummings J, et al: Tremors in Samoyed pups with oligodendrocyte deficiencies and hypomyelination, *Acta Neuropathol (Berl)* 71:267-277, 1986.

353. Mason RW, Hartley WJ, Randall M: Spongiform degeneration of the white matter in a Samoyed pup, *Aust Vet Pract* 9:11-13, 1979.

354. Sorjonen D, Cox N, Kwapien R: Myeloencephalopathy with eosinophilic refractile bodies (Rosenthal fibers) in a Scottish terrier, *J Am Vet Med Assoc* 190:1004-1006, 1987.

355. Meyers KM, et al: Hyperkinetic episodes in Scottish terrier dogs, *J Am Vet Med Assoc* 155:129-133, 1969.

356. Robert DD, Hitt ME: Methionine as a possible inducer of Scotty cramp, *Canine Pract* 13:29-31, 1986.

357. Meyers KM, et al: Muscular hypertonicity, *Arch Neurol* 25:61-67, 1971.

358. Meyers KM, Schaub RG: The relationship of serotonin to a motor disorder of Scottish terrier dogs, *Life Sci* 14:1895-1906, 1974.

359. Meyers KM, Padgett GA, Dickson WM: The genetic basis of a kinetic disorder of Scottish terrier dogs, *J Hered* 61:189-192, 1970.

360. Meyers KM, Dickson WM, Schaub RG: Serotonin involvement in a motor disorder of Scottish terrier dogs, *Life Sci* 13:1261-1274, 1973.

361. Andersson B, Andersson R: On the etiology of "Scotty cramp" and "splay"—two motoring disorders common in the Scottish terrier breed, *Acta Vet Scand* 23:550-558, 1982.

362. Clemmons RM, Peters RI, Meyers KM: Scotty cramp: A review of cause, characteristics, diagnosis and treatment, *Compend Cont Educ Pract Vet* 2:385-390, 1980.

363. Hargis A, et al: Post-mortem findings in a Shetland sheepdog with dermatomyositis, *Vet Pathol* 23:509-511, 1986.

364. Harari J, et al: Cerebellar agenesis in two canine littermates, *J Am Vet Med Assoc* 182:622-623, 1983.

365. Bichsel P, Vandevelde M: Degenerative myelopathy in a family of Siberian husky dogs, *J Am Vet Med Assoc* 183:998-1000, 1983.

366. Reinke JD, Suter PF: Laryngeal paralysis in a dog, *J Am Vet Med Assoc* 172:714-716, 1978.

367. Hartley WJ, Blakemore WF: Neurovisceral glucocerebroside storage (Gaucher's disease) in a dog, *Vet Pathol* 10:191-201, 1973.

368. Van De Water N, Jolly R, Farrow B: Canine Gaucher disease: The enzymatic defect, *Aust J Exp Biol Med Sci* 57:551-554, 1979.

369. Richards RB, Kakulas BA: Spongiform leukencephalopathy associated with congenital myoclonia syndrome in the dog, *J Comp Pathol* 88:317-320, 1978.

370. Johnson RP, et al: Myasthenia in Springer spaniel littermates, *J Small Anim Pract* 16:641-647, 1975.

371. Taylor R, Farrow B, Healy P: Canine fucosidosis: Clinical findings, *J Small Anim Pract* 28:291-300, 1987.

372. Abraham D, et al: The enzymic defect and storage products in canine fucosidosis, *Biochem J* 221:25-33, 1984.

373. Alroy J, Ucci AA, Warren CD: Human and canine fucosidosis: A comparative histochemistry study, *Acta Neuropathol (Berl)* 67:265-271, 1985.

374. Hartley WJ, Canfield PJ, Donnelly TM: A suspected new canine storage disease, *Acta Neuropathol (Berl)* 56:225-232, 1982.

375. Kelly WR, et al: Canine α-L-fucosidosis: A storage disease of Springer spaniels, *Acta Neuropathol* 60:9-13, 1983.

376. Littlewood JD, Herrtage ME, Palmer AC: Neuronal storage disease in English springer spaniels, *Vet Rec* 112:86, 1983.

377. Keller CB, Lamarre J: Inherited lysosomal storage disease in an English springer spaniel, *J Am Vet Med Assoc* 200:194-195, 1992.

378. Griffiths IR, et al: Shaking pups: A disorder of central myelination in the spaniel dog, Part 1: Clinical, genetic, and light microscopical observations, *J Neurol Sci* 50:423-433, 1981.

379. Slatter D: *Fundamentals of veterinary ophthalmology.* Philadelphia, 1981, WB Saunders.

380. Erickson F, Leipold HW, McKinley J: Congenital defects in dogs. Part 2, *Canine Pract* 14:51-61, 1977.

381. Hoover D, Little P, Cole W: Neuronal ceroid-lipofuscinosis in a mature dog, *Vet Pathol* 21:359-361, 1984.

382. Van der Velden A: Fits in Tervuren shepherd dogs: A presumed hereditary trait, *J Small Anim Pract* 9:63-70, 1968.

383. Cummings J, et al: Canine inherited hypertrophic neuropathy, *Acta Neuropathol (Berl)* 53:137-143, 1981.

384. Cooper BJ, et al: Defective Schwann cell function in canine inherited hypertrophic neuropathy, *Acta Neuropathol* 63:51-56, 1984.

385. Cooper BJ, et al: Canine inherited hypertrophic neuropathy: Clinical and electrodiagnostic studies, *Am J Vet Res* 45:1172-1177, 1984.

386. Cummings J, de Lahunta A: Hypertrophic neuropathy in a dog, *Acta Neuropathol (Berl)* 20:325-336, 1974.

387. Millichamp NJ, Curtis R, Barnett KC: Progressive retinal atrophy in Tibetan terriers, *J Am Vet Med Assoc* 192:769-776, 1988.

388. Geary JC, Oliver JE, Hoerlein BF: Atlanto-axial subluxation in the canine, *J Small Anim Pract* 8:577-582, 1967.

389. Oliver JE, Lewis RE: Lesions of the atlas and axis in dogs, *J Am Anim Hosp Assoc* 9:304-313, 1973.

390. Ladds P, et al: Congenital odontoid process separation in two dogs, *J Small Anim Pract* 12:463-471, 1970.

391. Cook JR, Oliver JE: Atlantoaxial luxation in the dog, *Compend Cont Educ Pract Vet* 3:242-252, 1981.

392. Downey RS: An unusual cause of tetraplegia in a dog, *Can Vet J* 8:216-217, 1967.

393. Bardens JW: Congenital malformations of the foramen magnum in dogs, *Southwest Vet* 18:295-298, 1965.

394. Parker AJ, Park RD: Occipital dysplasia in the dog, *J Am Anim Hosp Assoc* 10:520-525, 1974.

395. Gee B, Doige C: Multiple cartilaginous exostoses in a litter of dogs, *J Am Vet Med Assoc* 156:53-59, 1970.

396. Bichsel P, et al: Solitary cartilaginous exostoses associated with spinal cord compression in three large-breed dogs, *J Am Anim Hosp Assoc* 21:619-622, 1985.

397. Doige C: Multiple cartilaginous exostoses in dogs, *Vet Pathol* 24:276-278, 1987.

398. Acton CE: Spinal cord compression in young dogs due to cartilaginous exostosis, *Calif Vet* 41:7-26, 1987.

399. Vicini DS, et al: Peripheral nerve biopsy for diagnosis of globoid cell leukodystrophy in a dog, *J Am Vet Med Assoc* 192:1087-1090, 1988.

400. Kornegay JN: Dysmyelinogenesis in dogs. In Proceedings of the Third Annual Veterinary Medical Forum, American College of Veterinary Internal Medicine. San Diego, 1985.

401. Kornegay J: Hypomyelination in Weimaraner dogs, *Acta Neuropathol (Berl)* 72:394-401, 1987.

402. Comont PSV, Palmer AC, Williams AE: Weakness associated with myelopathy in a Weimaraner puppy, *J Small Anim Pract* 29:367-372, 1988.

403. McGrath JT: Spinal dysraphism in the dog, *Pathol Vet Suppl* 2:1-36, 1965.

404. Gieb LW, Bistner SI: Spinal cord dysraphism in a dog, *J Am Vet Med Assoc* 150:618-620, 1967.

405. Engel HN, Draper DD: Comparative prenatal development of the spinal cord in normal and dysraphic dogs: Embryonic stage, *Am J Vet Res* 43:1729-1734, 1982.

406. Engel HN, Draper DD: Comparative prenatal development of the spinal cord in normal and dysraphic dogs: Fetal stage, *Am J Vet Res* 43:1735-1743, 1982.

407. Botelho SY, et al: Electromyography in dogs with congenital spinal cord lesions, *Am J Vet Res* 28:205-212, 1967.

408. Confer AW, Ward BC: Spinal dysraphism: A congenital myelodysplasia in the Weimaraner, *J Am Vet Med Assoc* 160:1423-1426, 1972.

409. Osborne CA, Clifford DH, Jessen C: Hereditary esophageal achalasia in dogs, *J Am Vet Med Assoc* 151:572-581, 1967.

410. Bryant SH: Altered membrane potentials in myotonia. In Bolis L, Hoffman JF, Leaf A, editors: *Membranes and diseases.* New York, 1976, Raven Press.

411. Bryant SH: Myotonia in the goat, *Ann NY Acad Sci* 317:314-325, 1979.

412. Healy P, Sewell C: The use of plasma mannosidase activity for the detection of goats heterozygous for ß-mannosidosis, *Aust Vet J* 62:286-287, 1985.

413. Fankhauser R: Hydrocephalus Studien, *Schweiz Arch Tierheilkd* 101:407-416, 1959.

414. Healy PJ, et al: ß-Mannosidase deficiency in Anglo Nubian goats, *Aust Vet J* 57:504-507, 1981.

415. Robinson WF, et al: Atlanto-axial malarticulation in Angora goats, *Aust Vet J* 58:105-107, 1982.

416. Luttgen PJ, Storts RW: Ceroid lipofuscinosis in Nubian goats. In Proceedings of the Fourth Annual Veterinary Medical Forum, American College of Veterinary Internal Medicine. San Diego, 1987.

417. Fiske RA, Storts RW: Neuronal ceroid-lipofuscinosis in Nubian goats, *Vet Pathol* 25:171-173, 1988.

418. Mayhew J, Brown C, Trapp A: Equine degenerative myeloencephalopathy. In Proceedings of the Fourth Annual Veterinary Medical Forum, American College of Veterinary Internal Medicine. Washington, DC, 1986.

419. Mayhew IG, et al: Spinal cord disease in the horse, *Cornell Vet* 68 (Suppl 6):1-207, 1978.

420. Watson AG, Mayhew IG: Familial congenital occipitoatlantoaxial malformation (OAAM) in the Arabian horse, *Spine* 11:334-339, 1986.

421. Smith JM, DeBowes RM, Cox JH: Central nervous system disease in adult horses, Part II: Differential diagnosis, *Compend Cont Educ Pract Vet* 9:771-780, 1987.

422. Duncan I: Congenital tremor and abnormalities of myelination. In Proceedings of the Fifth Annual Veterinary Medical Forum, American College of Veterinary Internal Medicine. San Diego, 1987, pp 869-873.

423. Fraser H: Two dissimilar types of cerebellar disorder in the horse, *Vet Rec* 78:608-612, 1966.

424. Palmer AC, et al: Cerebellar hypoplasia and degeneration in the young Arab horse: Clinical and neuropathological features, *Vet Rec* 93:62-66, 1973.

425. Mayhew I: Seizures disorders. In Robinson NE, editor: *Current therapy in equine medicine.* Philadelphia, 1983, WB Saunders.

426. Scarratt WK, et al: Degenerative myelopathy in two equids, *J Equine Vet Sci* 5:139-141, 1985.

427. Bjorck G, et al: Congenital cerebellar ataxia in the Gotland pony breed, *Zentralbl Veterinarmed* 20[A]:341-354, 1973.

428. Mayhew IG, Watson AG, Heissan JA: Congenital occipitoatlantoaxial malformation in the horse, *Equine Vet J* 10:103-113, 1978.

429. Wilson WD, et al: Occipitoatlantoaxial malformation in two non-Arabian horses, *J Am Vet Med Assoc* 187:36-40, 1985.

430. Shupe JL, et al: Hereditary multiple exostoses, *Am J Pathol* 104:285-288, 1981.

431. Maciulis A, et al: High resolution chromosome banding analysis of horses with hereditary multiple exostosis, *J Equine Vet Sci* 5:284-286, 1985.

432. Powers B, et al: Pathology of the vertebral column of horses with cervical static stenosis, *Vet Pathol* 23:392-399, 1986.

433. Alitalo I, Karkkainen M: Osteochondrotic changes in the vertebrae of four ataxic horses suffering from cervical vertebral malformation, *Nord Vet Med* 35:468-474, 1983.

434. Wagner P, et al: Surgical stabilization of the equine cervical spine, *Vet Surg* 8:7-12, 1979.

435. Steel J, Whittem J, Hutchins D: Equine sensory ataxia ("wobbles"): Clinical and pathological observations in Australian cases, *Aust Vet J* 35:442-449, 1959.

436. Wagner P, et al: Evaluation of cervical spinal fusion as a treatment in the equine "wobbler" syndrome, *Vet Surg* 8:84-88, 1979.

437. Mayhew I, et al: Equine degenerative myeloencephalopathy: A vitamin E deficiency that may be familial, *J Vet Intern Med* 1:45-50, 1987.

438. Mayhew IG, et al: Equine degenerative myeloencephalopathy, *J Am Vet Med Assoc* 170:195-201, 1977.

439. Steinberg S, Bothelo S: Myotonia in a horse, *Science* 137:979, 1962.

440. Beech J: Neuroaxonal dystrophy of the accessory cuneate nucleus in horses, *Vet Pathol* 21:384-393, 1984.

441. Beech J, Haskind M: Genetic studies of neuroaxonal dystrophy in the Morgan, *Am J Vet Res* 48:109-113, 1987.

442. Roneus B: Glutathione peroxidase and selenium in the blood of healthy horses and foals affected by muscular dystrophy, *Nord Vet Med* 34:350-353, 1982.

443. Poss M, Young S: Dysplastic disease of the cerebellum of an adult horse, *Acta Neuropathol (Berl)* 75:209-211, 1987.

444. Grant B, et al: Surgical treatment of multiple level cord compression in the horse, *Equine Pract* 7:19-24, 1985.

445. Rooney J: Equine incoordination, I: Gross morphology, *Cornell Vet* 53:411-422, 1963.

446. Fraser H, Palmer A: Equine incoordination and wobbler disease of young horses, *Vet Rec* 80:338-355, 1967.

447. Falco M, Whitwell K, Palmer A: An investigation into the genetics of "wobbler disease" in thoroughbred horses in Britain, *Equine Vet J* 8:165-169, 1967.

448. Duncan I: Some aspects of the neuropathy of equine laryngeal hemiplegia. In Proceedings of the Fifth Annual Veterinary Medical Forum, American College of Veterinary Internal Medicine. San Diego, 1987.

449. Cole CR: Changes in the equine larynx associated with laryngeal hemiplegia, *Am J Vet Res* 7:69-77, 1946.

450. Duncan ID, et al: The pathology of equine laryngeal hemiplegia, *Acta Neuropathol* 27:337-348, 1974.

451. Hillidge C: Interpretation of laryngeal function tests in the horse, *Vet Rec* 118:535-536, 1986.

452. Cahill JI, Goulden B: The pathogenesis of equine laryngeal hemiplegia: A review, *N Z Vet J* 35:82-90, 1987.

453. Tulleners EP, Harrison IW, Raker CW: Management of arytenoid chondropathy and failed laryngoplasty in horses: 75 cases (1879-1985), *J Am Vet Med Assoc* 192:670-675, 1988.

454. Cahill JI, Goulden B: Equine laryngeal hemiplegia, Part II: An electron microscopic study of peripheral nerves, *N Z Vet J* 34:170-175, 1986.

455. Cahill JI, Goulden B: Equine laryngeal hemiplegia, Part I: A light microscopic study of peripheral nerves, *N Z Vet J* 34:161-169, 1986.

456. Cahill J, Goulden B: Equine laryngeal hemiplegia, Part V: Central nervous system pathology, *N Z Vet J* 34:191-193, 1986.

457. Cahill J, Goulden B: Equine laryngeal hemiplegia, Part IV: Muscle pathology, *N Z Vet J* 34:186-190, 1986.

458. Cahill J, Goulden BE: Equine laryngeal hemiplegia, Part III: A teased fibre study of peripheral nerves, *N Z Vet J* 34:181-185, 1986.

459. Baker GJ: Laryngeal hemiplegia in the horse, *Compend Cont Educ Pract Vet* 5:S61-S67, 1983.

460. Koch C: Diseases of the larynx and pharynx of the horse, *Compend Cont Educ Pract Vet* 2:573-580, 1980.

461. Vaala W: Diagnosis and treatment of prematurity and neonatal maladjustment syndrome in newborn foals, *Compend Cont Educ Pract Vet* 8:211-226, 1986.

462. Montali R, et al: Spinal ataxia in zebras: Comparison with the wobbler syndrome of horses, *Vet Pathol* 11:68-78, 1974.

463. Van den Berg P, Baker M, Lange A: A suspected lysosomal storage disease in Abyssinian cats, Part I: Genetic, clinical and clinical pathological aspects, *J S Afr Vet Assoc* 48:195-199, 1977.

464. Lange AL, Brown JMM, Maree CC: Biochemical studies on a lysosomal storage disease in Abyssinian cats, *Onderstepoort J Vet Res* 50:149-155, 1983.

465. Baker H, et al: Sphingomyelin lipidosis in a cat, *Vet Pathol* 24:386-391, 1987.

466. Sponenberg DP, Graf-Webster E: Hereditary meningoencephalocele in Burmese cats, *J Hered* 77:60, 1986.

467. Zook B, et al: Encephalocele and other congenital craniofacial anomalies in Burmese cats, *Vet Med Small Anim Clin* 78:695-701, 1983.

468. Rebillard M, Rebillard G, Pujol R: Variability of the hereditary deafness in the white cat, I, *Physiol Hear Res* 5:179-187, 1981.

469. Rebillard M, Pujol R, Rebillard G: Variability of the hereditary deafness in the white cat, II, *Histol Hear Res* 5:189-200, 1981.

470. Elverland HH, Mair IWS: Hereditary deafness in the cat, *Acta Otolaryngol (Stockh)* 90:360-369, 1980.

471. Faith RE, Woodard JC: Waardenburg's syndrome, *Comp Pathol Bull* 5:3-4, 1973.

472. Coulter DB, Martin CL, Alvarado TP: A cat with white fur and one blue eye, *Calif Vet* 34:11-14, 1980.

473. Delack JB: Hereditary deafness in the white cat, *Compend Cont Educ Pract Vet* 6:609-616, 1984.

442 Appendix

474. Creel D, Conlee JW, Parks TN: Auditory brainstem anomalies in albino cats, I: Evoked potential studies, *Brain Res* 260:1-9, 1983.
475. Saperstein G, Harris S, Leipold HW: Congenital defects in domestic cats, *Feline Pract* 6:18-41, 1976.
476. Watson AG, Hall MA, de Lahunta A: Congenital occipitoatlantoaxial malformation in a cat, *Compend Cont Educ Pract Vet* 7:245-254, 1985.
477. Carpenter M, Harter D: A study of congenital feline cerebellar malformations: An anatomic and physiologic evaluation of agenetic defects, *J Comp Neurol* 105:51-94, 1956.
478. Csiza C, et al: Spontaneous feline ataxia, *Cornell Vet* 62:300-322, 1972.
479. Herndon R, Margolis G, Kilham L: The synaptic organization of the malformed cerebellum induced by perinatal infection with the feline panleukopenia virus (PLV), *J Neuropathol Exp Neurol* 30:196-205, 1971.
480. Mesfin GM, Kuscwitt D, Parker A: Degenerative myelopathy in a cat, *J Am Vet Med Assoc* 176:62-64, 1980.
481. Cork LC, Munnell JF, Lorenz MD: The pathology of feline GM$_2$ gangliosidosis, *Am J Pathol* 90:723-734, 1978.
482. Cork LC, et al: GM$_2$ ganglioside lysosomal storage disease in cats with hexosaminidase deficiency, *Science* 196:1014-1017, 1977.
483. Johnson KH: Globoid leukodystrophy in the cat, *J Am Vet Med Assoc* 157:2057-2067, 1970.
484. Sandstrom B, Westman J, Ockerman PA: Glycogenosis of the central nervous system in the cat, *Acta Neuropathol (Berl)* 14:194-200, 1969.
485. Cribb A: Laryngeal paralysis in a mature cat, *Can Vet J* 27:27, 1986.
486. White R, et al: Outcome of surgery for laryngeal paralysis in four cats, *Vet Rec* 117:103-104, 1986.
487. Hardie EM, et al: Laryngeal paralysis in three cats, *J Am Vet Med Assoc* 179:879-882, 1981.
488. Fatzer R: Leukodystrophische Erschrankungen im Gehirn junger Katzen, *Schweiz Arch Tierheilkd* 117:641-648, 1975.
489. Hegreberg GA, Thuline HC, Francis BH: Morphologic changes in feline leukodystrophy, *FASEB J* 30:341, 1971.
490. Oliver JE, Hoerlein BF, Mayhew IG: *Veterinary neurology.* Philadelphia, 1987, WB Saunders.
491. Blakemore W: A case of mannosidosis in the cat: Clinical and histopathological findings, *J Small Anim Pract* 27:447-455, 1986.
492. Walkley SU, Blakemore WF, Purpura DP: Alterations in neuron morphology in feline mannosidosis, *Acta Neuropathol (Berl)* 53:75-79, 1981.
493. Braund KG, Ribas JL: Meningiomas of the central nervous system in dogs and cats. In Proceedings of the Fourth Annual Veterinary Medical Forum, American College of Veterinary Internal Medicine. Washington, DC, 1986.
494. Lawson DC, Burk RL, Prata RG: Cerebral meningioma in the cat: Diagnosis and surgical treatment of ten cases, *J Am Anim Hosp Assoc* 20:333-342, 1984.
495. Braund K, Ribas J: Central nervous system meningiomas, *Compend Cont Educ Pract Vet* 8:241-248, 1986.
496. Haskins ME, et al: Mucopolysaccharidosis in a domestic short-haired cat: A disease distinct from that seen in the Siamese cat, *J Am Vet Med Assoc* 175:384-387, 1979.
497. Haskins ME, et al: The pathology of the feline model of mucopolysaccharidosis: I, *Am J Pathol* 112:27-36, 1983.
498. Woodard JC, Collins GH, Hessler JR: Feline hereditary neuroaxonal dystrophy, *Am J Pathol* 74:551-560, 1974.

499. Vandevelde M, Greene C, Hoff E: Lower motor neuron disease with accumulation of neurofilaments in a cat, *Vet Pathol* 13:428-435, 1976.
500. Percy DH, Jortner BS: Feline lipidosis, *Arch Pathol Lab Med* 92:136-143, 1971.
501. Cuddon PA, Higgins RJ, Duncan ID: Feline Niemann-Pick disease associated polyneuropathy. In Proceedings of the Sixth Annual Veterinary Medical Forum, American College of Veterinary Internal Medicine. Washington, DC, 1988.
502. Kelly DF, Gaskell CJ: Spongy degeneration of the central nervous system in kittens, *Acta Neuropathol (Berl)* 35:151-158, 1976.
503. Clifford DH, et al: Congenital achalasia of the esophagus in four cats of common ancestry, *J Am Vet Med Assoc* 158:1554-1560, 1971.
504. Davidson AP: Congenital disorders of the Manx cat. *Southwest Vet* 37:115-119, 1986.
505. Kitchen H, Murray RE, Cockrell BY: Animal model for human disease, spina bifida, sacral dysgenesis and myelocele, *Am J Pathol* 68:203-206, 1972.
506. Hall JA, Fettman MJ, Ingram JT: Sodium chloride depletion in a cat with fistulated meningomyelocele, *J Am Vet Med Assoc* 192:1445-1448, 1988.
507. Leipold HW, et al: Congenital defects of the caudal vertebral column and spinal cord in Manx cats, *J Am Vet Med Assoc* 164:520-523, 1974.
508. Fyfe JC, et al: Familial glycogen storage disease type IV (GSD IV) in Norwegian forest cats (NWFC), *J Vet Intern Med* 4:127, 1990.
509. Maenhout T, et al: Mannosidosis in a litter of Persian cats, *Vet Rec* 122:351-354, 1988.
510. Jezyk PF, Haskins ME, Newman LR: Alpha mannosidosis in a Persian cat, *J Am Vet Med Assoc* 189:1483-1485, 1986.
511. Vandevelde M, et al: Hereditary neurovisceral mannosidosis with associated mannosidase deficiency in a family of Persian cats, *Acta Neuropathol* 58:64-68, 1982.
512. Green P, Little P: Neuronal ceroid-lipofuscin storage in Siamese cats, *Can J Comp Med* 38:207-212, 1974.
513. Cowell KR, et al: Mucopolysaccharidosis in a cat, *J Am Vet Med Assoc* 169:334-339, 1976.
514. Langweiler M, Haskins ME, Jezyk PF: Mucopolysaccharidosis in a litter of cats, *J Am Anim Hosp Assoc* 14:748-751, 1978.
515. Haskins ME, et al: Spinal compression and hindlimb paresis in cats with mucopolysaccharidosis: VI, *J Am Vet Med Assoc* 182:983-985, 1983.
516. Breton L, Guerin P, Morin M: A case of mucopolysaccharidosis VI in a cat, *J Am Anim Hosp Assoc* 19:891-896, 1983.
517. Jezyk P, Haskins M, Patterson DF: Mucopolysaccharidosis in a cat with arylsulfatase B deficiency: A model of Maroteaux-Lamy syndrome, *Science* 198:834-836, 1977.
518. Haskins ME, et al: The pathology of the feline model of mucopolysaccharidosis VI, *Am J Pathol* 101:657-674, 1980.
519. Haskins ME, Jezyk PF, Desnick RJ, et al: Animal model of human disease mucopolysaccharidosis VI. Maroteaux-Lamy syndrome arylsulfatase ß-deficient mucopolysaccharidosis in the Siamese cat, *Am J Pathol* 105:191-193, 1981.
520. Chrisp CE, et al: Lipid storage disease in a Siamese cat, *J Am Vet Med Assoc* 156:616-622, 1970.
521. Snyder S, Kingston R, Wenger D: Animal model of human disease: Niemann-Pick disease. sphingomyelinosis of Siamese cats, *Am J Pathol* 108:252-254, 1982.